Nurses' Handbook
of
Fluid Balance

THIRD EDITION

Nurses' Handbook
of
Fluid Balance

Norma Milligan Metheny, R.N., M.S.N., Ph.D.
Associate Professor of Nursing,
St. Louis Community College at Meramec, St. Louis, Missouri.

W. D. Snively, Jr., M.D., F.A.C.P.
Professor Emeritus of Life Sciences,
University of Evansville, Evansville, Indiana;
Clinical Professor of Pediatrics,
Indiana University School of Medicine,
Evansville Medical Center, Evansville, Indiana.

 J. B. Lippincott Company | Philadelphia   New York   Toronto

ISBN-0-397-54226-7
Library of Congress Catalog Card Number 78-24364
PRINTED IN THE UNITED STATES OF AMERICA

1 3 5 7 9 8 6 4 2

Library of Congress Cataloging in Publication Data

Metheny, Norma Milligan.
    Nurses' handbook of fluid balance.

    Includes bibliographies and index.
    1. Body fluid disorders—Nursing.   2. Body fluids.
I. Snively, William Daniel, 1911–   joint author.   II. Title.
[DNLM: 1. Body fluids—Nursing texts.   2. Nursing care.
3. Water-electrolyte balance—Nursing texts. WY150 M592n]

RB 144.M47 1979   612'.01522   78-24364
ISBN 0-397-54226-7

"Water . . . is the image of the ungraspable phantom of life; and this is the key to it all."

Herman Melville in *Moby Dick*

CONTENTS

PREFACE

Dr. Jose L. B. Montenegro, dedicated young pediatrician of Sao Paulo, Brazil, once told one of the authors, "Body fluid disturbances represent the common denominator of a host of illnesses." Increasingly, members of the healing professions are realizing that this is indeed the case. With this awareness has come rapidly mounting interest in these ubiquitous disorders and, as a result, increased knowledge in pathogenesis, in diagnosis, and in therapy. Another gratifying result of this development is the involvement, in depth, of members of the nursing and other allied health professions. For not only general duty nurses but also nurses in specialties, nurse practitioners, intravenous therapists, respiratory therapists, nurse anesthetists, and technicians in such crucial fields as nephrology and extracorporeal circulation are establishing themselves as indispensable allies of the physician. Aware of these facts, it appeared highly appropriate to both publisher and authors to do a thorough revision and expansion of the *Nurses' Handbook of Fluid Balance*.

As in the two previous editions, the text is divided into chapters on the fundamentals of body fluids and their imbalances and into chapters on clinical application of that knowledge. Some of the more significant changes include:

In the "fundamentals" area:
- Increased details on the body's homeostatic controls
- A comprehensive, entirely new chapter on the basics of nutrition, essential for in-depth understanding of body fluid disturbances
- Addition of numerous actual case histories of patients with diverse body fluid disturbances
- Explanation of the use of "Delta" (anion gap) in differentiating between organic and inorganic acid acidosis
- Useful methods for differentiating simple from mixed (nonrespiratory plus respiratory) acid-base disturbances
- A new section on magnesium excess, and one on its management

In the "clinical application" area:
- The latest information on elemental diets, tube feedings, and on starting and maintaining IVs
- Recent developments on protein, lipid, and hyperalimentation solutions
- Greatly enlarged coverage of the pathophysiology and treatment of renal failure
- A new section on hemodynamic monitoring
- Greatly expanded information on blood gases and their interpretation and on the nurse's responsibilities in obtaining samples for blood gas analysis
- New developments in treatment of near-drowned patients
- Expanded discussion of toxemia of pregnancy
- Description of CVP monitoring in children
- Many new figures and much innovative artwork by an experienced medical artist

The nurse and physician authors of this third edition of *Nurses' Handbook of Fluid Balance* were helped by able contributors in various fields, who importantly increased the worth of the text. The authors are grateful to them and also to Mr. David Miller, Managing Editor of J. B. Lippincott Company, who cheerfully gave needed counsel on innumerable occasions.

This edition has focused on significant new knowledge and on the expanding role of nurses and other members of the health team in the overall management of body fluid disturbances. It is a pleasure—and a privilege—to dedicate the third edition of *Nurses' Handbook of Fluid Balance* to them.

ACKNOWLEDGMENTS

We thank the following people for their contributions to this edition:

Donna R. Beshear, Medical Writer and Researcher, assisted in organization, research, and writing of chapters presenting basic material.

Darnell Roth, R.N., Intravenous Therapist, contributed to Chapter 16 in the area of starting and maintaining intravenous infusions.

Catherine A. Smith, R.N., M.S.N., Cardiovascular Nurse Specialist, contributed to Chapter 21 in the areas of hemodynamic monitoring and care of patients with congestive heart failure.

Ebert Westfall, Medical Artist, did most of the artwork throughout the text.

— 1 —
Body Fluid—
Our Heritage
from the Sea

"The sea never changes and its works, for all the talk of men, are wrapped in mystery." Joseph Conrad

Life on earth began in the ocean about two billion years ago. Scientists are far from certain as to the exact nature of that first form of life, but it may have been the single-celled organism that we know as the protozoan. Whether the protozoan was first or not, it most certainly appeared quite early in the development of life.

The ocean water surrounding that first microorganism and its infinite progeny contained everything necessary to maintain life. Dissolved in the sea water were oxygen and other gases besides various nutrients. The physical characteristics of the ocean—its ability to maintain a constant temperature, its volume, and its surface tension, among others—all suited the minuscule organism's needs.

The sea was a kind mother to the primitive organism that is the most ancient ancestor of our body cells. To this day, every one of us contains within his body a tight little pond that we might think of as a tiny, personal portion of the sea. We call it *body fluid*. Body fluid accounts for 60, 70, perhaps 80 per cent of our total body weight, depending upon age, sex, and body fat content. In general, the younger the

individual, the higher his percentage of body fluid. Women have a lower body water content than men, and a fat person contains less fluid than a thin person, since fat has little water associated with it.

But how did this sea water get into our bodies? Scientists explain it thus: over the course of millions of years, the single-celled organisms were joined to each other, forming many-celled metazoa. The metazoa were just as dependent on their physiochemical bath water, the ocean, for the maintenance of life as were the protozoa. Eons later certain sea creatures began to develop physical characteristics that would eventually enable them to exist on the continental land masses. An essential step in this evolutionary process occurred when some of the sea water was enclosed within their bodies. These creatures could never have left the ocean without some means of carrying their oceanic bath water along with them. James Gamble, a great physiologist, described the step in these words:

> Before our extremely remote ancestors could come ashore to enjoy their Eocene Eden or their

1

Paleozoic Palm Beach, it was necessary for them to establish an enclosed aqueous medium which would carry on the role of sea water.

These early animals contained two types of body fluid—the fluid within the individual cells, or *cellular fluid,* and an additional fluid that served to surround and bathe the cells, the *extracellular fluid.* These two types of fluid also occur in man. If the scientific consensus is correct, these fluids are the lineal descendants of sea water—in a real sense, our *heritage from the sea.*

BIBLIOGRAPHY

Gamble, J.: Chemical Anatomy Physiology and Pathology of Extracellular Fluid. Cambridge, MA: Harvard University Press, 1967.

Smith, H.: From Fish to Philosopher. Garden City, NY: Doubleday & Company, 1961.

Snively, W., and **Thuerbach, J.:** Sea of Life. New York: David McKay Co., 1969.

— 2 —

Cellular and Extracellular Fluid: Secretions and Excretions

The body fluid is divided into two major compartments. The first compartment, the *cellular fluid*, comprises the fluid contained within the billions of body cells and accounts for about three fourths of the total body fluid. We might think of it as a vast multitude of tiny, encapsulated droplets suspended in another type of fluid, the *extracellular fluid*. Extracellular fluid constitutes about one fourth of the total body fluid (Figs. 2-1 and 2-2).

During the evolutionary process, the extracellular fluid was further divided into two subdivisions. Once the sea water became enclosed within the body, it had to be circulated to carry nutrients and other substances to the cells and waste materials away from them. A heart and a circulatory system evolved, and part of the extracellular fluid—about a fourth of it—was appropriated for circulation through the system. This intravascular extracellular fluid is the *plasma*—the liquid fraction of the blood. The other three fourths of the extracellular fluid lies outside the blood vessels in the interstitial spaces between the body cells. This extravascular portion of the extracellular fluid is called *interstitial fluid*. Lymph and cerebrospinal fluid, while they have highly specialized and unique functions, are usually regarded as interstitial fluid. In some respects, lymph appears to be a sort of physiologic afterthought since it serves many purposes: it combats infection, traps tumor cells, serves important circulatory functions, and even transports nutrients—chiefly fatty acids—from the intestine to the venous circulation. Cerebrospinal fluid is the interstitial fluid of the central nervous system.

Consider what might be termed *microscopic anatomy of the body fluids* (Fig. 2-3). If one were to take a cross-section of a solid tissue, e.g., muscle, one might see something like this: extracellular fluid (including plasma, located within the blood vessels, and interstitial fluid, located outside the blood vessels) surrounding and bathing the cells. Cellular fluid would be seen inside body cells, including both the cells *inside* and those *outside* the blood vessels.

In addition to the two major divisions of body fluid, the cellular and extracellular fluid, there are other essential fluids—the *secretions* and *excretions*. The secretions include the juices manufactured in the stomach, pancreas, liver, and intestine. Urine and feces are excretions. Perspiration is also regarded as an excretion, although its primary purpose is not to rid the body of wastes but rather to aid in body heat regulation. Even though secretions and excretions are derived from extracellular fluid, they are not actually extracellular fluid.

A *topographic analogy of body fluids* (Fig. 2-4) might be helpful in understanding the relationships between the various body fluids. Cellular fluid can be regarded as a vast ocean that holds three fourths of the body fluid. It is fed by the extracellular fluid, which is pictured as a great river. The secretions and excretions represent streams and rivulets flowing from the extracellular fluid, which supplies them with all needed materials.

COMPOSITION OF BODY FLUIDS

Body fluid consists chiefly of *water* and certain dissolved substances sometimes referred to as salts, minerals, or crystalloids, but more correctly called *electrolytes*.

Water is the most essential nutrient to life. No known form of plant or animal life can exist for very long without it. Indeed, humans can live a long time without other nutrients, but only for a few days without water. Water possesses unique chemical and physical characteristics and there is no substitute for it in the living cycle. Water's boiling point (100° C.) and its freezing point (0° C.) enable the human body

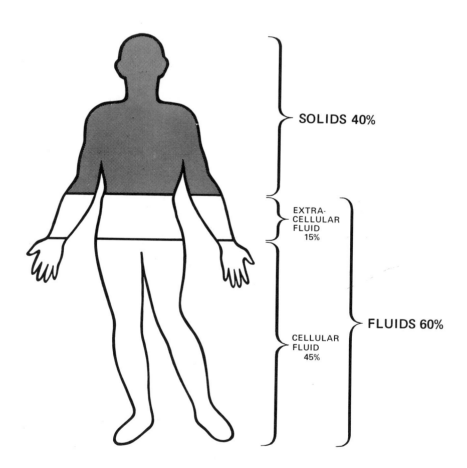

Figure 2-1.   Fluid and solid components of body weight in the adult.

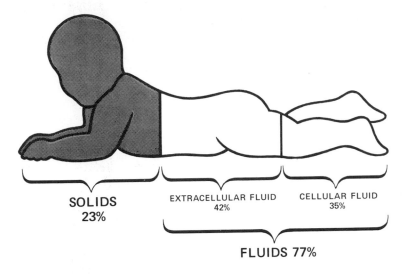

Figure 2-2. Fluid and solid components of body weight in the newborn.

to withstand all but the most drastic changes in heat or cold. Water is the closest substance known to a universal solvent. Since the adult body is from 60 to 70 per cent water, each one of us is, in a real sense, a bag of more or less solid materials dissolved in water. Water is required for the countless chemical reactions of the body; no major physiologic function can proceed without it.

Electrolytes are so named because they ionize—develop electrical charges—when they are dissolved in water. Some electrolytes, including sodium, potassium, calcium, and magnesium, develop positive charges; some, including chloride, bicarbonate, sulfate, phosphate, proteinate, carbonic acid, and other organic acids, develop negative charges.

One can determine which electrolytes carry positive charges and which carry negative charges by placing the electrolyte in question in a wet electric cell through which an electric current is conducted (Fig. 2-5). Such a cell has a negative pole called a

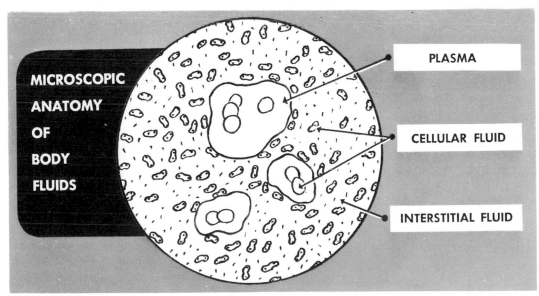

Figure 2-3. Microscopic anatomy of body fluids.

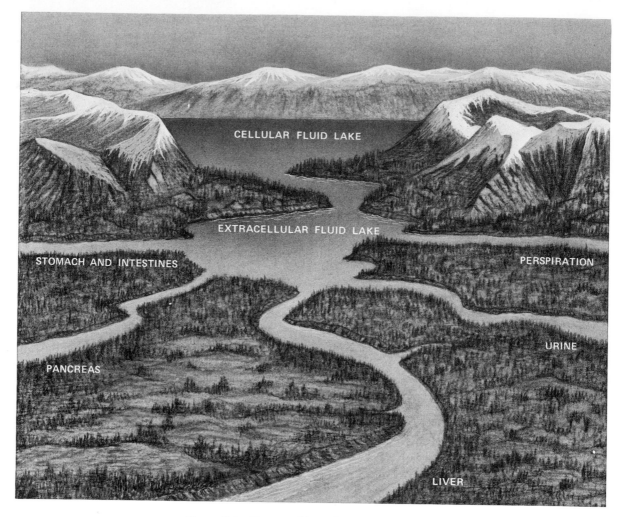

Figure 2-4. Topographic analogy of body fluid.

cathode and a positive pole called an *anode.* Since unlikes attract, positively charged particles travel to the negative pole, or cathode. Such particles, therefore, are designated as *cations.* Negatively charged particles, called *anions,* migrate to the positive pole, or anode. The term *ion* refers to both cation and anion. In all electrical systems, positive charges and negative charges balance each other. Cations and anions exist in equal strength and numbers when measured according to their chemical activity or ability to unite with other ions to form molecules (Fig. 2-6).

Each body fluid has its own normal composition of water and electrolytes. Cellular fluid contains large amounts of potassium, magnesium, and phosphate, and only small amounts of other electrolytes.

Don't think for a moment that these differences in composition between cellular and extracellular fluid are unimportant. Indeed, so important are they that the body uses up one fifth of its energy stored in adenosine triphosphate (ATP) in maintaining them. Scientists tell us that the cellular fluid originated in the pre-Cambrian seas—more than two billion years ago—in the single-cell organisms that were the first form of life. In apparent support of this theory, the composition of our cellular fluid resembles the composition of those ancient seas, as determined by paleogeologists. Extracellular fluid, on the other hand, is of relatively recent origin, being a mere 300 million years old. According to the consensus of science, it was brought ashore by the ancestor of the land vertebrates, a venturesome fish called the coelacanth, when he left his watery home for the land. His extracellular fluid reflected the composition of the seas of that time, the Cambrian seas. The composition of human extracellular fluid is said to resemble strikingly that of the Cambrian seas. The composition of sea water has changed over the years as the continental land masses have gradually dissolved and washed into it; hence, the two types of body fluid vary greatly in composition since they were enclosed within the body during two different geologic periods. Electrolytes in present-day sea water are several times as concentrated as they are in either of our body fluids, which explains why we are unable to drink it.

The chief difference between the plasma and the interstitial fluid is that plasma contains a much greater amount of proteinate, which acts as a sponge to prevent excess plasma from seeping into the interstitial fluid.

The composition of secretions and excretions varies considerably, particularly in illness. Therefore, the quantities of electrolyte per unit volume must be related to a constant, which consists of the levels of sodium, potassium, chloride, and bicarbonate in plasma. On this basis, we find that gastric secretions have about half the sodium concentration of plasma, about the same potassium, about half

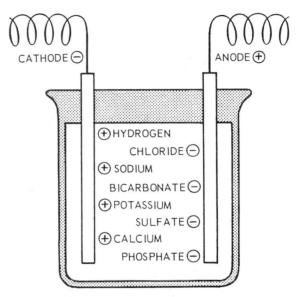

Figure 2-5. In a wet electric cell, cations go to the negative pole or cathode and anions go to the positive pole or anode.

again as much chloride, and a fraction of the bicarbonate. Pancreatic secretions have about the same sodium and potassium, about a third the chloride, and about three times the bicarbonate. Perspiration, a dilute secretion, has more than half the sodium and

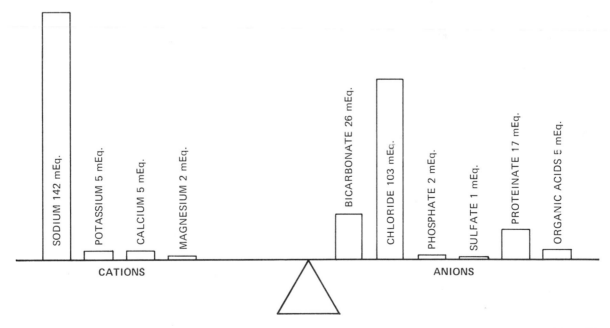

Figure 2-6. The cations and anions of the extracellular fluid (plasma) balance each other when expressed in milli-equivalents.

chloride and about the same potassium. Diarrheal stools in children have a fraction of the sodium, several times as much potassium, a fraction of the chloride, and probably much more bicarbonate.

FUNCTIONS OF BODY FLUIDS

The main function of body fluids is to maintain healthy living conditions for the body cells. Although we may regard ourselves as highly complex, highly civilized organisms, the cells remain the basic units of life. A living body could no more exist without cells than could a brick building exist without bricks. Unlike bricks, however, our cells are live, dynamic, working units that must be nourished. The cellular fluid, which normally contains all the nutrients the cells need, serves as the supply source to replenish nutrients as they are used up. In addition, the cellular fluid must be cleared of wastes, such as carbon dioxide and breakdown products of protein; the extracellular fluid performs these services. Nutrients and other materials seep from the plasma into the interstitial fluid at the arterial end of the capillary beds, which exist in every part of the body, and are carried to the cells via the interstitial fluid. Waste materials pass from the cellular fluid into the interstitial fluid and back to the plasma via the venous capillaries. The plasma then sorts the waste products for storage or excretion and carries them to their proper destinations.

In addition to transporting nutrients and wastes, extracellular fluid transmits enzymes and hormones, plus many additional substances. It carries red blood cells through the body and white blood cells to attack bacteria.

BIBLIOGRAPHY

Garrett, T. (ed.):   Baxter Guide to Fluid Therapy. Morton Grove IL: Baxter Laboratories, 1969.

Snively, W., and **Sweeney, M.:**   Fluid Balance Handbook for Practitioners. Springfield IL: Charles C Thomas, 1956.

Weisberg, H.:   Water, Electrolyte, and Acid-Base Balance, ed. 2. Baltimore: Williams & Wilkins, 1962.

— 3 —

Routes of Transport

Materials are transported between cellular and extracellular fluid via several routes, including osmosis, diffusion, filtration, active transport, pinocytosis, and phagocytosis, of which *osmosis* is the most important.

OSMOSIS A quick way of describing osmosis is to say, "Water goes where salt is." This means that if there are two solutions separated by a semipermeable membrane, the solution with the greatest concentration of electrolyte draws water from the solution with the lesser concentration of electrolyte (Fig. 3-1). It is almost as if there were an effort on the part of each electrolyte particle to surround itself with its fair share of the available water.

Osmosis is highly important in the body. If pure water not containing electrolytes were injected directly into the bloodstream, the red blood cells would absorb water and would swell and burst. If an extremely salty solution were injected into a vein, the red blood cells would lose water to their salty environment and would shrink, just as your fingers do if they have been in water too long. Osmosis occurs when the extracellular fluid develops an electrolyte content lower or higher than normal, because of disease or an accident such as drowning.

Osmotic pressure refers to the drawing power for water and depends on the number of molecules in solution. Electrolytes and substances such as mannitol with their low molecular weights exert ordinary osmotic pressure. Albumin and other substances with high molecular weights exert a special kind of osmotic pressure known as *colloid osmotic pressure*

or *oncotic pressure*. Colloids possess special importance since they cannot pass through the capillary wall, the barrier between plasma and interstitial fluid. Mannitol, with its low molecular weight, raises the osmotic pressure of plasma when given intravenously, whereas human albumin, having an extremely high molecular weight, exerts an oncotic pressure.

DIFFUSION The physical process of transport, called diffusion, occurs through the random movement of ions and molecules, which tend to become equally concentrated in all parts of a vessel. The molecules move incessantly, bump into each other, and bounce away. They scatter from regions where their concentration is high and pass to regions where the concentration is low. Exchanges of oxygen and carbon dioxide by the lung alveoli and capillaries occur through diffusion.

ACTIVE TRANSPORT When it is necessary for ions to move from areas of lesser concentration to areas of greater concentration, active transport occurs, whereby adenosine triphosphate (ATP) is released from a cell to enable certain substances to acquire the energy needed to pass through the cell membrane. This method of transfer, still not fully understood, may involve carrier systems located within cell membranes. Sodium ions, potassium ions, and amino acids are probably carried through all cell membranes by active transport, which also occurs in the transfer of chloride ions, hydrogen ions, phosphate ions, calcium ions, magnesium ions, creatinine, and uric acid through some cell membranes.

9

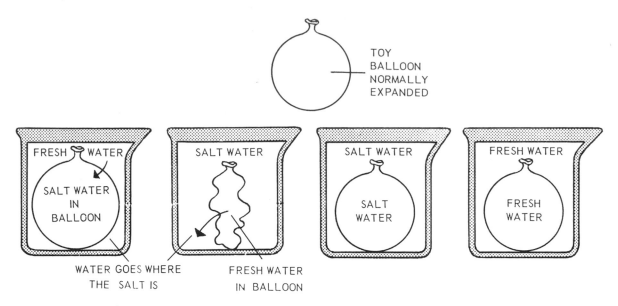

Figure 3-1. The principle of osmosis: "Water goes where the salt is."

FILTRATION   The transfer of water and dissolved substances through a permeable membrane from a region of high pressure to a region of low pressure is called filtration. The force behind filtration is *hydrostatic pressure,* produced by the pumping action of the heart. Examples of filtration include the passage of water and electrolytes from the arterial end of the capillary beds to the interstitial fluid and the passage of water and small molecules from the glomerular capillaries of the kidneys into the tubules. Opposing the hydrostatic pressure, which tends to force water and electrolytes out of the capillaries, is the oncotic pressure of the plasma proteins, which tends to hold them back.

PINOCYTOSIS AND PHAGOCYTOSIS   A form of movement by which large molecular weight substances, such as protein, enter body cells is pinocytosis (protein molecules are taken into the cell by invagination of the cell membrane). In phagocytosis, the microorganisms, cells, or foreign particles are engulfed or digested by phagocytes. Leukocytes employ phagocytosis in attacking bacteria.

COMMENT   It is via these methods of exchange that the body cells are nourished and excrete wastes, which greatly alters the composition of extracellular fluid. The effects would be catastrophic were it not for chemical regulatory activities that are carried out by the body. This enables the pond within the skin to maintain its compositional integrity and, at the same time, to keep the body cells just as healthy as if they were still floating in the wide blue Cambrian sea.

BIBLIOGRAPHY

Anthony, C., and Kolthoff, N.:   Textbook of Anatomy and Physiology, ed. 9. St. Louis: C. V. Mosby, 1975.

Ganong, W.:   Review of Medical Physiology, ed. 8. Los Altos, CA: Lange Medical Publications, 1977.

— 4 —

Organs of Homeostasis

For the maintenance of health, the body must maintain homeostasis—the normal state of the body fluids. The volume and electrolyte composition of extracellular fluid must be held very close to normal, in view of the many possible abnormalities involving water or electrolytes. Body cells constantly pour the results of chemical reactions into the extracellular fluid; they constantly withdraw from it substances needed for specific organ or cell activities. We eat and drink a wide variety of materials not needed by our body, and the digestive tract indiscriminately absorbs most of the substances offered it.

The volume of the liquids we drink would overcome us if there were no mechanism for maintaining a constant extracellular fluid volume. These problems in health are multiplied in disease, and this adds to the already gigantic task of maintaining homeostasis.

THE HOMEOSTATIC MECHANISM

Fortunately, nature has provided each of us with a system of automation, which demonstrates the wisdom of the body. In its handling of a complex task, this system, called the *homeostatic mechanism*, puts man-made automation to shame. Claude Bernard, with his amazing foresight, sensed the presence of these mechanisms even though he had no precise knowledge concerning them, for, in 1857, he said, "All the vital mechanisms, however varied they may be, have always but one end, that of preserving the constancy of the conditions of life in the internal en-

vironment." What he clearly meant by the internal environment was the body extracellular fluid. The homeostatic mechanism utilizes every body system and every body organ, with the possible exception of the reproductive organs. The lungs, kidneys, heart, adrenal glands, pituitary gland, and parathyroid glands are particularly involved, and because these organs are so important, we call them the *organs of homeostasis* (Fig. 4-1).

The lungs serve to regulate the oxygen level and carbon dioxide level of blood. Since carbon dioxide stems from the carbonic acid in the blood, the lungs help maintain the extremely important balance between acids and alkalies in extracellular fluid. As far as fluid balance is concerned, perhaps the chief role of the lungs lies in excreting CO_2 (an acid material) when there is an excessive concentration of hydrogen ions in the extracellular fluid or in retaining CO_2 when a deficit of hydrogen ion concentration exists.

Next, we have the great renocardiovascular mechanism. It includes the kidneys, the blood vessels, which bring blood to the kidneys, and the heart, which pumps the blood. How important the kidneys are! They might be called the master chemists of our body fluids (Fig. 4-2), for it is not what we eat and drink, but how the kidneys function that determines the volume and chemical composition of extracellular fluid. They excrete chemical wastes and remove from the extracellular fluid a great variety of foreign substances indiscriminately absorbed by the digestive tract. The kidneys further sort out electrolytes as they pass from the blood through their filtering beds, excreting all but those that the body needs. Consider:

Pituitary Mechanism
  • ADH from posterior pituitary
Parathyroid Mechanism
  • Parathormone
Renocardiovascular Mechanism
  • At least 8 cardinal functions
Pulmonary Mechanism
  • Hyperventilation/hypoventilation
Adrenal Mechanism
  • Cortex: aldosterone
  • Medulla: epinephrine

Figure 4-1. Key body homeostatic mechanisms.

the kidneys have an *excretory* function. They excrete the products of protein catabolism; they excrete powerful acids, such as phosphoric and sulfuric acids; they excrete certain drugs and toxins. They have a *regulatory* function, adjusting the concentration of electrolytes and the quantity of water in the extracellular fluid. In addition, they play an important role in regulating blood pressure through the secretion of renin from the juxtaglomerular apparatus of the kidneys. The kidneys also *regenerate*, for they produce bicarbonate when it is needed. They *convert* one form of vitamin D, which the body cannot use, to a form that the body can use. The kidneys even have a *manufacturing* function, for they synthesize erythropoietin, needed for normal red blood corpuscle function. We can exist for hours, days, or even longer without the use of our bones, muscles, digestive organs, nerves, endocrine glands, and even the cerebrum, but if the kidneys totally cease their chemical regulation of the extracellular fluid for an hour, physiologic deterioration promptly commences.

The kidneys are completely dependent on the heart, which pumps about 1,700 L. of blood to the kidneys for cleansing every day. Some 180 L. of this amount is filtered through the kidneys, and approximately 1.5 L. of this daily filtrate passes out as urine —the rest is reabsorbed.

The adrenal glands, located above the kidneys, secrete numerous hormones that influence the body in many ways, both in health and in disease. These glands function in the retention and excretion of water and electrolytes, especially sodium, chloride, and potassium. As far as body fluid disturbances are concerned, perhaps the key adrenal hormone is aldosterone. Secreted in the zona glomerulosa of the adrenal cortex, it is the great sodium saver. While conserving sodium, aldosterone saves chloride and

water as well and causes the excretion of potassium. Epinephrine, a hormone of the adrenal medulla, imitates the sympathetic nervous system in times of emergency. It increases the blood pressure, enhancing pulmonary ventilation, dilating blood vessels needed for meeting emergencies (e.g., those of the skeletal muscles), constricting those not needed (e.g., those of the gastrointestinal tract), and inhibiting the emptying of the contents of the gastrointestinal tract and bladder.

The pituitary gland, located within the brain, directly affects the body's conservation of water via its secretion of antidiuretic hormone (ADH). This water-conserving hormone is manufactured in the hypothalamus and then stored in the posterior pituitary gland, from where it is released when needed. ADH is the great water-controlling hormone, acting on the pores of the collecting ducts of the nephrons to determine the amount of water reabsorbed from the tubular urine.

The parathyroid glands are the last of the major organs of homeostasis. Located near or embedded in the thyroid gland, these pea-sized glands regulate the level of calcium in the extracellular fluid via their secretion of the important hormone parathormone, which acts to elevate the calcium level in the extracellular fluid. Without parathormone, one would die of calcium deficit within a few days' time.

The organs of body automation usually function efficiently; nevertheless, when any of the organs of homeostasis does malfunction, those persons caring for the patient face a formidable task.

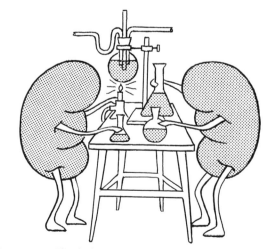

Figure 4-2. The kidneys are the master chemists of our *sea within.*

BIBLIOGRAPHY

Catt, K.:   An ABC of Endocrinology. Boston: Little, Brown & Co., 1971.

Chaffee, E., and **Greisheimer, E.:**   Basic Physiology and Anatomy, ed. 3. Philadelphia: J. B. Lippincott, 1974.

Garrison, F.:   An Introduction of the History of Medicine. Philadelphia: W. B. Saunders Co., 1929.

Snively, W. (ed.):   Body Fluid Disturbances. New York: Grune & Stratton, 1962.

Williams, R. (ed.):   Textbook of Endocrinology, ed. 4. Philadelphia: W. B. Saunders Co., 1968.

— 5 —

Essentials of Nutrition

Since this manual has as its chief goal the understanding of body fluid disturbances and their management, why inquire into the fundamentals of nutrition? There are compelling reasons. The constituents of body fluids that vary and so produce clinical disorders cut across chemical lines. Water (H^+OH^-) is a compound. Sodium (Na^+), potassium (K^+), calcium (Ca^{++}), and magnesium (Mg^{++}) are chemical elements and also minerals. Bicarbonate (HCO_3^-) is a molecule. Proteinate (proteinate$^-$) is a complex and gigantic molecule for which we have no abbreviation. Hydrogen (H^+) and carbon dioxide (CO_2) are gases except when they combine with other elements or molecules. All these substances develop electrical charges when dissolved in water, hence are electrolytes. *All actively influence and are influenced by other nutrients, such as carbohydrates, fats or lipids, vitamins, and other minerals.*

Repair of body fluid disturbances frequently involves correction of additional problems, such as vitamin deficits, major or minor mineral deficits, or caloric deficits (or, much less frequently, excesses of any of these nutrients). Whether an imbalance is a relatively simple one, such as sodium deficit, or a complex disturbance, such as protein-calorie malnutrition, the ideal route for intake is the enteral, either oral or by tube. Such correction might consist merely of supplying a well-balanced diet, or diet plus between-meal supplements, or oral feedings plus tube feedings, or even a precisely calculated diet, such as a chemically-defined diet. Any substance that can be given enterally usually can be infused intravenously when the former route is not feasible. In ad-

dition to simple parenteral solutions, all needed nutrients plus a surplus of calories to repair serious preexisting deficits can be injected. Such a solution is administered via a large central vein; this is called *hyperalimentation.* Or, similarly, a solution can be infused into a central vein to provide complete nutrition without an excess of calories over the daily need. This type of parenteral alimentation is called *complete parenteral* nutrition.

Now let us examine the physiology, not only of water and electrolytes, but of the *other minerals,* both major and minor; *vitamins;* and the *substance nutrients,* including carbohydrate, fat, and protein. (The latter is both an electrolyte and a substance nutrient.) By such a holistic approach to the body's needs, the groundwork can be laid for a theoretical and practical understanding of body fluid disturbances and related nutritional problems.

THE SUBSTANCE NUTRIENTS

One great class of nutrients comprises the overwhelming mass of our food, so we have given it the label of *substance nutrients,* meaning that they occupy space to a far greater extent than do other nutrients, such as vitamins. The substance nutrients include carbohydrates, fats, and proteins.

Carbohydrates

Carbohydrates are chemical compounds consisting of the elements carbon, hydrogen, and oxygen. The carbohydrate molecule contains hydrogen and oxygen in the same proportions as they occur in water—hence the name carbohydrate. The carbohydrate building block is called the *monosaccharide*, or simple sugar. Monosaccharides have a general formula of CH_2O and cannot be further broken down by the process of hydrolysis. These carbohydrates are colorless, crystalline substances and have a mildly sweet taste.

The monosaccharides are further classified according to the number of carbon atoms in the chain. Thus, a *diose* is $C_2H_4O_2$; a *triose*, $C_3H_6O_3$; a *tetrose*, $C_4H_8O_4$; a *pentose*, $C_5H_{10}O_5$; a *hexose*, $C_6H_{12}O_6$; and a *heptose*, $C_7H_{14}O_7$. Most of the important monosaccharides found in foods are either pentoses or hexoses. One hexose—glucose (or dextrose)—is by all odds the most important of the monosaccharides. When we refer to the *blood sugar*, we are referring to the glucose of the blood. Fructose, sometimes called fruit sugar, is another important hexose. The hexoses galactose and mannose do not occur in free form in foods. The pentoses ribose, xylose, and arabinose likewise are not found free in foods.

Disaccharides are sugars that yield two monosaccharides when they are hydrolyzed. They include sucrose, familiarly known as table sugar; lactose, also called milk sugar; and maltose, or malt sugar. *Polysaccharides* are carbohydrates that hydrolyze to more than ten monosaccharides. They include the indigestible carbohydrates cellulose, hemicellulose, and pectin; the partially digestible carbohydrates inulin, galactogen, and mannosans; and, finally, the digestible carbohydrates starch, dextran, and glycogen.

Carbohydrates constitute the chief mass of our food. Indeed, for the past seventy years, carbohydrate has consistently provided about 50 per cent of our total caloric intake. In primitive parts of the world, the proportion of carbohydrate in the diet is largely governed by the vegetation and animals in the area. Naturally, the proportionate intake of carbohydrate is high in tropical countries, where vegetation is plentiful and where the high temperature and humidity promote rapid deterioration of meats. But in the far north, where individuals live chiefly on meat and fish, carbohydrate intake is relatively low. Economic factors also influence carbohydrate intake. Many foods that are high in carbohydrate are relatively inexpensive. Hence, the proportion of carbohydrate in the diet tends to be higher in individuals of lower economic levels than in those of the higher levels.

Among the chief food sources of carbohydrate are vegetables, especially root vegetables (e.g., beets, potatoes, carrots, turnips, radishes, and onions), legumes (e.g., the various beans, lentils, and peanuts), and the stalks and leaves of vegetables (e.g., lettuce, cabbage, spinach, broccoli, asparagus, collards, rhubarb, celery, endive, and kohlrabi). Fruits, including apples, bananas, peaches, pears, cherries, oranges, grapefruits, lemons, limes, apricots, and berries of all kinds, also contain large amounts of carbohydrate. Other good sources include molasses and cane sugar, beet sugar, maple sugar, corn syrup, and dairy products, including milk and cheese. Meats and seafoods contain relatively small quantities of carbohydrate, hence are usually thought of in terms of their protein or protein and fat contribution.

The primary role of carbohydrate is to provide heat, or energy. The terms *heat* and *energy* are, of course, interchangeable. Heat, or energy, is measured in *kilocalories* (kcal). A kilocalorie can be defined as *the quantity of heat energy required to raise the temperature of one liter (L) of water one degree centigrade (C)*. (Most individuals use the term *calorie* instead of *kilocalorie*, but this is incorrect usage since a calorie really is a unit of measure used by physical scientists and is 1000 times smaller than the kilocalorie, the unit used by nutritionists.) A gram (Gm) of carbohydrate provides 4 kilocalories of heat when it is burned, or metabolized.

Carbohydrates not only constitute the *chief* source of energy but they also constitute the *preferred* source. In addition to being less expensive, carbohydrate calories are far more efficiently utilized by the body than are calories derived from fats and proteins, the other substance nutrients.

Fats or Lipids

Our second substance nutrient is fat, or lipid. The fats are enormously complex and cannot be defined in simple chemical terms as can carbohydrates and proteins. Indeed, their chemistry is so complex that some investigators devote their entire lives to its study. Fats are organic substances, which means that they were originally derived from living organisms and hence contain the element carbon. Fats do not dissolve in water but, in the laboratory, chemists can identify fats by their solubility in ether, chloroform, benzene, and similar solvents. It is via this solubility that fats are defined. In addition, fats have a greasy feel.

Fats have several important functions in the body. First, they serve as a storage form for excess kcals derived from carbohydrates, hence are an important reservoir of energy, available for use in time of need. The number of kcals that can be stored as fat appears to be limitless, as evidenced by the fat men and women who are featured in sideshows. But fat has other functions: it serves as an insulator and, hence, helps keep us warm on chilly days; it also serves as a protective covering for various organs, cushioning shocks transmitted to them from outside the body.

Fat plays an active role in metabolism. Under some circumstances, excessive intake of certain types of fats constitutes one of the risk factors in the development of the disorder of blood vessels termed *atherosclerosis*. This disease involves the deposit of cholesterol in the walls of arteries and can lead to serious disease of heart, brain, kidneys, and other organs. But the fat intake is only one of several etiologic factors in atherosclerosis. Others include hypertension, smoking (especially of cigarettes), inadequate exercise, and excessive psychic stress. In the blood, lipids may combine with protein and travel through the blood vessels as lipoproteins. If the lipoprotein level becomes too high, the individual has *hyperlipoproteinemia*, a condition that often leads to atherosclerosis.

Fats are found in many foods that come from animals and in some plant foods as well. When the fat is clearly visible, as in butter, margarine, and vegetable oils, or adjacent to the muscle in a cut of meat, we can clearly see that we are dealing with a source of food fat. Visible fats are prominent in the usual American diet. But there are many other food sources of fat, such as the cream of milk, cheeses (except those made with skim milk), avocados, nuts, chocolate, and a host of desserts, in which the fat, though part of the food, may not be recognized. Fat usually exists in liquid form, or oil, in vegetable substances. Examples are the oils from soybeans, cottonseed, olives, corn, coconut, peanuts, palm, sunflower, and safflower.

In foods, most fat consists of *triglycerides*, which are composed of one molecule of the compound glycerol and three fatty acid molecules (not necessarily the same fatty acid). The physical state of the triglyceride depends on the length of the chain and the degree of *saturation* of the fatty acid components. The more *unsaturated* a fatty acid is, the shorter the length of the chain and the lower the melting point of the fat. A compound that is said to be saturated has all its chemical affinities satisfied, i.e., it cannot unite with additional atoms or groups. On the other hand, a compound that is unsaturated can unite with other atoms or groups. If a compound has a high degree of unsaturation, it is said to be *polyunsaturated*. In edible fats or oils, fatty acids usually contain either sixteen or eighteen carbon atoms and may be saturated, unsaturated, or polyunsaturated. Most vegetable oils are unsaturated or polyunsaturated; exceptions to this rule are coconut oil and the oil of chocolate. However, if a polyunsaturated oil (e.g., peanut oil) is treated with hydrogen in order to make it firmer, it then becomes a saturated oil and loses the advantages that derive from its unsaturation. Thus, margarine is polyunsaturated in direct proportion to its softness. Margarines that consist of polyunsaturated fats are customarily kept in the freezer in grocery stores to maintain their firmness. If such margarines are treated with hydrogen (hydrogenated) to render them more firm, they are no longer polyunsaturated. A "good" fat has thus been changed to a "bad" fat.

The fats of meats—notably the red meats, such as beef, veal, pork, and lamb—are high in saturated fats. The total fat content of veal, however, is lower than that of the other red meats. The meat of fowl, such as chicken and turkey (but not ducks or geese), is lower in saturated fats than are red meats, especially if one removes the skin. The saturated fat content of seafoods requires additional research, although they are believed to be more unsaturated than the red meats. Olive oil is partially saturated, thus occupies a position intermediate between the saturated and polyunsaturated oils. The fat of milk and other dairy products is highly saturated.

Animal fats also contain *cholesterol*, either free or combined with a fatty acid in a compound called a cholesterol ester. Cholesterol has great physiologic importance: it acts as a structural element of the cell wall, and it serves as an intermediate in the synthesis of many physiologically active hormones. Vegetable oils have no cholesterol, but they do contain plant sterols. These are poorly absorbed by the body and may even interfere with the absorption of cholesterol. Edible fats also contain small quantities of phospholipids. These are important emulsifying agents, essential for the proper digestion of fats.

Some fatty acids either cannot be synthesized by the body or are synthesized in inadequate amounts for growth, maintenance, and proper functioning of many physiologic processes. These fatty acids are called *essential fatty acids* (EFA). Two fatty acids have been shown to be essential for many species of animals and for human infants: linoleic acid and arachidonic acid, both polyunsaturated. While animals cannot manufacture linoleic acid and must, therefore, obtain it from the diet, they can form arachidonic acid from linoleic acid in the body; hence, some nutritionists would not include arachidonic acid as an essential fatty acid. High concentrations of linoleic acid are found in the edible vegetable oils of corn, cottonseed, peanut, safflower, and soybean. Olive and coconut oils are not sources of the acid. Small amounts of arachidonic acid are found in animal fats.

Deficiency of fatty acids has been produced both in animals and in man by restricting the intake of essential fatty acids. When men were placed on diets virtually free of EFA, they developed dermatitis and derangements in lipid transport. Although deficiency has not been reported in human adults on ordinary diets, it has been observed in hospitalized patients maintained solely on fat-free intravenous alimentation for prolonged periods.

Essential fatty acids appear to play a role in the regulation of cholesterol metabolism. Diets high in polyunsaturated fatty acids, including the EFA, reduce the serum cholesterol both in experimental animals and in man; just what happens to the cholesterol removed from the blood is not known. EFA in phospholipids play a significant role in tissue metabolism: they help maintain the integrity and function of cellular and subcellular membranes. EFA have been demonstrated to be precursors of the hormone-like compounds called prostaglandins, which participate actively in a wide variety of physiologic processes.

Ingestion of sufficient quantities of EFA to prevent deficiency is not difficult: the intake need constitute only 1 to 2 per cent of the total kcals/day.

Protein

Proteins consist of large, complex molecules. Like carbohydrates and fats, they contain carbon, oxygen, and hydrogen; but, unlike them, they also contain the element nitrogen. In addition, some proteins contain sulphur, iron, phosphorus, and iodine. The building block of the protein molecule is a small compound called an *amino acid*. In a protein molecule, more than one hundred amino acid units are linked together by what is called the *peptide linkage*, in which the nitrogen of one amino acid is joined to the carbon of another.

Although forty different amino acids have been isolated from various proteins, only some twenty two are present in all proteins, though in varying amounts. The composition of each protein is highly specific, and every molecule of a given protein will have the same amino acids in precisely the same order. Combinations of amino acids joined by the peptide linkage form *peptides;* peptides combine to form *polypeptides*, and polypeptides unite to form proteins.

The body does not utilize proteins in the form in which they are eaten. Rather, it breaks the protein molecules down in the digestive tract to polypeptides, then to peptides, then to amino acids. Using these amino acids and others, which it manufactures itself, it then proceeds to build the specific proteins required for the many essential missions of protein within the body. Some of the amino acids the body uses in this process must be obtained from proteins that are eaten since they cannot be manufactured within the body. There are nine of these, and they are designated the *essential amino acids*. Other amino acids used by the body for protein synthesis need not be contained in eaten proteins, for they can actually be manufactured within the body from nonprotein chemicals. There are thirteen of these, and they are termed—somewhat misleadingly—*nonessential*. But they are "nonessential" only in the sense that they need not be obtained from ingested food. Amino acids "essential" for the human include histidine, isoleucine, leucine, lysine, methionine, phenylalanine, threonine, tryptophan, and valine. Although histidine is an essential amino acid for infants, it is not clearly established that it is essential for the adult. Obviously, the essential amino acids are the most critical components of dietary proteins. If they are provided, additional nitrogen can be supplied in a variety of forms. Two amino acids are sometimes called *semiessential:* cystine, which can be converted from methionine, and tyrosine, which can be converted from phenylalanine.

Proteins play a unique role in nutrition since they provide the structural building blocks for muscle, bone, enzymes, hormones, and other essential body constituents. Because of protein's unique role as a structural material, it is appropriately referred to as the *keystone nutrient,* forming in a sense a veritable keystone of the nutritional arch.

When one considers the cluster of essential functions performed by protein, it becomes clear that protein deficit can have catastrophic effects on the body. And the symptoms and findings in protein deficit are as numerous as the functions of protein: loss of appetite (which may have helped cause the deficit in the first place), loss of weight (chiefly from the muscle mass), emotional depression, reduced resistance to infection, lack of energy, and chronic fatigue—to name only a few. In severe protein deficit, the plasma albumin is below 4 Gm./100 ml. and may even drop below 3. How does one develop protein deficit? From failure to eat sufficient food of the proper type, from burns, from trauma, from surgical operations (especially repeated surgical operations), from disease of the gastrointestinal tract, and from malignant tumors. Protein deficit often comes on insidiously and may not be suspected until it is far advanced. To detect it early, you have to be aware of the possibility. (In the clinical section of this book, we'll examine protein deficit in considerably greater detail.)

Proteins vary greatly in their capacity to provide protein nutrition. Put another way, they differ in *quality.* And quality depends chiefly on whether the protein contains balanced amounts of the nine essential amino acids (EAA). In order to manufacture proteins, the body needs all of the EAA, and it needs them simultaneously; thus, they must all be ingested within a brief span of time, as at a meal. If one EAA is present in only a small amount or absent altogether, protein synthesis slows down or stops completely. EAA, of course, come from the protein foods we eat. Most food proteins contain all of the EAA, but, with a few exceptions, they contain inadequate quantities of one or more of them. Suppose the body is manufacturing a certain protein that requires a specific pattern of amino acids—and every protein does have its own specific pattern. So, you eat a meal consisting chiefly of a protein that provides balanced quantities of all the EAA except for tryptophan, which is present in only 50 per cent of the requirement. From the standpoint of protein synthesis, the quantity of all the EAA in that food protein is reduced to the 50 per cent represented by tryptophan. The tryptophan of that protein is a *limiting amino acid.* For if even one amino acid is partially missing in an ingested protein, all of the EAA of that protein are reduced in the same proportion. As we shall see, there is a way of getting around this by eating the proper combinations of protein foods in what is called *protein complementarity.*

How can we evaluate the nutritional worth of a protein? One useful index is the *biological value,* the percentage of absorbed protein that the body uses. Another important index is the *digestibility* of the protein, which refers to the proportion of the protein that gets absorbed by the digestive tract. Both these indices reveal the proportion of the protein that gets absorbed by the digestive tract. One term covers both: *net protein utilization* (NPU). You can readily see how valuable this characteristic of a protein is when you consider that it tells us just how much of a given protein is actually used by the body. The protein with the highest NPU is egg. Cheese and milk are not far behind, nor are meats and seafoods. Proteins with low NPU's include peanuts, corn, and gelatin.

How much protein does one need each day? The Food and Nutrition Board of the National Research Council has set the Recommended Daily Dietary Allowance (RDA) at 0.47 Gm./kg. body weight for the adult, with considerably more for children. This value assumes a protein with an almost perfect NPU that would be used completely by the body. But the total grams of protein eaten are never entirely used; the percentage used depends, of course, on the NPU of the proteins eaten. In view of these facts, nutritionists have come up with a useful formula for determining the actual desirable protein intake:

Protein allowance if eating fully usable protein (0.47 Gm./kg. body weight)	$\times$	$\dfrac{100}{\text{Net protein utilization characteristic of the national diet of the country}}$	$=$	Grams of total protein recommended for that population/person/kg. body weight/day

Suppose we have a 70-kg. individual with the NPU of the national diet at 70. Using the formula $0.47 \times 100/70 = 0.67$ Gm. protein/kg body weight. So, 0.67×70 (the weight in kg.) $= 46.9$ Gm. protein. These figures represent a diet moderately supplied with meat, poultry, seafood, or dairy products, along with plant proteins. Now let's consider a national diet consisting largely of plant proteins with an NPU of 50: $0.47 \times 100/50 = 0.94 \times 70 = 65.8$ Gm. protein required to meet the RDA.

Protein allowances are only approximate when applied to a given individual. The actual protein requirement can vary severalfold from one person to another, even though the individuals are healthy. Following injury, in sickness, or under conditions of severe stress, the variations may be even greater, with the requirement usually higher.

As you examine the tabulation showing the NPU for various food proteins (Table 5-1), note that proteins of animal and vegetable origin should not be regarded as in separate categories. For example, meat does not head the list; indeed, soybean and whole rice protein may equal—or in some instances exceed—the NPU for meat. One's protein nutrition depends on the correct assortment of amino acids regardless of the source. Hence, we can obtain the correct assortment of amino acids without eating meat or eggs or dairy products, or even without any of these. Thus, we can eat large amounts of the proper plant proteins so as to obtain a balanced cluster of amino acids. In choosing plant proteins, one should pick those whose amino acid patterns are complementary, eating these foods at the same meal. Dishes and meals are planned so that the protein of one food makes up for the EAA deficiencies of another food. This is what is meant by *protein complementarity.*

Look at specific examples: the lysine strength of seafood can be used to complement the protein of foods low in lysine, such as grains, peanuts, black walnuts, brazil nuts, sunflower seeds, and sesame seeds. Dairy products have excellent NPUs, but they are especially strong in isoleucine and lysine. So, milk or cheese can well be used with rice, wheat, corn + soybeans, peanuts, sesame seeds, and sesame seeds + wheat. Legumes, such as beans and peanuts, complement rice, wheat, corn, milk, sesame seeds, and sesame seeds + wheat. Nuts and seeds, such as sunflower seeds or meal, sesame seeds, black walnuts, or brazil nuts, complement soybeans, beans, peanuts + milk, and peanuts + wheat + milk.

Grains, cereals, and their products complement legumes, milk, and peanuts + milk. Fresh vegetables are quite low in the sulfur-containing amino acids methionine and cystine, except for mushrooms, which are high in these amino acids. Hence, mushrooms complement lima beans, green peas, and broccoli. Nutritional additives include dried, powdered egg white; brewer's yeast powder; and commercial wheat germ. Excellent complements include nutritional additives with sesame seeds, black walnuts,

Table 5-1. Net Protein Utilization (NPU) of Various Proteins

Food Protein	NPU in Percents
Egg	93
Milk	83
Fish	80
Cheese	70
Whole rice	68
Meat	67
Poultry	67
Tofu (soybean curd)	65
Cashews	57
Lima beans	52
Corn	52
Peanuts	43
Kidney beans	35

barley, oatmeal, and rice. Meats, poultry, and seafoods, even in small quantities, are rich in all EAA, hence are splendid in combination with grains, which are especially low in lysine. Turkey is especially useful for complementing plant proteins.

Native peoples appear to have sensed the importance of protein complementarity: Spanish-Americans have long eaten beans, rice, and corn at the same meal. The Chinese have been enjoying dishes made from soybean combined with other vegetables since long before history was recorded. Many foreign dishes involve excellent combinations of plant proteins.

How the Body Uses Nutrients

For a practical and thorough understanding of nutrition, we must examine how the body converts food (whether liquid or solid) into forms in which it can be used to provide heat, or energy, to carry out cellular work, as well as to construct bones, muscles, organs, hormones, enzymes, and the other substances that make up the body. With few exceptions, the foodstuffs we eat and drink are not ready for use by the body; their conversion to a usable form is accomplished by a series of processes: *digestion, absorption,* and *metabolism.*

Where do these processes, which represent the essentials of the great and continuing miracle of food utilization, do their work? *Digestion* occurs inside the gastrointestinal (digestive or alimentary) tract. *Absorption* is accomplished through the walls of the tract, really from the lumen through the mucosal cells of the intestinal villi into blood or lymph vessels coursing through the villi. *Metabolism,* the final stage of food utilization, involves the fates of the billions of tiny digested units of food after they enter the magical mini-factories we call the body cells.

DIGESTION   The digestive tract (Fig. 5-1) consists of the *digestive tube* and certain *auxiliary,* or *helping, organs.* The entrance to the tube is, of course, the mouth. Food progresses from the mouth into the oropharynx, then the laryngopharynx, esophagus, stomach, small intestine (it includes the short duodenum and the much longer jejunum and ileum), then into the large intestine (in order, the cecum, ascending colon, transverse colon, descending colon, sigmoid colon, and rectum). Auxiliary structures or organs include the teeth, tongue, salivary glands, pancreas, liver, gall bladder, and a sprinkling of tiny endocrine glands located in the walls of the stomach, duodenum, jejunum, and ileum.

Digestion encompasses all of the changes that foods undergo while they are inside the digestive tube. What digestion accomplishes is this: it converts food, by various mechanical and chemical actions, into units that can be absorbed through the wall of the digestive tube to be acted on outside the digestive tube by metabolic processes in the myriad cells of the body. Some foods, such as meat and bread, are changed drastically in the digestive process. Simpler —though just as essential—substances are altered little, if at all. Examples are water (HOH) and table salt, or sodium chloride (NaCl).

Mechanical Actions in the Digestive Tube Mechanical, or physical, actions change the physical form of food without altering its chemical composition and move it along the digestive tract.

First, the jaws, with the help of the teeth, cheeks, and tongue, carry out *mastication,* or *chewing.* This action decreases the size of food particles and mixes them with saliva, secreted by the salivary glands. Then various structures of the mouth cooperate with the teeth and tongue to cause *deglutition,* or *swallowing.* Food is propelled from the mouth into the oropharynx, then down into the laryngopharynx, on into the esophagus, and, finally, into the stomach. As the esophagus performs its role in swallowing, it utilizes a movement called *peristalsis.* This can be described as a wormlike movement that squeezes food down the digestive tube. A constriction, or narrowing, occurs at the upper portion of the esophagus and moves down into the next lower level, then to the next, and the next. As the waves of constriction

spread down the esophagus, they help push the food along to the stomach.

In the stomach, food is subjected to another movement—*churning.* In this movement, strong muscular action pushes the contents of the saclike stomach back and forth. Peristalsis also occurs in the stomach. This serves to move the food to the lower end toward the pyloric sphincter, the constricting muscle that leads into the duodenum. When this sphincter is closed, the descending food is stopped short, even pushed backwards. But then more peristalsis occur, and the stomach contents proceed—not all at once but in small portions—through the sphincter and into the duodenum.

The small intestine, of which the duodenum is a part, carries out churning within limited segments of intestine. Churning is of prime importance, for it mixes the food with the digestive juices and then serves to carry the digested food into close contact with the absorptive surface of the intestine, the intestinal mucosa. Thus is absorption facilitated. Peristalsis occurs throughout the small intestine; this is essential since unabsorbed food must keep moving through the jejunum and ileum and into the first portion of the large intestine, the cecum.

As food remnants enter the ascending and transverse colon, a unique type of churning occurs within the haustral sacs. It consists of rhythmic segmentation that shoves food forward and backward within the bounds of the haustral sacs before peristalsis moves the food mass farther along the tube.

As food materials reach the descending colon, a periodic form of peristalsis moves the entire contents of the descending colon into the S-shaped, or sigmoid (*sigma* is the Greek letter S) colon, then on into the rectum, which functions as a holding chamber. This massive peristaltic movement is appropriately called *mass peristalsis.* It normally takes place after a meal and serves to fill the rectal holding chamber. When fairly full, and with the voluntary cooperation of the individual, the rectum initiates *defecation*— the bowel movement or BM. Thus are food wastes, with their billions of usually harmless bacteria, expelled from the body.

Chemical Digestion Chemical digestion of foodstuffs depends on the action of a variety of digestive juices and enzymes. Enzymes, complex proteins produced in the body cells under the specifications laid down by DNA, are by nature catalysts: they promote chemical reactions without appearing in the

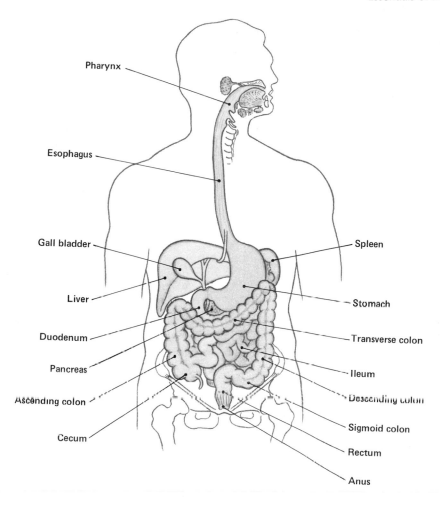

Figure 5-1 The digestive tract.

Labels on figure:
Pharynx
Esophagus
Gall bladder
Liver
Duodenum
Pancreas
Ascending colon
Cecum
Spleen
Stomach
Transverse colon
Ileum
Descending colon
Sigmoid colon
Rectum
Anus

final product of the reaction. When the modern system of naming enzymes is employed, the enzyme customarily ends in *ase*. We shall use *ase* with the root name of the nutrient or other substance whose chemical reaction is being catalyzed. Thus, *sucrase* catalyzes the breakdown of *sucrose* or cane sugar, *maltase* of *maltose*, and *lactase* of *lactose*. A protein-digesting enzyme is *protease* and a fat-digesting enzyme is *lipase*. If the protein-digestive enzyme is secreted by the stomach, it is called gastric protease and, if it is secreted by the pancreas, it is *pancreatic protease*. The logic of this system of nomenclature makes it far easier to remember the names of specific enzymes and where they are produced.

Chemical digestion begins with *saliva,* which contains the enzyme amylase (called ptyalin in the old terminology). Amylase hydrolyzes starch, a com-

plex carbohydrate (or polysaccharide). Amylase breaks down starch to form maltose, a disaccharide. Salivary amylase works only in a fairly alkaline environment. Hence, when amylase is swallowed and reaches the acid stomach interior, it becomes inactive. Thus, the food-digesting action of saliva is extremely limited.

Somewhat more active in chemical digestion are the *stomach juices*. They contain gastric protease (formerly called pepsin), which attacks protein, and hydrochloric acid, which aids gastric protease in its action. By gastric action, protein is broken down only to proteoses and polypeptides rather than to the true building blocks of protein, amino acids. The stomach also produces gastric lipase, a feeble fat-digesting enzyme, which helps convert emulsified fats to fatty acids and glycerol.

We now move down the digestive tube to the duodenum, which receives *bile,* produced in the *liver,* stored in the gall bladder, and released into the *duodenum* as needed. Although bile is not an enzyme and contains no enzymes, it does serve as a surface active agent that acts on large fat droplets to transform them into many tiny fat droplets in a physical state referred to as an emulsion. This transformation makes it possible for fat-digesting enzymes to act. (Homogenized milk is an emulsion.)

This brings us to the *pancreas,* unique in that it produces both *digestive juices,* which pour into the duodenum, and *hormones,* which are released directly into the bloodstream. Since they are released onto a surface—the duodenal mucosa—the digestive enzymes of the pancreas are examples of an *exocrine* secretion. The pancreatic hormones—insulin and glucagon—on the other hand, are released directly into the bloodstream and are examples of *endocrine* secretions. Indeed, all hormones are endocrine secretions. The importance of the pancreas in digestion cannot be overestimated: it produces powerful enzymes that act on all three of the bulk nutrients. The protein-digesting enzyme of the pancreas is called *pancreatic protease,* sometimes by the old name of *trypsin.* But it does not exist in the pancreas in an active form. The inactive form, trypsinogen, is converted to the active enzyme when it enters the duodenum. There it breaks down intact or partially digested protein into proteoses, polypeptides, and the ultimate building blocks of protein, amino acids. *Pancreatic lipase,* also called *steapsin,* converts fats previously emulsified by bile into fatty acids and glycerol. Pancreatic lipase is especially important since there exists no other important source of fat-digesting enzyme. A third pancreatic enzyme—*pancreatic amylase,* or *amylopsin*—changes starch to maltose.

Glands in the walls of the small intestine produce *intestinal juice,* also called succus entericus. It contains enzymes called peptidases. As the name tells us, they act on peptides, the last stage of protein breakdown before amino acids. Intestinal enzymes that act on carbohydrates include sucrase, which changes sucrose, or cane sugar, to glucose and fructose (both simple sugars, or monosaccharides); lactase, which converts lactose, or milk sugar, to glucose and galactose (also monosaccharides); and maltase, which transforms maltose, or malt sugar, into glucose (two molecules of glucose for each molecule of maltose). The small intestine secretes no fat-digesting enzymes.

The end products of digestion of the bulk nutrients (carbohydrate, fat, and protein) possess this enormous significance: they are the form in which the bulk nutrients are absorbed through the intestinal walls. They are also the chemical units on which the processes of metabolism go to work. For carbohydrate, the end products are *glucose* (also called dextrose and by far the most important), *fructose* (also called fruit sugar), and *galactose.* For the fats, or lipids, the end products are *fatty acids* and *glycerol.* For protein, the end products are the *amino acids* (there are at least twenty of them).

Control of Digestive Secretions   Many workings of the body originate in the great involuntary, or visceral, nervous system. The nerves, in part, control the secretion of digestive juices and enzymes. In sending out the efferent impulses that stimulate action, they are responding, in large part, to afferent messages which quite often originate in the very structures concerned. Thus, secretion of salivary juices is initiated by stimulation of taste buds on the tongue, by receptors located elsewhere in the mouth, by nerve endings in the esophagus, by sensory organs in the nasal cavity, and by visual receptors. This widespread sensory input activates the visceral nervous system, which in turn sends out the orders resulting in flow of juices.

The secretion of gastric juices arises from the same chain of events that starts salivary secretion. But it is also partly controlled by a hormone, or bloodborne messenger, called gastrin, formed by the gastric mucosa when the products of partial protein digestion are present. Another of the so-called gastrointestinal hormones, enterogastrone, is secreted by the duodenal mucosa when gastric contents pass from the stomach into the duodenum. It acts to inhibit both gastric secretory activity and motility. The presence of gastric contents in the duodenum also causes the secretion of two more gastrointestinal hormones that stimulate pancreatic secretion—pancreozymin, which causes the pancreas to release juices rich in pancreatic enzymes, and secretin, which nudges the pancreas to release a dilute juice low in enzymes and the liver to secrete bile. Finally, the gastrointestinal hormone cholecystokinin responds to the presence of fats in the duodenum by causing the gall bladder to eject some of its stored bile into the duodenum.

Just what factors bring about the secretion of the enzymes of the intestinal mucosa is not certain. The visceral nervous system and hormone are probably both involved.

It is within the small intestine that the overwhelming preponderance of digestion occurs. The mouth carries out only a tiny amount of digestion, with even that limited to starches; the stomach has some activity in relation to protein and fat, but it is distinctly minor; the large intestine has important functions, chief of which is the absorption of water, but it carries out no digestion. One might state the importance of the small intestine in digestion like this: if an individual had only his small intestine for digestion, he would get along adequately, perhaps well; without the digestive activities of the small intestine, he could not long stay alive.

ABSORPTION   By the term *absorption,* we mean the passage of the products of digestion through the intestinal mucosa and into the blood or lymph vessels. (In this chapter, we are focusing on the bulk nutrients. But vitamins, minerals, and water are also absorbed through the intestinal mucosa.) We shall see that several processes by which substances pass through the body's various membranes are involved.

Absorption of Carbohydrate End Products Glucose, the chief end product of carbohydrate digestion, moves into the cells of the intestinal mucosa by facilitated diffusion. Inside the cells of the mucosa, glucose is changed into a compound called glucose 6-phosphate. The transformation is catalyzed by the enzyme glucokinase. Because phosphate is added to glucose in the reaction, the whole process is designated *phosphorylation.* We can state the reaction in these words: glucose + adenosine triphosphate (ATP, the storage form of energy) *in the presence of glucokinase* reacts to form adenosine diphosphate (ADP) + glucose-6-phosphate. (Note that in the reaction, adenosine *tri*phosphate has lost a phosphate to glucose, changing it to a *di*phosphate.)

Now glucose-6-phosphate diffuses across the mucosal cell. Near the far border of the cell, adjacent to a blood capillary, another enzyme, *phosphatase,* reverses the phosphorylation, thus converting glucose-6-phosphate back to glucose. In short, what has happened? Phosphorylation has enabled glucose, as glucose-6-phosphate, to cross the mucosal cell from intestinal lumen to bloodstream. In the blood, it is back to glucose again.

Absorption of Lipid End Products   Absorption of lipid end products of digestion apparently requires active transport. Some fatty acids and glycerol enter the intestinal mucosal cells and there form *chylomicrons,* emulsified fat particles about 1 micron in diameter. The chylomicrons then leave the mucosal cells and enter the lymphatic capillaries of the intestinal villi. Some short chain fatty acids are absorbed into the blood capillaries of the villi, while some fats are absorbed as such without first being digested to fatty acids and glycerol. Uncertainties abound in regard to the exact details of fat absorption, including the question of whether active transport is involved in absorption into the mucosal cells.

Absorption of End Products of Protein Digestion Amino acids, the end products of protein digestion, are absorbed into the blood capillaries as amino acids by facilitated diffusion.

Fate of the End Products of Digestion   End products of fat digestion that pass into the lymphatic capillaries (lacteals) move through lymph channels to the thoracic duct, passing from it to the venous circulation and finally to the liver. Other fat end products and all carbohydrate and protein end products pass to the portal vein to be carried to the liver, the body's superb center of metabolic activities.

Rapidity of Digestion and Absorption of Nutrients   Nutrients not requiring digestion, such as water and electrolytes, are absorbed with great rapidity by the healthy gastrointestinal tract. Glucose is likewise absorbed rapidly since it does not require digestive action. It, therefore, represents a form of almost instant calories and, hence, energy. Disaccharides and other more complex carbohydrates have to undergo digestive action before absorption. The same holds for fat and protein. The rapidity of absorption of vitamins would depend largely on whether they were fat soluble or water soluble. The latter would be absorbed considerably more rapidly.

METABOLISM   The term *metabolism* includes the chemical changes that the end products of digestion undergo inside cells, as well as the uses to which the cells put these end products. Two general types of metabolism occur: *catabolism* and *anabolism.* Catabolism involves the breakdown of food molecules into simpler compounds, such as water (HOH), carbon dioxide (CO_2), and nitrogenous wastes. It also includes the transfer of some of the energy from the products of the catabolic reactions to be stored in the

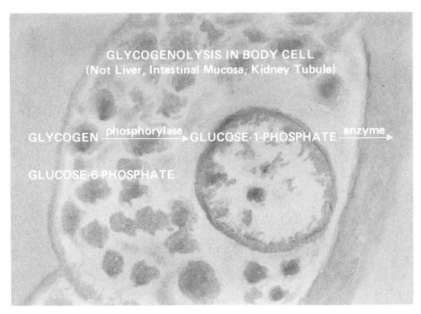

Figure 5-2. Glycolysis.

phosphate compound ATP or to be released as heat. While catabolism is in a sense destructive, it is in another sense constructive since it is essential for life. The second form of metabolism, anabolism, refers to the synthesis of complex compounds, such as glycogen, enzymes, hormones, tissues, and so on, from simple molecules, such as amino acids.

Metabolism of Carbohydrate   In the metabolism of carbohydrate within the body cells, glucose moves through the cell membrane with the help of phosphorylation. The hormone insulin promotes this process of converting glucose to glucose-6-phosphate, which is catalyzed by the enzyme glucokinase.

Catabolism of Carbohydrate. Catabolism of glucose consists of a complex series of chemical reactions within the cells of the body, which yield energy, carbon dioxide, and water. About half of the energy released from food molecules by catabolism is again stored in the high-energy, unstable bonds of ATP. The rest of the energy released is converted to heat. When ATP releases energy, it does so with explosive speed. Clearly, the purpose of the storage of energy in ATP is to provide cells with immediately available energy with which to do cellular work.

Glycolysis.   About 5 per cent of the total ATP generated during the catabolism of glucose is created by the process of glycolysis, simply defined as a series of *anaerobic* (non-oxygen using) chemical

reactions that change one molecule of glucose to two molecules of pyruvic acid (Fig. 5-2).

Citric Acid Cycle.   Closely following the reaction of glycolysis is a second series of chemical reactions that are aerobic (requiring oxygen). This, the *citric acid* or *Krebs cycle*, in a complex cascade of reactions, oxidizes two pyruvic acid molecules into six carbon dioxide molecules and six water molecules. The citric acid cycle yields more than 95 per cent of all the ATP produced during catabolism. We can summarize the citric acid cycle in words thus: 2 pyruvic acid molecules + 6 O_2 produce 6 CO_2 + 6 HOH + 36 ATP + heat (Fig. 5-3). The reaction is catalyzed by an orderly cluster of enzymes and constitutes the *sole reason* why the body requires oxygen. The enzymes that catalyze the cycle are located on the outer membrane of the cell mitochondria. The enzymes appear to be prearranged on that membrane in the precise order required for the sequential steps of the complicated reaction.

Early in the citric acid cycle, release of electrons from atomic hydrogen provides energy for the synthesis of ATP. This provides energy for subsequent stages of the reaction. At several stages of the cycle, oxygen enters the sequence of events. An end product of the cycle is citric acid, hence the cycle's name.

We can summarize what happens to a molecule of glucose ($C_6H_{12}O_6$) in glycolysis plus the citric acid cycle like this: $C_6H_{12}O_6 + 6\ O_2$ produces $6\ CO_2 + 6$ HOH + 38 ATP + heat.

Anabolism of Carbohydrate. Glucose anabolism involves the synthesis of larger compounds from glucose and represents one type of cellular work that utilizes energy made available through catabolism. *Glycogenesis,* for example, consists of the conversion of glucose to glycogen for storage (Fig. 5-4). It occurs chiefly in muscle cells and in the liver. When glucose is required for glycolysis or for the citric acid cycle, glycogen is broken down in the process of *glycogenolysis.* When glycogenolysis occurs in muscle cells, it involves the change of glycogen back into glucose-6-phosphate before it can be catabolized (Fig. 5-5). But in liver cells, in cells of the intestinal mucosa, and in the cells of the kidney tubules, glycogen is changed all the way to glucose because of the presence of phosphatase in these three types of cells (Fig. 5-6). The implication is clear: only from these three types of cells can glucose be released for transportation in the bloodstream to cells elsewhere in the body.

Only the liver carries on the process of *glyconeogenesis*—the manufacture of new glucose (from *gluco* = glucose, *neo* = new, *genesis* = formation). This chemical process can convert either fat or protein into needed glucose. Recall that the need for energy has first priority in the body economy. When fat is consumed in gluconeogenesis, the body usually profits; when protein is so consumed, the body's solid tissues are consumed, and the body is the loser.

Control of Glucose Metabolism. A complicated system of checks and balances regulates glucose metabolism. The immense importance of such controls becomes clear when we consider that glucose is the chief fuel of the human body. Of primary importance in glucose regulation are the hormones secreted by the islets of Langerhans in the pancreas. Insulin, manufactured by the beta cells of the islets, accelerates the use of glucose by the cells. It acts by speeding the transport of glucose through the cell membrane by the process of phosphorylation described above. It has the effect, then, of lowering the blood glucose, or, as it is termed, the blood sugar. When it is lowered below normal, we term it a *hypoglycemic* effect. Glucagon, manufactured by the alpha cells of the pancreatic islets of Langerhans, increases the activity of the enzyme phosphorylase, which cata-

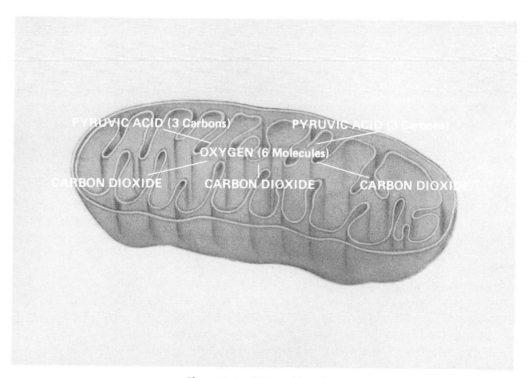

Figure 5-3. Citric acid cycle.

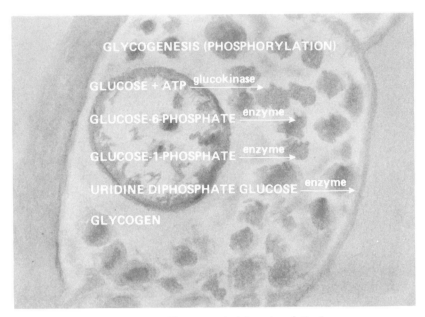

Figure 5-4. Glycogenesis (phosphorylation).

lyzes the breakdown of glycogen by the liver (glycogenolysis). This releases additional glucose into the blood and constitutes a *hyperglycemic* effect.

Other hormones, including those secreted by the anterior pituitary gland, adrenal cortex, and thyroid gland, also exert important effects on glucose metabolism. Growth hormone (GH) from the anterior pituitary gland decreases deposition of fat while increasing its mobilization and breakdown. It influences the body to shift from its preference for glucose as a source of energy to fat for provision of energy calories. (Fat must, of course, be converted to glucose before it can be utilized.) Adrenocorticotropic hormone (ACTH) of the anterior pituitary gland and the glucocorticoids of the adrenal cortex, such as cortisol, also exert important effects. ACTH stimulates the adrenal cortex to increase its secretion of glucocorticoids; these then speed up mobilization of tissue proteins and encourage gluconeogenesis in the liver from these mobilized proteins. Thus, both ACTH and the glucocorticoids increase the blood glucose and, therefore, exert a hyperglycemic effect. Thyrotropin (TSH), the thyroid-stimulating hormone of the anterior pituitary gland, stimulates the thyroid gland to increase its secretion of the thyroid hormones thyroxin (T^4) and triiodothyronine (T^3). Both accelerate catabolism, usually of glucose, thus producing a hypoglycemic effect. Finally, epinephrine, a hor-

mone secreted by the adrenal medulla, increases phosphorylase activity and, thus, accelerates muscle and liver glycogenolysis. Since it elevates blood glucose, epinephrine is a hyperglycemic agent.

Facts to Remember. Some fundamental facts should be kept in mind concerning the complex subject of carbohydrate metabolism: *carbohydrate is the most economical and usually the most readily available energy fuel. The cells appear to prefer it, sparing fats and proteins as long as carbohydrates are available. If insufficient glucose is available, fats are converted into glucose through the process of gluconeogenesis (manufacture of glucose from other substances, such as fat or protein); proteins are spared as long as sufficient fat is available for this purpose. If fat is not available, then proteins are catabolized, an unfortunate event since the breakdown of proteins means the destruction of solid tissues such as bone and muscle.* (If one is following a scientifically sound reducing diet, then fats are burned and proteins spared.)

When the level of glucose in blood carried to the liver by the portal vein exceeds 120 to 140 mg./100 ml., glucose enters the liver cells. There it forms glycogen in the process termed glycogenesis. When the blood glucose decreases below normal (120 to 140 mg./100 ml.), the liver breaks down glycogen through glycogenolysis. This tends to restore the blood glu-

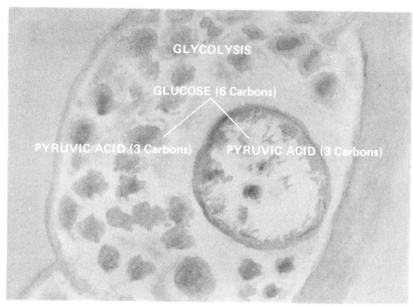

Figure 5-5. Glycogenolysis in body cell.

cose level to normal. If the liver does not contain adequate glycogen with which to combat hypoglycemia, then the liver resorts to gluconeogenesis, breaking down fat or protein or both, forming glucose from them and raising the blood glucose concentration.

When the blood glucose is elevated above normal, especially if there is an inadequate quantity of effective insulin, the glucose excess is converted to fat, chiefly by the liver cells. This fat is then carried to fat depots throughout the body for storage. Unfortunately, there appears to be almost no limit to the quantity of glucose that can be stored as fat.

Metabolism of Fat.   When carbohydrate is unavailable, fat is catabolized for energy purposes.

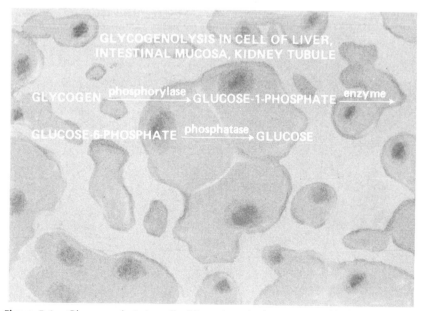

Figure 5-6. Glycogenolysis in cell of liver, intestinal mucosa, and kidney tubule.

Otherwise, it is anabolized and stored as adipose tissue.

Catabolism of Fat.   Catabolism of fat consists of hydrolysis (chemical reaction involving the addition of water) of fats to fatty acids and glycerol. It occurs primarily in the liver cells. Glycerol is then oxidized in the citric acid cycle in the same manner as carbohydrate. Fatty acids are converted to ketone bodies in the process called *ketogenesis,* which occurs chiefly in the liver (Fig. 5-7). Most ketones then leave the liver cells via the bloodstream to be transported to the tissues for oxidation to CO_2 and HOH in the citric acid cycle. When fat catabolism becomes excessive because of glucose shortage or defective metabolism of carbohydrate, as in diabetes mellitus, ketones accumulate and *ketosis* develops. Since ketones are acids, ketosis is a form of acidosis, specifically of nonrespiratory (metabolic) acidosis.

Anabolism of Fat.   Fat is anabolized for the synthesis of tissues and for the manufacture of various compounds; in some of these it is combined with protein (lipoproteins). When fats are deposited in connective tissue, they convert it to adipose tissue. Under the microscope, fat cells have a peculiar appearance, resembling a signet ring and, thus, earning the name of signet ring cells (Fig. 5-8).

Mobilization of Fat.   Fat is mobilized by being released from adipose tissue cells, after which it is catabolized. This release of fat occurs when hypoglycemia is present or when the quantity of effective insulin falls below normal.

Control of Fat Metabolism.   Fat metabolism is controlled by several factors, of which a chief determinant is the rate of glucose metabolism. Normal or elevated rates of glucose catabolism are accompanied by low rates of fat mobilization and catabolism and by high rates of fat deposition. Low rates of glucose catabolism, on the contrary, bring on high rates of fat mobilization and catabolism and low rates of fat deposition.

Insulin helps control fat metabolism through its effect on glucose metabolism. In general, normal amounts of insulin and normal levels of blood glucose depress fat mobilization and fat catabolism and increase fat deposition. Insulin deficit increases fat mobilization and catabolism. Excess of insulin has the opposite effect.

Growth hormone plays a role: it decreases fat deposition while increasing its mobilization and utilization. It, therefore, causes a shift from body utilization of glucose to that of fat. The glucocorticoids of the adrenal cortex also help control fat metabolism. With hypoglycemia or stress or both, secretion of glucocorticoids is increased. Mobilization of fat is accelerated, and gluconeogenesis of the mobilized fat occurs. With hyperglycemia combined

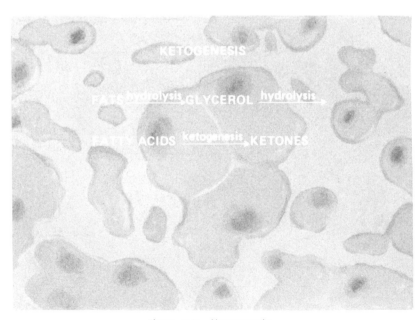

Figure 5-7.   Ketogenesis.

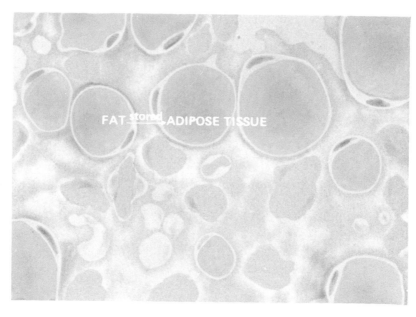

Figure 5-8. Fat anabolism.

with a low rate of glucose catabolism (as occurs in diabetes mellitus), glucocorticoids increase fat mobilization. The fat is not mobilized normally, and an excessive quantity of ketone bodies is produced. Ketosis then occurs. A time-honored way of describing the situation says, "Fats burn in the flame of the carbohydrates." When carbohydrate is not burning normally, then fats burn imperfectly and produce "smoke" in the form of ketones.

When hyperglycemia is combined with a normal quantity of effective insulin, glucocorticoids accelerate fat deposition.

Protein Metabolism   The primary "mission" of protein is to provide amino acids for the manufacture of a host of highly specialized proteins required by the body: enzymes, hormones, blood proteins, muscle cells, bone cells, antibodies, and so on. No wonder that protein has been called the *keystone nutrient*; it makes possible synthesis of the essential substances that not only make up the fabric of the body but that drive forward a virtually endless list of essential physiologic actions.

Catabolism of Protein.   When the body's carbohydrate and fat are depleted, protein is catabolized to provide energy. In the well-nourished individual, there is continuing catabolism and excretion of amino acids not required for protein synthesis. When this occurs, the amino acid molecule is broken down to form ammonia (NH_3) and ketoacids. (These are

chemical compounds containing the CO group and the COOH group, not to be confused with ketones or ketone bodies.) This first step in the catabolism of amino acids occurs chiefly within the cells of the liver; it is called *deamination*. The liver converts the ammonia, a substance extremely toxic to human beings, to urea, which is then released into the blood to be excreted by the kidneys in the urine. Ketoacids can be converted to glucose in the liver or to fat. Or, they can be oxidized in the citric acid cycle in any cell of the body (Fig. 5-9).

Anabolism of Protein.   The synthesis of the myriad proteins required for the healthy functioning of the body is one of the most important assignments of the body's living cells. Not all cells, of course, participate equally in this diversified manufacturing operation. The liver, headquarters for so many metabolic activities, synthesizes a large share of the proteins needed by the body. Without its protein anabolic activities, one cannot live long. For example, all the blood proteins except the globulins are manufactured by the liver.

Naturally, the proteins manufactured by the hepatic cells differ enormously from those put together by muscle cells, intestinal mucosal cells, or the cells of the parathyroids, adrenals, or ovary. But all cells, wherever located, have this in common: their protein anabolism is masterminded by the hereditary material of the cells, desoxyribonucleic

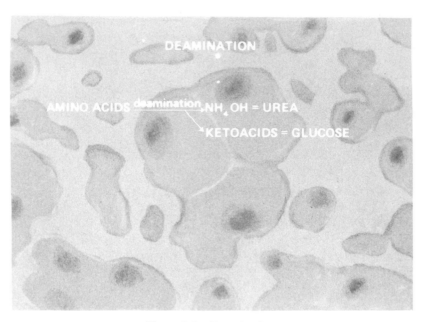

DEAMINATION

AMINO ACIDS → deamination → NH_4OH = UREA

KETOACIDS = GLUCOSE

Figure 5-9.   Deamination.

acid (DNA), residing in its "office," the cell nucleus. Like any good executive, DNA delegates: it splits off various types of ribonucleic acid (RNA), which enter the cytoplasm of the cells and there carry out the instructions received from the cell's DNA. Among the types of RNA are messenger RNA (m-RNA) and transfer RNA (t-RNA). They put together thousands of different proteins, using the twenty amino acids as building blocks.

Control of Protein Metabolism.   Hormonal controls of protein metabolism include growth hormone and testosterone (produced in the male testis). Both stimulate protein anabolism and are used in medicine to do just this. ACTH and the glucocorticoids have a catabolic effect on protein, accelerating tissue protein mobilization. They hydrolyze tissue proteins to amino acids and promote their release into the bloodstream. The liver can convert the amino acids to glucose through gluconeogenesis, or it can deaminate them. (The catabolic influence exerted by ACTH and glucocorticoids on protein are among the harmful side effects resulting from use of these valuable hormones in treatment.) In the presence of adequate thyroid hormone and good nutrition, protein anabolism is promoted. Thyroid hormone is essential for normal growth.

Caloric Yield from Catabolism of Bulk Nutrients   The complete catabolism of a gram of carbohydrate or of protein yields 4 calories. A gram of fat,

completely catabolized, provides 9 calories. The corresponding value for a gram of pure (200 proof) alcohol is usually given as about 7 calories. Alcohol is catabolized and provides energy. Hence, calories ingested as alcohol must be added to the caloric intake. Persons desiring to lose weight will find it difficult unless their consumption of alcohol is reduced along with calories from other sources. Since alcohol provides no protein, fat, vitamins, or minerals, and since, in addition, it actually promotes the loss of certain vitamins, such as thiamine, and the mineral magnesium (and probably others), alcohol calories deserve to be called *empty calories.*

REGULATION OF FOOD INTAKE   The exact mechanisms by which food intake is regulated have not been ascertained completely. Certainly the hypothalamus, which appears to supervise so many of the body's unconscious (or visceral) activities, plays a role in the regulation of food intake. There appears to be an appetite center in the hypothalamus and a satisfaction, or satiety, center as well. Stimulation of one center would cause one to want to eat; stimulation of the other would make him feel he had eaten enough. What activates these centers remains unknown. Some investigators believe that changes in the temperature in the blood passing through the hypothalamus would depress the appetite center, thus producing temporary anorexia. In cold weather, most people have hearty appetites; in hot weather or when one is feverish, the appetite is less, may even be absent. These bits of common knowledge lend credence to the blood temperature theory.

The glucostat theory holds that a low level of glucose in the blood stimulates the appetite, while a high level depresses it. Hypoglycemia is usually associated with an active appetite; hence, this theory, too, appears reasonable.

Psychologic factors undoubtedly play a role. Temporary or prolonged psychic stress causes loss of appetite in some persons and increased appetite (perhaps with the development of obesity) in others. Environmental factors, such as the eating habits of a given family, may influence the appetite heavily. Many additional factors, many as yet undiscovered, undoubtedly contribute to appetite.

THE "VITAL AMINES"

The substances we know as *vitamins* are organic compounds that do not fall into any one chemical category; rather, their chemical compositions vary widely. Vitamins are classified on the basis of their solubility, some being soluble in water, others only in fat. Water-soluble vitamins include vitamin C, or ascorbic acid, and the vitamin B complex, which includes thiamin, riboflavin, niacin, biotin, B_6, pantothenic acid, folacin, B_{12}, choline, and inositol. Vitamins soluble in fat include vitamins A, D, E, and K. All of these organic compounds serve as *catalysts,* which means that they participate in chemical reactions without being consumed in the process. They are needed only in tiny quantities, but they are absolutely necessary for reproduction, growth, and maintenance of life.

Vitamins were the last of the essential nutrients to be discovered. Funk, in 1912, recognized the existence of a cluster of chemical compounds that are essential for life. He named them *vital amines,* which later was shortened to *vitamines.* In the years following, it became clear that the substances Funk described are indeed vital; but it also became clear that not all of them are amines. Thus, the final *e* on the term *vitamine* was dropped, leaving *vitamin.*

Although vitamins were not recognized until the early part of the twentieth century, it had long been suspected that carbohydrate, fat, protein, minerals, and water could not of themselves sustain life. In-

deed, as early as 1824, Schutte, of Germany, was using cod liver oil to treat rickets; in the mid-1800s, a British naval surgeon discovered that citrus fruits both prevented and cured scurvy; and in 1858, physicians in the midwest were employing citrus fruits and cabbage to treat that disease. The early physicians did not realize, of course, that they were dealing with vitamin deficiencies. But they did observe that the conditions could be cured by the addition of a food substance to the dietary intake.

No one food provides the complete cluster of vitamins. On the other hand, the different vitamins are widely scattered among the foods we eat. For this reason, a varied diet that includes members of the four food groups will provide all the vitamins in the quantities required for robust health.

Water-Soluble Vitamins

The vitamins soluble in water include vitamin C, or ascorbic acid, and a cluster of B vitamins. The sequence of discovery of the several vitamins has led to what seems an illogical hodgepodge of names: some B vitamins have names, some have numbers, and some have both.

Given an adequacy of a water-soluble vitamin in the diet, there is practically no possibility that it will not be absorbed. Such is far from the case with the fat-soluble vitamins. This is all to the good. However, what is not so advantageous is the fact that the water-soluble vitamins leave the body more rapidly and, hence, are depleted more rapidly than are the fat-soluble vitamins.

THIAMIN (VITAMIN B_1) Thiamin (vitamin B_1), crystallized from food in 1926, is unusual in that it contains an atom of sulfur. It plays a crucial role as part of coenzymes essential for normal metabolism. In the catabolic breakdown of carbohydrates, carbon dioxide must be removed. This reaction is catalyzed by the coenzyme cocarboxylase, of which thiamin is a constituent. Thus, if insufficient thiamin is present, cocarboxylase is not formed, and intermediate metabolic compounds accumulate. Thiamin aids in the formation of ribose (a five-carbon sugar) from glucose (a six-carbon sugar) by activating an essential enzyme. Although only a small fraction of the body's glucose is converted into ribose, this transformation is of pristine importance since ribose is a necessary constituent of DNA and RNA. Normal activity within the erythrocytes is also directly related to the dietary adequacy of thiamin. Scientists of World War II vintage associated thiamin with the dread and often fatal deficiency disease beriberi. The eating of rice that has been polished so that the bran layer is removed causes beriberi. Numerous unpleasant symptoms occur: loss of appetite, nausea, vomiting, irritability, and depression. Cramps may afflict the legs, and walking may become quite difficult. One form of beriberi that affects adults is called *dry* beriberi because the patient appears "dried out," i.e., emaciated with severe weight loss. Mental confusion is also present. Another form of adult beriberi is the *wet* variety, in which there is edema caused by fluid retention. When the heart muscle becomes edematous, it is called *beriberi heart;* death may be imminent. Beriberi develops gradually in adults but, in infants under six months of age, the disease comes on rapidly and can kill in a short time unless thiamin is given.

Thiamin is available in generous quantities in pork, liver, brewer's yeast, wheat germ, whole-grain cereals and breads, enriched cereals and breads, soybeans, peanuts and other legumes, and milk. In order to retain the thiamin in foods, water losses in cooking should be held to a minimum. Much thiamin can be saved by avoiding the use of excessive quantities of water in food preparation and by using a low cooking temperature and a brief duration of cooking. Cooking water and meat drippings should be utilized, for these liquids frequently contain appreciable amounts of the water-soluble thiamin as well as other water-soluble nutrients. Since thiamin is less stable in an alkaline medium than in an acid medium, one should not use baking soda when cooking green vegetables, even though the soda greatly enhances the green color.

RIBOFLAVIN (VITAMIN B₂) Riboflavin, or vitamin B₂, is a fluorescent chemical, yellowish green in color. This fluorescent characteristic of pigments separated from milk whey was observed in the latter part of the nineteenth century, but the vitamin activity of riboflavin was not recognized until the 1930s. Then, American and British scientists discovered that, although the autoclaving of yeast for prolonged periods destroys its beriberi protective value, another growth factor contained in yeast remains active. This factor was later named riboflavin.

Riboflavin is an essential component of the coenzymes that occur in various flavoprotein enzyme systems. It combines with phosphoric acid to form flavin mononucleotide, or with adenine and phosphoric acid as flavin adenine dinucleotide. In these forms, riboflavin joins proteins to form the flavoprotein enzyme systems, essential for normal cellular respiration. The vitamin also functions in hydrogen transfer in protein metabolism and is required for the amino acid tryptophan to be converted into the B vitamin niacin.

Riboflavin deficiency is usually referred to as *ariboflavinosis.* It comes on gradually, heralded by angular stomatitis (deep cracks at both mouth corners), and cheilosis (cracking and soreness of both lips, especially where they meet). The papillae of the tongue atrophy, causing the tongue to appear abnormally smooth. In children, growth failure becomes manifest and the eyes feel irritated and become sensitive to light, watering readily. These symptoms may be followed by increased vascularity of the corneas and, later, complete opacity.

The outstanding food source of riboflavin is milk. Other excellent sources include liver, kidney, heart, eggs, green leafy vegetables, dried yeast, and various riboflavin-enriched foods. Riboflavin is stable to heat and acid and not readily oxidized, but it is highly susceptible to destruction by ultraviolet light and sunlight. For this reason, the riboflavin content of milk is reduced when milk marketed in clear glass bottles is directly exposed to sunlight. Despite the fact that this source of vitamin loss is well recognized, some milk is still marketed in clear glass rather than in brown glass or in opaque plasticized containers.

NIACIN Niacin, another of the B vitamins, is closely associated with the disease *pellagra* (from Italian, meaning "rough skin"). Early in this century, Joseph Goldberger, a physician with the U.S. Public Health Service, became convinced that a deficient diet was responsible for pellagra. Twenty years later, in 1937, scientists at the University of Wisconsin identified nicotinomide, closely related to niacin, as the cure for black tongue in dogs, a disease corresponding to pellagra in man.

Niacin is a key component in two coenzymes vital to the release of energy from foods in the body. Both of these coenzymes consist of ribose, a purine base, niacin, and phosphoric acid radicals. These coenzymes are important for the numerous reactions in tissue respiration involving the acceptance and release of hydrogen ions during metabolism. Niacin-containing coenzymes function in a cooperative manner with flavoproteins containing riboflavin and with other B vitamins.

The recommended daily dietary allowance (RDA) for niacin is expressed as niacin equivalents, which recognizes the relationship between dietary tryptophan and niacin. Tryptophan is an essential amino acid, which means that it must be included in the human diet for normal growth and maintenance. In the presence of pyridoxine (vitamin B_6), thiamin, and riboflavin, this essential amino acid can be converted in the body to niacin. But 60 mg of tryptophan are needed to provide 1 mg of niacin. For this reason, a niacin equivalent is defined as 1 mg of niacin or 60 mg of dietary tryptophan. When tryptophan is converted to niacin, it can no longer be used in the synthesis of protein. In the usual dietary intake in the United States, about half of the daily intake of niacin is consumed as the vitamin itself; the remainder is supplied as tryptophan.

When niacin is deficient for a long period, pellagra develops. Nursing and medical students were taught to remember the clinical picture of pellagra by the mnemonic of the "four Ds"—diarrhea, dermatitis, dementia, and death. Today the disease is extremely unusual except in severely malnourished persons, including alcoholics. Pellagra has a highly characteristic clinical picture: dermatitis develops in similar positions on both sides of the body, especially over areas exposed to sunlight. The skin becomes dry, scaly, and cracked. Whites develop discolorations of the skin resembling sunburn, while blacks tend to show hyperpigmentation. The tongue may become red and smooth, and abdominal cramps and diarrhea are often present. Mental symptoms include irritability, anxiety, memory defects, and insomnia. Indeed, many patients showed such severe mental symptoms that they were hospitalized for mental illness. Pellagra was once endemic in many parts of the southern United States, occurring in persons whose diet consisted largely of cornbread, molasses, and salt pork. Corn, low in tryptophan, did not provide adequate quantities of this important precursor of niacin, and the diet lacked proteins containing adequate amounts of tryptophan.

Among the good sources of niacin in the diet are beef, veal, pork, lamb, chicken, turkey, calf liver, tuna fish, swordfish, and peanut butter in the meat group; enriched rice and noodles in the bread and cereals group; and broccoli, collard greens, peas, baked potato, and ripe tomato in the vegetable and fruit group. Corn provides protein, but zein, the predominant protein in corn, is low in tryptophan, and the small amount of niacin in corn is largely unavailable. Enrichment of corn products with niacin effectively prevents pellagra. Niacin is more stable to heat, light, and oxidation and to variation in acidity than are many of the other vitamins.

VITAMIN B_6 (PYRIDOXINE)   The term vitamin B_6 includes pyridoxine, pyridoxal, and pyridoxamine. This vitamin is a recent arrival: its structure was first elucidated in 1939. Much research has been devoted to the vitamin during the past decade, particularly in relationship to amino acid metabolism. Vitamin B_6 plays a particularly important role in protein metabolism. For example, it makes it possible for the amino group of an amino acid to be transferred to new compounds in order to make amino acids that may be needed by the body for protein synthesis. Vitamin B_6 also participates in the conversion of tryptophan to niacin. During gestation, vitamin B_6 is stored in the fetus in sufficient quantity to enable the newborn to survive, even though his diet after birth is low in pyridoxine. Because of the reservoir of vitamin B_6, the newborn is able to metabolize the low quantities of protein found in human milk. If the pyridoxine store is inadequate, the infant may not be able to utilize the higher protein content of cow's milk formulas. Normal growth and development of young children, in both the physical and mental areas, requires an adequate intake of vitamin B_6.

Deficiency of pyridoxine, or vitamin B_6, is most unusual. When it does occur, hyperirritability, convulsions, and anemia are seen. The first two of these symptoms were observed in infants who were inadvertently fed a prepared formula deficient in vitamin B_6. Sophisticated medical sleuthing uncovered the cause of the symptoms, which occurred in a considerable number of infants fed on the formula in question. When adults have been experimentally depleted of vitamin B_6, they developed loss of appetite, weight loss, general weakness, and chronic fatigue.

Vitamin B_6 is obtained from liver, kidney, wheat

germ, whole-grain cereals, soybeans, peanuts, corn, bananas, lima beans, cabbage, potatoes, and spinach.

PANTOTHENIC ACID   The name *pantothenic acid* comes from Greek, meaning *everywhere*. And indeed, it does occur virtually everywhere. Pantothenic acid is fairly stable when food is prepared by moist heat and the pH is neutral. With dry heat, acid, or alkali, the vitamin is somewhat unstable. Supplements usually contain crystalline calcium pantothenate, not the acid.

Pantothenic acid is a component of coenzyme A, essential for the all-important citric acid cycle. The coenzyme is composed of pantothenic acid, a molecule of adenine, and a phosphate radical. By virtue of its presence in coenzyme A, pantothenic acid is involved in the release of energy from carbohydrate, fats, and proteins. It also functions in the synthesis of porphyrin (a step in hemoglobin formation), in some steroid hormones, and in cholesterol. In addition, the manufacture of fatty acids depends upon coenzyme A.

Pantothenic acid deficiency has not been described in humans. It is widely present both in plant and animal tissues. Especially good sources include liver, kidney, yeast, eggs, peanuts, whole-grain cereals, beef, tomatoes, broccoli, and salmon.

BIOTIN   Five active forms of biotin occur in food. In addition, it is synthesized in the intestine and is readily absorbed.

Biotin is required in small amounts for certain vital functions in the body: the formation of aspartate from pyruvate requires biotin. The vitamin functions in carboxylation and decarboxylation reactions and, therefore, is essential for the release of energy from carbohydrates and for synthesis and oxidation reactions involved in fatty acid metabolism. It is also required for the deamination of amino acids that must precede energy release from proteins. Biotin may be required to transform tryptophan into niacin and to form pancreatic amylase, an important carbohydrate-digesting enzyme.

Biotin deficiency is unknown in human beings. Excellent sources of the vitamin include egg yolks, milk, and meats of organs such as liver and kidney. Biotin is also obtained from cereals, legumes, and nuts.

FOLACIN   The chemical name of folacin is pteroylglutamic acid. The vitamin also may be called folic acid. But the term *folacin* suffices for our purposes and, indeed, fits the vitamin well since it is found in generous quantities in foliage-like vegetables.

Folacin can receive single carbon units from one compound and transfer the units to other molecules. The single carbon units can consist of methyl, formyl, or hydroxymethyl groups. The transfer mechanism is essential for the synthesis of numerous body compounds. Folacin serves as a coenzyme in various cellular reactions, including the synthesis of guanine, adenine, thymine, choline, and porphyrin. It plays a vital role in the formation of nucleic acids and, therefore, appears to be necessary for growth and reproduction of cells. It also helps in the degradation of amino acids and in the synthesis of some nonessential amino acids.

Deficiency of folacin or folic acid usually reflects an ailment such as sprue (a form of diarrhea), pellagra, or leukemia that impairs its utilization. Anemia occurs, characterized by abnormally large red blood corpuscles (macrocytic anemia). Lesions of the digestive tract and diarrhea are observed. The deficiency is frequently seen among chronic alcoholics.

Folacin is widely present in foodstuffs. Outstanding sources include liver, kidney, spinach and other dark-green leafy vegetables, mushrooms, and fruits. Storage of fresh produce for a few days is detrimental to folacin levels in the food; so is prolonged cooking, for losses may range as high as 90 per cent.

VITAMIN B_{12} (CYANOCOBALAMIN)   Vitamin B_{12}, the most recently isolated of the vitamins, is included among the B vitamins for which there is an RDA. The vitamin is red in color and consists of a large, unwieldy molecule containing an atom of cobalt.

When Doctors Minot and Murphy, of Boston, discovered that pernicious anemia can be arrested by feeding large quantities of raw liver, they concluded that some unknown substance in the liver corrected some deficiency in their subjects. Dr. Castle, one of their coworkers, called the substance *extrinsic factor* since it came from an external source. Researchers then discovered that normal individuals have an *intrinsic factor* as a regular component of gastric juice. (Intrinsic factor is a mucopolysaccharide or mucopolypeptide secreted from gastric mucosal cells; it combines with B_{12} and makes B_{12} available for absorption by the gut.) Additional research revealed that Castle's extrinsic factor was vitamin B_{12}, also known as cyanocobalamin.

Vitamin B_{12} is required by all cells but is particularly important for the nervous system, the digestive tract, and the bone marrow. If it is not present in adequate quantities, erythrocytes fail to mature, and the large, misshapen red blood cells of pernicious anemia are seen. In addition to the failure of erythrocytes to mature, nervous disorders occur, apparently due to a disruption of carbohydrate metabolism. Vitamin B_{12} is required for the synthesis of numerous complex biochemical compounds.

Pernicious anemia, of course, is the hallmark of B_{12} deficiency. Now readily treatable, it formerly was invariably fatal. Vitamin B_{12}, essential for normal development of red blood corpuscles, is not absorbed by the gastric mucosa unless intrinsic factor is present. Some persons, for reasons not discovered, lack intrinsic factor; they develop pernicious anemia despite what would ordinarily be an adequate dietary intake of vitamin B_{12}. However, if the diet is lacking in vitamin B_{12}, one can also develop pernicious anemia even though adequate intrinsic factor is present. Since vitamin B_{12} comes only from animal protein, an individual on a pure vegetarian diet (eating only foods of plant origin) can develop vitamin B_{12} deficiency and the disease pernicious anemia. In some "pure" vegetarians (such an individual is referred to as a vegans), pernicious anemia will not develop for a prolonged period of time because of vitamin B_{12} stored in the liver; in others, it may come on after a relatively brief period. The symptoms of vitamin B_{12} deficiency include generalized weakness, fatigue, smooth tongue, soreness and cracking of the lips and other mucous membranes, central nervous system symptoms—ultimately paralysis—and decreased or absent gastric hydrochloric acid. Pernicious anemia, for unknown reasons, rarely develops in pregnancy.

The treatment of pernicious anemia is through administration of vitamin B_{12} by deep subcutaneous or intramuscular injection. This has the effect of bypassing the stomach and passing directly to the liver. Maintenance injections are needed monthly except in the case of the individual whose pernicious anemia is caused by inadequate intake of vitamin B_{12}. In such an individual, restoration of an adequate intake of vitamin B_{12} by mouth should remedy the condition.

When folacin is given to an individual with pernicious anemia, the macrocytic anemia is corrected, but the nervous system changes progress to irreversible paralysis. It is, therefore, extremely dangerous to give more than 0.1 Gm. of folacin daily to a patient with an undiagnosed anemia. For this reason, by government edict, a prescription must be obtained from a physician if more than 0.1 Gm. of folacin are to be given daily.

Vitamin B_{12} comes only from animal protein such as meat, eggs, dairy products, or seafood. The daily requirement is amply met by a small quantity of animal protein, provided the individual does not lack intrinsic factor.

CHOLINE   Choline is required for the synthesis of an important component (phosphatidylcholine) of cell membranes and lipoproteins with a role in the transport of fat-soluble substances. Sphingomyelin, an important phospholipid of the brain, and acetylcholine, essential for transmission of nerve impulses, are composed of it in part. Although choline can be manufactured by the body, it is a dietary requirement for at least ten species of animals.

The requirement for choline depends upon the amounts of methionine, folic acid, and vitamin B_{12} in the diet and also on growth rate, energy intake and output, fat intake, and the type of fat in the diet. Choline deficiency has not been demonstrated in man, and it probably does not occur except in infants or young children who have been fed protein-poor diets rich in highly refined products. Food sources of choline include liver, egg yolk, brewers' yeast, wheat germ, nuts, milk, cereals, and green, leafy vegetables.

INOSITOL   Over a century ago, it was discovered that patients with diabetes mellitus, in contrast to those in good health, excrete large quantities of inositol in the urine. Neither this significant finding nor the fact that inositol is essential for yeasts and rodents has made possible an understanding of its metabolism or physiologic function in man. And while the true role of inositol in man is largely a mystery, the facts that it occurs widely in nature and that it is found in considerable quantities in the heart, brain, and skeletal muscle argue that it must have some important action.

Inositol appears to compete with glucose for reabsorption by the tubular cells. Both in diabetes mellitus and during glycosuria resulting from intravenous glucose, the reabsorption mechanism for inositol is overwhelmed by the quantity of glucose. Hence, large amounts of inositol are excreted in the urine. The significance of this loss is unknown.

Inositol deficiency has not been observed in man. The vitamin is found in organ meats, brewers' yeast, wheat germ, fruit, whole grains, and soybeans.

VITAMIN C Vitamin C, or ascorbic acid, is another of the water-soluble vitamins. The disease scurvy was known centuries, probably millenia, before vitamin C was ever heard of. But scurvy itself was not widely recognized until sailors began taking long ocean trips, made possible by the invention of the sail. On these trips, months from shore, there were no fresh vegetables or fruits, and the meat was dried and salted and virtually devoid of vitamin C. Scurvy was indeed a scourge to those early sailors. Sometimes an entire shipload would sail over the horizon, never to return because all aboard developed scurvy far out on the watery wastes. Scurvy was also a plague to navies. In the middle of the eighteenth century, a British naval physician, Dr. Lind, endeavored to find the cause of scurvy. He experimented with British sailors and discovered through modest but intelligent experiments that citrus fruit cured scurvy and, therefore, should prove useful in preventing it. The British navy finally agreed to implement Dr. Lind's recommendation that sailors be fed citrus fruits. They stored the fruits, called limes, in a certain district of London, which, thereafter, became known as the limehouse district. Sailors—and later, Englishmen in general—thus became known as Limeys. (If you really want to know what a dreadful disease scurvy was, read the narrative in the true story *Two Years Before the Mast* by Richard Henry Dana. It was 1838, and a sailor desperately ill with scurvy was quickly restored to health by eating raw potatoes and onions, excellent sources of ascorbic acid. Almost a hundred years later, in the early 1930s, a laboratory in Pittsburgh, Pennsylvania, and one in Szeged, Hungary, isolated ascorbic acid.)

One of the important roles of vitamin C is to form collagen, the connective tissue that cements cells and tissues together. It has been demonstrated repeatedly that surgical wounds simply do not heal if the patient has been on a diet deficient in ascorbic acid. Moreover, bone matrix fails to hold calcium and phos-

phorus normally when the formation of collagen is limited. The impaired calcification of the dentin of the teeth causes a weakening of tooth structure, followed by decay and breaking of teeth. Vitamin C is also essential for the maintenance of elasticity and strength of the capillary walls. With insufficient vitamin C for formation of collagen, blood vessels become fragile, and tiny hemorrhages occur under the skin, especially if a tourniquet is applied. Moreover, the conversion of folinic acid to folacin, the active form of the vitamin, is helped by the presence of ascorbic acid. Vitamin C also aids in the metabolism of certain amino acids. Conversion of both tyrosine and phenylalanine to the hormones thyroxin and adrenalin demand ascorbic acid. Recently, use of ascorbic acid in the treatment of colds has been the subject of heated controversy.

Ascorbic acid deficiency is called scurvy. Its devastating symptoms include muscular weakness, tenderness of the calves of the legs, depressed appetite, swollen gums, loosening of the teeth, hemorrhage under the skin, under the periosteum of the bones, and under the nasal mucosa, impaired wound healing, megaloblastic anemia, and shortness of breath.

With the taking of enormous doses of ascorbic acid in an effort to prevent the common cold, the possibility of toxicity from vitamin C must be considered. Quite safe in doses normally used for prevention of deficiency and even for cure of scurvy, reports in the medical literature indicate there may well be some instances of toxicity from ascorbic acid, i.e., hypervitaminosis C.

Fresh fruits (notably the citrus fruits, such as oranges, grapefruits, lemons, and limes, the acerola cherry—the cherry that grows in Puerto Rico—and strawberries), vegetables (such as potatoes, onions, green pepper, and cabbage), and even certain evergreen needles are all excellent sources of ascorbic acid. Synthetic ascorbic acid is available also; the body uses it just as well as it does the natural ascorbic acid from foods.

Fat-Soluble Vitamins

Since the fat-soluble vitamins—vitamins A, D, E, and K—dissolve only in fats or oils, they will not be absorbed when the fats or oils in which they are dissolved are not absorbed. Such failure of lipid absorption can occur under these circumstances:

1. In obstructive jaundice, bile is prevented from entering the duodenum. The emulsifying action of bile on fats is lost.
2. When excessive quantities of mineral oil are ingested, fat-soluble vitamins are carried out of the body with the oil.
3. When mucoviscidosis is present, fat absorption is impaired because the pancreas does not produce lipase.
4. Resection of the distal portion of the small intestine reduces the absorptive area for lipids.
5. Poor fat absorption occurs in malabsorption syndromes, including steatorrhea, nontropical sprue, adult celiac disease, and childhood celiac disease.
6. In pancreatic lithiasis, production of pancreatic lipase is greatly impaired.

Deficiency of one or more fat-soluble vitamins can occur in any state in which lipid absorption is impaired, such as those above listed, even though the quantity of vitamin ingested meets the normal requirement. But in the normal individual with adequate stores of fat-soluble vitamins whose intake of fat-soluble vitamins is interrupted, deficiency develops slowly because fats are broken down and excreted more slowly than are water-soluble substances.

Closely related to the fat-soluble vitamins and also necessary are the essential fatty acids linoleic acid and arachidonic acid.

VITAMIN A There are two forms of vitamin A—vitamin A_1 and vitamin A_2. We are primarily interested in vitamin A_1 since vitamin A_2 is found only in fresh water fish and in birds that eat these fish. In addition to the actual forms of vitamin A, there are substances known as *precursors* that are converted to vitamin A. The precursors of vitamin A, or provitamin A, are referred to as *carotenoids,* and they contribute importantly to the body's vitamin A content. The carotenoids, also called *carotene,* are yellow-colored compounds that give the yellow or yellow-orange coloration to many fruits and vegetables. The more intense the color of these foods, the higher the

provitamin A, or carotene, content. Dark green or leafy vegetables are also rich in provitamin A, but the green of their chlorophyl content masks the yellow color of the carotene. Tomatoes and watermelon also contain provitamin A, the red of their pigment masking the yellow of their provitamin A.

Vitamin A is an important component in the chemical cycle that enables one to see in a dim light; therefore, an adequate supply of vitamin A prevents night blindness. The ability to see in dim light rests in a substance called rhodopsin, also known as visual purple. Rhodopsin is used up in the process of seeing; a continuing supply of vitamin A is necessary for the formation of additional rhodopsin. Vitamin A also plays an important role in maintaining the external health of the eye. When it is present in adequate amounts, lacrimal secretions bathe the eye regularly and the cornea is healthy. In children, vitamin A is required for optimal growth. In the child who is deficient in vitamin A, the soft tissues grow more rapidly than bone. As a result, the spinal cord and brain are compressed and neurologic changes result. The epithelial cells that line the body surfaces and cavities require vitamin A for maintenance of health. A normal carbohydrate constituent of mucus fails to form if vitamin A is not present. Instead, another substance, keratin, is produced. The outer layer of cells dry out, or become keratinized. Cilia, which normally project from respiratory epithelial cells, are lost, and bacteria are more likely to enter the body and cause infection.

Vitamin A is absorbed through the wall of the small intestine, where it enters the lymphatics as a fatty acid ester; ultimately, it reaches the bloodstream. Provitamin A is converted to vitamin A in the intestinal wall; the absorbed vitamin A ultimately reaches the liver. There, surplus vitamin A is removed and stored for subsequent use. Since vitamin A is fat-soluble rather than water-soluble, it is not excreted in the urine; rather, it passes out with the bile salts in the feces. It is also excreted in the milk during lactation. Vitamin A is poorly absorbed when an individual has impaired bile formation, when the protein intake is severely restricted, when mineral oil is used to excess, or when there is impaired fat absorption as a result of disease.

The first manifestation of vitamin A deficiency is night blindness; it does not develop for several months after the vitamin intake is inadequate since vitamin A is stored in several tissues, notably the liver. In a severe prolonged deficiency, the health of the eye is endangered. First, inflammation of the eye occurs. In time, the cornea becomes keratinized and the eye dry. These findings are lumped together under the term *xerophthalmia*. If the deficiency is not corrected, the cornea ulcerates. The next stage is softening of the eye, or *keratomalacia*. Blindness results. Vitamin A deficiency is the chief cause of blindness of children suffering from protein-calorie malnutrition. Many cases of blindness were reported in Danish children during World War I, when they were deprived of cream and butterfat by the enemy. Skim milk, unfortified, contains no vitamin A.

Other findings in vitamin A deficiency include hyperkeratinization of the skin, epithelial changes in the urinary tract, and, as a result of the latter, urinary infection and kidney stones. Other findings in severe vitamin A deficiency include diarrhea, intestinal infections, and impairment of growth and of reproduction. Failure of absorption of the cerebrospinal fluid surrounding the brain may occur, resulting in paralysis of the extremities and blindness.

Excessive doses of vitamin A taken for a prolonged period—weeks or months—can increase pressure within the skull and mimic brain tumor. Other findings in hypervitaminosis A include retarded growth, dry cracked skin, and headaches. Bone pain and even bone deformities can occur. Because of the hazard of hypervitaminosis A, the Food and Drug Administration (FDA) has ruled that no more than 10,000 International Units (IU) of vitamin A can be ordered except by a physician.

Vitamin A is available only from animal sources, with the liver of all types of animals particularly rich in it. (Polar bear liver has a dangerously high concentration of vitamin A.) Milk and butterfat contribute vitamin A; its level in milk depends on the ration available to cows. Summer butter and milk have more vitamin A than do winter butter and milk. Vitamin A is also added to liquid skim milk, skim milk powder, and margarine. The richest sources of provitamin A include bright yellow and dark green vegetables.

VITAMIN D   Ten different forms of vitamin D have been identified; only two are of dietary significance, however. Vitamin D of animal origin is termed cholecalciferol, reflecting its cholesterol precursor.

Vitamin D performs a role in the absorption of calcium and phosphorus from the intestinal tract; the exact mechanism, though, is far from clear. Apparently, vitamin D is needed for the formation of the protein that acts as a carrier for calcium through the intestinal wall. Adequate vitamin D enhances the levels of phosphates in the body, chiefly because it increases resorption of phosphate from the kidney tubules. Various imbalances result from vitamin D deficiency, thus indicating the regulatory functions the vitamin performs in the body. The level of amino acids excreted in the urine increases when vitamin D is inadequate; it decreases when the vitamin is administered at normal levels. A low level of alkaline phosphatase results from vitamin D deficiency and is detrimental to phosphorus utilization (alkaline phosphatase is an enzyme that plays a major role in the release of phosphorus from compounds, thus making the mineral available for deposition as calcium phosphate).

Bile must be present in the intestine if the fat-soluble vitamins are to be absorbed; the factors that influence the absorption of these vitamins are the same as those for the absorption of fats. Under conditions of normal health, vitamin D is efficiently utilized by the body; limited excesses are stored in liver, bone, adrenal glands, and kidneys. Ultimately, vitamin D is excreted in the feces.

Vitamin D can be provided entirely from the diet, but it also can be produced in the body simply by exposing the skin to sunlight. Anything filtering sunlight, however, will impede the action of the sun in producing vitamin D in the skin. Vitamin D deficiency should be added to the long list of legitimate complaints against smog, for ultraviolet rays do not penetrate smog and smoke. Ordinary glass, screens, and clothing also inhibit irradiation of the skin. Thus, since most of us are not nudists, we don't bare enough skin to meet our total vitamin D requirement in this manner. Therefore, it is necessary to include the vitamin as a dietary constituent.

Vitamin D deficiency can cause rickets in children and osteomalacia in adults. In rickets, poor calcification of bone occurs because of inadequate absorption of calcium from the intestine. The anterior fontanel is slow to close. The epiphyses of the long bones swell, and beadlike protrusions develop on the ribs (these are referred to as the "rachitic rosary"). Pigeon breast, in which the chest of the child actually resembles the pointed breast of the pigeon, can appear. Usually the legs become bowed but, in some children, knock-knees develop. Children with rickets are slow in learning to sit, stand, and walk.

In the adult, vitamin D deficiency causes osteomalacia. The usual history is that of a series of pregnancies followed by lactation, combined with low vitamin D intake and minimal exposure to the sun. Pain occurs in the pelvis, lower back, and legs. Bones are tender on pressure. Fractures, involuntary twitching, and muscle spasms occur. There is extensive demineralization of the skeleton.

Hypervitaminosis D is the second established syndrome caused by excessive doses of a specific vitamin. It is considerably more serious than hypervitaminosis A since it can become irreversible soon after development. It can retard both physical and mental growth in children. Its train of untoward effects include nausea, weakness, stiffness, constipation, hypertension, and even death. Because of the hazard of hypervitaminosis D, the FDA has ruled that no more than 400 IU of vitamin D are to be taken daily.

The natural occurrence of vitamin D is limited to animal foods, with eggs, cheese, and butter providing limited amounts. Cod liver oil and other fish liver oils are among the richest dietary sources of vitamin D. (Although the German Schutte cured rickets with cod liver oil in 1824, it was not until 1922 that McCollum observed that fish liver oils retained their anti-rickets properties even after vitamin A was removed.) Today, milk is commonly fortified with 400 IU vitamin D per quart, a highly commendable practice rendering it a major food source of vitamin D.

VITAMIN E The usefulness of vitamin E for humans is limited and has been grossly overestimated by some individuals. The outstanding characteristic of vitamin E, also known as alpha tocopherol, is its antioxidant properties. Because alpha tocopherol is so readily oxidized, other oxidizable substances, such as ascorbic acid, vitamin A, and certain fats, must await oxidation until all vitamin E present has been oxidized. Therefore, vitamin E prevents oxidation of both of these vitamins and of unsaturated fatty acids and thus permits these essential nutrients to perform their specific functions in the body; once the substances are oxidized, they can no longer react. Vitamin E also serves as an antioxidant to protect the fat in red blood corpuscles from oxidation, thereby preventing undesirable hemolysis of erythrocytes. The vitamin E requirement is increased by a high consumption of polyunsaturated fatty acids and, possibly, by the presence of smog. Contrariwise, various other substances, such as selenium, spare vitamin E.

Vitamin E is present in a wide range of foods; it is particularly rich in fats and polyunsaturated oils of vegetable origin. It is also found in meats, various animal products, and in green vegetables. Vitamin E of fats and oils may be decreased by commercial processes involving excessive heat and exposure to air.

VITAMIN K Vitamin K, actually a group of compounds, is the only fat-soluble vitamin for which no RDA has been established. Its name signifies its role in coagulation, being spelled *koagulation* in Denmark, where the role of the vitamin was first observed. One way in which vitamin K aids coagulation is to promote the formation of prothrombin, which, in the presence of calcium, is converted to thrombin. Thrombin is required for fibrinogen, which is then transformed into the clotting substance known as fibrin. Although not a structural part of prothrombin, the entire cascade of reactions that terminate in coagulation requires the presence of vitamin K to initiate prothrombin formation. Another substance required for coagulation, proconvertin, also demands vitamin K for its synthesis.

Hemorrhage is the chief finding in vitamin K deficiency. Usually a disorder of infancy, the problem is more serious for the premature than for the full-term infant. Vitamin K deficiency can develop when fat absorption is impaired, as with disease of the liver. Adults who have been receiving anticoagulant drugs may develop bleeding because of vitamin K deficiency.

Although it is not an important food for man, alfalfa is an extremely rich source of vitamin K. Human food sources represent dark green and leafy vegetables (including spinach and cabbage), liver, and egg yolk. A deficiency in any normal individual more than a few days old is extremely unlikely, because bacteria in the intestine produce vitamin K beginning soon after birth. (Newborns will have a sufficient supply of vitamin K to prevent hemorrhagic disease until they are able to manufacture their own supply if the vitamin is administered to the mother just prior to delivery.) Indeed, the synthesis of vitamin K by the intestinal bacteria is the chief source of this vitamin; it explains why diseases characterized by chronic diarrhea or poor absorption cause vitamin K deficiency. For the same reason, prolonged use of certain antibiotics depresses the intestinal flora and prevents the synthesis of vitamin K.

MINERALS AND WATER

Minerals

An enormous amount of research has resulted in our current sophisticated knowledge concerning the *vitamins*. Our lack of in-depth information concerning the *minerals* is indicated by the fact that RDAs* have been established for only six—calcium, phosphorus, iodine, iron, magnesium, and zinc. Now, however, the focus of nutritional research has shifted in large part to the minerals. Much has been learned about the requirements for those for which RDAs are not yet established. It appears safe to predict that allowances for additional minerals will be forthcoming in the not-far-distant future. Perhaps some not-presently-deemed essential will be termed essential; some for which requirements can only be guessed at will have requirements determined; some for which we presently have requirements will have allowances determined. In future years, this period may be looked back upon as the *era of the minerals*. This part of Chapter 5 concerns itself with current knowledge concerning the minerals regarded as essential (or probably essential) for man, including those for which allowances have not yet been established.

* By virtue of years of intensive work by nutritional experts, the Food and Nutrition Board of the National Academy of Sciences/National Research Council has promulgated highly useful standards of requirements for specific nutrients, titled the *Recommended Daily Dietary Allowances*, usually called Rec-Daily Allowances, or RDAs. The purpose of the standards is stated succinctly: "Designed for the maintenance of good nutrition of practically all healthy people in the U.S.A." Tables of RDAs are usually based on the requirements for an individual of a certain weight in a certain age group. For example, the RDAs for an adult male aged 23 to 50 are usually expressed in the amounts needed by an individual weighing 70 kg. But since not all males aged 23 to 50 weigh 70 kg., the tables can be used only as general guides and cannot be applied specifically to individuals of widely varying body weight. Thus, we shall express the RDAs in terms of requirement/kg. body weight so that the amounts needed by any individual in a given age group can be easily calculated.

In discussing minerals, we shall use the quantitative classification employed by the National Academy of Sciences in *Recommended Dietary Allowances*, edition 8, 1974: "Mineral elements are treated in two groups: those needed in the diet at levels of 100 mg./day or more, and those needed in the diet in amounts no higher than a few mg/day (the trace elements)." On this basis, the larger mineral elements (we might well designate them the *macrominerals*) include calcium, phosphorus, magnesium, sodium, potassium, and chloride; trace elements (we can well call them the *microminerals*) encompass iron, copper, iodine, fluorine, zinc, chromium, cobalt, manganese, molybdenum, selenium, nickel, tin, vanadium, and silicon.

First, let us be certain that we know just what minerals are—and what they are not. They may be defined simply as *inorganic homogeneous substances*. A mineral can consist of either an element or a compound that occurs naturally as a result of, or as a product of, an inorganic process. When we say something is inorganic, we imply that it did not arise from living matter, hence does not contain the element carbon.

Closely related to minerals—in many cases identical with them—are the electrolytes. They are substances that bear or possess an electric charge, either positive or negative, when placed in water; they consist of minerals (e.g., sodium or Na) or molecules incorporating minerals (e.g., bicarbonate or HCO_3). Not all minerals are electrolytes, and not all electrolytes consist solely of minerals.

THE DYNAMIC HISTORY OF THE MINERALS
The minerals of the human body appear to represent an important portion of our heritage from the sea. Fabun, in the *Dynamics of Change*, presents (with tongue in cheek, we trust) the fantastic notion that the ocean is a great animal, so enormous that we earthlings cannot envision it as living. Fabun describes rivers as great tentacles of the ocean, the turbulent border between surf and shore as the sea animal's skin, the waves as the pulsations of a giant heart, and man himself as an emissary from the ocean who has invaded the land. However bizarre this fantasy, it is not fantasy that the sea that covers most of earth's surface would be as lifeless as the land-locked Dead Sea were it not for its endless stores of those dynamic active chemicals, the minerals. It is not fantasy that the ancestors of man carried small portions

of these minerals ashore when they left their ancient ancestral home. Even today, human body fluid contains that same varied cluster of minerals and electrolytes possessed by the primeval oceans, despite the fact that some of the minerals are not only useless, they are toxic. The stamp of the sea is an enduring one, and man bears it on every one of his trillions of cells.

Bear in mind that the minerals of the sea had their origin in the dissolving of the continents; they reflect, therefore, the composition of the planet earth. So, man's minerals are earth minerals, and man is indeed an *earthling*. Had he developed on another planet, his mineral legacy would have been different, and so would his basic physiology. So, the mineral profile of man's body carries a clarion message: *man cannot exist elsewhere in the universe*.

EXPRESSING QUANTITIES OF MINERALS In expressing quantities of minerals, we shall use the *gram* (Gm.), *milligram* (mg.), and *microgram* (μg). A milligram is 1/1000 of a gram, and a microgram is 1/1000 of a milligram and 1/1,000,000 of a gram. These are measures of weight. In discussing water and electrolytes, the measures customarily employed are the *milliequivalent* (mEq.) and the *millimole* (mM.). The milliequivalent is a measure of chemical combining power: 1 mEq. of an ion is equal to the atomic weight in mg. divided by the valence. A millimole is the molecular weight expressed in mg: 1 mEq. of sodium would be 23 mg., 1 mM. of sodium chloride is 58.5 mg.

CALCIUM The body's most abundant mineral, calcium, has phosphorus as its intimate working partner. The bones and teeth hold 99 per cent of the body's total calcium, with the remainder in the plasma and cells. Yet, even this relatively small quantity is crucial for life. Calcium and phosphorus share the responsibility for making our bones and teeth rigid, strong, and durable; after death, they remain intact long after all other body parts have succumbed to the erosion of time. Yet, bone contains far more than just calcium and phosphorus: living bone contains cells that produce a mother substance, collagen, a complex protein that incorporates fluorine, oxygen, carbon, and nitrogen along with calcium and phosphorus. In addition to its essential supportive function, bone constitutes a dynamic chemical system, holding in reserve minerals that can be called

upon for such special needs as milk production in mammals and egg laying in birds. Calcium of itself controls the excitability of peripheral nerves and muscles. Without it, blood could not coagulate, the myocardium could not function, muscles could not contract, and the integrity of intracellular cement substances could not be maintained. Calcium is required for absorption of vitamin B_{12} from the stomach and its utilization by body cells.

Frequently, the human diet is deficient in calcium, especially in countries where milk is scarce and where other food sources of calcium are lacking. Calcium deficit is especially serious during the rapid growth of early infancy, during puberty, and in pregnancy and lactation. Only from 20 to 30 per cent of the calcium in the diet is absorbed. If vitamin D intake is inadequate, even this per cent of absorption is reduced. The parathyroid glands, through their hormone parathormone, help maintain the plasma level of calcium: they stimulate bone breakdown and absorption when calcium is needed to maintain the plasma calcium level.

The RDA for calcium for formula-fed infants up to one year of age is 60 mg./day/kg. body weight. Breastfed infants' needs are fully met by breast milk. Other RDAs are as follows: children 1 to 3, 62 mg./day/kg.; children 4 to 6, 40 mg./day/kg.; children 7 to 10, 27 mg./day/kg.; adolescents 11 to 14, 27 mg./day/kg.; adolescents 15 to 18, 20 mg./day/kg. for males and 22 mg./day/kg. for females; adults 19 to 22, 12 mg./day/kg. for males and 14 mg./day/kg. for females; adults over 23, 11 mg./day/kg. for males and 14 mg./day/kg. for females.

The best food sources of calcium are milk and cheese. Less rich sources include dried beans, kale, brazil nuts, and bone. (While bone is largely made up of calcium, the absorption of calcium from bone is low.)

PHOSPHORUS Phosphorus teams up with calcium in contributing to the supportive and dynamic functions of bones and teeth, which contain about 75 per cent of the body's phosphorus; most of the rest resides in the cells, with a much smaller portion located in the plasma. As the chief anion of the cells, phosphorus participates in many important chemical reactions. Many of the B vitamins are effective only when combined with phosphorus. The mineral helps energy transfers within the body cells, promotes normal nerve and muscle action, helps maintain the acid-base balance of the body fluids, and participates in carbohydrate metabolism. Moreover, this busy mineral is required for cell division and for transmission of hereditary traits from parent to offspring.

Seventy per cent of dietary phosphorus is absorbed, in contrast to only 20 to 30 per cent of the calcium of the diet. Adequate intake of vitamin D promotes absorption of both calcium and phosphorus; hence, when vitamin D consumption is inadequate, intestinal absorption of both minerals drops precipitously. In renal failure, phosphates are abnormally retained; as a result, the calcium concentration of the plasma falls because of the reciprocal relationship between calcium and phosphorus. The parathyroid glands then secrete increased amounts of parathormone, causing excessive removal of calcium from bone and abnormal deposition of calcium in body tissues.

Because so many foods contain generous quantities of phosphorus, the human diet seldom is deficient in it. The RDAs for phosphorus closely resemble those for calcium, differing only in the RDAs for the first year of life. The RDA for formula-fed infants is 40 mg./day/kg. body weight for the first six months and 44 mg./day/kg. for the second six months. Breast-fed infants' needs are fully met by breast milk. RDAs for all other age groups are the same as those for calcium.

Foods especially high in phosphorus include beef, pork, dried beans, and dried mature peas.

MAGNESIUM The macromineral magnesium makes up 1.2 per cent of the earth's crust and 3.69 per cent of the ocean's solids. The mineral's physiologic action was first recognized by the villagers of Epsom, England, who discovered in 1618 that the bitter-tasting water from a village pool produced catharsis. The water from the pool gained a reputation—deserved or not—for promoting health, and people from all over Europe flocked to Epsom to drink it. Later, the active ingredient of the water was found to be magnesium sulfate and was named Epsom salts.

Magnesium and calcium appear to share several control mechanisms since renal reabsorption of magnesium varies inversely with that of calcium. When the dietary intake of calcium is reduced, excretion of magnesium in the feces falls. Second only to potassium as the predominant cation in living cells, magnesium's chief role in the body is that of activator, driving to completion a host of vital reactions related to enzyme systems. Systems activated by magnesium include those enabling B vitamins to function and those permitting utilization of potassium, calcium, and protein. It is important in maintaining electrical activity in nerves and muscle membranes. Although found both in bones and in soft tissues, magnesium is particularly important in heart, nerve tissues, and skeletal muscles.

Magnesium is absorbed in the small intestine, with magnesium and calcium appearing to share a common transport route across the intestinal membrane. The mechanism appears to prefer calcium, which may explain the occurrence of hypomagnesemia with high calcium intakes on a marginal magnesium diet. The kidney plays a key role in regulating the body's pool of magnesium. Depletion of magnesium promptly causes a decrease in urinary, but not in plasma, magnesium. Apparently, it is the proximal part of the distal convoluted tubule of the kidney that regulates magnesium. When renal function is impaired, magnesium should be given with great caution since under these circumstances, plasma magnesium rises sharply.

Thyroid hormone plays an important role in the control of magnesium. Magnesium deficiency can result from severe renal disease, toxemia of pregnancy, chronic alcoholism, hepatic cirrhosis, sustained losses of gastrointestinal secretions, drug-induced diuresis, and prolonged administration of magnesium-free parenteral fluids. Alcoholics can develop magnesium deficit even though their diets contain generous quantities of magnesium.

The RDA for magnesium is 10 mg./day/kg. body weight for infants during the first six months and 8 mg./day/kg. during the second six months. The child's RDA ranges from 12 mg./day/kg. for the 1 to 3 year old to 6 mg./day/kg. for the adolescent. For adults, the RDA for magnesium is 5 mg./day/kg.

Although nuts, legumes, fish, and whole grains provide much magnesium, the usual American diet, with its emphasis on meat, eggs, and dairy products, makes magnesium deficit a possibility. In contrast, the diet of most Orientals abounds in magnesium-rich cereals and vegetables.

SODIUM The English symbol for sodium, Na, comes from the term used by the Germans: *natrium*. Pure or elemental sodium is extremely unstable since it combines instantly with oxygen when exposed to it, either in air or water. For this reason, elemental sodium does not exist in nature. The most frequent combination of sodium with another element is sodium chloride, the familiar table salt. Sodium is the chief cation of our extracellular fluid and is also among the important cations of cellular fluid. While most of the body's sodium is to be found in the body fluids, some is stored in bone.

Sodium's prime function is simple but enormously significant: it is involved chiefly with the maintenance of osmotic equilibrium and body fluid volume. With potassium, it moves continuously across the cell membrane, propelled by a mysterious pump still only partially understood. Within the cell, it is required for numerous vital chemical reactions. It stimulates nerve action and plays a major role in maintenance of the acid-base balance of the body.

The body can tolerate only relatively minor deviations from the normal level of sodium in the extracellular fluid before serious disruptions in physiology occur. Potassium and hydrogen, for example, are permitted relatively greater deviations from the normal without disaster. For this reason, some clinicians speak of the "primacy of sodium." Not surprisingly, sodium conservation is energetic and tenacious: an individual placed on a sodium-restricted diet will lose virtually no sodium in the urine after the third or fourth day, assuming normal kidney function. Conservation of sodium is carried out in large part by an increase in the secretion of the mineralocorticoid aldosterone of the adrenal cortex. Its action is so formidable that destruction of the adrenal glands or their surgical removal will result in fatal sodium deficit in a few days unless replacement hormones are administered. Sodium deficit can be produced by any circumstances that cause a decreased intake or increased output of sodium or an increased intake or decreased output of water. Perspiring heavily and drinking plain water can cause sodium deficit; so can gastric suction with the water and electrolytes removed being replaced by plain water by mouth or dextrose in water intravenously. Sodium excess, on the other hand, can result from ingesting more sodium than the kidneys can excrete (an ancient form of execution consisted of forcing the victim to eat a cup of salt) or by excessive losses of water through diarrhea or prolonged rapid respiration.

Persuasive evidence indicates that persons who salt their food excessively or who are members of a culture that eats extremely salty food may stand a greater than average chance of developing hypertension. Heredity appears to play a determining role in who will and who will not develop high blood pressure from excessive salt intake. Most Americans eat from 2000 to 5000 or 10,000 mg. of sodium a day. For some, the figure probably tops 15,000 mg. In one area of Japan, where the average intake of sodium is 26,000 mg. daily, the number of persons who suffer from strokes and hypertension is startlingly high. Because of the possibility of harm from high sodium intakes, some nutritionists are convinced that the salt content of the infant's diet should be kept low so as not to accustom the baby to salty foods.

A diet restricted in sodium has proved effective in the treatment of various ailments, including hypertension, congestive heart failure, edema, excessive weight gain by otherwise healthy middle-aged women, and toxemia of pregnancy. At least a third, perhaps more, of patients with hypertension have their blood pressure reduced by a diet containing not more than 500 mg. of sodium a day.

The requirement for sodium has been stated as from 2.38 to 7.14 Gm. sodium, corresponding to 6 to 18 Gm. sodium chloride. The actual requirement, especially in individuals who have become accustomed to a low-sodium intake, is far less. Persons have been maintained in good health for indefinite periods on diets containing from 250 to 500 mg. of sodium daily. Certain primitive peoples have apparently done well on less than 100 mg./day.

Barring drug therapy or a stringent sodium-restricted diet, sodium deficit appears virtually impossible. In fact, most so-called low-sodium diets probably do not achieve effectiveness since it is so difficult to eliminate salt-containing foods in our society.

While most foods contain important quantities of sodium, those extremely high in it include ham, preserved meats (such as cold cuts), pretzels, salted nuts, almost all snacks, pickles, catsup, steak sauces —the list is almost endless.

POTASSIUM　The symbol for potassium is K, after the first letter of its German name, *Kalium*. A naturally radioactive element, potassium played a major role in the geologic development of the earth. Although potassium is closely related to sodium from the chemical standpoint, it differs strikingly from sodium in its physiologic behavior. Indeed, in many situations, potassium and sodium appear to be paired off against each other. Potassium also is a close chemical relative of lithium and rubidium. Potassium is a soft, bluish-silver metal that exists outside the test tube only when combined with other elements.

The primary function of potassium is its involvement with cellular enzyme activities. It plays a leading role in the intricate chemical reactions required to transform carbohydrate into energy and to convert amino acids into proteins. The difference in the concentrations of sodium and potassium across cell walls determines the electrical potentials of cell membranes, hence cell excitability and nerve impulse conduction. The cells require potassium to maintain their normal water content. It is essential for transmission of electrical impulses within the heart. Muscles cannot function normally without potassium.

The extracellular fluid contains about 70 mEq. of potassium, contained in a little more than a level teaspoonful of potassium chloride. But the body cells contain 4000 mEq. of potassium—the equivalent of more than 6 lb. of potassium chloride. Thus, although one cannot live long without potassium, each of us has enough in our body cells to kill dozens of persons if it were injected quickly into the bloodstream.

Body secretions and excretions are rich in potassium. Especially plentiful in this mineral are sweat (especially after one has become acclimatized to prolonged heat), saliva, stomach and intestinal secretions, and stools. The potassium content of urine varies with the intake, although it never approaches zero, even with depletion of body potassium. Scientists are baffled by the body's extremely negligent conservation of this essential mineral, which stands in striking contrast to the body's parsimonious husbanding of sodium. For even though the potassium intake is dangerously low, the urine may carry out as much as 40 to 50 mEq. daily. Why? Could it be that the body's conservation of sodium and lack of conservation of potassium reflects the theory that man's ancient ancestor was an herbivore, an exclusive plant eater? (Recall that meats are rich in sodium, while vegetables and fruits abound in potassium.) Physiologic "habits," even of one's extremely remote ancestors, have a way of perpetuating themselves.

In clinical medicine, potassium deficit occurs all too frequently, often in situations in which body secretions rich in potassium are lost in excessive quantities. Perhaps the most important cause of potassium deficit in the United States is the taking of powerful diuretics. Potassium deficit may also occur

as the undesirable side-effect of adrenocorticosteroid administration. Because surgical procedures often cause loss of large quantities of potassium-rich fluids (especially if gastrointestinal surgery is involved), potassium deficit is often associated with surgical procedures. There is also danger of it developing when gastric or intestinal juices are withdrawn through a suction tube or when an opening is made from the outside into the digestive tube. Diseases involving the intestinal tract, such as infections of the large or small intestine, tend to produce potassium deficit. Crushing injuries, broken bones, and extensive bruising induce cellular potassium loss through the release of potassium from damaged cell walls. (Recall that potassium is the chief mineral of the body's cells.)

Both emotional (psychic) and physical stress encourage potassium loss. Potassium deficit may occur during wound healing because the cells undergoing restoration rob the extracellular fluid of its potassium. Excessive sweating caused by high environmental temperatures, fever, or vigorous exercise help deplete the body's potassium. Potassium deficit can contribute to heat stress disease in hot weather, especially when elderly persons take medications that increase potassium excretion. Healthy young persons exposed to extreme heat for prolonged periods can develop potassium deficit. So, of course, can persons with aldosterone-producing tumors of the adrenal cortex.

Potassium excess can occur during the early period following a severe burn or after an injury in which there is massive crushing of body tissue. It can be caused by taking excessive quantities of potassium, either by mouth or intravenously. Oral potassium poisoning occurs only with ingestion of an enormous dose (perhaps 600 mEq. or more), provided the kidneys are normal.

While no RDA has been established for potassium, the daily requirement can be regarded as about 2.5 Gm. (64 mEq.), provided unusual stress, including prolonged high environmental temperature, is not present.

A well-balanced diet usually assures adequate potassium, provided no abnormal losses are occurring from vomiting, diarrhea, sweating, or diuresis. Leading food sources of potassium include apricots, bananas, dates, figs, oranges, peaches, prunes, raisins, tomato juice, orange juice, and vegetables in general. Meat and dairy products provide appreciable but lesser quantities of potassium. Pharmaceutical potassium supplements appear advisable if the individual is to receive a potent potassium-losing diuretic for a prolonged period.

CHLORIDE Chloride is by far the most important anion of the extracellular fluid. It is essential for formation of the hydrochloric acid of gastric juice. Loss of chloride usually parallels loss of sodium, with which it is normally paired. But chloride loss caused by vomiting may result in a chloride deficit apart from loss of sodium. In such an instance, the bicarbonate portion of the anion column is increased (since total anions must always equal total cations), and alkalosis results. Individuals whose sodium chloride intake is severely restricted because of disease of heart, kidney, or liver may need an alternative source of chloride, such as potassium chloride (provided the kidneys are relatively normal).

The requirement for chloride usually parallels that for sodium: 3.62 to 10.86 Gm. daily. Foods high in sodium are also high in chloride.

IRON Iron, a micromineral for which an RDA has been established, constitutes 4.7 per cent of the earth's crust. It is an essential constituent of hemoglobin, myoglobin, and various enzymes. It is required for healthy red blood corpuscles. Iron's role in oxygen transport and cellular respiration make it indispensable for man.

The average adult stores only 1 Gm. of iron, chiefly in the liver and spleen. Reservoir iron exists in the cells as a protein complex, either as a hemosiderin or as ferritin. Although the average person receives about 15 mg. of iron in his daily diet, usually only 1.5 to 2 mg. are absorbed. Ferrous iron is absorbed more efficiently than is ferric iron.

The nursing infant receives no iron from mother's milk; iron stores in his liver decrease progressively during the rapid growth of the first few months of life. Use of iron-supplemented feeding formulas and vitamin preparations help correct the iron deficit and forestall the development of iron deficiency anemia. Many pregnant women, especially multiparas, have iron deficiency. Women who experience heavy menstrual flow are also in danger of developing iron deficit. The adult male, on the other hand, rarely needs iron supplementation unless he is losing blood. Should a male develop iron deficiency anemia, a careful search should be carried out to determine the source of blood loss.

Excessive accumulation of iron can result from idiopathic hemochromatosis, transfusion, hemosiderosis, or prolonged excessive iron therapy, especially if the parenteral route of administration has been employed.

The RDA for iron varies from 10 mg./day for the first six months of life to a high of 18 or more mg./day for the pregnant woman—an amount that requires supplemental iron. For adolescents and females—except for the 51+ age group—18 mg./day is recommended.

Excellent sources of food iron include beef liver, lean meats, beans, oatmeal, spinach, egg yolk, peas, whole wheat bread, prunes, and dark molasses.

COPPER A micromineral from the standpoint of its role in the human body, copper was the first metal worked by man: the history of its use extends back seven or eight thousand years. Because it is such an excellent conductor of heat, it has long been used in cooking vessels. No micromineral from the viewpoint of its place in industry, some 3,000,000 tons are produced worldwide annually.

Copper is an essential component of various proteins and is required for healthy red blood corpuscles. It participates in the action of several essential enzymes; particularly important is copper's role in enzyme systems concerned with phospholipid synthesis.

The liver serves as the main storage organ for copper; bile acts as the primary vehicle in its excretion. Kidney, heart, and brain also contain large quantities of copper. Organ concentrations of copper are highest at birth, with the fetal liver containing five to ten times as much copper as that of the adult. The hepatic copper level shows an interesting geographical variation: Asiatics have higher levels than do citizens of the U.S. Since milk is low in copper, some clinicians believe that nutritional anemia in infants who have been restricted to a milk diet improves more rapidly when both iron and copper are given.

In a rare familial disorder involving copper metabolism—Wilson's disease or hepatolenticular degeneration—increased amounts of copper are found in brain, liver, and kidney. Treatment of this potentially fatal disorder centers around diets low in copper and agents that prevent intestinal absorption of copper.

Two mg. of copper daily appears sufficient to

maintain balance. Even generally poor diets appear to contain enough copper for the average person. Indeed, some writers suggest that death from caloric starvation would occur before overt clinical copper deficiency would develop.

Foods rich in copper include liver, kidney, shellfish, nuts, raisins, and dried legumes.

IODINE The micromineral iodine is best known for its role as a basic component of thyroid hormone. Often classified among the rarer elements, iodine constitutes 0.00000006 per cent of the earth's crust. A versatile mineral, it can be applied topically as a counterirritant, bactericide, and fungicide; it is also useful for disinfecting drinking water.

Iodine's prime function is as an essential component of the thyroid hormones thyroxin (T^4) and triiodothyronine (T^3). It is, therefore, required for normal growth and development and for maintenance of the metabolic rate.

The small intestine absorbs ingested iodine; the blood contains both inorganic iodide and protein-bound iodine. The iodine concentration of whole blood is about 1 part in 25 million; in the thyroid gland it is 1 part in 25 hundred. Drinking water contains varying quantities of iodine; estimates of the quantities of iodine in water provide a basis for determining the iodine concentration of nearby soil, as well as the iodine content of fruits, grains, grasses, and vegetables grown in the vicinity.

In the absence of sufficient iodine, the thyroid gland increases its secretory activity in a vain attempt to compensate for the deficit. The gland enlarges, causing an unsightly, uncomfortable mass on the anterior surface of the neck called *goiter*. In certain inland regions, including the Great Lakes area and the Alpine regions of Europe, water and soil provide inadequate iodine. The consequent high incidence of goiter can be diminished or eliminated by an iodine supplement, usually given as iodized table salt.

The drug propylthiouracil blocks the oxidation of iodide to iodine by the thyroid gland. Cabbage, rutabaga, and other members of the Brassica family contain goiter-causing substances.

Ingestion of iodine in therapeutic doses may cause skin lesions resembling acne in sensitive persons. Large quantities of iodine produce abdominal pain, nausea, vomiting, and diarrhea.

The RDA for iodine ranges from 5.83 μg./day/kg. body weight for the infant during the first six months of life to 2.95 μg./day/kg. for the adolescent male and lactating woman.

Outside of iodized salt, the best sources of iodine are seafoods, vegetables grown in iodine-rich soils, and iodine-rich drinking water.

FLUORINE The micromineral fluorine, discovered in 1771, constitutes 0.027 per cent of the earth's crust. It is widely, though sporadically, distributed. Traces of fluorine normally found in water can increase greatly when water passes through rocks and soils rich in fluorine.

Fluorine content of blood is about 0.2 parts per million (ppm), and of saliva, about 0.1 ppm. The largest amount of fluorine in the body is found in the teeth and bones. The element is a normal component of tooth structure. Its presence is required for maximal resistance to dental caries, especially in infancy and early childhood; however, it is of benefit later in life also. Although the precise mechanism by which fluorine inhibits the development of dental caries remains unknown, a theory is that during the formative years, fluorine reduces the solubility of tooth enamel in acids produced by bacteria, thus reducing dental caries. At any rate, addition of fluorine to drinking water at a level of slightly less than 1 ppm. gives remarkable protection against dental caries. Or, the fluorine can be given in a vitamin preparation, applied directly to the teeth by a dentist, or incorporated in toothpaste. Dentists properly emphasize that use of fluorine to prevent tooth decay is but one part of a broad preventive program designed to reduce dental caries.

Administration of sodium fluoride, in conjunction with vitamin D and calcium, has been suggested for the treatment of osteoporosis and Paget's disease of bone. Fluorides have also been suggested as one means of protecting the skeletal system from decalcification during space travel.

Intakes of fluorine in concentrations of more than 2 ppm. in water lead to mottling of the enamel of teeth. Endemic dental fluorosis occurs in communities in Texas and Colorado where the fluorine content of the water is above 2 ppm. Miners exposed to fluoride-containing dust for years develop hard, dense bones but no other physical abnormalities. While no RDA has been established for fluorine, it is the scientific concensus that drinking water with 1 ppm. of fluorine is advantageous for prevention of dental caries. When sodium fluoride is taken by mouth, the dose is usually 2.2 mg., which provides 1 mg. fluorine. Human beings excrete almost all ingested fluorine, up to 3 mg./day, via the urine. The degree of intestinal absorption depends upon the solubility of the ingested fluorine compound.

Sources of fluorine in addition to drinking water and pharmaceutical preparations are seafoods and seawater.

ZINC Although zinc comprises 0.2 per cent of the earth's crust, there is so little in seawater as to defy analysis. Only recently has zinc been shown to be essential for humans. Still, its presence in a variety of human tissues suggests its essentiality: its concentrations range from 16 to 50 ppm., with the highest values in the pancreas, liver, kidney, pituitary, adrenal, prostate gland, epididymis, seminal fluid, spermatozoa, bone leukocytes, hair, and the choroid of the eye.

Zinc is a constituent of enzymes involved in most major metabolic pathways. The function of the fairly consistent high concentration of zinc in nucleic acids is poorly understood. The blood zinc assists in carbon dioxide exchange. While relatively large amounts of zinc are located in bone, these stores are not readily available for use by the body.

Zinc metabolism is influenced by intestinal tract acidity, competing chemicals, hormones, and vitamins. Zinc conservation is good. Zinc deficiency appears in humans only in parts of the world where nutrition is extremely poor. The zinc levels in the neck hair of severely burned patients have been found to be depressed. When zinc toxicity occurs, it is usually associated with eating acidic foods stored in zinc-coated containers. Nausea, vomiting, and diarrhea result.

The zinc RDA for infants during the first six months is 3 mg./day. For all persons over 11 years of age, it is 15 mg./day, except for the pregnant (20 mg./day) and the lactating (25 mg./day).

Foods especially high in zinc include grain products, fish, and maple syrup.

CHROMIUM People in the United States have far lower chromium levels than Orientals, Africans, and persons from the Middle East. This may be explained by the fact that while raw sugars provide chromium in various quantities, refined sugars contain little or no chromium.

Chromium is required to maintain normal glu-

cose metabolism in experimental animals, probably acting as a cofactor for insulin. Cases of disturbances in glucose metabolism in man that responded favorably to administration of chromium have been described.

Chromium levels in tissues decline with age. The absorption and metabolism of chromium depend on the form in which the element is present. About 1 per cent of chromium in simple salts is absorbed, while the availability from some food sources appears to be between 10 and 25 per cent of a given amount.

A notion of the requirement for chromium can be obtained from the average daily loss, which is about 7–10 μg. and which occurs via the urine. Nevertheless, a meaningful recommendation for daily chromium intake is not currently possible, resulting chiefly from the great variation in availability of chromium in different foods.

Good sources of available chromium include most animal proteins but excluding fish, whole grain products, and brewers' yeast.

OTHER MICROMINERALS It is difficult to prove with direct evidence that the following microminerals are essential for man. However, their essential nature can be reliably assumed because they are essential for other mammals and also because they possess elements that are components of human enzyme systems.

Cobalt Cobalt, discovered in 1739, is thought to speed red blood corpuscle regeneration after destruction by radiation. Sheep grazing in pastures low in cobalt have developed weakness. The element is an integral part of vitamin B_{12}. This role appears to be its only contribution to normal nutrition.

A daily requirement of 15 μg. has been suggested; this need is amply met by an ordinary diet. The best source of cobalt is organ meats; muscle meats contain less generous quantities.

Manganese This micromineral was first isolated in 1774. It is needed for normal bone structure, reproduction, and normal function of the central nervous system. It is part of essential human enzyme systems. Like magnesium, it is an activator of enzymes. Manganese is concentrated in most organs and tissues, varying with different species.

The average human dietary intake of 2.5 to 7 mg./day appears to meet the requirement, as manganese deficiency has not been established in man.

Excellent sources of the element include nuts

and whole grains; vegetables and fruits also provide manganese.

Molybdenum   This element, discovered in 1778, is contained in highest concentration in the liver, skeleton, and kidneys. It contributes to bone formation, body growth, and normal metabolism. Excessive quantities interfere with copper metabolism.

The estimated daily intake in the U.S. is 45 to 500 μg, which probably meets the human need.

Beef kidneys, some cereals, and some legumes appear to be good sources of molybdenum. Dark green, leafy vegetables and animal organs also contain this micromineral.

Selenium   The selenium content of crops varies from one region to another; this fact is reflected in differences in the selenium content of pooled human blood from different areas. Although this element has been shown to be essential for several species, little is known about the human need. Selenium is found in the liver, heart, kidney, and spleen. It prevents various ailments in a variety of animals, including the rat, pig, lamb, and calf. It appears to prevent breakdown of polyunsaturated fatty acids in mammals.

A concentration of 0.1 μg./gm. in the diet prevents selenium deficit in animals; this concentration is present in the average mixed American diet.

Organ meats, such as liver, heart, kidney, and spleen, constitute a dietary source of selenium.

MICROMINERALS OF UNKNOWN IMPORT FOR HUMAN NUTRITION   Deficiencies of *nickel, tin, vanadium,* and *silicon* have been produced in experimental animals under rigidly controlled—and, hence, artificial—conditions. While the findings suggest that the elements are essential, their exact relationships to human nutrition are unknown.

CONCLUSION   New knowledge concerning the macro- and microminerals has opened up bright new vistas in the prevention and treatment of disease, as well as in the maintenance of optimal nutrition. While we may have reached a sort of impasse (however temporary) in our acquisition of facts concerning those marvelous catalysts we call vitamins, we have by no means achieved such a degree of sophistication in our understanding of minerals. They present a tantalizing treasure house of exciting opportunities for investigators, both in the basic and in the clinical sciences.

Water

Were you to ask a group of people what they regarded as the most essential nutrient, few of them would answer, "Water." Yet, if one were deprived of all liquid and solid nutrients, he would die of water deficit far sooner than he would die of deficit of any other nutrient. Doctor Thomas A. Dooley told one of the authors of his horrible experience of being forced to watch the sufferings of a boy imprisoned in a bamboo cage without food or water; the boy died—of water deficit —after eight days of agony. One needs lose only some 10 per cent of the body weight in water to be placed in danger of collapse and death.

Although we take water for granted, it is one of the most remarkable chemicals on earth. No known plant or animal can live without water in one form or another; it has no substitute. Fortunately, water is one of the most abundant and widely distributed chemicals on earth. (Of all the planets in the solar system, apparently only Earth has enough water to support human life.) Water can exist as a liquid, as solid ice or snow, or as gaseous vapor or steam. Snow is the purest natural source of water. Rain is second, although it contains dissolved atmospheric gases plus traces of other substances. Countless chemical compounds have water as part of the molecule, and few chemical reactions can occur unless water is present.

Among the mysteries of water that have constantly puzzled scientists is its unexpectedly high boiling point when compared to closely related chemicals such as hydrochloric acid (HCl) and ammonium hydroxide (NH_4OH). The boiling point of water, 100°C. (212° F.), and its freezing point, 0°C (32° F.), are ideally suited to the environmental temperatures in which we must live. These water constants enable us to withstand all but the most drastic changes in temperature. Suppose that instead of water, our body fluids had ammonia or hydrochloric acid as its solvent: the freezing point of ammonia is −77° C. and its boiling point a frigid −33° C. Or, look at hydrochloric acid: its freezing point is −114° C. and its boiling point −85° C!

By using sophisticated x-ray devices, investigators have finally solved one mystery associated with water: why does it take so much heat to change water into vapor? They found that, while the molecules of most liquids are closely packed, the molecules of water are widely separated. This loose chemical structure of water requires more heat for vaporization and boiling than does the tighter chemical structure of other substances. To clarify this, picture a room into which a large number of people are packed, contrasted to a room containing only a few people. It will obviously take more time and heat to reach a given temperature in the room with fewer people.

Living organisms contain more water than do most other substances. Water, therefore, exerts an enormous impact on our body's physiologic processes. Thus, we must examine both the distribution and regulation of body water, as well as the many substances dissolved in it, if we are to have any real understanding of the body's complex physicochemical mechanisms.

The percentage of fluid varies considerably from person to person, depending upon age, sex, and the amount of fat. A newborn infant is about 77 per cent fluid; the average adult is more like 60 per cent. While there is no important difference between the proportion of body fluid in the two sexes until about 16 years of age, after that the male accumulates more fluid, until he has some 17 per cent more. With advancing years, the total body fluid for both sexes decreases, but the sex difference remains. The average body fluid percentage of an elderly man is about 5 per cent more than that of an elderly woman.

The per cent of body fluid also varies with the fat content of the individual. Adipose, or fat, tissue is fairly free of water; hence, about 50 per cent of the obese adult's body weight is fluid; in the extremely lean adult, it is about 75 per cent. (Since females have more body fat than males, this explains why they have less body fluid in terms of percentage of body weight.) In disease states characterized by retention of excessive amounts of liquid (examples would be congestive heart failure or edema), the fluid percentage of the adult may approach that of the newborn.

As a solvent, water contains dissolved substances. Most of these substances are electrolytes, i.e., minerals that generate electrical charges when placed in water. The different locations of the body in which fluids are found are referred to as *compartments*. But this term may be misleading, for the compartments are by no means contiguous. The cellular compartment of body fluid, for example, is divided into trillions of tiny compartments consisting of the body cells. Yet, we refer to it as the *cellular compartment*. It is the largest compartment of our body fluid, about

three times the volume of the *extracellular compartment*. This compartment is divided into the fluid inside the blood vessels (the plasma) and the fluid outside the blood vessels (the interstitial fluid). This fluid has the missions of carrying nutrients to the body cells from the arterial capillary bed and of carrying waste materials from the body cells to the venous capillary bed and to the lymphatic capillary bed (which assists the venous capillary system in returning waste materials to the venous circulation). Lymph is usually regarded as a subdivision of the interstitial fluid. So is the cerebrospinal fluid; it is really interstitial fluid that has been specialized to meet the needs of the brain and spinal cord.

In addition to these major body fluids—the cellular and the extracellular fluid—there are other liquids in the body that usually are not classified as body fluids. Such are the secretions and excretions of organs and glands—saliva, gastric juice, intestinal juice, bile, perspiration, and urine. Then there are the fluids of the body cavities—the pleural cavity, which surrounds the lungs; the pericardial cavity, which surrounds the heart; and the peritoneal cavity, which surrounds the digestive organs. Since these "cavities" are really tightly packed with important organs, they are not really cavities at all. But they do contain small quantities of lubricating fluid, which can become excessive in disease. Then we have "pleural effusion" or "pericardial effusion" or "ascites," depending upon which cavity is involved.

Throughout the body, water serves a lubricating function, helping to protect the fragile body cells from injury. Water also acts as a temperature regulator, helping to maintain constant and within safe bounds the body temperature.

How do we gain water? We obtain it when we drink liquids, we obtain it from solid food (which, after all, is mostly water), and we gain it from chemical oxidation of foodstuffs and body tissues. We can also gain it—in combination with electrolytes and dextrose—from parenteral infusions. Water can also be given by rectal infusion.

How do we lose water? In a host of ways. We lose it through the skin both as insensible and sensible perspiration. While insensible perspiration consists only of water, sensible perspiration contains water plus sodium, potassium, chloride, magnesium, and even some urea. Then we lose important quantities of water in the moistened air we exhale; we lose it in the stools, and we lose a great amount in the urine. These are the normal losses that occur in health. When we become ill, we lose water in additional ways: as vomitus, in diarrheal stools, through excessive sweating if we have fever.

Considering all that water does, it appears logical that drinking generous quantities of it should be important for the maintenance of health. A generous intake of water is also indicated in most illnesses. Often the first order written for a newly admitted patient in the hospital order book is "force fluids" or "fluids freely." Physicians, nurses, nutritionists, and all members of the health team universally recognize the value of generous quantities of water.

BIBLIOGRAPHY

Anthony, C.: Basic Concepts in Anatomy and Physiology, A Programmed Presentation, ed. 3. St. Louis: C. V. Mosby, 1974.

Goodhart, R., and **Shils, M.:** Modern Nutrition in Health and Disease, ed. 5. Philadelphia: Lea & Febiger, 1973.

Indiana Diet Manual Committee: Indiana Diet Manual, 1976.

Labuza, T.: The Nutrition Crisis: A Reader. St. Paul: West Publishing Co., 1975.

Lappe, F.: Diet for a Small Planet. New York: Ballantine Books, 1971.

National Research Council, Food and Nutrition Board: Recommended Dietary Allowances, ed. 8. Washington, D.C: National Academy of Sciences, 1974.

Watt, B., and **Merrill, A.:** Composition of Foods. Washington, DC: U.S. Department of Agriculture, 1975.

Williams, S.: Nutrition and Diet Therapy, ed. 2. St. Louis: C. V. Mosby, 1973.

— 6 —

Disturbances of Water and Electrolytes

If the volume or chemical composition of the body fluid deviates even slightly from the safe bounds of normal, disease results. Diseases involving body fluids are called *body fluid disturbances* or *body fluid imbalances*. Such disturbances may be primary or they may occur secondarily to other conditions. Indeed, every patient with a serious illness is a potential candidate for body fluid disturbances, and even the patient who is only moderately or mildly ill may be stricken with one imbalance or a combination of two or more.

Despite the frequency and the importance of body fluid disturbances, probably no group of clinical problems has been so poorly understood.

Much of the early knowledge concerning imbalances of the body fluids originated with teachers who were biochemists first and clinicians second—if, indeed, they were clinicians at all. Quite naturally, they presented body fluid disturbances in the light of their own research. As a result, much of the early teaching about body fluid disturbances was concerned with detailed descriptions of all the possible imbalances that could occur in the one or two diseases on which the teacher had concentrated. Body fluid disturbances began to be regarded as *biochemical appendages* of disease states, rather than as a broad group of problems representing the common denominator of many ailments. No overall view of these disturbances was presented. The subject as taught was so complex, so specialized, and so sophisticated that most mem-

bers of the medical and nursing professions came to regard the subject as difficult, if not impossible. One student in the class of a famous pediatrician-biochemist described the subject: "as clear as if written backwards by Gertrude Stein in Sanskrit."

A completely different and enlightened approach to the study of body fluid disturbances might be termed the *clinical picture approach*. First introduced by Carl Moyer, it was enlarged upon considerably by Snively and Sweeney. Its basic breakthrough involved understanding that disturbances of water and electrolytes are produced by a fairly small number of mechanisms, most of which are simple and readily comprehensible.

Essential to the application of the clinical picture approach is a simple diagnostic classification, which divides body fluid disturbances into some sixteen basic imbalances or clinical pictures. Each has its own set of causative mechanisms; its own symptoms, subjective and objective; its own laboratory findings.

Since we don't have direct access to the cellular fluid except in highly sophisticated procedures, it is not practical to attempt to assess the state of the cellular fluid directly. However, we can determine the condition of the extracellular fluid directly (and, hence, of the cellular fluid indirectly) by examining plasma and other body liquids, such as sweat and urine. Thus, our diagnostic classification of body fluid disturbances is based on the extracellular fluid.

51

When we discover an imbalance, we correct it by correcting the composition of the extracellular fluid, knowing that the problems within the body's trillions of cells will also be corrected.

Two of the imbalances in our diagnostic classification involve changes in the *volume* of the extracellular fluid—either a deficit or an excess. Twelve imbalances involve alterations in the *concentrations* of electrolytes in the extracellular fluid in units of electrolytes per unit volume of body fluid. Bear in mind that what is important from the standpoint of a disturbance of body fluid is usually the concentration of the electrolyte per unit volume and *not* the total quantity of the electrolyte. The final two imbalances in our classification involve shifts of water and electrolytes from one extracellular fluid compartment to another.

There is nothing new to this pedagogic technique for studying disease. When ailments such as rheumatic fever, appendicitis, lobar pneumonia, or the contagious diseases are presented to nursing students, they are presented as clinical pictures, and the students analyze them as clinical pictures. Each picture includes the history, the symptoms—both subjective and objective—and the laboratory data. The student who studies body fluid disturbances by this method analyzes the underlying mechanisms responsible for the disturbances through clinical pictures.

Sometimes one of these disturbances exists by itself; at other times, it occurs in combination with one or more additional imbalances. Frequently, body fluid disturbances are associated with other disease states and, indeed, interact intimately with them. Sometimes a succession of body fluid disturbances occurs, one after another. Clearly, one must understand single imbalances if one is to understand the combinations.

BIBLIOGRAPHY

Berman, L.: Electrolyte games for rainy afternoons. J.A.M.A. 233:282, 1975.

Moyer, C.: Fluid Balance. Chicago: Year Book Publishers, 1952.

— 7 —

Units of Measure

Many years ago, a man named John Selden said,

> . . . if they should make the standard for the measure we call a "foot" a Chancellor's foot; what an uncertain measure would this be! One Chancellor has a long foot, another a short foot, a third an indifferent foot . . .

Master Selden was pointing out, quite correctly, that, without standard or invariable units of measure, we are severely limited. In the same light, we could never understand, diagnose, and treat body fluid disturbances without simple and accurate units of measure.

MEASUREMENT OF EXTRACELLULAR FLUID

Because of the constant exchanges between cellular and extracellular fluid, changes in either are reflected in the other. Therefore, imbalances in the extracellular fluid ultimately cause imbalances in the cellular fluid, and vice versa.

As explained in Chapter 6, because of its ready availability, we focus our chief attention upon the extracellular portion of the body fluid when we study imbalances of water and electrolytes.

MEASUREMENT OF VOLUME One of the most essential units of measure is the measurement of volume. The metric system of weights and measures is used universally in science. In the metric system, the *liter* (L.) is used for volume measurement. The liter is broken down into 1000 parts or milliliters (ml.), each milliliter representing 1/1000 of a liter. A milliliter virtually is identical to the cubic centimeter (cc.), but the milliliter is preferred in determining volume because the centimeter is a linear rather than a volumetric unit of measure. Expressed in terms of weight rather than volume, a liter of water weighs 1000 grams (Gm.), or about 2.2 pounds.

MEASUREMENT OF CHEMICAL ACTIVITY The electrolytes of the body fluid are dynamic, active chemicals. Since we are interested in their activity, we must have a unit that expresses *chemical activity*, or *chemical combining ability*, or the power of cations to unite with anions to form molecules. Virtually any cation can unite with any anion. The cation sodium, for example, combines with the anion chloride to form the molecule sodium chloride. Sodium united with proteinate forms the molecule sodium proteinate. Or, it may combine with nitrate, forming sodium nitrate. Similarly, the cations potassium, magnesium, and calcium can unite with any of the anions. Therefore, why could we not merely use as our unit of measure the weight of the ions in which we are interested? Unfortunately, this does not solve our problem, since the *weight* of a chemical bears no relation to its *chemical activity*. One mg. of sodium unites chemically with 180 mg. of proteinate to form the compound sodium proteinate, for example.

In searching for a unit of chemical activity, chemists have discovered the *milliequivalent* (mEq.). A traditional measurement of physical power in our civilization is the power of an imaginary average horse; our unit of chemical power, the milliequivalent, is *equivalent* to the activity of 1 mg. of hydrogen. In other words our *chemical horse is 1 mg. of hydrogen* (Fig. 7-1). One milligram of hydrogen exerts 1 mEq. of chemical activity; so do 23 mg. of sodium, 39 mg. of potassium, 20 mg. of calcium, 35 mg. of chloride, or 4140 mg. of proteinate. Each of these weights represents 1 mEq. of the ion in question, whether it is cation or anion.

When electrolytes are measured in milliequivalents, cations and anions always balance each other, and a given number of milliequivalents of a cation always reacts with exactly the same number of milliequivalents of an anion. Here is something useful to memorize:

> One Milliequivalent Of Any Cation
> Is Equivalent Chemically
> To One Milliequivalent Of Any Anion

It matters not a bit whether the cation is sodium, potassium, calcium, or magnesium, or whether the anion is chloride, bicarbonate, phosphate, sulfate, or proteinate.

The milliequivalent value of an element or molecule is determined by taking the *millimole* (mM.) (the atomic or molecular weight of the element or compound in milligrams) and dividing by the *valence* (the numerical measure of combining power for one atom of a chemical element). Valence also reflects the number of hydrogen atoms that can be held in combination or displaced in a reaction by one atom of an element. If a substance is *univalent* (e.g., chloride), *1 mM. equals 1 mEq.* If a substance is *bivalent* (e.g., calcium), *1 mM equals 2 mEq.* Therefore, *2mM. (2 mEq.)* of a *univalent* substance reacts chemically with only *1 mM. (2 mEq.)* of a *bivalent* substance.

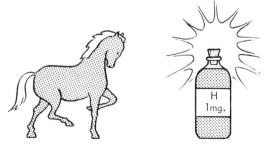

Figure 7-1. One milligram of hydrogen represents the unit for chemical combining power: it is the electrolyte horsepower.

MEASUREMENT OF OSMOTIC PRESSURE The milliequivalent also is a *rough* unit of measure for the osmotic pressure, or drawing power, of a solution. However, since not all substances that exert osmotic pressure can be measured in milliequivalents, a more accurate measure of osmotic pressure is the *milliosmole* (mOsm.). To determine the number of milliosmoles in a solution, we again refer to the millimole. *One millimole of a substance that does not dissociate into ions (e.g., glucose) equals 1 mOsm. However, a millimole of a compound that does dissociate into ions equals two or more milliosmoles,* depending on how many ions it dissociates into. Sodium chloride (NaCl), for example, dissociates into one sodium ion and one chloride ion, so 1 mM of this salt equals 2mOsm. A millimole of a more complex salt such as disodium phosphate (Na_2HPO_4) dissociates into two sodium ions and one phosphate ion, so it equals 3 mOsm. The osmotic pressure of a solution, therefore, is calculated by adding up all the ions, or milliosmoles, it contains.

The milliequivalents per liter and the milliosmoles per liter of plasma, interstitial fluid, and cellular fluid are as follows:

	mEq./L.	mOsm./L.
Plasma	308	296.50
Interstitial fluid	311	300.75
Cellular fluid	364	305.00

MEASUREMENT OF CHEMICAL REACTION The final unit of measure with which we shall concern ourselves is *pH*, which tells us whether the chemical reaction of a fluid is acid, neutral, or alkaline. Basically, the reaction of a fluid is determined by the number of hydrogen ions it contains. Hydrogen is present in the body fluid in only tiny amounts, between 0.0000001 and 0.00000001 Gm./L. of extracellular fluid. As a convenient way of expressing such minute hydrogen ion concentrations without resorting to decimals, the symbol pH was devised.

pH represents the reciprocal of the logarithm of the hydrogen ion concentration. Put more simply, pH is the power of 1/10, and it tells us the grams of hydrogen per liter of extracellular fluid. For example, pH 3 = $1/10^3$. As you probably recall from elementary arithmetic, power represents the product arising from the continued multiplication of a number by itself. Therefore, pH 3 = 1/10 × 1/10 × 1/10, or 1/1000 Gm. hydrogen per liter of extracellular fluid. Similarly, pH 7 = $1/10^7$, which, when multiplied, equals 1/10,000,000 Gm. hydrogen per liter of extracellular fluid.

It is not really necessary to do all that multiplying, however. All one has to do is put down 1/1 and add zeroes equal to the number of the pH. For example, if the pH is 3, you simply write down 1/1 and add three zeroes, and you see immediately that pH 3 = 1/1000 Gm. hydrogen per liter of extracellular fluid.

The more zeroes we have, of course, the smaller the amount of hydrogen. Since it is the amount of hydrogen in a fluid that determines its acidity, *as pH goes up the fluid becomes less acid and as pH goes down the fluid becomes more acid.* pH 7, for example, is ten times more acid than pH 8; pH 6 is ten times more acid than pH 7, and 100 times more acid than pH 8. The normal pH of extracellular fluid is between 7.35 and 7.45.

This unit of measure is extremely important in understanding acid-base (or acid-alkali) balance, which we shall discuss in Chapter 10.

Another value used for expressing the hydrogen ion concentration in body fluids is the nanomole (nM.), which is 1/1,000,000,000 Gm., or 1/1,000,000 mg. of hydrogen. (Recall that in the case of hydrogen—and only in the case of hydrogen—1 mg. = 1 mEq.) Now, nM. are not difficult to understand. They are *linear*, which means that when the number of nM. of H+/L. rises, so does the acidity; when it goes down, so does the acidity. Nanomoles are an arithmetic rather than a *logarithmic* measurement. Nanomoles are measured, first, by using a pH meter and, second, a simple conversion table (Table 7-1).

Table 7-1. Nanomoles of Hydrogen for Varying pH values

pH		Nanomoles
7.0	=	100.0
7.1	=	79.4
7.2	=	63.0
7.3	=	50.1
7.4	=	39.8
7.5	=	31.6
7.6	=	25.1
7.7	=	20.0
7.8	=	15.8
7.9	=	12.5
8.0	=	10.0

The extreme ranges for nM. H+/L. of human body fluid start with a high of 100 nM./L.—extremely severe acidosis, as acidic as one can become and still live. The other end of the range of 10 mM./L. is about as alkalotic (or alkaline) as one can become and survive. The normal value is about 40 nM. H+/L.; 50 represents acidemia, 30 represents alkalemia—but neither is really extreme.

BIBLIOGRAPHY

Snively, W.; Leitch, G.: and **Beshear, D.:** Acid-base disturbances, a programmed text. Am. J. Intravenous Therapy 1:22–40, 1977; 5:26–41, 1978; 5:36–56, 1978; and 5:26–34, 1978.

Stedman's Medical Dictionary, ed. 23. Baltimore: Williams & Wilkins, 1976.

— 8 —

Gains and Losses of Water and Electrolytes

Whether they be primary or secondary to other conditions, all body fluid disturbances are caused by abnormal differences between gains and losses of water and electrolytes.

A comparison of the routes by which we gain water and electrolytes and the routes by which we lose them is in order. The body gains water and electrolytes in various ways: water alone is gained by

GAINS

Ingested water ●
Ingested food ●
Tube feedings ●
Oxidation of foodstuffs ●
(water only)
Oxidation of body tissues ●
(water only)
Parenteral feedings ●
Rectal feedings ●

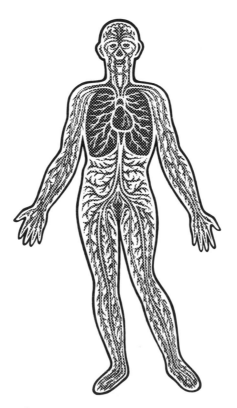

LOSSES

● Vomiting
● Lungs—water vapor and carbon dioxide
● Burn exudate
● Gastric suction
● Perspiration
● Insensible loss of water
● Internal pooling & fixation
● Paracentesis
● Colitis
● Intestinal suction
● Draining intestinal fistula
● Stools
● Urine
● Ulcer exudate
● Wound exudate
● Loss into injured areas

Figure 8-1. Gains and losses of water.

drinking distilled water and by oxidation of food-stuffs and body tissues; softened water, well water, mineral water, and most city water supplies provide both water and electrolytes. Food also supplies both, for although it consists largely of water, it is rich in electrolytes and other nutrients, such as protein, fat, carbohydrate, and vitamins. Hospitalized patients frequently gain water and electrolytes, as well as other materials, via nasogastric tube, intravenous needle, or, though not often used, rectal tube.

Normal losses of both water and electrolytes occur through the lungs in breath, through the eyes in tears, through the kidneys in urine, through the skin in perspiration, and through the intestines in feces. In addition, water alone is lost through the skin in insensible perspiration, which goes on constantly. Abnormal losses can occur during illness or injury, as in burn or wound exudate, hemorrhage, vomiting, and diarrhea. Rapid breathing, suction via gastric or intestinal tube, enterostomy, colostomy, and cecostomy also cause great losses of water and electrolytes. Drainage from sites of surgical operations or from abscesses contains both water and electrolytes, as does fluid extracted via paracentesis. Fluids sur-

rounding the brain and spinal cord can be lost if there is an abnormal opening to the outside. Indeed, fluids may be lost even inside the body, since when abnormal closed collections of fluid develop, as in intestinal obstruction, *these fluids are just as useless to the body economy as if they were outside the body* (Fig. 8-1).

Now, what is important about these gains and losses is this: when one becomes ill, his gains decrease (may cease altogether) and his losses almost invariably increase. So it is no wonder that every seriously ill person is a logical candidate for a body fluid disturbance. In the healthy adult, the volume of urine excreted is approximately equal to the volume of fluid ingested as fluid; and water derived from solid food and from chemical oxidation in the body approximately equals the normal losses of water through the lungs and skin and in the stool (Fig. 8-2). Thus, in health, gains approximately equal losses whereas, during illness, gains and losses are not always equal. Intake of food and fluids may cease or diminish, while the normal losses continue, and the losses may outweigh the gains by as much as one half liter or more a day. The daily losses are cumula-

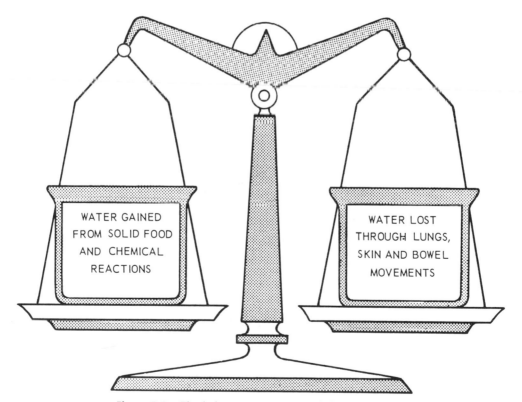

Figure 8-2. The balance portrays water balance in health.

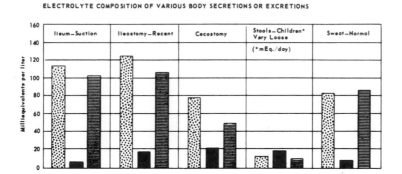

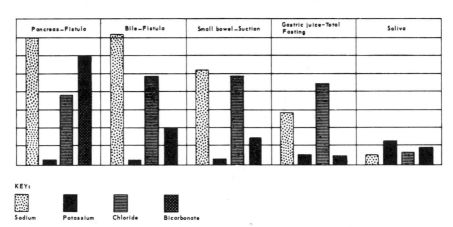

Figure 8-3.   Electrolyte composition of various body secretions or excretions.

tive, so a serious deficit can develop in a short time. If abnormal losses are occurring in addition, as in vomiting or diarrhea, the patient may become gravely ill within a matter of hours. The type of imbalance caused depends upon the kind of fluid lost, since body secretions and excretions vary greatly in electrolyte compositions and concentrations (Fig. 8-3).

Serious imbalances also occur when the gains are greater than the losses, as when the kidneys are not functioning properly. Excesses are just as dangerous as deficits and can prove fatal in a short period of time.

Thus, abnormal differences between gains and losses cause all of the sixteen basic imbalances in our diagnostic classification; these imbalances involve changes in volume, composition, and position of the extracellular fluid.

BIBLIOGRAPHY

Kintzel, K. (ed.):   Advanced Concepts in Clinical Nursing, ed. 2. Philadelphia: J. B. Lippincott Co., 1977.

— 9 —

Volume Changes in Extracellular Fluid

Both extracellular fluid volume deficit and extracellular fluid volume excess are fascinating to study. One of them (volume deficit) has caused more death than all the wars in history. Even today, it is a massive problem for countries without modern medical facilities.

Volume disturbances of the extracellular fluid represent either deficits or excesses of both water and electrolytes—not water alone—in approximately the same proportions as they are found in the normal state. Thus, although the extracellular fluid changes in volume, the percentages of water and electrolytes remain about the same. It is also important to note that, when volume changes occur in the extracellular fluid, there are corresponding changes in the cellular fluid. An uncorrected volume deficit of extracellular fluid, for example, will ultimately cause a volume deficit of cellular fluid as well.

EXTRACELLULAR FLUID VOLUME DEFICIT

Among the terms frequently used to describe this imbalance are fluid deficit, hypovolemia, and dehydration. The term dehydration is incorrect, however, since it involves the loss of water only.

Volume deficit results from an abrupt decrease in fluid intake, from an acute loss of secretions and excretions, or from a combination of decreased intake and increased loss (Fig. 9-1). It usually begins with

one of the following: a loss of secretions and excretions, as occurs in vomiting; diarrhea; fistulous drainage; a systemic infection, with its attendant fever and increased utilization of water and electrolytes; or intestinal obstruction. As secretions and excretions are depleted, they are replenished by water and electrolytes of the extracellular fluid, thus reducing the volume of the extracellular fluid. With continued depletion of the extracellular fluid, water and electrolytes are drawn from the cells, thus causing a deficit in the cellular fluid as well, although not immediately.

A volume deficit can develop slowly or with great rapidity, in which case it may cause death within hours after onset. In epidemics of Asiatic cholera, thousands upon thousands died of an extracellular fluid volume deficit produced by the severe vomiting and purging associated with the disease. Fortunately, increased knowledge concerning body fluids has virtually eliminated deaths caused by cholera, and today's cholera victim usually survives with no aftereffects if given prompt treatment for the extracellular fluid volume deficit that occurs during the initial period.

Diagnosis of Extracellular Fluid Volume Deficit

Extracellular fluid volume deficit frequently is difficult to diagnose since so many of its clinical symptoms appear in any seriously ill patient. In the infant,

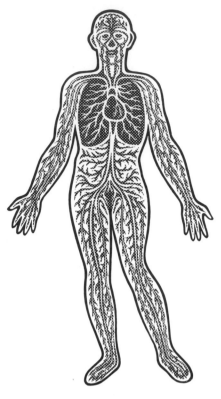

PRECEDING EVENTS

- Loss of water and electrolytes
- Decreased intake of water and electrolytes

CLINICAL OBSERVATIONS

- Depressed fontanel in infant
- Longitudinal tongue wrinkles
- Urine flow rate under 40 ml./hr.
- Systolic blood pressure 10 mm. Hg less standing than supine
- Temperature subnormal
- Body weight loss

LABORATORY FINDINGS

- Little help

RELATED PROBLEMS

- Kidney tubules deteriorate rapidly
- Quickly leads to other deficits

Figure 9-1. Extracellular fluid volume deficit.

depression of the anterior fontanel is diagnostic. In others, observations that are generally useful include longitudinal wrinkles in the tongue (one of the most valuable); dry skin and mucous membranes; fatigue; a urine flow rate of less than 20 to 40 ml./hr. in an adult, and materially lower in children, in proportion to body surface area. A systolic blood pressure of 10 mm. Hg less for the patient in the standing position than in the supine is also indicative of the imbalance in the adult. Characteristically, the pulse is rapid, the temperature is normal or subnormal (unless infection is present, as it often is), the respiratory rate is elevated, and the venous pressure (which can be measured either centrally or peripherally) is decreased. Acute body weight loss is enormously helpful in diagnosis. For a mild deficit weight loss might be 2 per cent, for a pronounced deficit 5 per cent, and for a severe deficit 8 per cent or more, with the loss considerably more alarming if it is acute. Unfortunately, the patient often does not know his pre-illness weight.

The laboratory offers us little, if any, help in diagnosing volume deficit, although findings of hemoconcentration may be present in a severe deficit. Thus, diagnosis must be based on a careful history and searching physical examination.

One of the great hazards of a severe extracellular fluid volume deficit is inadequate perfusion of the kidney, since there is not enough extracellular fluid to bring the requisite amount of plasma to the glomeruli. When this imbalance is permitted to exist for more than a short period of time (minutes, if the imbalance is severe), the kidney tubules deteriorate and may soon become permanently damaged. The reason for this deterioration is not clear at present.

Extracellular fluid volume deficit frequently is followed by other body fluid disturbances, including bicarbonate deficit and potassium deficit. If excessive water is lost in watery stools or with rapid breathing, sodium excess also may develop.

The goal of therapy for extracellular fluid volume deficit is to restore the volume to normal without altering the electrolyte composition of the fluid. This is accomplished by oral or parenteral administration of a solution formulated to provide electrolytes in quantities balanced between the patient's minimal needs and maximal tolerances. It also provides free water to form urine and to carry out metabolic functions. Such a solution is called a *balanced solution,* or a *Butler-type solution.* When this type of solution is used, the homeostatic mechanisms selectively retain or excrete water and electrolytes according to the patient's individual needs.

CASE HISTORIES Eight-year-old R.S. was admitted to the hospital following two days of severe vomiting and diarrhea, which started after a school picnic (where the sanitation had been poorly supervised). He had not been able to keep anything down for 36 hours and had not voided for 24 hours. His weight before he became ill was about 60 lb. (27 kg.). Physical examination revealed lethargy, a rectal temperature of 101° F., pulse 105, respirations deep and regular at 24/min., blood pressure 110/80, dry skin and mucous membranes, an acetone odor to his breath, increased intestinal peristaltic sounds, weight 55 lb. (25 kg.), and a height of 50 in. Laboratory tests showed hemoglobin 15 Gm., plasma sodium 148 mEq./L., plasma potassium 5 mEq./L., plasma bicarbonate 12 mEq./L., plasma chloride 108 mEq./L., pCO_2 28 mm.Hg, and plasma pH 7.25. A catheterized urine specimen revealed a bladder urine volume of 10 ml., pH 5, specific gravity 1.032, a trace of albumin, and the presence of acetone. Nausea, vomiting, and diarrhea persisted throughout the first day. Estimated fluid lost from vomiting and diarrhea was 500 ml. in the first 12 hours and 400 ml. during the second 12 hours.

Commentary The increased respirations and the depressed pCO_2 (indicating hyperventilation) in this clearcut case of extracellular fluid volume deficit are revealed as compensatory for HCO_3 deficit since the pCO_2 was depressed 1 mm. Hg from the normal of 40 for each 1 mEq./L. depression of the bicarbonate from the normal 24 mEq./L. (If the pCO_2 had been depressed more than 1 mm. Hg for each mEq./L. depression of the bicarbonate from the normal of 24 mEq./L., one must suspect a complicating carbonic acid deficit since such a change would indicate that something more than simple compensatory decrease of pCO_2 was occurring. If, on the other hand, the pCO_2 was depressed less than 1 mm. Hg for each mEq./L. depression of the bicarbonate from the normal of 24 mEq./L., then carbonic acid excess must be superimposed on the compensatory decrease of pCO_2 since such depression of pCO_2 would be less than normally occurs

as compensation for bicarbonate deficit. For detailed explanation, refer to the section on acid-base disturbances in Chapter 10.)

E.D., age 57, was admitted to the hospital at 9 A.M. Her husband stated that she had become nauseated two days before after a day or two of just "not feeling up to par," with loss of her usual excellent appetite. The day before admission, she complained of intermittent pain centering around the umbilicus. She vomited occasionally, usually when she was having pain. On physical examination, her skin felt dry, her tongue showed definite longitudinal wrinkles. Her blood pressure was found to be 130/90 in the supine position and 115/75 when she was held upright. Her abdominal wall was tight but not rigid. There was slight distention. Peristaltic sounds could be heard with the stethoscope, louder during periods when there was pain. No gas or feces were passed. On admission to the hospital, a Foley catheter was inserted; her urine flow rate in the ensuing 2 hours was 20 ml./hr. Urine specific gravity was 1.020 (concentrated), but the specimen was otherwise normal. All electrolytes and blood gases (pCO_2, pO_2, pH) were within limits of normal. Red and white blood counts and hemoglobin were normal. The weight was 130 lb. (59 kg.), which represented no change from recent weights (patient had been on a reducing diet and had been weighing regularly). A diagnosis of complete intestinal obstruction was made, later found to be caused by obstruction of the small intestine by a tumor. The body fluid imbalance diagnosis was extracellular fluid (ECF) volume deficit. Of key importance in making this diagnosis was the physician's recognition of the fact that as much as 8 L. of fluid that closely resembles ECF can accumulate daily within an obstructed intestine without any weight loss. Yet, this accumulated fluid, still within the confines of the body, is just as much lost to the body as if it were outside. The "lost" fluid was replaced immediately, before surgical intervention was carried out.

Commentary The various causes of intestinal obstruction can be divided under headings of *mechanical* (e.g., pressure on the intestine from adjacent tumors), *vascular* (e.g., thrombosis of a splancnic artery or vein), or *neurogenic* (e.g., as occurs in pneumonia). Essential to remember in ECF volume deficit caused by intestinal obstruction is the fact that one cannot rely on acute weight changes to give a clue to the diagnosis. This truth holds, regardless of what portion of the intestine is obstructed. Important clues to the diagnosis in this type of ECF volume deficit are orthostatic hypotension, decreased urine flow rate (under 40 ml./hr. in an adult), increased urinary specific gravity, and longitudinal wrinkles in the tongue.

EXTRACELLULAR FLUID VOLUME EXCESS

This imbalance is frequently called *fluid excess* or *overhydration*, but the latter term is incorrect since it represents an excess of water only.

A volume excess develops when the kidneys are unable to rid the body of unneeded water and electrolytes. This inability may result from simple overloading of the body by oral or parenteral administration of excessive quantities of an isotonic solution of sodium chloride. Somewhat paradoxically, it is the quantity of sodium in the body that determines the volume of the extracellular fluid; therefore, excess sodium from any cause may well precede extracellular fluid volume excess. The imbalance may occur in diseases

that affect the function of the homeostatic mechanisms, such as chronic kidney disease, chronic liver disease with portal hypertension, congestive heart failure, and malnutrition. In all of these conditions, there is abnormal retention of water and sodium and, whether the volume excess is caused by simple overloading or by diminished function of the homeostatic mechanisms, the result is the same: the extracellular fluid becomes excessively salty. Therefore, in an attempt to maintain its normal composition, the extracellular fluid draws water from the cells.

Diagnosis of Extracellular Fluid Volume Excess

Expanding volume of extracellular fluid produces numerous clinical symptoms which contribute far more in diagnosing this imbalance than they do in the case of extracellular fluid volume deficit (Fig. 9-2). Clinical observations include puffy eyelids; peripheral edema, which may actually be pitting; ascites (accumulation of fluid in the abdominal cavity); pleural effusion; pulmonary edema (often visible by roentgenography when undetectable by stethoscope); elevated central or peripheral venous pres-

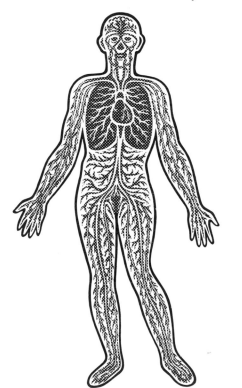

PRECEDING EVENTS
- Any cause of retention of excessive sodium and water

CLINICAL OBSERVATIONS
- Puffy eyelids
- Peripheral edema
- Ascites
- Pleural effusion
- Pulmonary edema
- Moist rales in lungs
- Acute weight gain

LABORATORY FINDINGS
- Little help

RELATED PROBLEMS
- Patient may succumb from pulmonary edema
- Imbalance may occur with remobilization of edema fluid third postburn day
- If BUN and potassium are elevated, kidneys may be failing

Figure 9-2.   Extracellular fluid volume excess.

sure; acute weight gain, sometimes as much as 10 per cent of the normal body weight; and moist rales in the lungs (late in the imbalance). In many patients, this imbalance occurs without frank edema because of the mysterious third factor, which causes diuresis before frank edema supervenes; in a severe excess, the patient may succumb from the pulmonary edema.

The laboratory gives little help in diagnosing extracellular fluid volume excess, except that the formed elements of the blood may be decreased because of plasma dilution. If renal impairment has occurred, both the blood urea nitrogen (BUN) and the plasma potassium may be elevated. An x-ray picture of the lungs will detect fluid accumulation long before it can be detected by auscultation.

Considering related problems, we should recall that the patient may succumb from pulmonary edema. The imbalance can occur with remobilization of edema fluid on the third day following a severe burn, if the patient has been given, or permitted, excessive fluids during the first two days of the burn. If the cause of the excess is kidney failure, the blood urea nitrogen (BUN) and potassium (K) would be elevated, thus providing a valuable clue to the cause of the accumulation.

The goal of therapy in extracellular fluid volume excess is to rid the body of excess water and electrolytes without altering the electrolyte composition of the fluid. Primary treatment is directed toward the causative factors. Diuretics are often helpful in providing symptomatic relief and, in addition, it may be necessary to withhold all liquids for a time.

CASE HISTORIES Eight-year-old J.D. was unable to retain liquids by mouth following appendectomy and, therefore, was provided needed water and electrolytes by the intravenous route. For two days, he was given a continuous intravenous infusion of 5 per cent dextrose in isotonic solution of sodium chloride in the amount of approximately 4 L./day. Early on the morning of the third day, he complained of shortness of breath; his eyelids were puffy, his cheeks appeared full, and moist rales were heard in the lungs. He was found to have gained about 6 per cent over his admission weight. His RBC was 4,000,000 and his hemoglobin was 10 Gm.

Commentary Isotonic solution of sodium chloride is sometimes called *normal saline* or *physiological solution of sodium chloride*. It is not *normal* from the chemical standpoint, and it is certainly not physiologic. It provides 154 mEq. of Na/L., somewhat in excess of the normal 142 mEq./L. And it also contains 154 mEq. of Cl, far in excess of the normal 105 mEq./L. Thus, it forces a considerable excess of chloride on the kidneys. Moreover, it contains no K, Ca, Mg, or PO_4, all required for a solution to meet both the extracellular and cellular needs of the body. Finally, since it is isotonic with plasma, it provides no free water for renal function and metabolic processes. Because of its chloride excess, isotonic solution of sodium chloride tends to favor bicarbonate deficit (metabolic acidosis).

H.F., a 45-year-old male, visited his physician because of episodic weakness, paresthesias, tetany, polyuria, and polydipsia. In the course of a complete workup for hypertension, it was found that the patient's aldosterone excretion on a sodium intake of more than 10,000 mg./day exceeded 200 μg daily. The patient was given spironolactone, an aldosterone antagonist, and all manifestations of the disease were reversed in six weeks. Adrenal adenoma or adenomata were suspected. At surgical operation, the patient was found to be suffering from bilateral adrenal hyperplasia, rather than from adrenal adenoma. No corrective surgery was carried out; instead, the patient was placed on mild sodium restriction, low doses of chlorthalidone, and supplementary potassium.

Commentary Adrenal hyperplasia, as does an adrenal adenoma, causes the production of excessive aldosterone, which is not responsive to the body's need for sodium conservation, volume conservation, and potassium excretion. Even when a large quantity of sodium is given, as in the above example, the patient continues to secrete large quantities of aldosterone. The symptoms of excessive aldosterone are due chiefly to the excessive retention of sodium, chloride, and water, and the excessive excretion of potassium. While spironolactone reverses the effects of aldosterone, its side effects are often undesirable. The patient with an adrenal adenoma is fortunate since removal of the tumor can be expected to cure the hypertension.

BIBLIOGRAPHY

Daly, W.: Papper, S.: and Whang, R. (eds.): Clinical Fluid and Electrolyte Management. Washington, DC: Veterans Administration, 1976.

— 10 —

Concentration Changes
of Major
Extracellular Electrolytes

"Nothing but a cloud of elements organic . . . such as man is made of." Oliver Wendell Holmes

Each electrolyte has special bodily functions and, although some play larger roles than others, all are necessary for the maintenance of life. Their normal concentrations are precisely geared to the body's needs, so they must be maintained at proper levels if the body is to remain healthy. Also vitally important are the concentrations of carbonic acid and base bicarbonate.

Discussed in this chapter are disturbances involving alterations in the normal concentration of the extracellular fluid's electrolytes, as expressed in mEq./L. of extracellular fluid. A change in the concentration of an electrolyte can be produced either by a change in total quantity of the electrolyte or in the total volume of water in extracellular fluid. For example, one could develop a sodium deficit either because of decreased intake or increased loss of sodium, or because of excessive intake or decreased loss of water. Similarly, one could develop an excess of sodium in extracellular fluid either because of increased intake or decreased loss of sodium, or because of decreased intake or increased loss of water.

These mechanisms apply not only to changes in sodium concentration but also to all the other extracellular electrolytes.

SODIUM

Sodium is the most abundant cation of extracellular fluid and the second most important cation of cellular fluid. Chemically, sodium is a metallic element, and its chemical symbol, Na, stems from the Latin word *natrium*, meaning sodium. In pure form, the element is extremely unstable since it readily combines with oxygen either in air or in water. In nature and in body fluids, it exists only in combination with various anions, usually chloride; the compound sodium chloride is more commonly called table salt.

Sodium affects many vital functions of the human body. It is largely responsible for the osmotic pressure of extracellular fluid; inside cells, sodium is a factor in numerous vital chemical reactions. The kidneys regulate body water and electrolytes, based in part on sodium concentration in the extracellular fluid. Therefore, when sodium concentration rises, the kidneys retain water in an effort to maintain the normal composition of the extracellular fluid. When the amount of water increases, the kidneys retain sodium. Other functions of the element are as follows: probably through some type of chemical-electrical action, sodium stimulates reactions within nerve and muscle tissues; as a component of sodium bicarbonate, it is highly important in maintaining the delicate balance between the acids and alkalies of the body fluid.

Since sodium plays such a vital role, it is not surprising that the body possesses a highly efficient mechanism for regulating the electrolyte so that its normal concentration of 142 mEq./L. of extracellular fluid can be maintained. During periods of decreased intake or increased loss, the mechanism acts to conserve sodium. Important in sodium conservation is the hormone aldosterone, secreted by the adrenal cortex, which promotes potassium loss and sodium retention via a complex and little understood feedback mechanism involving the afferent arterioles, the juxtaglomerular apparatus, and the macula densa of the distal tubule. When fluid volume deficit occurs, a resultant decrease in glomerular filtration aids in sodium conservation simply because there is less sodium in the tubular urine to be exchanged for potassium and hydrogen in the peritubular capillaries of the distal tubules. Body sodium conservation is usually so effective that patients being maintained on a low sodium diet for control of certain diseases, such as essential hypertension, are seldom in danger of developing sodium deficit as a result of the decreased intake.

When sodium intake increases, the regulating mechanism acts to rid the body of excesses, and there is a prompt increase both in sodium excretion and in the glomerular filtration rate. For many years, it was believed that the increased filtration of sodium through the glomeruli was responsible for the increased urinary excretion of the ion. Recent studies, however, indicate that the increase in sodium excretion is related to decreased reabsorption of sodium from the proximal tubules of the kidneys. A similar sodium loss occurs when salt-retaining hormones, such as aldosterone, are administered over a prolonged period to normal human subjects. It is believed that tubular excretion of sodium is controlled by a third factor, perhaps a hormone, whose chemi-

cal structure and site of origin are unknown. This mysterious third factor may explain why patients with primary hyperaldosteronism do not develop marked edema.

Although the sodium regulating mechanism is quite effective, an *acute* decrease or increase in the sodium level of extracellular fluid produces severe reactions.

Sodium Deficit of Extracellular Fluid

Sodium deficit of extracellular fluid occurs when the concentration of sodium in extracellular fluid falls below normal. Other names for this imbalance are *electrolyte concentration deficit, low sodium syndrome, hypotonic dehydration,* and *hyponatremia.*

Sodium deficit can result either from losses of sodium without corresponding water loss—as with overzealous administration of diuretics, especially thiazide diuretics or furosemide, or in mucoviscidosis (pancreatic fibrosis), in which excessive sodium is lost by way of sweat. Sodium deficit also results from gains of water in excess of sodium—as when one perspires profusely and replaces the fluid lost with plain water, or in persons who are compulsive drinkers of water. Inappropriate secretion of ADH (SIADH) caused by brain tumor, brain injury, or certain lung tumors causes excessive conservation of water and produces this imbalance. Other clinical causes include chronic lung disease, intracranial disease, myxedema (adult hypothyroidism), and hypodermoclysis of dextrose in plain water (the fluid pools under the skin and draws sodium into it). Sodium deficit may develop when a severely burned patient—or one who is undergoing gastric or intestinal suction—is permitted to drink plain water in large amounts. In addition, the use of repeated tap water enemas causes sodium deficit, as does parenteral administration of electrolyte-free solutions. Inhalation of fresh water, as occurs in fresh water drowning, also produces this imbalance.

The clinical findings in sodium deficit are virtually identical with those of so-called heat prostration, often the result of sodium deficit in unacclimatized persons. (Because of the body's sodium conservation mechanism, the properly acclimatized individual is remarkably resistant to heat stress disease caused by sodium loss.) The patient first suffers apprehension or anxiety, followed by a bizarre, undefinable feeling of impending doom. He is weak, confused, and perhaps even stuporous, and may suffer abdominal cramps or muscle twitching, diarrhea, and, in severe deficit, convulsions. In an effort to counterbalance the deficit, the adrenal glands secrete increased amounts of aldosterone, which stimulate the kidneys to conserve water, sodium, and chloride. This action results in depressed urinary output (oliguria) or complete absence of urinary output (anuria). If the deficit is severe, there is vasomotor collapse, with the following symptoms: hypotension; rapid, thready pulse; cold, clammy skin; and cyanosis. An interesting finding that may be observed is fingerprinting over the sternum, consisting of a visible fingerprint apparent after pressure is applied with a finger or thumb on the skin overlying the sternum. Fingerprinting is due to increased plasticity of the tissues, which results from the transfer of water from the abnormally dilute extracellular fluid into the cells. As a result of this osmotic transfer of water, an abnormally large portion of the body fluid lies within the confines of the cells, and the fluid volume of the extracellular fluid—both plasma and interstitial fluid—is decreased. Consequently, tissues become more plastic than normal and tend to retain any shape attained by pressure deformation.

Laboratory findings are helpful in diagnosis of sodium deficit, as the plasma sodium is below 137 mEq./L.—it may be as low as 110, 100, or even 90— and plasma chloride is below 98 mEq./L. The specific gravity of the urine is below 1.010.*

There are related problems: heat exhaustion in unacclimatized persons may develop because of sodium deficit. One takes a long walk on a hot day, sweats profusely, and drinks plain water. Having replaced lost water, sodium, and chloride with plain water only, the individual, therefore, develops sodium deficit. The low-sodium syndrome (another term for sodium deficit) can occur when diuresis is excessive. (One patient we know of took four times the dose of a potent diuretic, appeared in the hospital emergency room with a plasma sodium of 90 mEq./L., and could not be saved even by energetic treatment.)

The goal of therapy in sodium deficit of the extracellular fluid is to restore the sodium concentration to normal as quickly as possible without producing a fluid volume excess. If the fluid volume is normal or excessive, a 3 per cent or 5 per cent solution of sodium chloride is administered. This type of solution is hypertonic, so it will provide the needed sodium in a minimal amount of water. If the extracellular fluid volume is below normal, an isotonic solution of sodium chloride may be administered (Fig. 10-1).

CASE HISTORIES The day following the removal of her gallbladder, a 35-year-old woman, L.B., complained repeatedly of gas and abdominal discomfort. A gastric tube was inserted through the nose and suction drainage started. Since the woman complained of thirst, she was given ice chips to suck. It seemed to the student nurse that she was consuming an inordinate quantity of these. During the following two days, a little more than 2 L. of fluid were removed from her stomach, replaced only by the plain water of ice chips. On the morning of the third day, the woman complained of being "nervous" and of having abdominal cramps, considerably more painful than the discomfort she had complained of on the first postoperative day. Examination of the intake-output records showed that the patient had passed only some 400 ml. of urine during the previous 24 hours. Physical examination revealed an apprehensive, jittery patient with definite fingerprinting over the sternum. The serum sodium was determined to be 128 mEq./L., and the chloride 86 mEq./L. Other electrolytes were within limits of normal, except for the potassium, which bordered on a deficit. A catheterized specimen of urine revealed a specific gravity of 1.002, with no other abnormal findings.

Commentary All extracellular electrolytes were being removed via the gastric tube with no replacement since only plain water was consumed. Since sodium is the chief cation of the ECF, and since the body tolerates relatively slight variations in sodium, the clinical syndrome that developed was that of sodium deficit. This sensitivity of the body to relatively modest deficits or excesses of sodium has been referred to as *the primacy of sodium.* (The maximal hydrogen tolerated by the body is ten times the minimum, as is also the case with potassium. But the maximal sodium that the body can tolerate is only about twice the minimum.)

Apprehensiveness and the more severe and even fatal neurologic symptoms of severe sodium deficit appear due to the absorption of water by the cerebrospinal fluid from the relatively hypotonic ECF by

---

* In SIADH, the urine specific gravity does not reflect the extracellular sodium deficit and may well be in excess of 1.010. In fact, this elevated specific gravity of the urine is a diagnostic hallmark of SIADH.

PRECEDING EVENTS
- Loss of sodium in excess of water
- Gain of water in excess of sodium

CLINICAL OBSERVATIONS
- Vary greatly but often include:
  - Apprehension
  - Abdominal cramps
  - Diarrhea
  - Convulsions

LABORATORY FINDINGS
- Plasma sodium below 137 mEq./L.
- Specific gravity of urine below 1.010

RELATED PROBLEMS
- Heat exhaustion in unacclimatized persons may result in sodium deficit
- Sodium deficit may occur with excessive drug diuresis

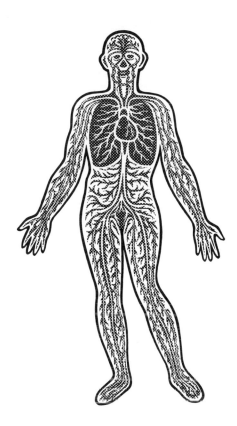

Figure 10-1. Sodium deficit.

osmosis. Recall that a lag exists in the response of the cerebrospinal fluid to changes in the ECF. This lag is the reason why abnormalities of the ECF should be corrected slowly, to allow the cerebrospinal fluid time to "catch up."

On a rainy morning, a 30-year-old housewife was driving down a slippery highway to a nearby shopping center. Her car skidded off the road as she rounded a curve and careened into a tree. Passersby, observing the mishap called an ambulance. The ambulance log indicated that the woman, C.T., was freed from the wreckage and taken to a nearby hospital at 9:30 A.M. In the emergency room of the hospital, the patient was found to be conscious, rational, and oriented as to time, place, and person. She was found to have sustained fractures of her mandible, maxilla, and left zygomatic arch. She also had extensive facial contusions. Blood was drawn for baseline electrolyte values, and a urine sample was obtained. She was prepared for operation and, under general anesthesia, underwent surgical procedures in which her fractures were aligned and immobilized. Initial electro-

lyte values were found to be normal, and urinalysis revealed no abnormalities. Intake-output measurements were started because of the tendency of patients with head injuries to develop body fluid disturbances. The following morning, the patient appeared to be in good spirits. Serum electrolytes revealed a sodium of 130 mEq./L. and a chloride of 90 mEq./L. Urine specific gravity was 1.010. The next morning, after a restless night, the patient's blood and urine were again tested. On ward rounds, the patient impressed her physician as apprehensive and jittery. The serum sodium was found to be 114 mEq./L. and the chloride 79 mEq./L. Specific gravity of urine was 1.016. A repeat sodium was 115 mEq./L. and chloride 80 mEq./L. Intake-output records indicated that the patient was not excreting water normally; moreover, she weighed 4 pounds more than on admission. The pronounced depression of the serum sodium and chloride plus the unduly high specific gravity of the urine indicated that the patient was suffering from sodium deficit (hyponatremia) caused by inappropriate secretion of ADH (syndrome of inappropriate secretion of ADH, or SIADH) caused by the trauma to the skull and its contents. On the basis of this diagnosis, fluids were greatly restricted, and small quantities of a 5 per cent solution of sodium chloride in water were slowly administered.

Commentary   Note that this patient's urinary specific gravity was 1.016. Hyponatremia not caused by SIADH is characterized by a dilute urine with a specific gravity of 1.001 to 1.003. The excessively secreted ADH, while conserving water inappropriately, also appears to inhibit secretion of aldosterone, the chief sodium-conserving hormone. This probably explains the relatively high output of sodium in the urine, despite the severe deficit of sodium in the ECF. SIADH not only occurs in various forms of trauma to the central nervous system but it also has been reported to occur with several malignant tumors, nontraumatic disorders of the central nervous system, pulmonary disease, the postoperative state, and with most anesthetics and a wide variety of drugs. It has been seen in some patients in whom no cause could be discovered.

Sodium Excess of Extracellular Fluid

Sodium excess of extracellular fluid, sometimes called *hypernatremia, salt excess, oversalting,* or *hypertonic dehydration,* is one of the most dangerous of all body fluid disturbances. It occurs when the sodium concentration of extracellular fluid rises above the normal level. The imbalance, which may be acute or chronic, results from decreased intake or increased output of water or from increased intake or decreased output of sodium.

Acute sodium excess may follow excessive administration of concentrated oral electrolyte mixtures. A tragic example of this occurred when salt instead of sugar was mistakenly used in preparing infant formulas. The infants fed the mixture developed sodium excess so severe that even the most vigorous therapy failed to save several of the babies. The imbalance also may occur in any condition in which more water is lost than electrolytes, as in tracheobronchitis—in which excessive water losses occur through the lungs as a result of fever and deep, rapid breathing, leaving an abnormally high concentration of sodium in the ECF—or in profuse watery diarrhea when treatment has been inadequate. Some sodium is lost in diarrheal stools, but the concentration of the remaining sodium is so high as to produce hypernatremia, emphasizing the fact that it is the *concen-*

tration of sodium in mEq./L.—not the total quantity of sodium in the body—that is all important. Sodium excess can also develop because of a hypothalamic tumor. In this condition, ADH is no longer produced, and the individual loses excessive water (having lost the water-conserving action of ADH), leaving an excessive sodium concentration. Unconscious patients may develop sodium excess simply because they cannot drink water. The individual who has inhaled ocean water frequently develops a sodium excess, which must be corrected if the patient is to recover; indeed, sodium excess is often the actual cause of death in salt water drowning. Infants are particularly prone to develop acute sodium excess, and the mortality rate is quite high—about 50 per cent in hospital-treated infants with diarrhea and sodium excess.

Clinical findings in sodium excess include dry, sticky mucous membranes, flushed skin, intense thirst, and rough, dry tongue. Body tissues are firm and rubbery because water from the cellular fluid, following the law of osmosis, flows into the more concentrated extracellular fluid. Oliguria or anuria is present, and the patient may have fever. He appears agitated and restless, may develop mania or convulsions, and his reflexes are decreased.

Laboratory findings are helpful in diagnosis, since the plasma sodium is usually above 147 mEq./L. —but may range far higher—plasma chloride is above 106 mEq./L., and the specific gravity of urine is above 1.030.

Long-term or chronic ingestion of large amounts of sodium, as when one salts his food excessively or eats extremely salty foods, also can cause sodium excess and may lead to hypertension. Although the daily requirement for sodium is probably below 100 mg. in acclimatized persons, most individuals ingest from 3000 to 5000 mg. daily, and inhabitants in certain areas of Japan have an average daily intake in excess of 20,000 mg. Hereditary factors largely determine whether this type of sodium excess will cause hypertension in a given individual, but researchers have induced uninherited but life-long hypertension in experimental animals by feeding them highly salted foods. Fairly recently, researchers questioned a group of Americans about normal use of salt and learned that only 1 per cent of those who never salted their food at the table suffered from hypertension, as compared to 8 per cent of those who salted to taste, and 10 per cent of those who salted before tasting.

Another study revealed that a large segment of the population in areas of Japan where the usual diet is extremely salty suffers from hypertension.

The goal of therapy in sodium excess is to reduce the sodium concentration of the extracellular fluid before it reaches a critical level. Treatment involves administration of a Butler-type solution, which is only one third to one half as concentrated as plasma and which provides free water for formation of urine. Hypertension can often be controlled by use of a sodium-restricted diet (Fig. 10-2).

CASE HISTORIES   Six-year-old S.W. was admitted to the hospital because of extreme agitation and inability to sleep. The mother asserted that the little girl had "not slept a wink" for the past 48 hours. The history revealed that for the past six days, the child had been suffering from a mild, nonbloody diarrhea. Her mother had been treating her with a home remedy consisting of a solution of salt and soda in water. She had added a tablespoon of salt and a tablespoon of baking soda to each pint of water and had forced the child to drink about a pint of this mixture every day. On physical examination, the child was found to have dry, sticky mucous membranes and a rough, dry tongue. Her skin was flushed, and she complained of thirst. Her tissues had a firm, rubbery feel to them. The mother stated that the child had not urinated for the past 24 hours. The plasma sodium was 165 mEq./L. and the chloride 117 mEq./L. The potassium was 3 mEq./L. The child could not urinate.

Commentary   This patient represents a simple example of sodium excess of the ECF caused by administration of an excessive quantity of sodium, both as NaCl and $NaHCO_3$. It demonstrates that the body does not tolerate sodium excess well. Discontinuance of the salt and soda mixture and oral administration of water could probably remedy the imbalance.

Four-year-old J.M. was admitted to the emergency room of the hospital, obviously extremely ill. His mother stated that he had had profuse watery diarrhea for the past week. He had been given sips of

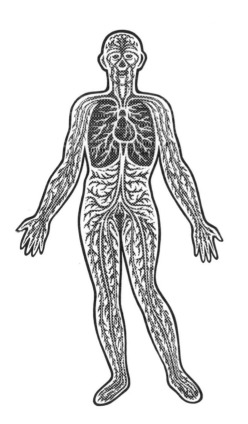

PRECEDING EVENTS
- Intake of sodium in excess of water
- Loss of water in excess of sodium

CLINICAL OBSERVATIONS
- Agitation, which may progress to mania or convulsions
- Dry, sticky mucous membranes
- Oliguria
- Firm, rubbery tissue turgor

LABORATORY FINDINGS
- Plasma sodium above 147 mEq./L.
- Specific gravity of urine above 1.030

RELATED PROBLEMS
- Drowning in ocean water
- Often occurs on fifth or sixth day after onset of diarrhea

Figure 10-2.   Sodium excess.

water and a soft drink but had vomited part of this. The child appeared surprisingly alert. His cheeks were flushed, mucous membranes dry and sticky, and his tongue rough. His subcutaneous tissues felt firm and rubbery. While being examined, he had a watery stool not containing blood. His serum electrolytes were sodium 180 mEq./L., chloride 137 mEq./L., bicarbonate 16 mEq./L., potassium 3.8 mEq./L., and pCO_2 33 mm. Hg. A urine specimen could not be obtained.

Commentary   This patient demonstrates that what is important in concentration disturbances of ECF is not the total quantity of an electrolyte in the body but its concentration in units per liter. This child had a life-threatening excess concentration of sodium, yet his total body sodium was partially depleted since some sodium had passed out in the watery stools. In treatment of such a patient, therefore, it is important to give a hypotonic solution of water and electrolytes plus dextrose so as to resupply not only the badly depleted water but also the sodium. Obviously, close observation of the body electrolytes is essential as the deficits are repaired.

POTASSIUM

Potassium, a soft, silver-white metal that exists outside the test tube only in combination with other elements, is the chief cation of cellular fluid. Its chemical symbol, *K*, is derived from the German word *kalium*. Potassium is indispensable in the human body, as it is necessary for the intricate chemical reactions needed for transformation of carbohydrate into energy and for reassembling amino acids into proteins. The ion helps maintain the normal water and electrolyte content of cellular fluid, and it is also needed for transmission of nervous impulses within the heart. Skeletal muscles and the muscles of the heart, intestines, and lungs could not function normally without potassium.

Ironically, although one cannot live without potassium, the human body contains enough of the electrolyte to kill dozens of people were it injected quickly into them. The extracellular fluid normally contains 5 mEq./L., or about 70 mEq.; the cellular fluid contains a total of 4,000 mEq. Secretions and excretions, especially sweat, saliva, gastric juice, and feces, are rich in potassium. The potassium content of urine varies with the intake but it amounts to at least

40 to 50 mEq. daily. In the kidneys, along with water and other electrolytes and small molecules, potassium is completely filtered at the glomerulus and is then completely reabsorbed in the proximal convoluted tubules. Excretion occurs only in the distal convoluted tubules, and then in exchange for sodium.

Potassium Deficit of Extracellular Fluid

While the human body has an efficient mechanism for conserving sodium, it has no such mechanism for conserving potassium. Even in times of great need, the kidneys continue to pour out 40 to 50 mEq. of potassium daily in the urine, and, with such continuing losses, potassium deficit or *hypokalemia* can develop quickly when the patient's intake is inadequate, as in starvation. This imbalance occurs frequently, not only as a result of prolonged inadequate intake of potassium, but also as a result of excessive losses of potassium-rich secretions or excretions, as occurs in prolonged diarrhea.

Probably the leading cause of potassium deficit is administration of powerful diuretics, particularly the thiazides or furosemide, without adequate potassium supplementation. Surgical operations often cause losses of potassium-rich fluids, especially if the procedure involves the digestive tract. The imbalance also is often associated with gastrointestinal suction, diseases involving the intestinal tract, familial periodic paralysis, pyelonephritis, thyroid storm, aldosterone-secreting tumor of the adrenal cortex, crushing injuries, broken bones, extensive bruising, and wound healing. Even emotional or physical stress can cause the imbalance. Excessive sweating, fever, and high environmental temperatures are further causes. Indeed, potassium loss plays a major role in the development of heat stress disease, which affects people of all ages who are subjected to high environmental temperatures, especially if they are exercising. Factory workers, athletes, and others who are exposed to high environmental temperatures often use salt tablets to replace the sodium lost in sweat, but, since the body conserves sodium and continues to lose potassium, potassium supplementation, at least as important as sodium supplementation, is often neglected.

Potassium deficit is frequently associated with metabolic alkalosis, as discussed later in this chapter.

The clinical findings in potassium deficit can be remembered easily if one recalls that potassium is essential for the normal functioning of muscle cells; thus symptoms of potassium deficit are caused largely by muscle weakness. Early, symptoms are nonspecific, as the patient has malaise, or is simply not feeling well. In some patients, potassium deficit damages renal tubules, and thus impairs the concentrating ability of the kidney, the result of which is polyuria and thirst. Later, the skeletal muscles become weak, and the reflexes are decreased or absent, and eventually muscle weakness leads to flabbiness, with the patient lying flat, like a cadaver. Cardiac disturbances accompanying potassium deficit may include atrial and ventricular arrhythmia, diminution of the intensity of heart sounds, weak pulse, falling blood pressure, and heart block. Degeneration of the myocardium with loss of cellular striations may follow prolonged potassium deficit, and the intestinal muscles, too, are affected. The patient suffers anorexia, vomiting, gaseous intestinal distention, and paralytic ileus. Weakness of the respiratory muscles produces shallow respiration, and death in potassium deficit apparently results from apnea and respiratory arrest rather than from cardiac standstill.

Laboratory findings helpful in diagnosis include repeated serum potassium determinations of below 4 mEq./L. (a single determination can be seriously misleading). The plasma chloride is often below 98 mEq./L., and plasma bicarbonate is above 29 mEq./L. Potassium deficit also induces specific EKG findings, including low, flattened T wave, depressed S-T segment, and prominent U wave.

There is a pertinent note: after the potassium of the blood coursing through the glomeruli of the kidneys is filtered, all of the potassium (or almost all) is reabsorbed into the peritubular arterioles. Then, in the distal convoluted tubules, it is exchanged for the sodium of the tubular urine, under the influence of aldosterone. Recall, there are 4,000 mEq. of potassium in the cellular fluid and 70 mEq. in the extracellular fluid; yet, it is the extracellular potassium that is all-important in causing symptoms and findings. Metabolic alkalosis is frequently associated with potassium deficit. The reasons for this are complex, and even leading authorities are not in full agreement on just what these reasons are. *Bear in mind: in considering potassium deficit, one of the most frequent of all body fluid disturbances, that the body conserves potassium poorly, in striking contrast to its parsimonious hoarding of sodium.*

Fortunately, potassium deficit is not difficult to correct. Abnormal potassium losses may be counteracted by oral administration of a potassium salt or by providing a high potassium diet. A frank potassium deficit is best treated by oral administration of potassium chloride or other potassium salts or by parenteral infusion of a potassium-containing solution. A balanced, or Butler-type, solution is often used (Fig. 10-3).

CASE HISTORIES   J.K., a 55-year-old businessman, was found to have an elevated blood pressure on his first annual physical examination, with his reading 190/120. A thorough workup ruled out an obvious cause for his hypertension, and a diagnosis of essential hypertension was made. He was given a thiazide diuretic, and his sodium intake was restricted to about 1,000 mg./day. His pressure responded well and was maintained at about 140/88. He checked with his internist every two months. Five months after starting therapy, he began to notice that he was short of breath on climbing stairs, he was exceedingly fatigued, he was constipated yet troubled with gas, and he felt that his heart was beating irregularly. On reporting the symptoms to his physician, blood was drawn for electrolyte studies. His sodium was 142 mEq./L., potassium 2.6 mEq./L., bicarbonate 36 mEq./L., and serum pH 7.6. A pCO_2 on arterial blood was 55 mm. Hg. The electrocardiogram showed low, broad T waves with a double summit caused by superimposition of the U wave on the T wave. The P-R interval was prolonged. Treatment of the hypokalemia consisted of a potassium supplement, 100 mEq./day, plus the addition of generous quantities of orange juice and bananas to the diet. In five days, the sodium was 142 mEq./L., potassium 4.5 mEq./L., bicarbonate 24 mEq./L., serum pH 7.4, and the pCO_2 40 mm. Hg. The patient was advised to discontinue the potassium supplement and instead to use a KCl salt substitute in palatable quantities on his food.

Commentary   Although the electrocardiogram is useful in making a diagnosis of potassium deficit, it may be impossible to determine the exact degree of hypopotassemia from the tracing. Potassium deficit and alkalosis, both nonrespiratory (bicarbonate excess) and respiratory (carbonic acid deficit), are closely interrelated. Either tends to cause the other. Probably the chief reason is the twin facts that potassium and hydrogen are exchanged for sodium in the distal convoluted tubule of the nephron and, similarly, across the cell membrane. Suppose potassium

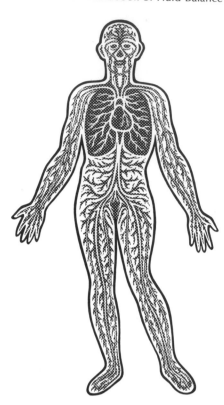

PRECEDING EVENTS

- Prolonged inadequate intake
- Excessive losses from body
- Hyperaldosteronism
- Drug therapy
- Prolonged heat stress

CLINICAL OBSERVATIONS

- Symptoms stem from muscle weakness
- Cause of death: apnea

LABORATORY FINDINGS

- Repeated plasma potassium below 4 mEq./L.
- Specific EKG findings: low voltage, flattening of T waves, depression of ST segment

RELATED PROBLEMS

- Metabolic alkalosis frequently associated

Figure 10-3.   Potassium deficit.

deficit of the ECF exists. Then hydrogen will preponderantly exchange for sodium in the distal convoluted tubules and across the cell membrane. A relative deficit of hydrogen will develop in the ECF, resulting in alkalosis. On the other hand, suppose that alkalosis exists. Then there will be a dearth of hydrogen in the ECF, and potassium will preponderantly exchange for sodium in the two locations. Potassium deficit will develop.

_____

M.J., 23-years old, told her physician of periodic attacks of complete paralysis, usually brought on by rest after exercise, exposure to cold, overeating in the evening, or on waking. The attacks were sometimes preceded by thirst, sweating, or muscular cramps. Not all attacks proceeded to complete paralysis; some consisted only of great weakness. Family history revealed similar attacks in her mother's family. On physical examination during an attack, no sensory changes were found, but the deep reflexes were lost and electrical excitability of muscle was absent. Examination was performed during a prolonged attack (attacks lasted from a few minutes to several

days). Two serum potassium readings were 2.6 mEq./L. and 2.7 mEq./L.

Commentary   This unusual form of potassium deficit of ECF appears to be caused by passage of extracellular potassium into the body cells. It remains one of the many diseases of mystery. Strangely enough, some patients have similar attacks with *hyper-* rather than *hypo*kalemia. Immediate ingestion of a potassium salt appears to help in hypokalemic periodic paralysis.

Potassium Excess of Extracellular Fluid

Because the kidneys so efficiently rid the body of potassium, potassium excess or *hyperkalemia* does not develop as often as potassium deficit. However, this does not mean that excesses are any less dangerous than deficits; indeed, they can be extremely hazardous. In most cases, potassium excess is caused by leakage of the electrolyte from the body cells, and so following a severe burn or crushing injury, the extracellular fluid may be flooded with potassium from the damaged cells. If the kidneys are not functioning properly, the imbalance can result from excessive oral ingestion of potassium. Intentional excessive oral ingestion, as in a suicide attempt, is another cause. The imbalance also may result from overzealous parenteral administration of potassium-containing solutions. Mercuric bichloride poisoning, which damages the kidneys, can lead to potassium excess, since the imbalance is inevitable following renal failure (end-stage renal disease) and may be the cause of death. Severe excesses also result from cellular hypoxia, uremia, adrenal insufficiency—as in Addison's disease, in which aldosterone is lacking—and administration of spironolactone, which opposes aldosterone (recall that aldosterone promotes excretion of potassium). Metabolic acidosis may be associated with potassium excess, as discussed later in this chapter.

The clinical findings in potassium excess include irritability, nausea, diarrhea—a result, not a cause, of the imbalance—and intestinal colic. If the condition becomes severe, there is weakness and flaccid paralysis, perhaps difficulty in phonation and respiration, and there is oliguria, which may progress to anuria. Because transmission of stimuli through the heart muscle is slowed or prevented, intraventricular conduction disturbance occurs, with or without atrioventricular dissociation, and finally, ventricular fibrillation and cardiac arrest develop. Death in potassium excess results from poisoning of the heart muscle.

A repeated plasma potassium above 5.6 mEq./L. indicates potassium excess, and a test for renal function usually will show renal impairment. The imbalance also presents specific EKG findings: early, T waves are peaked and elevated; later, P waves disappear; finally, there are biphasic deflections resulting from fusion of the QRS complex, RS-T segment, and the T wave.

When the kidneys are functional, an uncomplicated potassium excess can be corrected simply by avoiding additional intake of the electrolyte, either orally or parenterally. Should kidney function be drastically impaired, as in anuria, a diet that supplies fat and carbohydrates but not protein or potassium should be administered, or carbonic anhydrase inhibitors, insulin and dextrose, or ion exchange resins can be used. In some cases, hemodialysis or peritoneal dialysis may be necessary (Fig. 10-4).

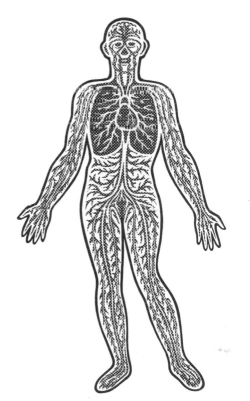

PRECEDING EVENTS
- Kidney failure
- Excessive ingestion of potassium
- Excessive parenteral administration of potassium
- Leakage of potassium from cells
- Lack of aldosterone because of drug antagonism or disease

CLINICAL OBSERVATIONS
- Oliguria progressing to anuria
- Intestinal colic
- Diarrhea
- Cardiac muscle failure

LABORATORY FINDINGS
- Repeated plasma potassium above 5.6 mEq./L.
- Specific EKG findings

RELATED PROBLEMS
- Follows kidney failure
- Metabolic acidosis frequently associated

Figure 10-4. Potassium excess.

CASE HISTORIES P.T. was admitted to the hospital with a history of chronic renal disease resulting from acute glomerulonephritis. Recently, the symptoms had become more severe, with dyspnea, pallor, weakness, and fatigue from the slightest exertion. The physical examination revealed hypertension in the supine position, hypotension when upright. There was generalized muscle weakness, a pericardial friction rub, and mild flank tenderness on both sides. The patient vomited during the examination. Slight edema of the ankles was detected. Laboratory findings included serum creatinine 4 mg./100 ml. (normal, 0.6–0.7), sodium 130 mEq./L., potassium 7 mEq./L., bicarbonate 16 mEq./L., pCO$_2$ 32 mm. Hg, Delta 16 mEq./L., calcium 7 mg./100 ml. (3.5 mEq./L.), phosphate 8 mg./100 ml. (4.8 mEq./L.). Proteinuria was calculated at 15 Gm./day; no red blood cells were seen, and finely and coarsely granular tubular cell and hyaline casts were present in moderate numbers in the urinary sediment.

Commentary This is presented as a frequent cause of potassium excess of the ECF, although other findings of end-stage renal disease are present. Note the elevated creatinine, the depressed sodium, the evidence of bicarbonate deficit (metabolic acidosis), with a Delta of 16. This indicates the acidosis is due to accumulation of organic acids titrating bicarbonate. One would expect the calcium to be depressed and the phosphate to be elevated in end-stage renal disease, and this is the case. The elevation of the potassium is only moderate. It would be more severe with oliguria and less severe—even normal or subnormal—with copious urine flow. Note the urine findings, indicating chronic nephritis. The loss of protein accounts for the edema observed. (For details concerning the values for calcium and phosphorus, refer to the section on calcium. For details on the acid-base disturbance, refer to the section on acid-base disturbances.)

E.H., a 44-year-old business executive, was admitted to the hospital with a history of blood pressure averaging about 190/120, which had failed to respond to chlorthalidone, 50 mg. b.i.d., plus propranolol, 40 mg./day. He had been on a sodium-restricted diet, estimated at 1000 mg. (43 mEq.) daily and had been using a salt substitute consisting largely of KCl in quantities estimated at 2925 mg. (75 mEq.) daily. He brought the salt substitute with him to the hospital and, unknown to the nurses, began using it on his food. The physician ordered a new vasodilator plus a potassium-sparing diuretic for the patient. Inadvertently, 40 mEq. of supplemental potassium was administered daily to E.H. On the fourth hospital day, the patient began complaining of tingling about the mouth and in the fingers and toes. He stated he felt extremely weak. Upon examination, his muscles proved to be hyperirritable and his heart rate irregular. A battery of electrolyte determinations revealed serum potassium 8 mEq./L., bicarbonate 16 mEq./L., and pCO$_2$ 32 mm. Hg. Other serum electrolytes were normal; urine pH was 5, but otherwise the specimen was normal. An electrocardiogram revealed no P waves. The physician made a firm diagnosis of potassium excess and discontinued the salt substitute and the potassium supplement. The potassium dropped to normal within four days, and all symptoms disappeared.

Commentary Totaling the patient's dietary intake of potassium (about 75 mEq.), that from the salt substitute (about 75 mEq.), and that from the potassium supplement (40 mEq.), it was obvious that he had been ingesting about 190 mEq. of potassium daily. An individual with normal kidneys can tolerate about 135 mEq. without developing potassium excess. Both the serum potassium and the electrocardiogram indicated potassium excess. Potassium excess is usually associated with acidosis (bicarbonate deficit), and this was the case in this instance, with the bicarbonate and the pCO$_2$ both depressed. Depression of the pCO$_2$ was of such extent as to indicate that it was compensatory in nature. (See section on acid-base disturbances for details.) The error above cited has been reported from numerous institutions.

CALCIUM

The cation calcium (Ca) is the most abundant electrolyte in the body; about 99 per cent is concentrated in bones and teeth, the remainder throughout the plasma and body cells. The normal concentration of calcium in the extracellular fluid is 5 mEq./L. Calcium is closely associated with phosphorus; together, they make bones and teeth rigid, strong, and durable. The plasma levels of calcium and phosphorus are regulated by the parathyroid glands, and normally, an increase or decrease in the serum phosphate concentration is associated with the opposite decrease or increase in the plasma calcium level, and vice versa. Vitamin D promotes intestinal absorption of calcium and increases kidney excretion of phosphate.

The element is also a necessary ingredient of cell cement, which holds the body cells together, and, in addition, it determines the strength and thickness of cell membranes. Calcium exerts a sedative effect on nerve cells, and, thus, is important in maintaining normal transmission of nerve impulses. The electrolyte also aids in the transfer of energy and in the absorption and utilization of vitamin B_{12}. It activates enzymes that stimulate many essential chemical reactions in the body and plays a role in blood coagulation. Since only the ionized calcium is physiologically active, calcium bound to protein, which depends on the concentration of the plasma protein, is inactive. Usually from 50 to 75 per cent of the serum calcium is ionized and most of the rest is bound to serum albumin; when the total protein of the blood falls, more of the calcium becomes bound.

The normal adult needs about 1 Gm. of calcium daily, and pregnant or lactating women require additional amounts. Vitamin D and protein are required for absorption and utilization of calcium.

Calcium Deficit of Extracellular Fluid

Calcium deficit of extracellular fluid, also called hypocalcemia, can result from abnormalities in body metabolism, from inadequate dietary intake of calcium, or from excessive losses of calcium in diarrheal stools or wound exudate. The imbalance is often associated with sprue, acute pancreatitis, hypoparathyroidism, surgical removal of the parathyroids, massive subcutaneous infections, burns, and generalized peritonitis. Excessive infusion of citrated blood, as in an exchange transfusion in an infant, may bring about calcium deficit, and the imbalance can also result from rapid correction or overcorrection of acidosis, wherein calcium ionization is increased. When the plasma pH returns to normal, or above normal, calcium ionization decreases, and unless adequate calcium is provided, the decreased ionization may cause hypocalcemia. Magnesium excess also tends to cause calcium deficit, possibly because magnesium plays a role in parathyroid function. Renal failure also looms large as a cause of calcium deficit for this reason: phosphorus is reciprocal with calcium; in early renal failure, the kidneys

aren't able to dispose of phosphorus normally. Hence, the phosphorus rises and the calcium falls. Subsequently, added secretion of parathormone stimulates the calcium to rise. But because of kidney malfunction, the body is unable to utilize this calcium normally. Finally, in the late stages of renal failure, the calcium falls again in a final decline.

The clinical findings in calcium deficit are as follows: tingling of the ends of the fingers and of the circumoral region; muscle cramps, affecting both abdominal and skeletal muscles; carpopedal spasms; tetany; and convulsions. If calcium deficit is prolonged, calcium will be drawn from the bones to replenish the extracellular fluid, after which the bones become porous and break at the slightest provocation.

Laboratory findings helpful in diagnosis include a plasma calcium determination below 4.5 mEq./L., or below 10 mg./100 ml. However, plasma calcium determinations can be misleading since only the ionized calcium is physiologically active. The ionized calcium can be measured by determining calcium levels before and after treatment with dextran gel or by ultrafiltration. In the simple and sometimes useful urinary Sulkowitch test, Sulkowitch reagent is added to urine and urinary calcium is precipitated as calcium oxalate. If no precipitate forms, hypocalcemia is present, whereas a fine white precipitate indicates normal plasma calcium, and a dense precipitate indicates calcium excess. The Sulkowitch test results do not correlate well with urinary calcium excretion, but the test is valuable in tetany, in hyperparathyroidism, and for regulation of vitamin D intake in a patient with hypoparathyroidism. And finally, a specific abnormal EKG finding in calcium deficit is a prolonged Q-T interval.

An interesting manifestation of prolonged calcium deficit is a condition called osteomalacia. In this condition, bones lose their calcium, phosphorus, and other electrolytes, becoming soft and pliable, and the patient actually shrinks in height. In the first recorded case of osteomalacia, the physician reported that his patient had shrunk some 17 inches. Fortunately, osteomalacia is rare, yet it is seen during famines and among pregnant and lactating women in countries where calcium intake is grossly inadequate.

A not so rare manifestation of calcium deficit is osteoporosis, which has a high incidence among women over 45 and men over 55; 25 per cent of women and 20 per cent of men over the age of 70 have osteoporosis. In this condition, the bones maintain their chemical composition but become thinner, lighter, and more porous. The ailment reveals itself in back pains, decreased height, and frequent and painful fractures of the vertebrae, ribs, and the bones of the arms, legs, hands, and feet.

Problems related to calcium deficit include the elevated phosphate in end-stage renal disease. In health, the kidneys convert a nonusable form of vitamin D to one that the body can use. But in serious renal disease, this conversion does not take place: calcium is not utilized and may precipitate out in tissues as harmful concretions. Recently, a usable form of vitamin D that can be administered to patients with end-stage renal disease was developed. Dietary deficiency of vitamin D causes inadequate absorption and utilization of calcium. Insufficient exposure to ultraviolet light from the sun, in the absence of oral vitamin D, causes calcium deficit.

Acute calcium deficit is treated by intravenous administration of a 10 per cent solution of calcium gluconate—of crucial importance if tetany or convulsions have occurred. Milder deficits may be corrected by a high calcium diet plus oral supplements of calcium lactate. In osteoporosis, no treatment has proved entirely successful, but physical therapy is useful to keep the bones active, and a high protein diet, plus generous supplements of vitamin D and calcium, is essential. Administration of parathormone is often helpful (Fig. 10-5).

CASE HISTORIES   A.G., 70-years old, was admitted to the hospital because of sprue of some two-months' duration. The attack had followed ten years spent in the tropics, in the Amazon Valley of Brazil. During his first two weeks in the hospital, the patient had numerous large, foul-smelling stools daily. Because of the frequent bowel movements, he was given a potassium supplement in addition to the regular diet. During the third week in the hospital, he complained of tingling of the ends of his fingers and of abdominal cramps. Physical examination revealed hyperactive deep reflexes and bilateral carpopedal spasms. A

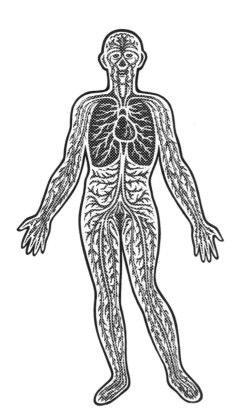

PRECEDING EVENTS
- Loss of calcium-rich intestinal secretions
- Immobilization of calcium
- Parathormone deficit
- Phosphate reciprocity

CLINICAL OBSERVATIONS
- Tingling of fingers
- Muscle cramps
- Tetany
- Convulsions

LABORATORY FINDINGS
- Plasma calcium below 4.5 mEq./L. or 10 mg./100 ml.
- Urinary Sulkowitch test: no precipitation
- Specific EKG findings

RELATED PROBLEMS
- Elevated phosphate
- Vitamin D deficiency
- Inadequate ultraviolet exposure

Figure 10-5.   Calcium deficit.

Sulkowitch test on the urine revealed no precipitation, and the serum calcium was found to be 7 mg./100 ml. (3.5 mEq./L.).

Commentary The impaired fat digestion of sprue causes large quantities of calcium to be excreted in the stools as calcium soaps. Calcium deficit of ECF can readily develop under such circumstances. The clinician showed good judgment in this case in giving potassium, but he should have added a calcium and vitamin D preparation. (Vitamin D promotes the absorption of calcium from the intestine.)

D.A., an energetic sales executive, had been in robust health as far back as he could remember. In his thirtieth year, he was visiting the home office to have a conference with his superior. Sitting in the latter's office, he suddenly fell from his chair to the floor and immediately began convulsing violently. So severe was the convulsion that he became cyanotic, as observed by a company physician with an office nearby. Steps were taken to prevent him from swallowing his tongue. By the time an ambulance arrived, his convulsion had subsided. He was taken to a local hospital and was admitted. His previous history was noncontributory. The patient had used alcohol only moderately. Upon admission to the hospital, he complained of severe abdominal pain—continuous, boring, and partially relieved by sitting up. He was nauseated and vomited. His temperature was 102° F. He had epigastric tenderness and moderate abdominal distention. After two days in the hospital, ecchymoses appeared about the umbilicus. Laboratory tests revealed a white blood cell count of 16,000, and serum amylase 700 Somogyi units (normal 50 to 200). Serum calcium was 5 mg./100 ml. (2.5 mEq./L.). There were no positive x-ray findings. The diagnosis was acute hemorrhagic pancreatitis with calcium deficit.

Commentary Despite the serious illness this patient experienced, he made an uneventful recovery and ten years later was still in good health. Such a result is unusual in acute hemorrhagic pancreatitis. How does pancreatic infection cause calcium deficit? The current theory, which has been recently reviewed and corroborated, is that somehow, calcium is removed from the ECF in considerable quantities by the exudate surrounding the inflamed pancreas. The same phenomenon appears to occur in massive infections in other areas.

Calcium Excess of Extracellular Fluid

Calcium excess of extracellular fluid, or *hypercalcemia,* can develop from drinking too much milk— as an ulcer patient might do to soothe his pain—or too much hard water with a high calcium content. The imbalance may be caused by tumor or overactivity of the parathyroid glands, multiple myeloma, or excessive administration of vitamin D (over 50,000 units daily) in the treatment of arthritis. Multiple fractures, bone tumors, and prolonged immobilization also produce symptoms of calcium excess when calcium stores released from bone flood the extracellular fluid. Osteomalacia and osteoporosis, although manifestations of calcium deficit, cause symptoms of hypercalcemia during the early stages when calcium is moving out of bones and into the extracellular fluid. Thus, while the bones may be dangerously deficient in calcium, there still exists calcium excess of the extracellular fluid. In idiopathic hypercalcemia, the cause is unknown.

The clinical observations in calcium excess include relaxed skeletal muscles, deep bony pain (caused by honeycombing of bones), flank pain (caused by kidney stones, which form from the excess calcium presented to the kidneys for excretion), and pathologic fractures (caused by weakening of bone by leeching away of calcium). (This symptom was formerly the first inkling that the patient had calcium excess. Recall that the "excess" refers to the ECF, not to the bony tissues from which calcium has been removed.)

The plasma calcium concentration is above 5.8 mEq./L. or above 11 mg./100 ml., the urinary Sulkowitch test shows dense precipitation, and calcium excess is indicated by x-ray examination revealing generalized osteoporosis, widespread bone cavitation, or radiopaque urinary stones. (X-ray examination early reveals rarefaction, or thinning, of the bone just under the periosteum of long bones, a most valuable early test that becomes positive before serious and perhaps irreparable damage has been done to the kidneys.) An elevated blood urea nitrogen (BUN) indicates that the urinary stones have damaged the kidneys.

Hypercalcemic crisis is the most important syndrome of calcium excess, for it represents an emergency situation requiring immediate attention to prevent cardiac arrest. The symptoms include intractable nausea and vomiting, dehydration, stupor, coma, and azotemia.

Medical management of hypercalcemic crisis has generally been unsatisfactory, since, owing to slow action or inherent toxicity, none of the many regimens tried has been consistently successful. Sulfate solutions and inorganic phosphate solutions are among the most frequently used, and in less critical situations, therapy is directed toward correcting the underlying cause. If the patient is also being treated for other fluid imbalances, only calcium-free solutions should be used (Fig. 10-6).

CASE HISTORIES A.W., 35-years old, had commented to her friends how "poorly" she had been feeling for the past several weeks. On their urging, she consulted her family physician. Her current symptoms included weakness, anorexia, nausea, polyuria, and thirst. Her past and family histories made no contribution. The physical examination revealed only that the patient looked ill and had lost some 22 lb. (10 kg.). But x-ray and laboratory findings were more revealing: the x-ray study showed subperiosteal resorption of the cortex of the phalanges of the fingers but no evidence of renal calcinosis. The serum calcium was 16 mg./100 ml. (8 mEq./L.), and the phosphorus was 2 mg./100 ml. (1.18 mEq./L.). At operation, a moderate sized parathyroid adenoma was discovered.

Commentary A parathyroid adenoma elaborates excessive quantities of parathormone, which mobilizes calcium from the bony skeleton. If the process has gone on long enough, fractures can occur, or stones can form in the renal pelves, in time destroying the substance of the kidney. Early roentgenography of phalanges should be carried out in anyone even remotely suspected of suffering from a parathyroid tumor because it reveals subperiosteal resorption of the cortex. Diagnosis because of the presence of kidney stones is tragically late. In about half the patients with calcium excess of the ECF, the serum phosphorus is normal. Hypercalcemia may be masked by the effect of high phosphate intake but can be made evident by phosphate deprivation.

W.T., 54-years old, reported to his family physician because of a train of symptoms that had developed within the past three weeks. His first symptom was that of excessive dryness of the mouth, accompanied by thirst and excessive urination. After about ten days, he began to experience nausea and occasional vomiting. Then he began to become drowsy

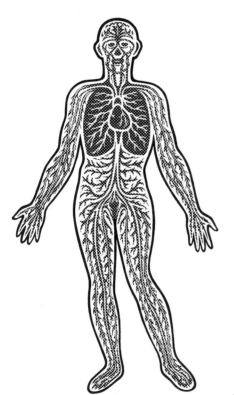

PRECEDING EVENTS
- Excessive parathormone
- Excessive vitamin D
- Tumor

CLINICAL OBSERVATIONS
- Relaxed muscles
- Flank pain
- Deep thigh pain
- Pathologic fractures
- Nausea and vomiting
- Stupor
- Coma
- Cardiac arrest

LABORATORY FINDINGS
- Plasma calcium above 5.8 mEq./L. or 10 mg./100 ml.
- Urinary Sulkowitch test: increased precipitation
- X-ray examination shows generalized osteoporosis, widespread bone cavitation, radiopaque urinary stones
- Elevated BUN

RELATED PROBLEMS
- Kidney damage caused by stones

Figure 10-6.   Calcium excess.

and lethargic. His wife was particularly disturbed by his brief periods of disorientation and confusion. Prior to the present illness, the patient had enjoyed robust good health. The physical examination revealed exaggerated deep reflexes, some questionable muscle weakness, and definite tenderness in the right upper quadrant of the abdomen and somewhat less tenderness in the right lower quadrant of the abdomen and the right lumbar region.

The patient was admitted to the hospital for a thorough workup. Examination of the serum electrolytes revealed a serum calcium of 7.5 mEq./L. (15 mg./100 ml.), bicarbonate 26 mEq./L., parathyroid hormone normal, alkaline phosphatase normal, and other serum electrolytes normal. The urine revealed numerous red cells but was otherwise normal. X-ray examination revealed a mass in the right kidney about the size of a small potato. An intravenous pyelogram confirmed this finding. X-rays of the long bones, skull, and lungs revealed no significant findings. A diagnosis of carcinoma of the right kidney, probably without metastasis, was made, with secondary hypercalcemia, or calcium excess, responsible for the symptoms. Appropriate therapy of the hypercalcemia was instituted and surgical removal of the carcinoma contemplated.

Commentary About 20 per cent of patients with malignant disease develop hypercalcemia. Among the tumors known to cause it are carcinoma of the lung, carcinoma of the kidney, ovarian tumor, bony metastases, and sarcoidosis. Unlike hypercalcemia caused by hyperparathyroidism, the parathyroid hormone and alkaline phosphatase are not elevated. Other causes of hypercalcemia include diseases involving immobilization and ingestion of an antacid. In arriving at a diagnosis of hypercalcemia, it is wise to obtain two serum calciums to avoid the chance of laboratory error. One or more of three mechanisms operate to produce calcium excess of the ECF: (1) increased bone resorption, (2) increased intestinal resorption of calcium, and (3) decreased excretion of calcium via the kidneys. In the case of W.T., the most likely mechanism would be 3, although 1 is a possibility.

MAGNESIUM

Magnesium, known chemically as Mg, is the fourth most abundant cation in the human body. The average adult contains about 20 Gm., about half of which

is stored in bone cells; 49 per cent is distributed throughout the specialized cells of the liver, heart, and skeletal muscles. The extracellular fluid contains only 1 per cent, most of which is in the cerebrospinal fluid, and the normal serum level is 1.67 mEq./L.

The minimum daily requirement for magnesium is a matter of controversy, but most medical authorities agree on 250 mg. for the average adult, 150 mg. for the infant, and 400 mg. for the pregnant or lactating woman. The usual American diet provides from 180 to 300 mg. daily.

Calcium and magnesium, both of which are regulated by the parathyroid glands, share a common route of absorption in the intestinal tract and appear to have a mutually suppressive effect on one another. If calcium intake is unusually high, calcium will be absorbed in preference to magnesium, and, conversely, if magnesium intake is high, more of it will be absorbed and calcium will be excluded. A normal intake of both allows for adequate absorption of both.

The body's magnesium content also directly affects the potassium concentration because, if magnesium is deficient, the kidneys tend to excrete more potassium. Consequently, potassium deficit may also develop.

Magnesium's importance was not understood until its recent recognition as the activator of numerous vital reactions related to enzyme systems. Among the systems that magnesium activates are those that enable the B vitamins to function and those associated with utilization of potassium, calcium, and protein. Magnesium is particularly important in nervous tissue, in skeletal muscle, and in the heart, having considerable therapeutic value in correcting arrhythmias and in counteracting the toxic side effects of certain powerful drugs used in the treatment of heart disease. When used in conjunction with hypotensive agents, magnesium is a useful therapeutic agent in treatment of hypertension. And lastly, toxemia of pregnancy, which formerly had a high mortality rate, responds to magnesium therapy.

Magnesium Deficit of Extracellular Fluid

Magnesium deficit of extracellular fluid, also referred to as *hypomagnesemia*, develops when the magnesium concentration of that fluid decreases.

Alcoholism looms high on the list of factors causing magnesium deficit and, indeed, ingestion of alcohol appears to promote the imbalance, even in the face of what normally would be an adequate intake. The combination of liver disease and sustained losses of gastrointestinal secretions is almost certain to produce magnesium deficit. Diabetes mellitus appears to predispose to magnesium deficit, and so does a high intake of calcium since absorption of magnesium from the intestinal tract varies inversely with calcium absorption. Other causes are primary hyperaldosteronism, severe renal disease, toxemia of pregnancy, diseases of the small intestine that impair gastrointestinal absorption, vigorous drug-induced diuresis, or prolonged administration of magnesium-free solutions. Severe malnutrition, such as kwashiorkor or pluricarencial syndrome (perhaps better designated protein/calorie malnutrition) is also a cause of magnesium deficit. This condition affects countless infants and young children in developing countries in both hemispheres.

Although magnesium deficit is relatively simple to diagnose, a review of the literature suggests that many persons die of undiagnosed magnesium deficit. Perhaps the reason the imbalance is so frequently overlooked is that it is easily mistaken for potassium deficit, with which it is often associated. Magnesium deficit should always be considered a possible imbalance when a patient being treated for potassium deficit does not respond to appropriate therapy, or in the alcoholic with a body fluid disturbance.

While the clinical picture of magnesium deficit varies from patient to patient, certain symptoms are frequently seen. These include tremor, athetoid or choreiform movements, tetany, a positive Chvostek or Trousseau sign, excessive neuromuscular irritability, painful paresthesia, and—an ominous symptom—convulsions. The patient usually is confused and may hallucinate. Another symptom is tachycardia; when it occurs, the blood pressure rises. A therapeutic test consisting of administration of a 1 per cent solution of magnesium sulfate or magnesium citrate by mouth may prove of great value in diagnosing magnesium deficit. If the imbalance is present, there will be an immediate response; all symptoms, however, may not disappear for some 60 to 80 hours.

The most useful laboratory test in magnesium deficit is the plasma magnesium determination, since, if it is below 1.4 mEq./L., magnesium deficit is probably present.

Magnesium deficit is treated by administration of magnesium as magnesium sulfate or other salt, and when excessive amounts of magnesium-rich secre-

tions or excretions are being lost, appropriate replacement solutions should be administered to prevent a deficit (Fig. 10-7).

CASE HISTORIES R.S., 27 years of age, was admitted to the hospital with regional enteritis. Diarrhea was severe. He was given the usual hospital diet plus a potassium supplement. After a month in the hospital, the patient began to have periods of disorientation. Physical examination revealed a tremor of the fingers, hyperactive deep reflexes, and a positive Chvostek sign (twitching of facial muscles when zygoma is tapped). On one occasion, the patient had a brief convulsion. When serum electrolytes were determined, the plasma potassium was 5 mEq./L., but the magnesium was found to be .9 mEq./L. When magnesium sulfate was administered orally as a therapeutic test, improvement was immediate.

Commentary Deficit of potassium and of magnesium result from much the same causes. Therefore, when a patient with potassium deficit does not improve when the potassium is raised to normal, magnesium deficit should be suspected. Magnesium deficit is especially important in the alcoholic, since persons with this problem appear to have a tendency to develop magnesium deficit even when receiving a diet containing generous quantities of magnesium.

J.G., a 20-month-old child, was brought into a clinic because of emaciation and failure to thrive. He had been fed only cola drinks, corn syrup, and palatable (empty) snacks. He had never been breastfed, nor had he had a milk formula. Examination revealed generalized edema; scaly, irritated skin; thin, reddish hair; an enlarged fatty liver; and apathy so extreme that it was pitiful to see him. The laboratory findings were as follows: potassium 2 mEq./L., magnesium 0.8 mEq./L., hemoglobin 6 Gm./100 ml., RBC 3,000,000, serum albumin 2.7 Gm./100 ml. He was given a high-protein diet (it was no easy task devising one that he would eat), an iron preparation, a potassium supplement, and a vitamin supplement containing all essential vitamins. He failed to improve. After three weeks, a magnesium supplement was added to the therapeutic program, after which he improved rapidly.

Commentary The child described was suffering from kwashiorkor, also called pluricarencial syndrome in Latin America and protein/calorie malnutri-

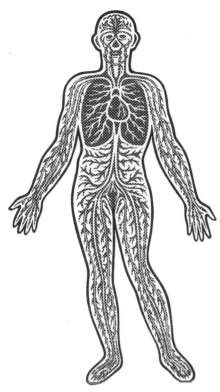

PRECEDING EVENTS

- Usually a combination of liver malfunction and loss of intestinal contents
- Alcoholism
- Severe malnutrition

CLINICAL OBSERVATIONS

- Tremor
- Hyperactive deep reflexes
- Neuromuscular irritability
- Disorientation
- Convulsions
- Improvement with magnesium sulfate

LABORATORY FINDINGS

- Plasma magnesium below 1.4 mEq./L.

RELATED PROBLEMS

- This an easy imbalance to miss; think of it when preceding events are suggestive
- If potassium deficit is present and improvement fails to occur with its correction, suspect magnesium deficit
- Alcoholics may develop magnesium deficit on a well-balanced diet

Figure 10-7. Magnesium deficit.

tion in the United States. It was discovered in Africa in 1957 that infants with this severe form of malnutrition frequently do not improve until magnesium is added to their therapeutic program. Magnesium is extremely important from its promotion of cellular enzymatic reactions. It deserves its name of the *activator*.

Magnesium Excess of Extracellular Fluid

Magnesium excess, or *hypermagnesemia*, represents a rare imbalance, hence we have not included it in our diagnostic classification. It can occur when magnesium is not being excreted normally, as in chronic renal disease or untreated diabetic acidosis. Administration of excessive quantities of magnesium, as in a child with congenital megacolon who is given magnesium sulfate rectally, can cause an excess, and the imbalance has also been reported when perfusion fluid used in hemodialysis contained excessive magnesium. Deficiency of aldosterone, as in Addison's disease, can cause it, as can hyperparathyroidism.

Symptoms of magnesium excess, including lethargy, coma, and impaired respiration, can termi-

nate in death and appear when the plasma magnesium exceeds 6 mEq./L. (Fig. 10-8).

CASE HISTORIES B.N., a 26-year-old male, was admitted to the hospital with hopelessly infected kidneys. Following bilateral nephrectomy, he was put on hemodialysis pending availability of a transplant. Following the third hemodialyzing session, he became extremely lethargic and appeared to have some difficulty in breathing. Complete serum electrolyte studies revealed a magnesium concentration of 3 mEq./L. The source of the excess was sought without success until one of the nurses recalled that water from a new supplier had been used for the last perfusion bath. When analyzed, the water was found to be unduly high in several electrolytes, including magnesium. The supplier of water for the perfusing equipment was immediately changed, and the patient's next hemodialyzing session was uneventful.

W.B., a 52-year-old female, was suffering from advanced chronic glomerulonephritis. (Such patients are unable to excrete magnesium normally.) Because

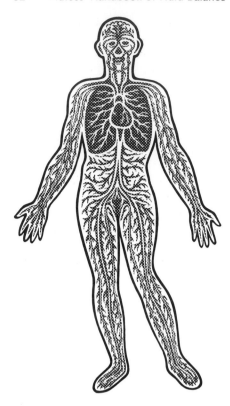

PRECEDING EVENTS

- Chronic renal disease, including uremia
- Untreated diabetic acidosis
- Parenteral or oral administration of magnesium, especially to patients with the above conditions
- Addison's disease (due to lack of mineralocorticoids)
- Hyperparathyroidism
- Administration of antacids containing magnesium salts (e.g., Maalox) to patients with renal impairment

CLINICAL OBSERVATIONS

- Ventricular premature contractions
- Lethargy
- Coma
- Respiratory failure
- Death

LABORATORY FINDINGS

- Plasma magnesium above 6 mEq./L.
- EKG shows prolonged P-R interval, prolonged QRS interval, tall T waves, A-V block, evidence of ventricular premature contractions

RELATED PROBLEMS

- Hypermagnesemia is rarely seen except in the case of patients who have impaired kidneys or are on dialysis

Figure 10-8. Magnesium excess.

of gastric discomfort, the patient was given a magnesium-containing antacid (e.g., Maalox). She immediately developed EKG abnormalities, including ventricular premature contractions, and central nervous system symptoms and signs, including lethargy, which progressed to coma. Her serum magnesium was 7.5 mEq./L. Since dialysis is far from efficient in removing magnesium, patients on dialysis should not be given magnesium-containing medications.

PROTEIN

Protein has been called the *keystone* of the nutritional arch. Because all living matter is composed largely of proteins, there would be no life without protein. Through its drawing power for liquids—oncotic pressure—protein helps prevent leaking of plasma from the blood vessels. In addition, the amino acids of which proteins are composed are the building blocks for the growth of new tissue. Protein is also required for the elaboration of enzymes, for the fabrication of those blood-borne messengers we call

hormones, for the manufacture of some vitamins, and in the immune mechanism since many antibodies are proteins. Since it is practically impossible to develop protein excess, this imbalance is not included in our diagnostic classification and will not be discussed.

Protein Deficit of Extracellular Fluid

Since protein is an anion (e.g., Ca^+ caseinate$^-$), we have included protein deficit of extracellular fluid in our diagnostic classification. The imbalance is also known as *hypoproteinemia* and *protein malnutrition;* Kwashiorkor, or the pluricarencial syndrome, and hypoproteinosis are closely related clinical states.

Protein deficit, which develops slowly, frequently does not attract the attention of the attending physician, and can be deadly. The imbalance can result from decreased intake, increased loss, or impaired utilization of protein. Naturally, the individual on an inadequate diet—for whatever reason—will develop protein deficit, most extreme in starvation, which causes wasting and internal cannibalization of the body tissues. Bleeding, whether severe, repeated, or of long duration, drains the body's protein stores, sooner or later causing a deficit, as does infection. Burns, fractures, and surgical procedures help deplete protein stores through the destruction and apparently purposeless wastage of tissues; this is called *toxic destruction of protein.* Diseases that affect the digestive tract interfere with protein intake and cause protein poverty. Protein deficit is often associated with potassium deficit since adequate potassium is essential for protein synthesis. Indeed, every patient with any disturbance of the body fluids is a candidate for protein deficit, particularly if he has been ill for a long time, since the sort of conditions that cause body fluid disturbances can also cause protein deficit.

The clinical findings of protein deficit include weight loss and wasting of the muscles; body tissues become flabby and soft. The patient complains that he is always tired and becomes chronically depressed. His poor appetite becomes still poorer and he may vomit repeatedly. If he is injured, his wounds will not heal. His recuperative powers are greatly decreased; he may experience one infection after another. Lastly, the protein deficient patient frequently suffers from anemia, which may be either microcytic or macrocytic.

Laboratory aids in diagnosis of hypoproteinemia are limited; they include depressed hemoglobin, depressed hematocrit, and low red blood cell count—these findings are significant only when iron intake is adequate. In severe imbalances, the plasma albumin may drop below 4 Gm./100 ml. However, there is no accurate test for mild or moderate deficits. Bear in mind that it is the albumin that is significant; the total protein can actually be elevated in the face of a protein deficit, provided the globulin has risen in response to an infection or allergic disturbance. When the hemoglobin is depressed, it probably indicates a protein deficit *provided* the patient has been receiving adequate iron. If iron deficiency anemia is present, the depressed hemoglobin would be due—in part, at least—to that.

Under related problems, we should mention that clinicians often neglect to consider protein deficit since it is so slow to develop. Its onset can often be well described as insidious. Protein deficit is likely to develop with fad diets. Several persons at a prominent western university developed protein deficit

when they were following macrobiotic diets. A "pure" vegetarian diet (i.e., a vegetarian diet without milk or eggs) can induce protein deficit if protein complementarity is not achieved. (Recall that protein complementarity refers to a wise choice of protein so as to achieve a satisfactory amino acid mixture.)

The most desirable method of treating protein deficit is via a mixed diet providing high-quality protein, adequate calories, and sufficient amounts of vitamins and minerals. If the deficit must be corrected rapidly, either a high protein diet alone or one supplemented with high protein oral electrolyte mixtures can be used. If the patient cannot take nourishment by mouth, partial or complete feeding via nasogastric tube may be necessary. When oral or nasogastric feedings are impossible, difficult, or contraindicated, then protein may be administered parenterally (Fig. 10-9).

CASE HISTORIES S.G. was a 28-year-old female admitted to the hospital following an automobile accident in which she was severely injured. She had sustained multiple fractures, one of which was compound, and had lost considerable blood. She received several blood transfusions during the first few days in the hospital. After this initial period, her only nutrition consisted of the usual hospital diet, at which she only nibbled. Both fractures and flesh wounds healed slowly. She was emotionally and mentally depressed, she was pale, she had almost no appetite, her muscles were soft and flabby, and she lost 22 lb. (10 kg.) during the first month in the hospital. Her serum potassium was 3.2 mEq./L., albumin 3 Gm./100 ml., hemoglobin 8 Gm., and RBC 3,000,000. After the diagnosis of protein deficit was made, numerous steps were taken to restore her protein nutrition.

Commentary Protein has been called the *keystone nutrient* and, indeed, it is. It provides amino acids, the building blocks of growth and repair; it provides oncotic pressure for the cardiovascular system; it defends the body against infection; and it is required for the formation of enzymes and hormones. The severely injured patient not only is prone to eat far less protein than normal, there is also an enormous loss of protein in the form of nitrogen in the urine—the so-called toxic destruction of protein. Protein deficit usually comes on insidiously and is often recognized quite late, as was the case with this patient.

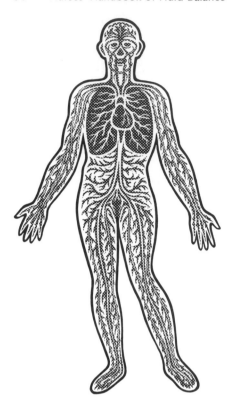

PRECEDING EVENTS

- Prolonged loss of protein

CLINICAL OBSERVATIONS

- Mental and emotional depression
- Anorexia
- Loss of muscle mass and tone
- Weight loss
- Reduced resistance to infection

LABORATORY FINDINGS

- Plasma albumin below 4 gm./100 ml.

RELATED PROBLEMS

- Easy to fail to think of protein deficit since it develops so slowly
- May develop with fad diets; pure vegetarian diet may cause deficit if protein complementarity is not achieved

Figure 10-9. Protein deficit.

R.H. was a 20-month-old boy brought to the doctor because he had almost no appetite, was underweight and underheight, was pale (his mother called him a "pastel child"), had poor posture, was irritable, and developed one upper respiratory infection after another. He was an only child, reared in a home in which the grandparents were living. According to the history, the first year of life was uneventful, except that there was some resistance to weaning. The infant, therefore, was subsisting largely on the bottle well past the end of the first year. Trouble began about the fourteenth month. This is a time when growth slows drastically, and so does appetite. Many mothers do not understand this, hence they are greatly disturbed when the formerly voracious eater loses much of his interest in food. This happened with R.H. His mother reacted by trying to force him to eat, by one means or another. The child resisted, and the mother forced all the more. In this, she was enthusiastically supported by Grandma. So, the infant resorted to the formula bottle and rejected the introduction of new solid foods. By the time the child was taken to the physician, he was living primarily on milk—a splendid food when taken in moderation and in conjunction with other foods, but never intended as the sole food for the preschool child.

The physical examination showed that all was not well. It revealed all that the mother had complained about; in addition, the muscles were flabby and there was a moderately severe hypochromic microcytic anemia. Serum albumin was 3.8 Gm./100 ml. Electrolytes were within limits of normal. The diagnosis was moderate protein deficit. Drastic revision of the child's eating program was indicated if serious future trouble was to be avoided.

Commentary   The hazard of an exclusive milk diet for children was highlighted by Dr. Joseph Brennemann (whom many regard as the father of modern pediatrics) when he protested: "Milk, the great 'protective food,' has been crammed down our and our children's throats, in season and out of season, although the observing, practical pediatrician has long known that even in the use of milk, children should be dealt with as individuals and that the slogan of 'a quart of milk or more every day' originated in the laboratory, and has a sweeter sound to the milk producer than to the pediatrician." Meat, fish, eggs, and cheese are solid, concentrated sources of high-quality protein and should be included in the preschool child's diet, provided he does not have an allergy to one of them.

ACID-BASE BALANCE

The normal composition of the body fluid depends not only upon the concentration of the various electrolytes but also upon the concentration of acids and alkalies. Acids are substances that contain hydrogen ions that they can release to other substances, whereas alkalies possess no hydrogen ions of their own but are able to accept them from acids. The strength of an acid is determined by the number of hydrogen ions it contains per unit of weight, and the power of an alkali is measured by the number of hydrogen ions it can accept per unit of weight.

Together, the acids and alkalies of the body fluids produce the chemical reactions necessary for life, and, in order for such reactions to proceed normally, the body must maintain a precarious balance between the burning acids on the one side and the corrosive alkalies on the other. This is called *acid-base balance*. When acid-base balance is maintained, the reaction of the body fluid is neutral, or normal, and if the balance becomes upset, the body fluid becomes either acid or alkaline in its reaction. *It is the number of hydrogen ions present in the body fluid that determines whether its reaction is acid, neutral, or alkaline.*

Recall that we use the term pH to express the reaction of the body fluid (see Chapter 7, Units of Measure). A pH scale ranges from 1 to 14; 7 is neutral, below 7 is acid, and above 7 is alkaline. The normal pH of extracellular fluid ranges from 7.35 to 7.45 (slightly alkaline). If the plasma pH drops below 7.35, acidosis, or acidemia, is said to be present—even though in the technical sense, a true acid reaction must be below 7. Rarely does plasma pH drop below 7, although it may be as low as 6.8 in extremely ill acidotic patients. If plasma pH rises above 7.45, alkalosis, or alkalemia, is said to be present. Death occurs when the plasma pH is below 6.8 or above 7.8. Hydrogen could be measured simply and logically in nanomoles (nm.) per liter. (A nanomole of hydrogen is

one billionth of a gram, or one millionth of a milligram, of hydrogen.) But by tradition and usage, we still measure hydrogen by pH. pH is defined as "the reciprocal of the logarithm of the hydrogen ion concentration." However, it isn't necessary to understand the mathematics of pH to have a working knowledge of the measure. But it is important to remember two facts: (1) as the pH figure becomes larger the number of H^+ ions becomes fewer; and (2) pH values move by tens, thus, pH 7 is ten times as acid as pH 8 and one tenth as acid as pH 6. If we were to convert pH 7 to nanomoles of H^+, we would find it equals 100 nm.; if we convert pH 8 to nanomoles, we find it equals only 10 nm. Notice that as the nanomoles of H^+ figure goes up, the number of H^+ ions goes up; as the nanomoles of H^+ figure goes down, the number of H^+ ions goes down. So, pH 7 = 100 nm. H^+; pH 8 = 10 nm. H^+; and pH 7.4 (approximately normal) = 40 nm. H^+. Unfortunately, the laboratories aren't ready for the simpler and more forthright nanomole measure. One day (perhaps soon) it will come to all hospitals, while at the present it is confined to a few teaching centers. In the meantime, we shall employ the time-honored pH method of expressing H^+ ion concentration.

How does the body control H^+ ion concentration of the body fluids? It accomplishes this monumental task by the help of the body fluid buffers, the lungs, and the kidneys. Buffers tend to prevent changes in H^+ ion concentration when acid or alkali is added to the body from the environment or generated within the body. Buffers occur in pairs; each pair consists of a weak acid and the salt of that acid. There are four major buffer pairs: the *bicarbonate pair*, active in ECF; the *hemoglobin pair*, active in blood; the *plasma protein pair*, exerting its effect on plasma; and the *phosphate pair*, which does its work within the cells. Of primary importance for clinical acid-base disturbances is the bicarbonate pair, which consists of carbonic acid and base bicarbonate. Basically, it is the ratio of carbonic acid to base bicarbonate that determines the H^+ ion concentration of the ECF.

Carbon dioxide (CO_2) unites with water in the ECF to form carbonic acid (H_2CO_3). Thus, H_2CO_3 is equivalent to CO_2. There is a good reason for this: everywhere in the body, CO_2 is being given off from cells. Water is everywhere in the body. Everywhere in the body is carbonic anhydrase, the enzyme that catalyzes the combination of CO_2 and water (HOH) to make carbonic acid. This means that everywhere in the body there is CO_2 and, in equilibrium with it, H_2CO_3. Therefore, from the practical (if not from the strict chemical) standpoint, the two are equivalent. Now, H_2CO_3 ionizes to provide H^+ ions. Since CO_2 is the equivalent of H_2CO_3, it too must be regarded as an acid substance. Base bicarbonate is formed when the cations sodium, potassium, calcium, and magnesium unite with the anion bicarbonate.

The normal ratio of carbonic acid to base bicarbonate is 1:20, and so, as long as there is 1 mEq. of carbonic acid for every 20 mEq. of base bicarbonate in the extracellular fluid, the hydrogen ion concentration lies within normal limits. Normally, there are 1.2 mEq. of carbonic acid to every 24 mEq. of base bicarbonate.

It is important to note that *absolute* quantities of carbonic acid and base bicarbonate are not important in maintaining the balance; it is the *relative* quantities that are important. For example, acid-base balance will not be disturbed if base bicarbonate is increased, perhaps doubled, as long as the carbonic acid is also increased by the same factor; or, both can be decreased by the same factor without upsetting the balance. Imbalances result only when the normal 1:20 ratio is upset.

Think of acid-base balance as a teeter-totter, with carbonic acid on one end and base bicarbonate on the other. In health, the teeter-totter is level, but any condition that increases carbonic acid or decreases base bicarbonate tilts the teeter-totter toward the carbonic acid side and causes acidosis, or acidemia, and any condition that increases base bicarbonate or decreases carbonic acid tilts the teeter-totter toward the base bicarbonate side and produces alkalosis, or alkalemia.

The balance can be tilted by two general types of body disturbances: one type adds or subtracts base bicarbonate and the other type adds or subtracts carbonic acid. Body metabolism affects the base bicarbonate side of the balance and, for this reason, imbalances caused by alterations in base bicarbonate concentration are called *metabolic disturbances* of acid-base balance. The kidneys largely regulate base bicarbonate concentration. When the H^+ ion concentration is excessively high (*low* pH) the kidneys increase the excretion of hydrogen by several ingenious chemical mechanisms, and they save and regenerate bicarbonate. When the H^+ ion concentration drops to an abnormally low level, the kidneys cease their excretion of hydrogen and permit excessive bicarbonate to pass out in the urine.

The amount of carbon dioxide blown off by the lungs affects the carbonic acid side of the balance, since by speeding up or slowing down respiration, the lungs increase or decrease the level of carbonic acid in the extracellular fluid. When hydrogen accumulates excessively in the body, the lungs simultaneously speed up respiration and blow off carbon dioxide. Recall that CO_2, being the equivalent of H_2CO_3, is an acid material. When, on the other hand, the body lacks hydrogen, the lungs slow down respiration and retain CO_2. The lungs' action in blowing off CO_2 is more vigorous than its role in retaining CO_2. Neither may occur in newborns, whose homeostatic controls are imperfectly developed. Pulmonary ventilation has a rapid effect on the pH of the body fluids. If you hold your breath for one minute, your ECF will become acidotic. If, on the contrary, you hyperventilate actively for one minute, your ECF will become alkalotic. When lung function is abnormal, acid-base balance is disturbed, causing the resultant imbalances referred to as *respiratory disturbances* of acid-base balance.

To determine the status of one's acid-base balance, it is necessary to study the blood gases. Usually when one speaks of blood gases, he is referring to oxygen and carbon dioxide. However, sometimes two additional laboratory values—pH and bicarbonate—are referred to as blood gases since they are intimately involved in acid-base balance: pH, of course, represents the value for H^+, which is a gas and which deserves to be designated a blood gas. Bicarbonate, on the other hand, represents the chief alkaline, or basic, constituent of ECF and is a chemical, not a gas. Nevertheless, bicarbonate is so intimately concerned with the three blood gases already mentioned that it is convenient (if incorrect) to classify it among the blood gases.

The pH of the plasma, of course, tells us whether we have acidosis or alkalosis, although it does not indicate the nature of the imbalance, i.e., whether it is metabolic or respiratory. pH can be measured directly by a pH meter or with a colorimeter, using either heparinized arterial blood or "arterialized" blood from a warmed ear lobe or fingertip. Blood from a vein can be used if it is promptly drawn and kept stoppered under oil.

Carbonic acid—really CO_2 + HOH—can be measured by a pCO_2 meter and, from this, the amount of carbonic acid can be determined by use of a nomogram. Normal pCO_2 values range from 38–42 mm. Hg if arterial blood is used, and from 40–41 mm. Hg if venous blood is used.

Various laboratory tests can be used to measure the bicarbonate level of the plasma, including the carbon dioxide (CO_2) content, CO_2 capacity, and CO_2 combining power. The names of these tests can be misleading unless one recalls that what is being measured is not the carbon dioxide of plasma but, rather, the bicarbonate. In all these tests, bicarbonate is treated with sulfuric acid, which causes it to release carbon dioxide. The carbon dioxide is then measured and, after an adjustment has been made to allow for the amount of carbon dioxide dissolved in the plasma, the bicarbonate concentration is calculated on the basis of the carbon dioxide released from the bicarbonate as a result of the chemical treatment.

The test for CO_2 content measures the total carbon dioxide freed when plasma is acidified, representing not only the carbon dioxide derived from bicarbonate—which is a measure of plasma alkali—but also carbon dioxide in the form of dissolved CO_2 or carbonic acid—which measures the acid portion of the plasma. The normal CO_2 content ranges from 24–33 mEq./L. If there is a respiratory acid-base disturbance, the CO_2 content will not represent an accurate measure of the bicarbonate. In carbonic acid excess (respiratory acidosis), because of the CO_2 retention by the lungs, the carbonic acid is elevated; in carbonic acid deficit (respiratory alkalosis), because of the blowing off of CO_2, it is depressed. But there are tests that give one a more accurate estimate of the plasma bicarbonate, even in the presence of a respiratory disturbance, and these include the CO_2 capacity test and the CO_2 combining power test.

In these tests, the actual carbonic acid and carbon dioxide concentration of the plasma is adjusted to normal either by bubbling a 5.5 per cent carbon dioxide gas mixture through the plasma (CO_2 capacity test) or by having the laboratory technician blow his breath through it (CO_2 combining power test). Thus, if the test plasma's CO_2 is elevated because of respiratory acidosis, bubbling the normal concentration of CO_2 through it will reduce it to normal, a process known as *equilibration*. If the plasma's CO_2 is depressed because of respiratory alkalosis, then

equilibration will raise it to normal. In essence, equilibrating plasma amounts to recirculating the plasma through the lungs of a normal person so that it will achieve its normal CO_2-carbonic acid level. The result is that either the CO_2 capacity test or the CO_2 combining power test gives a fairly close approximation of the test specimen's bicarbonate. Normally, CO_2 capacity varies from 24 to 33 mEq./L., and CO_2 combining power varies from 24 to 35 mEq./L. (depending on reference source).

The CO_2 content, bicarbonate, pH, pCO_2, and carbonic acid content can all be calculated by use of a nomogram if two of the values are known. A straight line is drawn between the two known points and the desired value read from the other three scales.

Considerably more complex and somewhat more accurate methods of measuring acid-base disturbances have been introduced by Astrup, by Siggard-Andersen, and by Kintner, all involving logarithmic relationships, neither easy for the nonmathematician to visualize nor necessary for the usual clinical purposes.

Primary Base Bicarbonate Deficit of Extracellular Fluid

A primary deficit in the concentration of base bicarbonate in the extracellular fluid is usually called *metabolic acidosis or acidemia*, and is caused by any clinical event that decreases the concentration of base bicarbonate in the extracellular fluid. Thus, any condition that floods the extracellular fluid with acid metabolites (either organic or inorganic), such as diabetic acidosis, infection, renal insufficiency, or salicylate intoxication, can cause this imbalance. When one or more other etiologic factors is present, metabolic acidosis can be caused by the parenteral infusion of an isotonic solution of sodium chloride (normal saline) since this imposes an excessive chloride load on the kidneys. A ketogenic diet can produce the imbalance. Metabolic acidosis is frequently associated with potassium excess, whereby the kidneys attempt to reduce the potassium concentration of the extracellular fluid by excreting the excess potassium in the urine. Therefore, potassium rather than hydrogen is exchanged for sodium in the distal convoluted tubules, and the hydrogen ion concentration of the extracellular fluid, thus, is elevated. To make matters still worse, treatment of potassium excess is directed toward forcing the excess potassium from the extracellular fluid back into the cells. When potassium enters the cells, hydrogen leaves them, further contributing to acidosis; conversely, metabolic acidosis promotes potassium excess. In metabolic acidosis, the kidneys exchange hydrogen rather than potassium for sodium in the distal convoluted tubules, and hydrogen replaces potassium in the cells, causing an excess of potassium in the extracellular fluid.

Among the clinical findings in metabolic acidosis are deep, rapid breathing (Kussmaul) and shortness of breath on exertion, each caused by the body's effort to rid itself of carbon dioxide—and, hence, of carbonic acid—and thus restore the acid-base balance to normal. However, these findings may be absent in a young infant or in extremely severe acidosis. Other symptoms include weakness, disorientation, and coma. Ultimately, metabolic acidosis, as well as the other acid-base disturbances, can lead to death if not corrected.

What help does the lab give us? In *uncompensated* metabolic acidosis, the urine pH is usually below 6 and plasma pH is below 7.35. Plasma bicarbonate is below 24 mEq./L. The CO_2 combining power is roughly equivalent to the plasma bicarbonate. The pCO_2 is below 40 mm. Hg because of hyperventilation. If the acidosis is caused by an organic acid, the Delta, or anion gap, will be high; if the acidosis is caused by an inorganic acid, Delta would be normal. A high Delta really represents a large quantity of organic acid anions in the ECF. It is simple to determine Delta: Delta = the Na of the ECF − (the Cl + the HCO_3 of the ECF). Suppose we had, in mEq., Na 142, Cl 105, and HCO_3 16. Then 142 − (105 + 16) = 21 (high Delta, or high anion gap). Suppose we had, in mEq., Na 142, Cl 106, and HCO_3 26. Then 142 − (106 + 26) = 10 (normal Delta, or normal anion gap). Delta is said to be abnormal, and, hence, to indicate acidosis caused by organic acids if the figure for it is greater than 13 (some clinicians say 14 or 15). A Delta of less than 13 indicates acidosis caused by inorganic acids. In *compensated* metabolic acidosis, whereby the carbonic acid concentration may be decreased by the lungs blowing off of CO_2, the plasma pH is about 7.35. The kidneys aid in compensation by retaining bicarbonate, but renal compensation is slower than pulmonary compensation.

If the compensatory efforts of the lungs and kidneys do not restore balance, metabolic acidosis may be treated by administration of bicarbonate or lactate

parenterally or an alkaline solution by mouth (Figure 10-10).

CASE HISTORIES S.T., 18 years old and suffering from diabetes, was admitted to the hospital because of uncontrolled diabetes mellitus. Two days before admission, she had developed a fever and sore throat. At the same time, she found glucose when she tested her urine. The day before admission, she had ingested little except water but kept up her usual insulin dose. During the eight hours before admission, she complained of abdominal pain, vomited several times, and became increasingly lethargic. She had urinated at frequent intervals. Physical examination revealed a lethargic young woman with rectal temperature 103° F.; pulse 110; respirations 30, of Kussmaul type (deep and labored); blood pressure 110/75; acetone odor to the breath; dry skin and mucous membranes; acute pharyngitis; weight 115 lb. (52.5 kg.), usual weight 120 lb. Laboratory tests revealed WBC 20,000, with 85 per cent polymorphonuclear cells; blood sugar 300 mg./100 ml. Serum electrolytes: sodium 138 mEq./L., potassium 5 mEq./L., chloride 98 mEq./L., bicarbonate 10 mEq./L. pCO_2 26 mm. Hg. Urine: pH 5.5, specific gravity 1.035, sugar 4+, acetone present, acetoacetic acid present. The diagnosis was bicarbonate deficit (metabolic acidosis or diabetic ketoacidosis) and ECF volume deficit. Calculating the Delta, we arrive at a figure of 30, indicating acidosis caused by organic acids.

Commentary As is so often the case, we have not just one, but two fluid imbalances—bicarbonate deficit and ECF volume deficit. In treatment, they are managed simultaneously. In this instance, insulin and antibiotics would be used in addition. In this case, we see how extremely useful Delta can be in telling us whether the acidosis is due to inorganic or organic acids.

———

Two-and-one-half-year-old R.T. drank an undetermined quantity of oil of wintergreen (methyl salicylate). He vomited and screamed, holding his hands over his abdomen. In the emergency room of the hospital, he was immediately gavaged, then admitted to the hospital. Admitted to a pediatric ward, he perspired profusely, held his head as if in pain, became restless and excited, then went into convulsions. His pulse was 120/min., and feeble. He was pale and appeared short of breath. Blood pressure was 100/60.

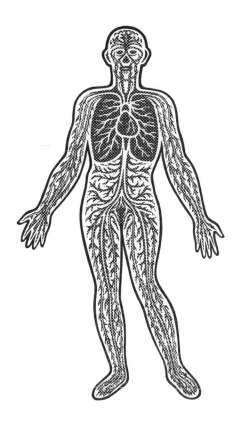

PRECEDING EVENTS

- Flooding of ECF with acid, endogenous or exogenous
- Clinical situations: high Delta
  - Diabetic ketoacidosis
  - Uremic acidosis
  - Ingestion of toxins or drugs
  - Lactic acidosis
  - Starvation ketoacidosis
  - Alcoholic ketoacidosis
- Clinical situations: normal Delta
  - Diarrhea
  - Renal tubular acidosis
  - Dilutional acidosis
  - Acidifying drugs
  - Hyperalimentation
  - Acetazolamide
  - Acid-producing tumor

CLINICAL OBSERVATIONS

- Hyperventilation
- Weakness
- Disorientation
- Coma
- Death

LABORATORY FINDINGS

- Urine pH often below 6
- Plasma pH below 7.35
- Plasma bicarbonate below 24 mEq./L
- pCO_2 below 40 mm. Hg

RELATED PROBLEMS

- Body correction, both renal and pulmonary
- Often associated with K excess

Figure 10-10. Primary base bicarbonate deficit (metabolic acidosis).

His serum HCO_3 was 12 mEq./L., pCO_2 26 mm. Hg, pH 7.2. Urine pH was 5, and the urine tested positive for salicylates. The diagnosis was severe bicarbonate deficit caused by salicylate poisoning.

Commentary   Salicylate poisoning is usually seen in infants and children, but it can be observed in adults. Salicylates produce two opposed acid-base disturbances. First, stimulation of the respiratory center of the brain produces pronounced hyperventilation and primary carbonic acid deficit (respiratory alkalosis). Within one hour or longer, the salicylate disrupts carbohydrate metabolism and causes depletion of liver glycogen. Lactic and pyruvic acids accumulate and cause primary base bicarbonate deficit (metabolic acidosis). Thus, there is a shift from respiratory alkalosis to metabolic acidosis, especially pronounced in children under 5 years of age. Treatment is directed at removing the salicylates from the stomach, if possible, and in correcting the body fluid disturbances. In severe salicylate intoxication, hemo- or peritoneal dialysis can prove lifesaving.

Primary Base Bicarbonate Excess of Extracellular Fluid

A primary excess of base bicarbonate, usually referred to as *metabolic alkalosis* or *alkalemia*, can result from any clinical event that increases the amount of base bicarbonate in the extracellular fluid. This imbalance is frequently preceded by a loss of chloride-rich secretions, such as the gastric juice lost in vomiting or in gastrointestinal suction. Bear in mind that the total anions in the extracellular fluid must always equal the total cations, and so, if one anion decreases, another anion must increase to maintain the balance. Hence, with excessive losses of chloride, bicarbonate rises precipitously and produces alkalosis. Excessive intake of alkalies, such as baking soda, can also cause this imbalance, as can administration of adrenocortical hormones. Infusion of potassium-free solutions, administration of a potent diuretic, or any other condition that leads to potassium deficit can also produce metabolic alkalosis. Indeed, there is a close association between metabolic alkalosis and potassium deficit since, although potassium deficit does not cause alkalemia, it leaves the body peculiarly vulnerable to the imbalance should chloride loss occur. In potassium deficit, hydrogen rather than potassium is exchanged for sodium in the distal convoluted tubules and, in addition, hydrogen moves into cells so that cellular potassium can enter the extracellular fluid to raise its potassium concentration. If chloride has already been lost, with a resultant increase in base bicarbonate, the decrease in hydrogen concentration that occurs in potassium deficit only exaggerates the alkalosis; conversely, metabolic alkalosis promotes development of potassium deficit. In alkalosis, potassium enters the cells in exchange for hydrogen, which leaves the cells, lowering the pH of the extracellular fluid. In addition, potassium rather than hydrogen is exchanged for sodium in the distal convoluted tubules.

Among the clinical observations in metabolic alkalosis are hypertonicity of the muscles, tetany, and depressed respiration, the latter of which retains carbon dioxide, thus causing an increase in the carbonic acid concentration of extracellular fluid and helping to restore the acid-base balance to normal. Correction of metabolic acidosis to normal or to metabolic alkalosis may precipitate tetany or convulsions for the following reason: a latent calcium deficit of the extracellular fluid becomes active and causes hyperirritability, manifesting itself in tetany and convulsions if the deficit is severe. The effective calcium of the extracellular fluid is the ionized portion, with the degree of ionization directly proportional to the acidity of the fluid. In the acid body fluid of acidosis, calcium ionization is high, even if the total calcium con-

centration is decreased, and for this reason, tetany and convulsions from calcium deficit do not occur in acidosis, even though muscle twitching may. In the alkaline fluid of alkalosis, ionization is greatly decreased, and so with the correction of the acidosis to normal, or with its overcorrection to alkalosis, the latent calcium deficit becomes manifest and symptoms of hyperirritability occur.

Laboratory findings are helpful in diagnosis of metabolic alkalosis. The urine pH is often above 7, but it may actually be 6 or below if the imbalance is associated with potassium deficit—because hydrogen rather than potassium is being exchanged for sodium in the distal convoluted tubules, causing the urine to be acid. The venous plasma pH is above 7.45 and in severe alkalosis may approach 7.8; plasma bicarbonate is above 24 mEq./L., and the plasma potassium is below 4 mEq./L. If the alkalosis is hypochloremic, the plasma chloride will be below 98 mEq./L. The above findings obtain in uncompensated metabolic alkalosis. Should there be sufficient retention of carbonic acid (compensated metabolic alkalosis), the plasma pH may be within the limits of normal. The pCO_2 is usually above 40 mm. Hg, revealing the lungs' efforts to hold back CO_2. Such compensation rarely carried the CO_2 above 62 mm. Hg.

Body correction is both renal and pulmonary, with the kidneys excreting the excessive bicarbonate as rapidly as they can. If these efforts fail, chloride should be administered (Figure 10-11).

CASE HISTORIES   L.K., 20-years old and 4-months pregnant, was admitted to the hospital because of severe vomiting, with a presumptive diagnosis of hyperemesis gravidarum. She was fed a general diet, most of which she vomited. About all she was able to keep down was a little water. She was given a vitamin-mineral supplement but no parenteral fluid therapy. On day 4 in the hospital, she exhibited tetanic movements of the fingers. Physical examination revealed that her muscles were hypertonic, and the physician believed that her respirations were suppressed. Laboratory tests revealed normal urine and these serum findings: sodium 135 mEq./L., potassium 3.3 mEq./L., HCO_3 38 mEq./L., pCO_2 30 mm. Hg, pH 7.65, and chloride 94 mEq./L. Diagnosis was bicarbonate excess (metabolic alkalosis) with sodium deficit and potassium deficit. The bicarbonate excess can be explained on the basis of the loss of chloride and potassium in the vomitus.

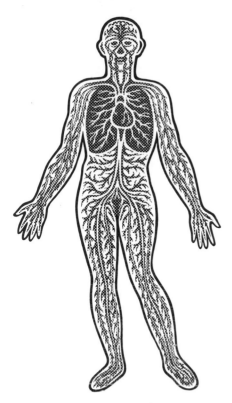

PRECEDING EVENTS

- Loss of chloride, with compensatory bicarbonate rise
- Excessive intake of alkalies

CLINICAL OBSERVATIONS

- Muscles hypertonic
- Tetany
- Depressed respiration
- Death

LABORATORY FINDINGS

- Urine pH sometimes above 7
- Plasma pH above 7.45
- Plasma bicarbonate above 24 mEq./L.
- pCO_2 above 40 mm. Hg

RELATED PROBLEMS

- Body correction, both renal and pulmonary
- Often associated with potassium deficit

Figure 10-11.   Primary base bicarbonate excess (metabolic alkalosis).

Commentary   Chloride loss promotes bicarbonate excess since the bicarbonate rises in compensation as chloride is lost. (Total cations must always equal total anions.) Potassium deficit always tends to favor alkalosis. Gastric juice, you will recall, contains generous quantities of potassium and bicarbonate.

J.S., age 45, felt he could cure his peptic ulcer by taking generous doses of bicarbonate of soda (baking soda) several times a day. After a few weeks on this program, he became so tense and jittery that he consulted his physician. The doctor found him to be a tense, jittery person with hyperactive deep reflexes, suppressed respiration, and x-ray evidence of a large gastric ulcer. Laboratory findings were as follows: urine pH 7, otherwise normal. Serum electrolytes: sodium 146 mEq./L., chloride 93 mEq./L. HCO_3 36 mEq./L., potassium 3.6 mEq./L., pCO_2 57 mm. Hg, and pH 7.65. The HCO_3 was elevated because of the ingestion of baking soda, the pCO_2 was elevated as a

pulmonary compensatory measure (which was why respirations were suppressed), chloride was lowered because the bicarbonate was elevated (total cations must always equal total anions), potassium was lowered because of the effect of alkalosis in causing potassium deficit, and the serum pH indicated alkalosis.

Commentary   Baking soda now sees little use as an antacid since it is absorbed and causes systemic alkalosis. Rather, nonabsorbable alkalies are employed for oral treatment of pepetic ulcer.

COMMENT   While the acid side of the acid-base balance goes up and down in the two imbalances just described, it is important to remember that base bicarbonate is the cause, and changes in the carbonic acid side occur only secondarily to alterations in the concentration of base bicarbonate. In the next two imbalances, the carbonic acid side becomes the cause, whereby changes in the base bicarbonate side become secondary to alterations in the concentration of carbonic acid.

Primary Carbonic Acid Deficit of Extracellular Fluid

Any condition that produces an increased rate and depth of respiration, thereby accelerating carbon dioxide loss, can cause a primary deficit of carbonic acid in the extracellular fluid. This imbalance is usually called *respiratory alkalosis* or *alkalemia*. Its principal cause, *hyperventilation,* may be voluntary, as is the case with the individual who overbreathes so that he can swim a long distance underwater; or it may be caused by oxygen lack, as in high altitudes, or by fever, anxiety, or hysteria. It is also seen in the early stages of salicylate intoxication and in encephalitis.

The clinical observations of respiratory alkalosis include deep breathing or deep and rapid breathing, light-headedness, circumoral paresthesia, tetany, convulsions, and finally, unconsciousness. (The clinical picture of this imbalance, with the exception of the hyperventilation, can be experimentally induced in normal subjects by an intravenous infusion of sodium lactate.) Following hyperventilation, a period of apnea frequently occurs. One can anticipate that the patient will start breathing again as the CO_2 builds up in the blood and stimulates the respiratory center in the medulla, but cases have been reported where individuals did not resume breathing.

As for laboratory findings, the urine pH is characteristically above 7 and the plasma pH above 7.45. Plasma bicarbonate is depressed below 23 mEq./L. This depression, of course, represents a body compensatory measure designed to maintain the normal acidity of the body fluid. pCO_2 is below normal.

For obvious reasons, the lungs are unable to participate in correction of respiratory alkalosis, and so compensation must depend upon the kidneys alone, which excrete bicarbonate and retain acid. Therapy is directed toward correcting the condition that initially caused the overbreathing (Figure 10-12). Parenteral infusion of a solution containing chloride ions to neutralize bicarbonate may be helpful in restoring balance while the pulmonary problem is being corrected.

Related problems include voluntary hyperventilation before swimming underwater, an exceedingly dangerous practice often resorted to by swimmers trying to set distance records. Why is it so dangerous? When one hyperventilates, he blows off CO_2, the chief stimulus to respiration (it is not oxygen lack, as

is widely believed). Therefore, he can go a long time (perhaps a minute or two or three) without receiving an impelling urge to breathe. Obviously, this makes long swims underwater possible. So, the hyperventilated underwater swimmer moves along blissfully, quite pleased with his ability to stay under so long. But in many instances (hundreds? thousands?), the swimmer's brain becomes anoxic before he has a strong urge to breathe; he becomes unconscious, yet still swims automatically along—until, that is, his CO_2 builds up and stimulates the medulla to cause inhalation. Then he inhales water, not air. If the swimmer is observed and rescued at this point, he has a 50 per cent chance of being resuscitated; the chances are not greater because his lungs are full of water. (Some believe that the vigorous expulsion of water from the lungs by the justly famous "hug of life," or Heimlich maneuver, might improve the swimmer's chances, and this impresses us as reasonable.) The moral: *don't hyperventilate before swimming underwater!*

CASE HISTORIES   Eighteen-year-old M.S. was admitted to the hospital for study because of tetanic spasms of the fingers and occasional convulsions. The medical history revealed that she had been extremely apprehensive because of her fear of failing in school. Her mother had noticed that she had been breathing deeply and rapidly for several weeks. Physical examination revealed a tense young woman with hyperactive reflexes. Laboratory tests showed a serum with pH 7.6, HCO_3 20 mEq./L., pCO_2 25 mm. Hg, and urine normal. The serum pH indicated alkalosis, the HCO_3 indicated compensatory lowering of the HCO_3 by the kidneys, and pCO_2 was lowered by the hyperventilation.

Commentary   By having a patient with suspected neurotic hyperventilation to deliberately hyperventilate, one can usually reproduce the symptoms of which the patient has been complaining and, thus, corroborate the diagnosis.

J.N., age 16 years, was a victim of bulbar poliomyelitis and was placed in a respirator because he was unable to breathe unaided. About the second day in the respirator, he began complaining of a "tense" feeling and of spasmodic twitchings of his fingers. Serum pCO_2 was found to be 28 mm. Hg, HCO_3 21 mEq./L., and pH 7.6. The respiratory rate of the ma-

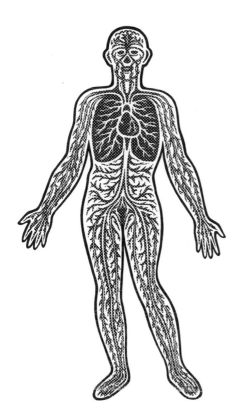

PRECEDING EVENTS

- Hyperventilation from any cause

CLINICAL OBSERVATIONS

- Deep, rapid breathing
- Tetany
- Unconsciousness
- Death

LABORATORY FINDINGS

- Urine pH above 7
- Plasma pH above 7.45
- Plasma bicarbonate below 24 mEq./L.
- pCO_2 below 40 mm. Hg

RELATED PROBLEMS

- Body compensation must depend on kidneys alone; therefore, slow
- Voluntary hyperventilation before swimming underwater *deadly*

Figure 10-12.   Primary carbonic acid deficit (respiratory alkalosis).

chine was slowed, and the symptoms disappeared. The conclusion was that the patient had been suffering from respirator-induced carbonic acid deficit (respiratory alkalosis).

Commentary   Either carbonic acid excess or carbonic acid deficit can occur when the respiratory rate on a respirator is not adjusted to fit the needs of the patient.

Primary Carbonic Acid Excess of Extracellular Fluid

Primary carbonic acid excess of extracellular fluid, commonly called *respiratory acidosis* or *acidemia*, is caused by any condition that obstructs respiratory exchange. Such conditions as emphysema, asthma, pneumonia, occlusion of the respiratory passages, barbiturate poisoning, and morphine poisoning cause respiratory depression, with impaired expiration of carbon dioxide. Inspiration of excessive carbon dioxide, as in spaces with poor ventilation, can also cause respiratory acidosis. Other causes include acute pulmonary edema, atelectasis, pneumothorax, poliomyelitis, and even hypoventilation (as can occur in the extremely obese patient).

The clinical observations in this imbalance include weakness, respiratory embarrassment, giddiness, disorientation, and coma.

Laboratory findings include a urine pH below 6, and a plasma pH below 7.35. As a body compensatory measure, plasma bicarbonate rises to above 24 mEq./L., pCO_2 is elevated to above normal. It may exceed 65, or even 70 mm. Hg. As it rises, the pO_2 must descend since the total pCO_2 + the total pO_2 can never exceed 140 mm. Hg unless oxygen is being administered.

The lungs, of course, are unable to participate in compensation, but the kidneys help by retaining bicarbonate and excreting hydrogen, although with the kidneys working alone, compensation is slow. Therapy is directed primarily toward correcting the condition that is responsible for the impaired lung function, and administration of bicarbonate or lactate

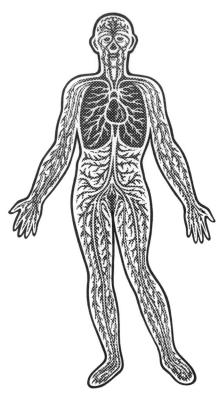

PRECEDING EVENTS

- Respiratory obstruction

CLINICAL OBSERVATIONS

- Impaired respiration
- Disorientation
- Coma
- Death

LABORATORY FINDINGS

- Urine pH below 6
- Plasma pH below 7.35
- Plasma bicarbonate above 24 mEq./L.
- pCO_2 above 40 mm. Hg

RELATED PROBLEMS

- Body compensation must depend on kidneys alone, therefore slow

Figure 10-13.   Primary carbonic acid excess (respiratory acidosis).

may also be necessary to restore balance while the lung ailment is being corrected. (Fig. 10-13).

CASE HISTORIES   An intern, impatient with 84-year-old M.O., who had been upsetting his entire ward in a chronic disease hospital, foolishly ordered ½ grain of morphine for him. The intern then left for a date. The patient quieted down immediately but soon became so lethargic and difficult to arouse that the nurse on night duty became alarmed. She called the intern on duty, who found that the patient could be aroused only with considerable effort. The patient's muscles were relaxed, his deep reflexes were unobtainable, his skin was pale, he was perspiring profusely, and his respirations were down to 2 to 3/min. Even these respirations were shallow, irregular, and heavy. Resuscitative measures were immediately started without waiting to obtain a blood specimen for analysis. Had one been obtained, it would undoubtedly have revealed a carbonic acid excess (respiratory acidosis), with a pCO_2 in excess of 65 mm. Hg. The HCO_3 would not have been elevated since the kidneys had not had time to swing into action. The serum pH would probably have been about 7.1 or 7.2.

Commentary   Both the elderly and the very young have poor tolerance to narcotics. One-fourth grain of morphine would have been dangerous for this oldster; ½ grain was nearly lethal. Fortunately, the patient did survive and was again joyfully keeping the ward upset the next day.

P.K., age 40, came from a family afflicted with a cluster of allergies. His past history revealed that he had been shown to be allergic to pollens, molds, horse dander, ragweed, and various medications. On this admission to the hospital, he was suffering from status asthmaticus that had been preceded by a severe attack of bronchitis that had simply not let up. Instead, it had gradually worsened: for the past several days and nights, the patient had sat on the edge of his bed propped up with his arms in a desperate effort to expand his airway. On physical examination there was evident prolongation of expiration with rales throughout the chest. Respiration was labored, and the patient was slightly cyanotic. The laboratory findings were as follows: HCO_3 36 mEq./L., pCO_2 65 mm. Hg, pH 7.2. The urine pH was 5.5; otherwise, urine was normal. The pCO_2 clearly indicated carbonic acid excess, supported by the serum pH of 7.2. The HCO_3 was elevated as a renal compensatory measure. Diagnosis: carbonic acid excess resulting from status asthmaticus.

Commentary In mild status asthmaticus, carbonic acid deficit (respiratory alkalosis) prevails. When the status worsens, the carbonic acid deficit changes to carbonic acid excess, or respiratory acidosis. This change represents an unfavorable prognostic sign. Urgent action is required, with ventilation, oxygen, and other measures judiciously applied.

Trends in uncompensated and compensated acid-base disturbances are shown in Tables 10-1 and 10-2.

Many clinicians regard the term acidosis as any clinical situation tending to produce acidemia, even though it has not produced it. Similarly, they regard the term alkalosis as any clinical situation tending to produce alkalemia, whether or not it has succeeded in so doing.

Using this terminology, one might encounter such a paradoxical situation as alkalemia (caused by carbonic acid deficit, or respiratory alkalosis) coexisting with base bicarbonate deficit (metabolic acidosis). In this instance, the respiratory alkalosis would, in effect, overpower the effects of the metabolic acidosis. Similarly, one might conceivably find acidemia (caused by carbonic acid excess, or respiratory acidosis) coexisting with base bicarbonate excess (metabolic alkalosis). In this instance, the respiratory acidosis would overpower the metabolic alkalosis.

Some would refer to the former situation as a compensated metabolic acidosis coexisting with a respiratory alkalosis, and to the latter as a compensated metabolic alkalosis coexisting with a respiratory acidosis. Obviously, mixed metabolic and respiratory acid-base disturbances can be enormously complex.

One important clue to whether we are dealing with a mixed nonrespiratory and respiratory imbalance is the pCO_2. (We'll see shortly how this can help us.) Another help, which cannot be overemphasized, is the clinical history. Also important is knowing what the more frequent combination acid-base disturbances are. As we proceed, we'll use our "etiologic" classification of acid-base disturbances—i.e., bicarbonate deficit, bicarbonate excess, carbonic acid deficit, and carbonic acid excess.

CARBON DIOXIDE ALTERATIONS: COMPENSATORY OR PRIMARY? In examining the laboratory values for a given patient with an acid-base disturbance, one must ask these questions concerning alterations in the pCO_2 (CO_2 or H_2CO_3):

Table 10.1. Early Uncompensated pH Disturbances

Imbalance	HCO_3	Arterial pCO_2	Arterial Plasma pH
Metabolic alkalosis	Above 25 mEq./L.	Normal	Above 7.42
Metabolic acidosis	Below 23 mEq./L.	Normal	Below 7.38
Respiratory alkalosis	Normal	Below 38 mm. Hg	Above 7.42
Respiratory acidosis	Normal	Above 42 mm. Hg	Below 7.38

Table 10-2. Partially Compensated pH Disturbances

Imbalance	HCO_3	Arterial pCO_2	Arterial Plasma pH	Urine pH
Metabolic alkalosis	Above 25 mEq./L.	Above 42 mm. Hg	Still above 7.42, but closer to normal	Above 7
Metabolic acidosis	Below 23 mEq./L.	Below 38 mm. Hg	Still below 7.38, but closer to normal	Below 6
Respiratory alkalosis	Below 23 mEq./L.	Below 38 mm. Hg	Still above 7.42, but closer to normal	Above 7
Respiratory acidosis	Above 25 mEq./L.	Above 42 mm. Hg	Still below 7.38, but closer to normal	Below 6

1. Is the alteration primary, hence responsible for a respiratory acid-base disturbance, namely H_2CO_3 deficit or H_2CO_3 excess? Or, is the alteration in pCO_2 secondary—i.e., does it represent respiratory compensation for a metabolic or nonrespiratory disturbance, namely bicarbonate deficit or bicarbonate excess?

2. Are there simple guidelines by which we can tell? Yes. First, there is a simple method by which we can tell whether a depression of pCO_2 in a patient with bicarbonate deficit is compensatory or caused by a complicating carbonic acid excess: if the pCO_2 is compensatory, then the pCO_2 will be lowered about 1 mm. Hg for each mEq./L. depression of the HCO_3. Or, one can use a somewhat more complicated formula, thus, in compensatory lowering of pCO_2:

$$pCO_2 = 1.54 \times HCO_3 + 8.36 \pm 1.1$$

(a range either way of 1.1). If, on the other hand, the pCO_2 is higher than the pCO_2 predicted by the formula, then a complicating carbonic acid excess (respiratory acidosis) is present. If the pCO_2 is lower than the value predicted by the formula, then the pCO_2 is too low for compensation (hyperventilation is just too vigorous) and a primary complicating carbonic acid deficit (respiratory alkalosis) is present. However, under any combination of circumstances, the pCO_2 does not fall below 10 mm. Hg, barring laboratory error.

3. We have a second useful guideline that helps tell us when an elevation of the pCO_2 is compensatory, such as occurs in bicarbonate excess, or whether it is due to a complicating carbonic acid excess. The rule is simple: if the pCO_2 rises as high as 60 mm. Hg (at most, 62 mm. Hg), we must be seeing a carbonic acid excess, or respiratory acidosis, rather than a CO_2 rising in compensation for a bicarbonate excess, or nonrespiratory alkalosis.

Do we have similar simple and useful rules of thumb applying to the bicarbonate? None that we know of.

Now let us examine the clinical conditions that are especially likely to produce combination nonrespiratory and respiratory acid-base disturbances:

1. Cardiac arrest tends to produce carbonic acid excess because of impairment of breathing and bicarbonate deficit because of the production of lactic acid in anoxia. (This would be a high Delta acidosis.)

2. Septic shock, salicylate intoxication, and hepatorenal syndrome produce carbonic acid deficit because of hyperventilation induced by these states and bicarbonate deficit because of alkali-neutralizing toxins released into the circulation.

3. A patient with bronchial asthma who is on a sodium-restricted diet tends to develop carbonic acid excess because of inadequate respiration and bicarbonate excess because of deficient chloride intake with compensatory rise in bicarbonate generated by the kidneys.

4. Suppose we have a patient with carbonic acid excess who had already developed an elevated plasma HCO_3 because of renal compensation. We give the patient assisted ventilation, which converts the carbonic acid excess to a carbonic acid deficit. The already elevated bicarbonate would swing the patient over into a bicarbonate excess.

A SYSTEMATIC APPROACH FOR DIAGNOSIS OF ACID-BASE DISTURBANCES Donna McCurdy, M.D., of the University of Pennsylvania, has presented a logical and systematic approach to the diagnosis of acid-base disturbances. It makes such eminent good sense that we are presenting it here:

1. Examine the clinical history for processes that might lead to simple acid-base disturbances.

2. Note findings on physical examination that suggest an acid-base disturbance.

3. Study the laboratory reports on the electrolytes, the HCO_3, the Na, the K, the pH, the pCO_2, and the Cl. Calculate the Delta.

4. Examine other laboratory data for disease processes associated with acid-base disorders.

5. As you examine the pCO_2, determine whether any change stems from compensatory action or whether it signals a complicating primary respiratory acid-base disturbance.

BIBLIOGRAPHY

Aldinger, K., and **Samaan, N.:** Hypokalemia with hypercalcemia. Ann. Intern. Med. 87: 571–573, 1977.

DeGowin, E., and **DeGowin, R.:** Bedside Diagnostic Examination, ed. 3. New York: Macmillan Publishing Co., 1976.

Duke, M.: Thiazide-induced hypokalemia, association with acute myocardial infarction and ventricular fibrillation. J.A.M.A. 239: 43–46, 1978.

Goldberger, E.: A Primer of Water, Electrolyte and Acid-Base Syndromes, ed. 5. Philadelphia: Lea & Febiger, 1975.

Holvey, D. (ed.): The Merck Manual of Diagnosis and Therapy, ed. 12. Rahway NJ: Merck Sharp & Dohme Research Laboratories, 1972.

McCurdy, D.: Mixed metabolic and respiratory acid-base disturbances: diagnosis and treatment. Chest 62:35S–44S, 1972 Supplement.

Silver, H., Kempe, C., and **Bruyn, H.:** Handbook of Pediatrics, ed. 12. Los Altos CA: Lange Medical Publications, 1977.

Snively, W., and **Thuerbach, J.:** Voluntary hyperventilation as a cause of needless drowning. J. Indiana State Med. Assn. 65: 493–497, 1972.

— 11 —

Position Changes of Water and Electrolytes of Extracellular Fluid

Normally, about one fourth of the extracellular fluid exists as plasma, and about three fourths as interstitial fluid. These two fluids are quite similar in composition, except for the amount of protein they contain: plasma has about 18 mEq./L., and interstitial fluid only 1 mEq./L. It is the oncotic pressure exerted by the plasma protein that prevents large amounts of the plasma's water and electrolytes from being forced into the interstitial fluid by the hydrostatic pressure produced by the pumping action of the heart. However, under certain circumstances, water and electrolytes do shift into the interstitial fluid, and, in other cases, water and electrolytes of interstitial fluid shift into the plasma.

We can readily understand why such shifts occur when the plasma protein content is altered. However, shifts also take place when plasma protein is normal, although the mechanisms for these shifts are obscure and appear to be of little value.

Before we study these shifts, we would do well to review what we learned about the delivery of water, electrolytes, glucose, amino acids, fatty acids, vitamins, and so on to the cells. This all occurs in the area of the arterial capillary bed. Indeed, the capillary bed is the whole reason for the existence of the cardiovascular system.

In the arterial capillaries, we have some 22 mm. Hg force exerted by the plasma albumin, holding liquids in the capillaries; however, we have 32 mm. Hg of force (hydrostatic pressure transmitted from the heart pump) pushing liquids from the capillaries. The net force propelling liquids from the capillaries, then, is $32 - 22 = 10$ mm. Hg. This force is sufficient for water, electrolytes, and other nutrients to leave the capillaries, pass into the interstitial fluid, and, ultimately, to enter the cell. There are forces opposing and favoring this movement within the interstitial fluid, but their net force is negligible (Figure 11-1).

Now let's turn our attention to the venous capillaries. They possess that same 22 mm. Hg exerted by plasma albumin in the arterial capillaries, again acting as a sort of sponge, pulling materials into the capillaries. But the venous capillaries have only some 12 mm. Hg hydrostatic pressure pushing liquids from the capillaries, the force of the cardiac contraction having greatly dissipated itself by the time it reaches the venous capillaries. We have, therefore, a net movement from the cells into the venous capillaries. Urea, CO_2, and other wastes leave the cells and enter the venous capillaries to return to the large veins. In this return of wastes from the cells, the venous capillaries are assisted by the lymph capillaries, blind capillaries that help carry the cellular wastes through lymph channels to the thoracic duct, where they are poured into the left subclavian vein (Figure 11-2). With this brief review of the capillary bed, and recalling the essential role played by the plasma albumin, let us consider the great shifts.

PLASMA-TO-INTERSTITIAL FLUID SHIFT

In plasma-to-interstitial fluid shift, sometimes called *hypovolemia*, abnormal quantities of water and electrolytes move from plasma into the interstitial fluid. This decreases the volume of plasma and increases the volume of interstitial fluid; the normal three to one ratio is upset. The imbalance is closely related to shock and to edema and is almost invariably seen on the first or second day following a severe burn. The shift is also often seen following a massive crushing injury, severe trauma, or perforation of a peptic ulcer and may be observed with intestinal obstruction or following the acute occlusion of a major artery. Plasma-to-interstitial fluid shift may occur in the patient undergoing surgery, producing the condition known as *surgical shock.*

The clinical symptoms of plasma-to-interstitial fluid shift include pallor, tachycardia, low blood pressure, weak pulse—perhaps undetectable—cold extremities, disorientation, and, finally, coma. The clinical picture usually suffices for diagnosis of this imbalance, but laboratory tests are helpful, as the red blood cell count, hemoglobin, and packed cell volume will be elevated because of the decrease in plasma volume.

Hypovolemia appears similar, if not often identical, to the condition known as *shock.* The exact mechanism of shock is not known, but certainly a shift of water and electrolytes from plasma to interstitial fluid can cause it. Pooling of blood in dilated blood vessels of the abdomen may play a role. Shock is a frequent aftermath of injury, and even patients with minor injuries, such as a sprain, broken finger, or a small cut, sometimes suffer severe shock and die from it before reaching the hospital.

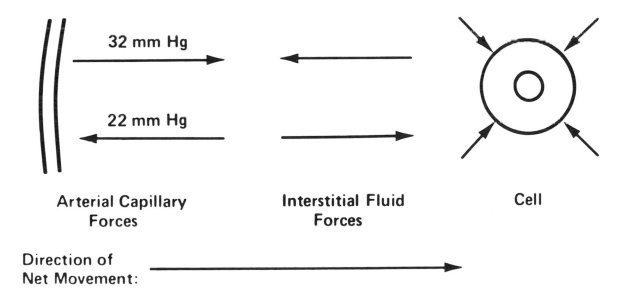

Figure 11-1. Delivery of water, electrolytes, and other nutrients to cells.

Area is the venous capillary bed

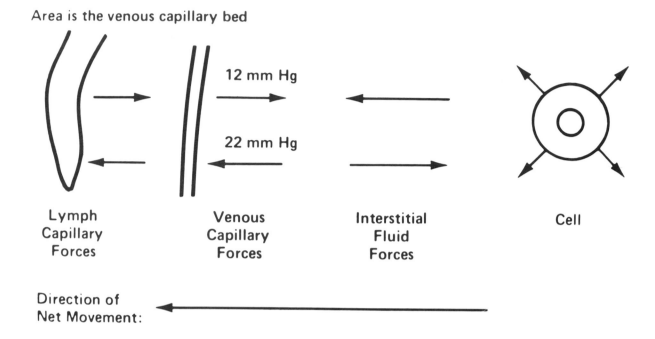

12 mm Hg

22 mm Hg

Lymph
Capillary
Forces

Venous
Capillary
Forces

Interstitial
Fluid
Forces

Cell

Direction of
Net Movement:

Figure 11-2. Transport of urea, carbon dioxide, and other wastes away from cells.

When plasma-to-interstitial fluid shift develops slowly over a long period of time, as in starvation, the patient displays a huge belly, as well as swollen ankles, legs, wrists, and arms—a condition known as *starvation edema.*

In general, treatment of plasma-to-interstitial fluid shift is directed toward the underlying cause of the shift and toward replacing the shifted fluid with solutions given by mouth or vein. Localized shifts may be relieved by application of a binder, and mild or moderate shifts caused by depletion of plasma protein can be corrected via a high protein diet plus commercially prepared protein supplements. In severe protein deficiency, plasma volume is restored by parenteral administration of plasma, dextran, or an electrolyte solution that has approximately the same composition as plasma. Injured persons should be given emergency treatment for shock *at the scene of the accident* (Fig. 11-3).

CASE HISTORIES Eleven-year-old D.G. was admitted to the hospital with two thirds of her body covered with second- and third-degree burns suffered when a flammable party dress caught fire as she danced near the open fire in the fireplace. The burn team of the hospital immediately took charge and carried out their customary excellent routine for severe burns. Nevertheless, during her second 24 hours in the hospital, her hemoglobin and red blood cell count rose rapidly as her blood pressure fell to 90/70 and her pulse increased to 125. She complained of cold hands and feet. The burned area appeared boggy, as if filled with fluid, as indeed it was, from a plasma-to-interstitial fluid shift. As with all severely burned patients, she was permitted no fluids—not even ice chips—by mouth for the first 48 hours of her hospital stay. All fluids permitted were monitored carefully and given by the intravenous route.

Commentary Just why a plasma-to-interstitial fluid shift should occur during the first 48 hours of a severe burn remains an unanswered mystery. If it accomplishes anything, one is hard put to see what it accomplishes. It makes the burned patient thirsty—desperately thirsty. If they are permitted to drink water (they used to be), they are prone to develop sodium deficit and plasma fluid overload when the interstitial fluid-to-plasma shift of the third day begins. Many severely burned patients used to die of sodium deficit because they were permitted water ad libitum. But their deaths were mistakenly attributed to "burn poisoning."

Eight-year-old T.B. was suffering from childhood nephrosis, an ailment of unknown cause and largely unknown pathophysiology, which involves the loss of enormous quantities of plasma albumin in the urine. Because of the loss of the albumin, the oncotic pressure of the plasma is decreased, and water and electrolytes are allowed to escape from the plasma and accumulate in the interstitial space, causing edema so severe that sometimes the child's eyes are swollen shut. On one occasion when the child was given a checkup, her plasma albumin was 2.6 Gm./

100 ml. The urine is, of course, loaded with albumin since this is the route of loss.

Commentary Fortunately, most children recover from childhood nephrosis and may never have a recurrence. Treatments vary widely, but several appear effective. This ailment provides a striking example of the function of albumin in maintaining the oncotic pressure of the plasma.

INTERSTITIAL FLUID-TO-PLASMA SHIFT

In interstitial fluid-to-plasma shift, or *hypervolemia*, water and electrolytes from interstitial fluid flow into the plasma. This imbalance always occurs during the recovery phase of a condition that previously caused a plasma-to-interstitial fluid shift, such as burn or fracture. In this case, the shift is called *remobilization of edema fluid*. If too much fluid is administered during the initial shift, the secondary shift may endanger life. Following hemorrhage, water and electrolytes

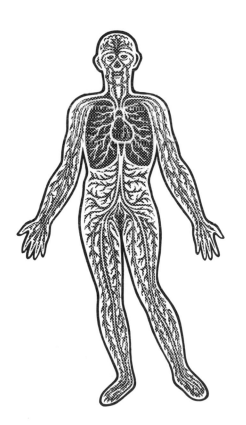

PRECEDING EVENTS
- Severe trauma
- Critical abdominal event
- Depression of plasma albumin

CLINICAL OBSERVATIONS
- Pallor
- Rapid pulse
- Low blood pressure
- Cold extremities
- Disorientation
- Coma

LABORATORY FINDINGS
- Formed elements of blood elevated

RELATED PROBLEMS
- Invariable occurrence during first two days of severe burn
- Closely related to surgical shock

Figure 11-3. Plasma-to-interstitial fluid shift.

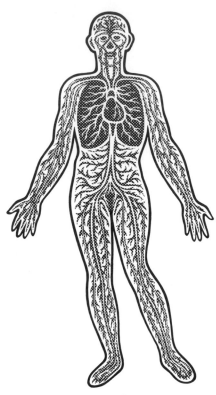

PRECEDING EVENTS

- Occurs during recovery from plasma-to-interstitial fluid shift
- Compensatory shift following hemorrhage

CLINICAL OBSERVATIONS

- Bounding pulse
- Engorgement of peripheral veins
- Moist rales

LABORATORY FINDINGS

- Formed elements of blood depressed

RELATED PROBLEMS

- Begins on third day after severe burn; can be fatal if too much fluid given first two days

Figure 11-4.   Interstitial fluid-to-plasma shift.

move from interstitial space to plasma in an effort to replace those that were lost in blood. The shift also can occur when the oncotic pressure of the plasma has been increased by administration of excessive amounts of blood, plasma, dextran, or hypertonic solutions.

In many respects, the clinical observations of interstitial fluid-to-plasma shift are just the opposite of those seen in plasma-to-interstitial fluid shift. They include a bounding pulse, engorgement of the peripheral veins, moist rales in the lungs, pallor, weakness, and air hunger. Cardiac dilatation and ventricular failure may occur as well. Laboratory findings helpful in diagnosis include a decrease in the red blood cell count, hemoglobin, and packed cell volume.

Treatment of interstitial fluid-to-plasma shift varies according to the cause and, of course, is directed toward lowering plasma volume. If the shift is severe, phlebotomy may be necessary, and application of tourniquets is helpful in other cases. If the shift develops as a compensatory effort to replace water and electrolytes lost in blood, then transfusion of whole blood is the proper treatment. If the shift is

not large enough to require urgent therapy, a balanced diet supplemented by iron tablets will correct it (Fig. 11-4).

CASE HISTORIES   Fourteen-year-old K.B. was admitted to the hospital suffering from second- and third-degree burns over 60 per cent of his body. His initial water and electrolyte therapy was overzealous. On his third postburn day, he complained of being unable to get his breath, and physical examination at that time revealed a bounding pulse, with engorgement of the peripheral veins. Moist rales were heard in both lungs, and the RBC was found to be 3,500,000, with a hemoglobin of 9 Gm./100 ml. He was clearly suffering from the remobilization of edema fluid that occurs during the third to fifth day following a severe burn. The shift can be hazardous, even fatal, if administration of water and electrolytes during the first two days postburn has not been carefully controlled, which usually means given entirely by the intravenous route.

Commentary   This shift and the plasma-to-interstitial fluid shift that preceded it do not appear to serve a useful purpose. They may well have a purpose but, to date, it has eluded discovery. In order to prevent such dangerous remobilization of shifted fluid, several useful formulas for administration of fluid to burned patients have been developed. All are excellent if used in accordance with the patient's ever-changing condition. Perhaps the most useful gauge for fluid therapy is the urine output per hour, as measured from an indwelling catheter. This is ideally 40 ml./hr. in an adult, proportionately less in children and in infants.

D.L., a 24-year-old medical student, contributed 850 ml. of his blood to a desperately injured friend, both of whom had a relatively rare blood type. For several days following the donation of blood, the student experienced a bounding pulse, noticed some engorgement of his peripheral veins, and was short of breath. But within a week, and with no treatment, he felt his normal self. The symptoms were due to a shift of water and electrolytes from interstitial fluid to plasma, a compensatory effort on the part of the body to restore the normal viscosity of the circulating blood, rendered unduly viscous by the release of large quantities of red blood cells into the circulation by the spleen.

Commentary   This case history illustrates at least one potential function of the spleen, which is certainly not necessary for life. It also demonstrates a useful shift of water and electrolytes from one ECF compartment to another. The other shifts described in this section serve no obvious useful purpose and may, indeed, prove fatal.

COMMENT   The clinical examples of body fluid disturbances were chosen so as to represent relatively pure examples of single disturbances. Actually, these examples are not uncommon. Sometimes, one sees combined imbalances, and in some patients a considerable number of imbalances can be present simultaneously. Usually, however, one or two imbalances dominate the clinical picture. The infant with an acute onset of vomiting and diarrhea, for example, early has volume deficit of extracellular fluid, and shortly thereafter, if not properly treated, will develop primary base bicarbonate deficit. If potassium is not given and the diarrhea continues, he will, after three or four days, develop potassium deficit. If he continues to have loose, watery stools and, particu-

larly, if he is also given salt mixtures by mouth, he may well develop a sodium excess.

The addition of each one of these fluid balance disturbances has the effect of increasing, perhaps doubling, the mortality. Various disease states are characterized by a wide variety of body fluid disturbances, depending upon the severity of the disease. Among these conditions might be mentioned burns, severe trauma, diabetes mellitus, gastrointestinal disease and intestinal obstruction. As an example, obstruction of the large intestine can manifest the following disturbances:

1. Extracellular fluid volume deficit, caused by decreased intake of water and electrolytes, and by losses through vomiting and through secretion of intestinal juices into the dilated obstructed bowel.
2. Extracellular fluid volume excess, caused by administering excessive quantities of isotonic saline following surgical intervention.
3. Sodium deficit, resulting from failure to supply water and electrolytes when gastric or intestinal suction tubes are functioning.
4. Sodium excess, caused by cessation of eating and drinking and the resultant loss of water in excess of electrolytes—may also occur when isotonic saline is given without adequate quantities of electrolyte-free solutions.
5. Potassium deficit, an imbalance that results when potassium is not supplied to the patient with intestinal obstruction.
6. Potassium excess, resulting from extensive tissue damage caused by gangrenous bowel, as in volvulus, by the administration of excessive potassium, or by impaired renal function.
7. Calcium deficit, seen with strangulating obstruction of the small intestine, much less frequently in large bowel obstruction, but massive repeated transfusions of blood can precipitate it.
8. Primary base bicarbonate excess, seen when gastric juice has been lost in considerable amounts through vomiting; there is a compensatory rise in bicarbonate since the body's anions must always equal the cations. In some instances, loss of gastric juice is counterbalanced by loss of alkaline intestinal secretions.

Table 11-1. Terminology Chart for Physicochemical Imbalances and Related Clinical States

Physicochemical Imbalance	Conventional Terminology	Closely-Related Clinical States
Extracellular fluid volume deficit	Fluid deficit Dehydration (incorrect term, since ECF volume deficit means loss of water *and* electrolytes) Hypovolemia	
Extracellular fluid volume excess	Fluid volume excess Overhydration (incorrect term, since this imbalance means an excess of both water *and* electrolytes)	
Sodium deficit	Electrolyte concentration deficit Hyponatremia Low sodium syndrome Hypotonic dehydration	Heat exhaustion Sodium-losing kidney Severe muscle cramps
Sodium excess	Hypernatremia Hypertonic dehydration Salt excess Oversalting	
Potassium deficit	Hypokalemia Potassium deficiency	Potassium-losing kidney Muscle necrosis
Potassium excess	Hyperkalemia	
Calcium deficit	Hypocalcemia	Calcium deficiency leg cramps
Calcium excess	Hypercalcemia	Pathologic fractures
Primary base bicarbonate deficit	Metabolic acidosis Acidemia	Diabetic ketosis Renal acidosis
Primary base bicarbonate excess	Metabolic alkalosis Alkalemia	Milk-alkali syndrome
Primary carbonic acid deficit	Respiratory alkalosis Alkalemia	Hyperventilation
Primary carbonic acid excess	Respiratory acidosis Acidemia	Impaired ventilation
Protein deficit	Hypoproteinemia Protein malnutrition	Kwashiorkor Pluricarencial syndrome Hypoproteinosis
Magnesium deficit	Hypomagnesemia	
Shift of water and electrolytes from plasma to interstitial space	Hypovolemia	Shock Edema
Shift of water and electrolytes from interstitial space to plasma	Hypervolemia	Remobilization of edema fluid

It cannot be overemphasized that if one is to understand either combined or complex body fluid disturbances, one must understand the single imbalances, the mechanism of their development, plus their relationships to each other and to disease.

TERMINOLOGY PROBLEMS

Understanding body fluid disturbances is made considerably more difficult by the fact that so many terms frequently apply to the same condition. In an attempt to resolve this problem, we are including in this chapter a table showing in parallel columns each

chemical imbalance, then the conventional term applied to the imbalance, and, finally, the related clinical term, if any. A careful study of Table 11-1 will help to resolve apparent conflicts in terms.

BIBLIOGRAPHY

Richardson, D.: Basic Circulatory Physiology. Boston: Little, Brown, and Co., 1976.

Snively, W., and **Beshear, D.:** Textbook of Pathophysiology. Philadelphia: J.B. Lippincott Co., 1972.

— 12 —

Help from the Lab

"The causes of all diseases are to be found in the blood." Hebrew Proverb

For some years there hung on the office wall of a friend, Dr. Alex Steigman (then Professor of Pediatrics at the University of Louisville School of Medicine), an editorial that told of a pilot who was attempting to land his airplane at a coastal airport during a heavy fog. Unknown to the pilot, the airplane's instruments, by which he was attempting to land the plane, were out of kilter. The instrument readings, therefore, conflicted with what his senses told him. He was faced with an awesome choice: believe the instruments or believe his own God-given faculties. He chose to place his faith in the instruments; the plane plunged into the sea, and all aboard were killed. The moral that the editor drew from the tragedy was this: modern mechanistic aids are wonderful, and they frequently help us enormously, but now and then we must choose between believing the robot and believing our own impressions.

Certainly this lesson applies to the use of laboratory findings in body fluid disturbances. We must always direct our attention to the recovery of the patient, rather than to the manipulation of his biochemical findings. The famous pediatrician, Dr. Edward Park, used to tell of the nurse whose grief over the death of an infant with diarrhea was considerably eased by the fact that, before the baby died, he had had a "beautiful stool." The "beautiful stool" was no more satisfaction to the baby than the correc-

tion of an abnormal biochemical finding would be to the patient who does not live to enjoy it. We must view the clinical picture as being of primary importance; we must regard the laboratory findings as confirmatory rather than diagnostic; we must always treat *patients* rather than *biochemical findings*. In short, we must place the clinical Dobbin before the biochemical cart, which is, of course, where he belongs. Dr. Robert E. Cooke stated the matter well when he said: "Regardless of the multiplicity of laboratory determinations, proper interpretation and therapy depend nonetheless upon frequent and accurate clinical evaluation."

LIMITATIONS OF THE LABORATORY

What are some of the limitations of the laboratory? First of all, many of the usual test procedures have difficulties inherent in them that make consistently accurate results difficult to attain, even though the tests are performed by highly skilled technicians. Moreover, physicians do not always know the "normal" laboratory values for ill persons, since our tables of values are based on those found in healthy persons. It may sometimes be undesirable—even dangerous—to attempt to restore the "abnormal" value of a patient to "normal," since what we regard as an abnormal value may be the result of a defensive action on the part of the body. For example, in primary carbonic acid deficit (respiratory alkalosis), the body lowers the level of base bicarbonate in order to maintain the carbonic acid-base bicarbonate balance. The plasma level of base bicarbonate is, therefore, lower than normal; but the normal referred to is the normal for health, not for this particular imbalance. The normal level of base bicarbonate for carbonic acid deficit is much lower than the level for health, and so, to bring this properly low base bicarbonate level up to the normal level for health by the injection of base bicarbonate into the blood would make the disturbance worse and might well kill the patient.

We can cite many other examples showing why we must take the laboratory reading with the proverbial grain of salt. For example, the level of potassium in plasma is but one indication of the cellular stores. For the long-term survival of the patient, these are vastly important but, for the acute situation, the plasma level of potassium determines whether there will be an ECF deficit or excess of the cation. And, it is the ECF status of potassium that largely determines symptoms and findings. It also determines whether the patient requires measures to increase or decrease the plasma potassium level, which will be reflected both by the serum potassium and by the EKG.

Another example is the state of urine, ordinarily acid in acidosis, but sometimes alkaline even though acidosis is present. This fact is demonstrated in several clinical conditions, such as chronic renal disease, in which the infecting organism converts urea in newly formed urine to ammonia. And, although the urine is usually alkaline in alkalosis, we may find an acid urine when alkalosis is accompanied by a severe potassium deficit. Nevertheless, the physician can almost always improve diagnosis and treatment of body fluid disturbances when he has laboratory aids available. In short, he must learn to use the aids intelligently.

LABORATORY AIDS AVAILABLE

In addition to the chemical methods for determining the plasma levels of calcium, chloride, phosphorus, magnesium, proteinate, albumin, bicarbonate, nonprotein nitrogen and urea, the *flame photometer* has been immensely useful in determining the level of sodium and potassium in body fluids. The flame photometer reading depends upon the color of the flame given out when the electrolyte in question is burned.

The *electrocardiograph* is useful in diagnosing potassium deficit, potassium excess, calcium deficit and calcium excess, although, like other laboratory tests, it is confirmatory rather than primarily diagnostic. *Roentgenography*, too, is a useful diagnostic aid, helping to diagnose certain imbalances in the calcium level. An important development in laboratory techniques is the number of tests that can be performed on a small quantity—for example, a few drops of blood. These *microchemical determinations* are particularly useful in the case of the small baby, who does not have much blood to spare for laboratory tests. The use of *radioisotopes* is becoming more and more important in medicine and may soon be of value to the practicing physician as he diagnoses abnormalities of the body fluid. In addition to laboratory tests that require complex equipment, there are many tests that physicians can do in their offices, including tests to determine the acidity or specific gravity of the urine, the hemoglobin level of the blood, the red blood cell count, and the packed cell volume.

There are other measurements which are not strictly laboratory tests but which are extremely valuable, including the determination of body weight and measurements of fluid intake and fluid output. Indeed, a careful measurement of both the kind and quantity of fluids going into and passing from the patient is of utmost importance for the proper treatment of body fluid disturbances. Since the nursing staff has responsibility for the 24-hour supervision of the patient, the important duty of measuring intake and output falls to them. Basic knowledge of body fluid disturbances and their treatment makes it apparent to nurses that accurate intake-output records can only be described as invaluable for the welfare of the patient. There is usually no substitute for them, as they are often the chief basis for accurate diagnosis and effective treatment. Knowledge of intake-output figures is vital to the physician treating a patient with an imbalance of the body fluids.

EVALUATION OF TEST RESULTS

Variations in laboratory values for individuals of different ages are important considerations when evalu-

Table 12-1.   Laboratory Values

I. Normal Ranges

*Blood Formed Elements**

	Birth	3 mo.	1 yr.	5 yr.	12 yr.	Women	Men
RBC—million/cu. mm.	4.1–5.7	3.1–4.7	3.9–4.7	4.0–4.8	4.3–5.1	4.2–5.0	4.8–6.0
Hemoglobin—Gm./100 ml.	14–20	9–13	11–12.5	12–14.7	13.4–15.8	13–16	15–18
Hematocrit—% vol. of packed RBC/100 ml.	43–63	28–40	32–40	36–44	39–47	39–47	44–52

Plasma Chemical Constituents

Plasma Na^+	137–147 mEq./L.
Plasma K^+	4.0–5.6 mEq./L.
Plasma Ca^{++}	4.5–5.8 mEq./L.
Plasma Cl^-	98–106 mEq./L.
Plasma Mg^{++}	1.4–2.3 mEq./L.
Plasma protein	6–8 Gm./100 ml.
Plasma HCO_3^-	Adults: 25–29 mEq./L. venous; 23–25 mEq./L. arterial
	Children: 20–25 mEq./L.
Plasma Cl^- plus plasma HCO_3^-	123–135 mEq./L.
Plasma pH	7.35–7.45 venous; 7.38–7.42 arterial
Plasma HPO_4^-	1.7–2.6 mEq./L.
Plasma pCO_2	38–42 mm. Hg (arterial or arterialized blood)
Plasma pO_2	95–100 mm. Hg (arterial or arterialized blood)
Delta (anion gap) = Na^+ (mEq./L.) − (Cl^- (mEq./L.) + HCO_3^- (mEq./L.))	13 or below = normal, or if acidosis caused by inorganic acids above 13 = acidosis due to organic acids

Urine Values

Urine pH	4.5–8.2
Urine specific gravity	1.010–1.030

II. Average Values in Health

Blood Formed Elements

	Birth	3 mo.	1 yr.	5 yr.	12 yr.	Women	Men
RBC—million/cu. mm.	4.9	3.9	4.3	4.4	4.7	4.6	5.4
Hemoglobin—Gm./100 ml.	17.1	11.1	11.7	13.3	14.5	14.5	16.5
Hematocrit—% vol. of packed RBC/100 ml.	53	43	36	40	43	43	48

Plasma Chemical Constituents

Plasma Na^+	142 mEq./L.
Plasma K^+	5 mEq./L.
Plasma Ca^{++}	5 mEq./L.
Plasma Cl^-	103 mEq./L.
Plasma Mg^{++}	1.67 mEq./L.
Plasma protein	7.0 Gm./100 ml. (16 mEq./L.)
Plasma HCO_3^-	Adults: 27 mEq./L. venous; 24 mEq./L. arterial
	Children: 23 mEq./L.
Plasma pH	7.4
Plasma HPO_4^-	2 mEq./L.

Urine Values

Urine pH	6.0
Urine specific gravity	1.015

* Covers 94% of normal population.

ating the results of laboratory tests. Normal values for the red cell count, hemoglobin, packed cell volume and plasma bicarbonate differ in infants, children and adults. This is true not only for *average values* but *normal ranges* as well; both are presented in Table 12-1. Plasma levels are best reported as milliequivalents per liter (mEq./L.), but when they are reported as milligrams (mg.), they can be quickly converted by reference to a conversion table.

A reasonable minimal daily program for laboratory surveillance of the patient should include, if facilities are available, plasma sodium, plasma potassium, plasma magnesium, plasma bicarbonate, and plasma chloride. Initially, the hemoglobin, urinary pH and urinary specific gravity should be tested, and measurement of the plasma pH is always helpful if facilities are available for its determination. Blood gases, especially the pCO_2, are essential in evaluating body fluid disturbances. When tests are abnormal, they should be repeated daily until they return to normal. Although body weight and fluid intake-output measurements are not strictly laboratory procedures,

they do provide important objective information, which helps to guard against gross over-provision or under-provision of water and electrolytes. If possible, these measurements should be performed daily until fluid balance is achieved.

The ancient Hebrews must have been interested in something akin to modern laboratory diagnosis, since they had a proverb that states: "The causes of all diseases are to be found in the blood." Today, the examination of blood, particularly of plasma, and of other body fluids is invaluable in the management of the patient with body fluid disturbances.

BIBLIOGRAPHY

Harper, H., Rodwell, V., and **Mayes, P.:**   Review of Physiological Chemistry, ed. 16. Los Altos CA: Lange Medical Publications, 1977.

Meyers, F., Jawetz, E., and **Goldfien, A.:**   Reivew of Medical Pharmacology, ed. 4. Los Altos CA: Lange Medical Publications, 1974.

Tietz, N. (ed.):   Fundamentals of Clinical Chemistry. Philadelphia: W. B. Saunders Co., 1976.

— 13 —

The Role of Nursing Observations in the Diagnosis of Body Fluid Disturbances

"Regardless of the multiplicity of laboratory determinations, proper interpretation and therapy depend nonetheless upon frequent and accurate clinical evaluation."
Robert E. Cooke

FORMULATION OF NURSING DIAGNOSIS

Although her role is not diagnostic in a medical sense, the nurse must possess enough knowledge of body fluid disturbances to make an intelligent nursing diagnosis in order to locate pertinent nursing problems. Once the problems (or potential problems) are identified, the nurse can plan for meaningful observations, measures to prevent imbalances, intelligent execution of medical directives, and other effective nursing care measures. The emphasis of this chapter is the observations of the nurse.

The nurse must be a careful observer in all areas of nursing—fluid balance is no exception. Changes in

the patient who is developing a fluid imbalance are often subtle and perceptible only to those familiar with him and his condition. Thus, observations made by the nurse are particularly valuable, because she spends more time with the patient than does the physician. The observations must be planned and based on an understanding of basic physiologic processes; otherwise, they are of little or no value.

To assist in nursing diagnosis formulation, the nurse should answer the following:

1. Is there present any disease state that can disrupt body fluid balance? (For example: diabetes mellitus, emphysema, or fever) What type of imbal-

ance does this condition usually result in? (See Table 13-1.)

2. Is the patient receiving any medication or treatment that can disrupt body fluid balance? (For example: steroids or thiazide diuretics) If so, how might this therapy upset fluid balance? (See Table 13-2.)

3. Is there an abnormal loss of body fluids and, if so, from what source? What type of imbalance is usually associated with the loss of the particular body fluid or fluids? (See Table 13-3 and Table 13-4.)

4. Have any dietary restrictions been imposed? (For example: low sodium diet) If so, how might fluid balance be affected or altered in this case?

5. Has the patient taken adequate amounts of water and other nutrients orally or by some other route? If no, how long?

6. How does the total intake of fluids compare with the total fluid output?

The nurse should remember that the symptoms seen in an imbalance, and their severity, depend on how long the imbalance has been present, its magnitude and rapidity of onset, and how efficiently the homeostatic mechanisms compensate for it. Also, remember that imbalances rarely occur alone; usually more than one imbalance is present and this makes identification more difficult.

Table 13-1. Imbalances Likely to Occur in Various Clinical Conditions

ILLNESSES		
Condition	Imbalances Likely to Occur	Reason
Uncontrolled severe diabetes mellitus	Metabolic acidosis	Increased utilization of fat for energy needs causes accumulation of ketone bodies (acids)
	Fluid volume deficit	Hyperglycemia causes osmotic diuresis
Adrenal insufficiency	Sodium deficit Potassium excess	Inadequate amounts of adrenal cortical hormones produced, causing the body to retain potassium and release too much sodium
Acute pancreatitis	Calcium deficit	Fixation of calcium by fatty acids liberated from necrotic mesenteric fat deposits
Perforated viscus and chemical peritonitis	Plasma-to-interstitial fluid shift	Loss of fluid into peritoneal cavity as result of inflammatory process
	Calcium deficit	Fixation of calcium by fatty acids liberated from necrotic mesenteric fat deposits
Occlusion of breathing passages, bronchial pneumonia, pneumothorax, hemothorax	Respiratory acidosis	Inability to exchange carbon dioxide
Tracheobronchitis	Sodium excess	Excessive water vapor loss caused by very rapid breathing
Hysteria (psychogenic hyperventilation)	Respiratory alkalosis	Overbreathing, resulting in excessive loss of carbon dioxide
Oxygen-lack with hyperpnea	Respiratory alkalosis	Overbreathing results in excessive loss of carbon dioxide
Fever	Fluid volume deficit	Increased loss of water from lungs, and loss of water and electrolytes from kidneys and skin
	Respiratory alkalosis	Increased respirations resulting from overstimulation of respiratory center

Table 13-1. (Continued)

Condition	Imbalances Likely to Occur	Reason
Severe diarrhea	Metabolic acidosis Potassium deficit Fluid volume deficit	Excessive loss of potassium-rich, alkaline intestinal fluid (increased peristalsis shortens absorption period)
Emphysema, asthma, pulmonary edema	Respiratory acidosis	Inability to exchange carbon dioxide
Congestive heart failure	Fluid volume excess	Increased retention of sodium and water by kidneys caused by: • decreased renal perfusion secondary to failing pumping action of heart • increased aldosterone secretion
Renal disease	Metabolic acidosis Potassium excess Fluid volume excess	Inability of the kidneys to adequately excrete acid metabolites, potassium, and fluid
Hyperparathyroidism	Calcium excess	Increased secretion of parathyroid-hormone causes calcium to be released from bone matrix into extracellular fluid
Hypoparathyroidism	Calcium deficit	Decreased bone resorption causes depressed plasma calcium level
Hyperaldosteronism	Fluid volume excess Potassium deficit	Excessive secretion of aldosterone by adrenal cortex causes the body to retain sodium, chloride, and water and to lose potassium
Meningitis and encephalitis	Respiratory alkalosis	Overstimulation of respiratory center in medulla produces overbreathing
Gastric outlet obstruction with repeated loss of gastric juice through vomiting	Metabolic alkalosis	Loss of acid gastric juice
Vomiting with greater loss of alkaline intestinal juice than of gastric juice	Metabolic acidosis	Loss of alkaline fluid exceeds loss of acidic fluid
Chronic alcoholism	Magnesium deficit	Alcohol produces magnesium diuresis; also, dietary intake of magnesium is often low

BURNS OR INJURIES

Condition	Imbalances Likely to Occur	Reason
Burn, early	Potassium excess	Increased cellular destruction results in release of potassium from cells into extracellular fluid
	Plasma-to-interstitial fluid shift	Plasma leaks out through the damaged capillaries at the burn site
Burn after third day	Potassium deficit	Excracellular potassium shifts back into cells
	Interstitial fluid-to-plasma shift	Edema fluid shifts back into intravascular compartment as capillaries heal
Massive crushing injury	Potassium excess	Cellular damage results in release of potassium from the cells into the extracellular fluid
	Plasma-to-interstitial fluid shift	Plasma leaks out through damaged capillaries at injury site

Table 13-2. Imbalances Caused by Medical Therapy

Condition	Imbalances Likely to Occur	Reason
Excessive administration of adrenal gluco-cortical hormones	Fluid volume excess Potassium deficit	Adrenal cortical hormones cause the body to retain sodium and water and to lose potassium
	Metabolic alkalosis	Potassium deficit is frequently associated with metabolic alkalosis
	Negative nitrogen balance	Adrenal glucocorticoids are catabolic
Administration of potent potassium-losing diuretics: (thiazides, furosemide, ethacrynic acid, mercurials)	Potassium deficit	These agents promote potassium loss
Administration of potassium-conserving diuretics (spironolactone, triamterene) to patients with oliguria	Potassium excess	These agents promote potassium retention
Morphine, meperedine or barbiturates in exccessive doses	Respiratory acidosis	These agents depress respirations and thus decrease the elimination of carbon dioxide
Excessive or too rapid parenteral administration of potassium-containing fluids	Potassium excess	Kidneys unable to excrete potassium rapidly enough to prevent buildup in bloodstream
Early salicylate intoxication (children and adults)	Respiratory alkalosis	Toxic salicylate level stimulates respiratory center and causes overbreathing
Salicylate intoxication (not early) in young children	Metabolic acidosis	Toxic salicylate level results in inadequate utilization of carbohydrate and, thus, increased metabolism of body fats (ketosis)
Excessive administration of vitamin D	Calcium excess	Increased resorption of bone induced by excessive doses of vitamin D
		Increased intestinal absorption of calcium
Excessive parenteral administration of calcium-free solutions	Calcium deficit	Dilution of plasma calcium level by calcium-free fluids
Excessive parenteral administration of magnesium-free solutions	Magnesium deficit	Dilution of plasma magnesium level by magnesium-free fluids
Excessive infusion of large molecular fluids	Interstitial fluid-to-plasma shift	Large molecular substances pull fluid into intravascular space
Excessive administration of citrated blood (particularly to patients with liver damage)	Calcium deficit	Citrate ions combine with ionized calcium in bloodstream
Excessive ingestion of sodium chloride	Sodium excess (if water intake is inadequate)	Sodium level increased as result of excessive intake
	Fluid volume excess (if water intake is adequate)	Large sodium intake causes body to retain water
Gastric suction plus drinking plain water	Sodium deficit Metabolic alkalosis Potassium deficit	Washout of gastric electrolytes
Recent correction of acidosis	Calcium deficit	Increased alkalinization of plasma causes calcium to ionize less freely than in acidosis

Table 13-2. (Continued)

Condition	Imbalances Likely to Occur	Reason
Mechanical respirator inaccurately regulated (causing too deep or too rapid breathing)	Respiratory alkalosis	Excessive loss of carbon dioxide
Mechanical respirator inaccurately regulated (causing too shallow or too slow breathing)	Respiratory acidosis	Retention of carbon dioxide
Prolonged immobilization	Calcium excess	Disuse osteoporosis (absence of weight bearing causes calcium to be resorbed from bone matrix into extracellular fluid)
	Respiratory acidosis	Decreased chest expansion and stasis of secretions
	Negative nitrogen balance	Nitrogen losses exceed intake (increased protein catabolism)
Inhalation anesthesia	Respiratory acidosis	Respiratory depression
Tight abdominal binders or dressings	Respiratory acidosis	Decreased respiratory excursions cause retention of carbon dioxide
Elemental diets and high protein tube feedings (with inadequate water intake)	Sodium excess	Water drawn from tissues to supply the needed volume for urinary excretion of the increased solute load
	Elevated blood urea nitrogen level	Eventually inadequate fluid is available to excrete the high solute load and metabolites are retained
Excessive use of phosphate-binding antacids, especially when combined with maintenance hemodialysis	Phosphorus depletion	Excessive loss of phosphorus (phosphorus depletion can occur under these circumstances although renal failure is more commonly associated with phosphate retention)

ANTICIPATION OF FLUID IMBALANCES ASSOCIATED WITH SPECIFIC BODY FLUID LOSSES

Because the anticipation of an imbalance makes its appearance easier to detect, the nurse should learn to anticipate imbalances. It is extremely difficult to recognize significant changes in the patient when one does not know what to look for, and prevention is easier to practice when one knows which imbalance is likely to occur.

The type of imbalance (or imbalances) that accompanies the loss of a specific body fluid varies with the content of the lost fluid. The nurse can learn to anticipate most specific imbalances when she knows the chief constituents of the lost fluids and how they function. Table 13-4 lists the sodium, chloride, potassium, and bicarbonate concentration of many of the body fluids. A brief discussion of some

of the body fluids and types of imbalances associated with their loss may help to clarify how the nurse can learn to anticipate fluid disturbances.

Gastric Juice

The usual daily volume of gastric juice is 2500 ml. and the pH is usually 1 to 3, but the amount of gastric fluid can vary from 100 to 6000 ml. in abnormal states. Gastric juice contains hydrogen (H^+), chloride (Cl^-), Sodium (Na^+), and potassium (K^+) ions. Imbalances that may result from severe vomiting or prolonged gastric suction include:

1. *Extracellular Fluid Volume Deficit:* This imbalance is due to the loss of both water and electrolytes.
2. *Metabolic Alkalosis (Primary Base Bicarbonate Excess):* Alkalosis develops because

H^+ and Cl^- are lost from the body. The loss of H^+ from the body causes the pH to become more alkaline. The carbonic acid-base bicarbonate buffer system compensates for Cl^- loss by increasing the amount of HCO_3^-; thus, base bicarbonate excess develops. Because both Cl^- and HCO_3^- are anions, as the amount of Cl^- decreases, the body releases more HCO_3^- to keep the total number of anions equal to the total cations. Because HCO_3^- is basic, however, the pH becomes more alkaline.

3. *Sodium Deficit:* Note in Table 13-4 that sodium is rather plentiful in gastric juice.
4. *Potassium Deficit:* There is sufficient potassium in gastric juice to result in a potassium deficit if vomiting or gastric suction is prolonged. Potassium deficit is also associated with alkalosis.

Sodium is more plentiful in gastric juice than is potassium (see Table 13-4). Recall that sodium is the chief extracellular ion and that potassium is the chief cellular ion. The loss of sodium occurs more rapidly because extracellular ions move easily out of the body.

5. *Tetany (if metabolic alkalosis is present):* Although there is no loss of calcium in gastric juice, the patient may develop tetany from a deficit of *ionized* calcium. Since calcium ionization is readily influenced by pH and calcium ionization is decreased in alkalosis, the tetany accompanying alkalosis is corrected when the pH is restored to normal, unless there is a severe calcium deficit.
6. *Ketosis of Starvation:* Patients with gastric suction or with prolonged vomiting are usually allowed nothing by mouth. The parenteral route may supply only a fraction of the

Table 13-3. Imbalances Likely to Result from Loss of Specific Body Fluid

	Gastric Juice	Intestinal Juice	Sensible Perspiration	Insensible Water Loss	Ascites	Wound Exudate	Bile	Pancreatic Juice	Blood
ECF Volume Deficit	X	X	X		X	X		X	
ECF Volume Excess									
Sodium Deficit	X	X	X		X	X	X	X	
Sodium Excess				X					
Potassium Deficit	X	X							
Potassium Excess									
Calcium Deficit						X		X	
Calcium Excess									
Magnesium Deficit	X								
Protein Deficit					X	X			
Metabolic Acidosis		X					X	X	
Metabolic Alkalosis	X								
Respiratory Alkalosis									
Respiratory Acidosis									
Plasma-to-Interstitial Fluid Shift					X	X			
Interstitial Fluid-to-Plasma Shift									X

Table 13-4. Electrolyte Content of Body Fluids Expressed in Milliequivalents per Liter

Body Fluid	Na+	K+	Cl-	HCO3-
Saliva	9	25.8	10	10–15
(fasting) Gastric juice	60.4	9.2	84	0–14
(suction) Small bowel	111.3	4.6	104.2	31
(recent) Ileostomy	129.4	11.2	116.2	..
(adapted) Ileostomy	46	3.0	21.4	..
(fistula) Bile	148.9	4.98	100.6	40
(fistula) Pancreatic juice	141.1	4.6	76.6	121
Cecostomy	79.6	20.6	48.2	..
Urine: normal	40–90	20–60	40–120	..
abnormal	0.5–312	5–166	5–210	..
(normal) Perspiration	45	4.5	57.5	..
Plasma*	137–147	4–5.6	98–106	..
Transudates**	130–145	2.5–5	90–110	..

Adapted from Weisberg, H.: Water, Electrolyte, and Acid-Base Balance, ed. 2. Baltimore: Williams & Wilkins, 1962, p. 143.
* Also contains protein, 6–8 Gm./100 ml.
** Protein content is similar to plasma.

caloric need; hence the patient undergoes starvation. Ketosis results from the excessive catabolism of body fat during starvation. The accumulation of ketone bodies in the blood stream may tend to counteract metabolic alkalosis caused by loss of gastric juice (the accumulation of sufficient ketones can convert the alkalosis into acidosis).

7. *Magnesium Deficit:* Although this imbalance is rare, it can occur with the loss of gastric juice, particularly when prolonged nasogastric suction is used and magnesium-free parenteral fluids are given. There is 1 mEq./L. of magnesium in gastric juice.

Intestinal Juice

The daily volume of intestinal juice is usually about 3000 ml. and its pH is usually alkaline. Diarrhea, intestinal suction, or fistulas can result in the loss of Na+ and HCO3- in excess of Cl-. Losses from these sources can lead to:

1. *Extracellular Fluid Volume Deficit:* This imbalance is due to the loss of both water and electrolytes.
2. *Metabolic Acidosis (Primary Base Bicarbonate Deficit):* The loss of HCO3- is compensated for by an increase in the number of Cl-. (As mentioned earlier, this change occurs to keep the total number of anions equal to the total number of cations in the body). The loss of HCO3-, which is basic, results in acidosis.
3. *Sodium Deficit:* The amount of sodium lost from the intestines in diarrhea or intestinal suction can be great.
4. *Potassium Deficit:* This imbalance develops because relatively large amounts of potassium are lost in the secretions.

Bile

The normal daily secretion of bile is 500 ml. and the pH is alkaline. Abnormal losses of bile can occur from fistulas or from T-tube drainage following gallbladder surgery. Imbalances that can result from excessive loss of bile include:

1. *Sodium Deficit:* Note in Table 13-4 that the sodium content of bile is quite high.
2. *Metabolic Acidosis:* This imbalance develops because of the loss of HCO3- and the compensatory increase of Cl-.

Pancreatic Juice

The normal daily secretion of pancreatic juice is 700 ml. and the pH is 8 (alkaline). Losses of pancreatic juice result in depletion of Na+, HCO3- and Cl-. The loss of HCO3- exceeds the loss of Cl- because it is more plentiful in pancreatic juice (see Table 13-4), which is an integral part of intestinal secretions; thus, loss of pancreatic juice is accompanied by losses of other intestinal secretions. Imbalances that can result from pancreatic fistulas include:

1. *Metabolic Acidosis:* This imbalance occurs because the basic ion, HCO_3^-, is lost in excess of Cl^-.
2. *Sodium Deficit*
3. *Calcium Deficit*
4. *Decrease in Extracellular Fluid Volume*

Sensible Perspiration

Excessive sweating caused by fever or high environmental temperature can result in large losses of water, sodium, and chloride. Normally, sweat is a hypotonic fluid containing sodium, chloride, potassium, magnesium, ammonia, and urea. Severe perspiration can lead to:

1. *Sodium Deficit:* This is especially likely to occur when plain water is ingested in large amounts after profuse sweating, replacing the lost water but not the electrolytes.
2. *Sodium Excess:* This imbalance can occur if the heavily perspiring individual has an inadequate water supply. The sodium concentration in sweat averages around 50 to 80 mEq./L. (considerably less than the sodium content of plasma). Still, proportionately more water than sodium is lost in sweat and results in a relative plasma sodium increase. If water intake is deficient, plasma sodium elevates further.
3. *Extracellular Fluid Volume Deficit:* Both water and electrolytes are lost in sweat, and an imbalance may result if there is no provision for fluid (water and electrolytes) intake.

Insensible Water Loss

The insensible loss of water without solute through the lungs and skin is normally about 600 to 1000 ml. daily and is increased by anything that accelerates metabolism. For example, the increase in insensible water loss is roughly 50 to 75 ml. per degree of Fahrenheit temperature elevation for a 24-hour period.

Increased respiratory activity causes an increased loss of water vapor by way of the lungs. Damage to the skin's surface also results in loss. Increased insensible water loss either via lungs or skin can lead to:

1. *Sodium Excess:* A loss of water alone results in an increased concentration of sodium in the extracellular fluid, that is, water deficit or dehydration.

Large Open Wounds

Considerable quantities of water, electrolytes, and protein are lost in the drainage from large open wounds. Such drainage has a composition similar to plasma. (Note the similarity between transudates and plasma in Table 13-4.) Severe losses from wound drainage can lead to:

1. *Protein Deficit*
2. *Sodium Deficit*
3. *Fluid Volume Deficit*

Ascites

Ascites is the accumulation of fluid within the abdominal cavity. The composition of ascitic fluid is similar to plasma; the amount varies, but occasionally as much as 20 L. can form in a week, creating an enormous loss of protein. The accumulation of large quantities of ascitic fluid requires periodic paracentesis, which can result in considerable losses of protein and electrolytes, sometimes leading to sodium deficit. Ascites can lead to:

1. *Protein Deficit*
2. *Sodium Deficit*
3. *Plasma-to-Interstitial Fluid Shift:* This imbalance may be serious if the formation of ascites is rapid.
4. *Fluid Volume Deficit*

PLANNED NURSING OBSERVATIONS RELATED TO BODY FLUID DISTURBANCES

The following summary of familiar nursing routines will show how meaningful observations can reveal a wealth of information concerning the patient's fluid balance status. When the nurse detects significant symptoms, she can relay them to the physician, thus facilitating early diagnosis and treatment. *The ability to sort out observations demanding urgent action comes with a working understanding of fluid balance and experience in applying this knowledge. The* tables presented in this section refer to symptoms and the diagnoses that they may possibly indicate.

Body Temperature

Usually the body temperature is checked at least twice daily, and when indicated, every four hours or oftener. Fever causes an increase in metabolism and, thus, in formed metabolic wastes, which require fluid to make a solution for renal excretion; in this way, fluid loss is increased. Fever also causes hyperpnea, an increase in breathing resulting in extra water vapor loss via the lungs. Because fever increases loss of body fluids, it is important that temperature elevations be reported and appropriate orders be sought.

It is important to remember that regulation of body temperature is disturbed by lack of water. The body requires at least 800 ml. of water daily to maintain normal temperature control.

Changes in the temperature of the extremities may be noted by touch; external skin temperature gives some insight into the state of peripheral circulation. Any of these changes in body temperature can indicate an imbalance (Table 13-5).

Pulse

The pulse should be evaluated in terms of rate, volume, regularity, and ease of obliteration. The average rate for the adult at rest is 70 to 80 beats per minute. When abnormalities are noted, the pulse should be checked for a full minute. It is wise to observe it for no less than 30 seconds even though the patient does not appear to be seriously ill; a shorter period might not reveal an irregularity. (Variables that may have influenced the pulse, such as activity and emotional upsets, should be considered.)

The pulse should be checked whenever the temperature is taken, more often if indicated; indeed, the nurse should check the pulses of all seriously ill patients whenever she makes rounds.

Because the nurse often delegates TPRs to auxiliary personnel, it is important to teach them the importance of observing pulse volume and regularity as well as pulse rate. See Table 13-6 for possible implications of pulse variations.

Respiration

The nurse should become skilled in observing respiration for indications of body pH changes, because

Table 13-5. Significance of Body Temperature Variations

Symptom	Imbalance Indicated by Symptom
Depressed body temperature	Fluid volume deficit (if infection not present) Sodium depletion
Elevated body temperature	Sodium excess (excessive water loss)
Extremities cold to touch	Plasma-to-interstitial fluid shift Profound sodium depletion Profound fluid volume deficit

the lungs play a major role in regulating body pH by varying the amount of carbon dioxide retention. In order to detect variations from normal, the nurse must evaluate respiration in terms of rate, depth, and regularity and be familiar with the respiratory changes accompanying both metabolic alkalosis and metabolic acidosis.

Severe metabolic alkalosis affects all aspects of breathing: (1) the rate is decreased; (2) the depth is shallow; (3) the respiratory pattern is disrupted by

Table 13-6. Significance of Pulse Variations

Symptom	Imbalance Indicated by Symptom
Weak, irregular, rapid pulse	Severe potassium deficit
Weak, irregular, slowing pulse	Severe potassium excess
Increased pulse rate	Sodium excess Magnesium deficit Hypovolemia (due to plasma-to-interstitial fluid shift or fluid volume deficit)
Decreased pulse rate	Magnesium excess
Bounding pulse (not easily obliterated)	Fluid volume excess Interstitial fluid-to-plasma shift
Bounding, easily obliterated pulse	Impending circulatory collapse
Rapid, weak, thready pulse, easily obliterated	Circulatory collapse Sodium deficit Hemorrhage Plasma-to-interstitial fluid shift
Irregular pulse	Magnesium deficit

periods of apnea lasting from 5 to 30 seconds. Note that the lungs attempt to compensate for the alkalosis by retaining carbon dioxide, hence carbonic acid and, of course, hydrogen ions. (Slow, shallow respiration favors carbon dioxide retention.)

Severe metabolic acidosis affects primarily the rate and depth of breathing: (1) the breathing rate is increased and may be as fast as 50 per minute; (2) depth is greatly increased. The increased volume of lung ventilation is striking; all of the respiratory accessory muscles are used to increase the capacity of the thorax. Note that the lungs attempt to compensate for the acidosis by "blowing off" carbon dioxide. (Fast, deep respiration favors a loss of carbon dioxide from the lungs.)

Usually, respiration is observed for 30 seconds and multiplied by two for a full minute's count; when abnormalities are noted, respiration should be observed for two full minutes. More accurate results are obtained if the patient is unaware that his breathing is being observed. Variable factors, such as increased activity or emotional upsets, may influence respiration.

Respiration is checked routinely when temperatures are taken and more often if indicated. Again, because auxiliary personnel frequently take TPRs, the importance of observing depth and rhythm as well as rate should be impressed upon them. The nurse should make it a practice to observe the respiration of seriously ill patients when she makes rounds.

Other factors related to fluid balance may also influence respiration (Table 13-7). Rales in the absence of pulmonary disease indicate accumulation of alveolar fluid and imply an increased plasma volume or heart failure or both. If rales are due to fluid volume excess, the acute increase in volume is at least 1500 ml.

Blood Pressure

Normal adults have an average systolic pressure of 90 to 140 mm. Hg and an average diastolic pressure of 60 to 90 mm. Hg. The pulse pressure (difference between systolic and diastolic pressures) is usually between 30 to 50 mm. Hg. The systolic pressure indicates the pressure within the blood vessels when the heart is in systole, whereas the diastolic indicates the pressure when it is in diastole. Pulse pressure varies directly with cardiac output.

Table 13-7. Significance of Variations in Breathing

Symptom	Imbalance Indicated by Symptom
Shallow, slightly irregular, slow breathing (compensatory attempt of lungs to correct alkalosis by retaining CO_2)	Metabolic alkalosis
Shortness of breath on mild exertion (in absence of cardiopulmonary disease)	Mild metabolic acidosis
Deep rapid breathing—close observation reveals an effort with expiration (compensatory attempt of lungs to correct acidosis by blowing off CO_2)	Metabolic acidosis
Shortness of breath (in absence of cardiopulmonary disease)	Fluid volume excess
Moist rales (at first, heard only with stethoscope)	Fluid volume excess Interstitial fluid-to-plasma shift Pulmonary edema
Shallow breathing (secondary to weakness or paralysis of respiratory muscles)	Potassium deficit (severe) Potassium excess (severe)
Respiratory stridor	Calcium deficit (severe)
Severe dyspnea	Acute pulmonary edema
Hyperventilation	Phosphorus depletion
Decreased respirations	Magnesium excess (respiratory center paralyzed at a plasma level of 10–15 mEq./L.)

When blood pressure changes are due to blood loss, the systolic pressure falls more rapidly than the diastolic, resulting in diminished pulse pressure. A fall in systolic pressure exceeding 10 mm. of Hg from the lying to the standing or sitting position (postural hypotension) is a cause for concern and usually indicates fluid volume deficit. Symptoms such as dizziness while standing, sudden apprehension, or a weak pulse are indications to check the blood pressure.

Blood pressure variations are immensely helpful in evaluating body fluid disturbances and should be used often as a means of evaluation when there is a real or potential water and electrolyte balance problem. When an abnormal reading is obtained, it is wise to check the pressure in both arms. Variables that may influence blood pressure such as increased activity, position change, and emotional upsets should be considered.

Infrequently the nurse may notice an unusual reaction while checking the blood pressure of a patient with calcium deficit, wherein tightening of the blood pressure cuff to systolic pressure for 3 minutes may elicit a spasmodic reaction in which the hand assumes a clawlike position. See Table 13-8 for possible implications of blood pressure variations.

Peripheral Veins

JUGULAR VEINS The jugular veins provide a built-in manometer for following changes in central venous pressure. Examination of these veins requires no invasive technique and can be highly reliable when done correctly. Changes in fluid volume are reflected by changes in neck-vein filling, provided the patient is not in heart failure. Recall that central venous pressure is elevated by an increased plasma volume or by heart failure and is lowered by a decreased plasma volume.

Normally, with the patient supine, the external jugular veins fill to the anterior border of the sternocleidomastoid muscle. Flat neck veins in a supine patient indicate a decreased plasma volume. In a healthy person positioned sitting at a 45 degree

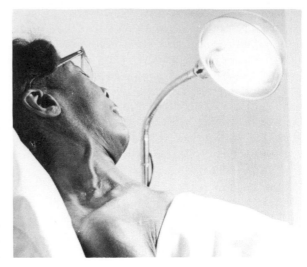

Figure 13-1. When lying in a semireclined position, this patient has distended neck veins, which indicates that the heart is incapable of receiving and pumping adequately all the incoming venous blood. (Reproduced with permission of the American Heart Association)

angle, the venous distentions should not extend higher than 2 cm. above the sternal angle. High venous pressure is manifested by neck veins distended from the level of the manubrium (top portion of sternum) up to the angle of the jaw (Fig. 13-1). To estimate cervical venous pressure the nurse should:

1. Position the patient in semi-Fowler's (head of bed elevated to a 30 to 45 degree angle), keeping the neck straight.
2. Remove any clothing that could constrict the neck or upper chest.
3. Provide adequate lighting to effectively visualize the external jugular veins on each side of the neck.
4. Measure the level to which the veins are distended up the neck above the level of the manubrium.

HAND VEINS Observation of hand veins can be helpful in evaluating the patient's plasma volume. Usually, elevation of the hands causes the hand veins to empty in 3 to 5 seconds; placing the hands in a dependent position causes the veins to fill in 3 to 5 seconds. (See Figs. 13-2 and 13-3.)

A decreased plasma volume causes the hand veins to take longer than 3 to 5 seconds to fill when the hands are in a dependent position. The decreased plasma volume may be secondary to an extracellular

Table 13-8. Significance of Blood Pressure Variations

Symptom	Imbalance Indicated by Symptom
Hypotension	Sodium deficit Plasma-to-interstitial fluid shift Contracted plasma volume due to hemorrhage Severe potassium deficit or excess Magnesium excess (3 to 5 mEq./L.)
Hypertension	Early interstitial fluid-to-plasma shift Fluid volume excess Magnesium deficit
Normal blood pressure while patient is flat in bed—systolic pressure drops in excess of 10 mm. Hg when head of bed elevated	Contracted plasma volume Impending circulatory collapse Sodium deficit

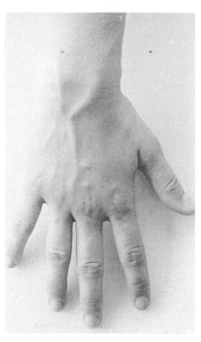

Figure 13-2. Appearance of hand veins when the hand is held in a dependent position.

fluid volume deficit or to a shift of fluid from the plasma to the interstitial space. The veins are not readily apparent when plasma volume is reduced. The slow filling of hand veins often precedes hypotension when the patient is in the early stage of shock.

An increased plasma volume causes the hand veins to take longer than 3 to 5 seconds to empty when the hands are elevated. The increased plasma volume may be secondary to an increased extracellular fluid volume or to a shift of fluid from the interstitial space into the vascular compartment. When this is the case, the peripheral veins are engorged and clearly visible.

Skin and Mucous Membranes

Changes in skin elasticity and in mucous membrane moisture are important for evaluation of changes in fluid volume and electrolyte concentration, as pointed out in previous chapters. (However, skin turgor is less reliable than tongue turgor in older individuals because their skin is less elastic.)

A dry mouth may be due to a fluid volume deficit or may be due to mouth breathing. When in doubt, the nurse should run her finger along the oral cavity and feel the mucous membrane where the cheek and gum meet; dryness in this area indicates a true fluid volume deficit. Dry mouth is relieved by gargling a small amount of water but thirst is not. (See Table 13-9 for possible implications of skin and mucous membrane variations.)

In a normal person, pinched skin will fall back to its normal position when released. In an individual with fluid volume deficit, the skin may remain slightly raised for many seconds (Fig. 13-4). In part A of Figure 13-4, the skin of the forearm is picked up; in part B, 30 seconds later, the skin has not returned to its normal position. The patient in this instance is a young man with moderately severe extracellular fluid volume deficit.

Normally, there is some degree of moisture constantly present in the axilla and groin areas because of action of the apocrine sweat glands; complete dryness may indicate a major fluid deficit (unless a skin disorder has caused malfunction of the sweat glands). Absence of moisture in the axilla or groin probably is indicative of a fluid volume deficit of at least 1500 ml

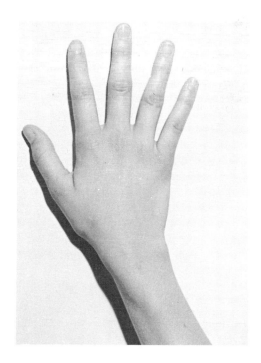

Figure 13-3. Appearance of hand veins when the hand is held in an elevated position.

Table 13-9.   Significance of Skin and Mucous Membrane Variations

Symptom	Imbalance Indicated by Symptom
Poor skin turgor (best tested over forehead and sternum)	Fluid volume deficit
Dry mucous membranes with longitudinal furrows on tongue	Fluid volume deficit
Dry but otherwise normal axilla or groin (normally a small amount of moisture should be present in these areas)	Fluid volume deficit
Decrease in tearing and salivation	Fluid volume deficit
Warm flushed skin (peripheral vasodilatation)	Metabolic acidosis
Flushed dry skin	Sodium excess
Pale, cold, and clammy skin (peripheral vasoconstriction to compensate for hypovolemia)	Decreased plasma volume
Pitting edema	Fluid volume excess
Fingerprinting on sternum	Sodium deficit
Coarse dry skin and alopecia	Chronic calcium deficit

Edema

Edema is the presence of excess interstitial fluid in the tissues. Clinically, edema is not usually apparent until 5 to 10 lb. of excess fluid have been retained. It is sometimes gauged on a scale of plusses, ranging from +1 to +4 (+1 indicating barely perceptible edema, up to +4 indicating severe edema). Among the types of edema seen in clinical practice are pitting edema, dependent edema, and refractory edema.

Pitting edema is a phenomenon manifested by a small depression when one's finger is pressed over an edematous area (Fig. 13-5). Gradually, within 5 to 30 seconds after the pressure is removed, the "pit" disappears. Usually, pitting edema is not evident until a 10 per cent increase in weight has occurred. It is often tested for over a bony prominence, such as the pretibial area. Dependent edema refers to the flow of excess fluid by gravity to the most dependent por-

tion of the body (feet and ankles if standing, back and buttocks if lying down). Refractory edema refers to edema that persists despite treatment with low sodium diet and diuretics.

Besides the subcutaneous tissues, excess body fluid may accumulate in the lung tissue (pulmonary edema), peritoneal cavity (ascites), pleural cavity (hydrothorax), and pericardial cavity (hydropericardium).

Phonation

Speech variations can be significant in the evaluation of the patient's state of water and electrolyte balance, and so the nurse should observe for the presence of subtle changes in quality, content, and formation of speech.

Hoarseness may indicate extracellular fluid volume excess, whereas irrelevant, hyperactive speech may be indicative of potassium deficit. Difficulty in forming words may be secondary to dry mucous membranes, or it may be due to a generalized muscular weakness. (See Table 13-10 for possible implications of speech changes.)

Fatigue Threshold

Many factors contribute to a low fatigue threshold, but those related to fluid balance may include deficits in extracellular fluid volume, potassium, sodium, and protein. The nurse should compare the patient's activities and fatigue level with that of previous days to detect significant changes. Episodes of muscular weakness, fatigability, and diminution of stamina and endurance should be noted—the latter symptoms are particularly descriptive of potassium deficit.

Facial Appearance

A patient with a severe extracellular fluid volume deficit has a drawn facial expression; the eyes are sunken and feel much less firm than normal.

A patient with an excess of extracellular fluid may have puffy eyelids and the cheeks may appear fuller than usual.

Behavior

Behavior changes may be indicative of water and electrolyte disturbances. (See Table 13-11 for pos-

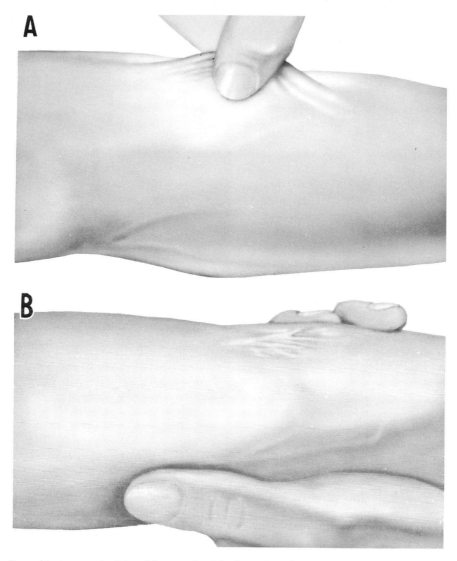

Figure 13-4.   Poor skin turgor: *A,* Skin of forearm is picked up; *B,* it does not return to its normal position 30 seconds later. (From Moyer, C. A.: Fluid Balance, A Clinical Manual. Copyright © 1952 by Year Book Medical Publishers, Inc., Chicago. Used with permission)

sible implications of behavior changes.) These changes are subtle at first and often the patient's family is the first to notice them. The attitude of the patient toward his illness is significant; a severely depleted patient is usually aware that he is seriously ill. Aged patients are particularly prone to develop personality changes and impaired mental function with fluid imbalances, because their homeostatic mechanisms do not function as efficiently as those of younger persons.

Disturbances in plasma pH manifest themselves primarily as central nervous system (CNS) changes.

In acidosis, the major problem is depression of the CNS; a sharp decrease in plasma pH toward 7.0 or below causes disorientation and finally coma. In alkalosis, the major problem is overexcitability of the CNS; symptoms may manifest themselves as nervousness or, in susceptible persons, as convulsions.

Skeletal Muscles

Usually the condition of skeletal muscles is readily observable by the nurse. Subjective complaints from

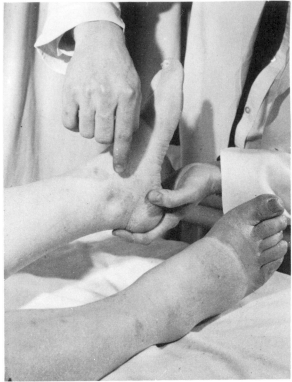 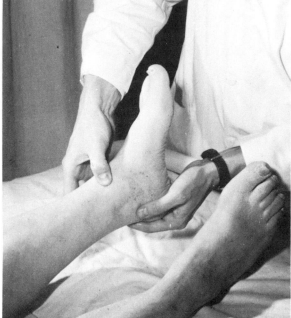

Figure 13-5. *Left,* Pitting edema of feet and lower legs; *Right,* The same patient after edema has been relieved by treatment. (Courtesy of CIBA Pharmaceutical Co., Summit, New Jersey)

the patient, such as weakness or cramping, should be noted.

Muscle weakness is prominent in most electrolyte disturbances and, thus, by itself, is not diagnostic. Neuromuscular symptoms are prominent in severe hypokalemia (usually when the plasma potassium level is below 2.5 mEq./L). Usually the weak-

Table 13-10. Significance of Speech Changes

Symptom	Imbalance Indicated by Symptom
Difficulty in forming words without first moistening mouth	Sodium excess Fluid volume deficit
Hoarseness	Fluid volume excess
Hyperactivity of speech with tendency to irrelevancy	Potassium deficit
Difficulty in speaking due to muscular weakness or paralysis	Severe potassium deficit Severe potassium excess
Voice change—progresses to a crowing noise associated with dyspnea (laryngospasm)	Severe calcium deficit

ness is most prominent in the quadricep muscles of the legs; muscles innervated by cranial nerves are almost never affected. Fatigability is common in chronic hypokalemia and may be present for months. Muscle cramps, tenderness, and paresthesias may be pronounced in the patient with hypokalemia. With profound potassium deficit, the respiratory muscles become involved; "fishmouth" (pursed-lip) breathing may occur as respiratory failure ensues. Death may be caused by respiratory failure.

Seizures may commonly occur in sodium imbalances, hypocalcemia, hypomagnesemia, and alkalosis. They less commonly occur in hypokalemia, hypercalcemia, and respiratory acidosis. Seizures do not occur in metabolic acidosis, hyperkalemia, or hypermagnesemia. (See Table 13-12 for possible implications of symptoms related to skeletal muscles.)

Sensation

Patients with water and electrolyte imbalances frequently report changes in sensation. Some of the more common sensation changes are listed in Table 13-13.

Table 13-11. Significance of Behavior Changes

Symptom	Imbalance Indicated by Symptom
Lassitude and indifference	Fluid volume deficit
Irritability and restlessness	Potassium excess Sodium excess in children Phosphorus depletion
Carphologia (picking at bedclothes)	Potassium deficit Magnesium deficit
Apprehension and giddiness	Sodium deficit Plasma-to-interstitial fluid shift
Hallucinations and delusions	Magnesium deficit Severe sodium deficit or excess
Disorientation and confusion	Acidosis or alkalosis Severe potassium deficit Magnesium deficit
Stupor progressing to unconsciousness	Profound acidosis or alkalosis Late calcium deficit or excess Late magnesium deficit or excess Late potassium deficit (occasionally) Late sodium deficit or excess

CARPOPEDAL ATTITUDE OF HANDS

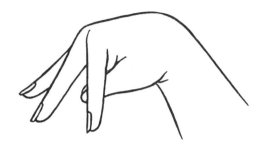

Figure 13-6. Carpopedal spasm.

Table 13-12. Significance of Skeletal Muscle Changes

Symptom	Imbalance Indicated by Symptom
Muscle weakness (particularly in legs)	Chronic potassium deficit Phosphorus depletion
Flabbiness (like half-filled hot water bottles)	Potassium deficit
Flaccid paralysis of respiratory muscles and extremities	Severe potassium deficit or excess
Hypertonus: a. Chvostek's sign* may be positive	Calcium deficit
b. carpopedal spasm (Trousseau's sign**) (Fig. 13-6)	Alkalosis (decreased calcium ionization)
c. Tremors in mild deficit d. convulsions in severe deficit	Magnesium deficit
Painful tonic muscle spasms	Calcium deficit
Muscle rigidity (particularly in limbs and abdominal wall)	Calcium deficit

* Chvostek's sign is a local spasm of the lip, nose, or side of the face following a tap just below the temple where the facial nerve crosses the jaw.
** Trousseau's sign refers to the hand assuming a position of palmar flexion after circulation to the hand is constricted for several minutes.

Desire for Food and Water

ANOREXIA The patient's interest in food and water is useful in evaluating his body fluid status. Anorexia is common in potassium deficit and in protein deficit. Many fluid imbalances are accompanied by nausea, vomiting, and anorexia.

THIRST Thirst is a subjective sensory symptom and has been defined as an awareness of the desire to drink. The sense of thirst is so strong a defender of the plasma sodium level in normal persons that hypernatremia never occurs unless thirst is impaired or rendered ineffective because the patient is unconscious or is denied access to water.

The desire to drink can be initiated by cellular dehydration, which may accompany (1) a decreased extracellular water volume or (2) a hypertonic extracellular fluid such as occurs with intravenous administration of excessive amounts of hypertonic salt solution, with or without extracellular fluid volume excess.

Table 13-13. Significance of Sensation Changes

Symptom	Imbalance Indicated by Symptom
Numbness and tingling of fingers and toes; circumoral paresthesia	Calcium deficit Alkalosis (decreased calcium ionization)
Light-headedness and tinnitus	Respiratory alkalosis
Abdominal cramps	Sodium deficit Potassium excess
Painful muscle cramps	Potassium deficit Calcium deficit
Numb, dead feeling, particularly in extremities (precedes flaccid paralysis)	Severe potassium deficit and excess
Nausea	Calcium excess Potassium excess Potassium deficit
Deep bony pain (decalcification of bones)	Calcium excess
Flank pain (calcium deposits in kidneys)	Calcium excess
Abnormal sensitivity to sound	Magnesium deficit
Paresthesia	Phosphorus depletion
Warm sensation throughout body	Magnesium excess
Dizziness when turned quickly in bed	Sodium deficit

Cellular dehydration will occur when the body's water needs are not met. Gamble has estimated the daily water requirement of the adult at rest as 1500 ml. Butler and his associated cite a somewhat higher figure, 1500 ml. per square meter of body surface per day. These figures are minimal, since the average active adult, not ill, requires from 2000 to 3000 ml. of water per day, including 1000 to 1500 ml. for insensible perspiration and 1000 to 1500 ml. for urine excretion. Among the condition that can increase the requirement for water are:

    Fever
    Excessive perspiration
    Abnormal loss of fluids from vomiting, diarrhea, intestinal suction, and fistulas

    Hyperthyroidism or any other cause of increased metabolic rate
    Diminished renal concentrating ability, such as occurs in old age

Of interest in this connection is the comparison of the water needs in patients with no complications with those of patients with increased water loss, as shown in Table 13-14.

The nurse should constantly remember how important it is to meet the daily water requirement of the patient, by keeping accurate records of his intake and output and by carefully observing the patient for signs of water deficit.

Thirst is often caused by dryness of the mouth resulting from decreased salivary flow, which can be caused by extracellular fluid volume deficit. In this case, true thirst exists. Decreased salivary flow can also be caused by administration of atropine, in which case, there is a desire to relieve the unpleasant dry sensation, but no true thirst.

Thirst is not always a reliable indicator of need and should not be the sole factor influencing fluid intake. The aged patient often does not recognize thirst and, even if he does, may be too weak to reach his water supply. Confusion or aphasia may stop him from making known his desire to drink. Patients with fluid volume excess caused by cardiac and renal damage are sometimes quite thirsty; a problem in this situation is to meet their need without adding to their fluid overload, and the nurse must use caution in allowing patients to ingest as much water as they desire. Seriously burned patients experience great thirst; if allowed to drink all the water they desire, serious sodium deficit will develop. Thirst in the burned patient should be met with specially prepared oral electrolyte solutions with the quantity carefully calculated or with intravenous infusion of fluids. (See Table 13-15 for implications of changes in desire for food and water.)

Character and Volume of Urine

SPECIFIC GRAVITY OF URINE To maintain fluid and osmolar balance, the kidneys must be able to dilute and concentrate urine. The specific gravity test is a convenient and simple method for evaluation of the kidney's ability to perform this function.

The specific gravity of urine is its weight compared with the weight of an equal volume of distilled

Table 13-14. Calculation of Daily Water Requirements

	Average Variation
Uncomplicated Cases:	
For vaporization	1000–1500
For urine	1000–1500
	2000–3000
Complicated Cases (sepsis, elevation of temperature, humid weather, renal disease):	
For vaporization	2000–2500
For urine	1000–1500
	3000–4000
Seriously Ill Patients With Drainage:	
For vaporization	2000
For urine	1000
For replacement of body fluid losses:	
1000 ml. bile	1000
3000 ml. Wagensteen	3000
	7000

Reprinted from Wohl, M., and Goodhart, R.: Modern Nutrition in Health and Disease, ed. 3. Philadelphia: Lea and Febiger, 1964, p. 1055, with permission.

water; it indicates the amount of dissolved solids in the urine. The specific gravity of distilled water is 1.000; the specific gravity of urine, in health, ranges from 1.003 to 1.030. The higher the solute content of urine, the higher the specific gravity.

The chief urinary solutes are nitrogenous end products (urea), sodium, and chloride; others include potassium, phosphate, sulfate, and ammonia. Urinary solutes are mainly derived from ingested foods and from metabolism of endogenous protein and other substances. Diet, then, influences specific gravity of the urine. The usual diet supplies approximately 50 Gm. of urinary solutes in 24 hours. Patients on low sodium or low protein diets cannot concentrate urine to high levels because they are ingesting an inadequate amount of solute. The inability of the patient eating a normal diet to concentrate urine is an indication of renal disease. Renal function is easily assessed by measuring the specific gravity of the first morning urine specimen. If the patient is able to concentrate a protein and glucose free urine to a level of 1.016 or higher, renal function probably is adequate.

The patient's state of hydration can be assessed by measuring specific gravity, provided the kidneys are healthy. A highly concentrated urine implies

water deficit; a dilute urine implies adequate hydration or possibly over-hydration.

Urine specific gravity measurement can help differentiate between the scanty urinary output of acute renal failure and that of water deficit. In acute renal failure, the specific gravity is fixed at a low level (1.010 to 1.012); in water deficit, the specific gravity is high. (Specific gravity persistently below 1.015 is a sign of significant renal disease.)

The nurse may be asked to measure the urinary specific gravity of patients with burns, renal disease, cardiovascular disease, febrile conditions, and general surgical conditions. She should keep the following points in mind:

1. The nurse should be familiar with the equipment used to test the specific gravity of urine:
   a. The apparatus used for the test consists of two parts—the cylinder to contain the urine, and the urinometer (Fig. 13-7).
   b. Note that the urinometer is calibrated in units of .001, beginning with 1.000 at the top and progressing downward to 1.060. A urinometer is read from top to bottom (Fig. 13-8).
   c. New urinometers should be checked for accuracy against distilled water before use, and rechecked from time to time thereafter —even a slight discrepancy can be significant.
2. The urine sample must be fresh.

Table 13-15. Significance of Changes in Desire for Food and Water

Symptom	Imbalance Indicated by Symptom
Anorexia	Potassium deficit Protein deficit Calcium excess
Thirst	Sodium excess (hypertonic extra-cellular fluid) Blood volume deficit due to hemorrhage Blood volume deficit due to acute heart failure Calcium excess (hypertonic extra-cellular fluid)
Absence of thirst	Sodium deficit (hypotonic extra-cellular fluid)

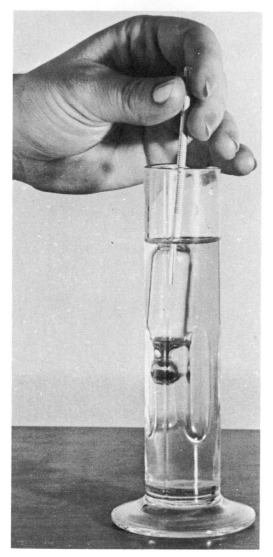

Figure 13-7. Urinometer.

7. To read specific gravity, it is necessary that the urinometer be at eye level (Fig. 13-9). It is read by imagining a line where the lower portion of the meniscus crosses the scale on the urinometer.

The results of specific gravity tests are evaluated in relation to other clinical signs shown by the patient. (See Table 13-16 for conditions that may cause low or high specific gravity of urine.)

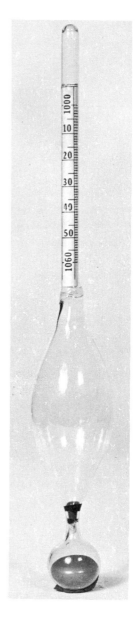

3. The urine sample must be well mixed—remember, the specific gravity test measures solute concentration and a uniform solution must be used to yield an accurate reading.
4. The cylinder should be filled ¾ of the way with urine.
5. After the urinometer is placed in the cylinder, it is given a gentle spin with the thumb and forefinger to prevent it from adhering to the cylinder's sides. (See Fig. 13-7.)
6. Should there be an insufficient amount of urine to float the urinometer, the reading cannot be made. In such an event, q.n.s. (quantity not sufficient) is charted.

Figure 13-8. Urinometer Scale.

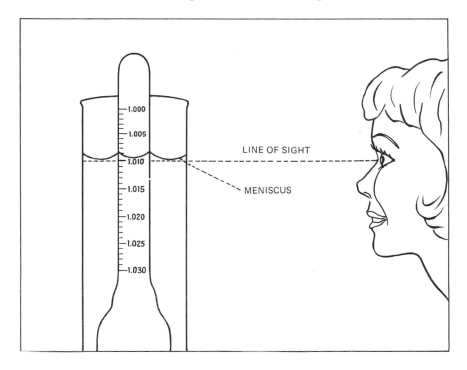

Figure 13-9. The urinometer must be at eye level for an accurate reading of specific gravity.

Table 13 16. Conditions Associated With Persistently Low or High Urinary Specific Gravity

Low Specific Gravity (1.010 or less)	Sodium deficit:
	  Drinking large quantities of water
	  Excessive parenteral administration of electrolyte-free solutions
	  Severely restricted dietary intake of sodium chloride
	  Diuresis from potent diuretics
	Diabetes insipidus (deficiency of antidiuretic hormone)
	Renal disease:
	  Acute renal failure
	  Pyelonephritis
	  Hydronephrosis
	  Severe potassium deficiency
	  Calcium excess

High Specific Gravity (1.030 or higher)	Sodium excess:
	  Decreased water intake
	  Excessive loss of water
	  Excessive ingestion of sodium chloride
	Glycosuria

pH OF URINE. The kidneys play a major role in maintaining the acid-base balance in the body, by excreting electrolytes that are not required and by retaining those that are needed in the body. When an acid factor is in excess, the kidneys excrete hydrogen ions and conserve basic ions; when an alkaline factor is in excess, the kidneys excrete basic ions and retain hydrogen ions.

Urinary pH tests measure the hydrogen ion concentration in urine and, because the excreted electrolytes vary according to the body's need, the urinary pH can range widely (from 4.5 to 8.0) and still be within normal limits. However, the pooled daily urine output averages around 6.0 (acidic) because more acid than alkali are formed in the body during metabolism, and these acids must be removed continually by the kidneys. Several factors may cause normal fluctuations in urinary pH.

1. Sleep causes urine to become highly acid, as respiration is depressed during sleep and a

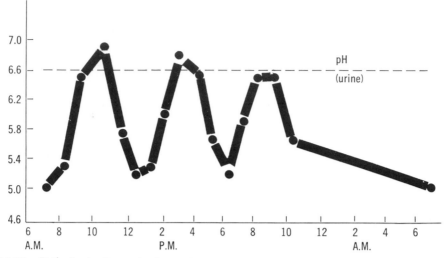

Figure 13-10.   Daily fluctuations of urinary pH. (Pictoclinic 9:6, No. 6, Ames Co., Elkhart, Indiana, 1962)

mild state of respiratory acidosis is induced. (Shallow respiration favors retention of carbon dioxide and an increase in the acid side of the carbonic acid:base bicarbonate ratio.) Note the low pH during the night hours in Figure 13-10. A rise in pH usually occurs upon awakening.

2. A rise in pH usually occurs following meals, since they stimulate the production of hydrochloric acid, a process causing hydrogen ions to be extracted from the blood. The type of food ingested affects pH. (See Table 14-5 for the acid-base reactions of various foods.) Note the rise in pH following meals in Figure 13-10.

3. Certain drugs significantly alter urinary pH. Drugs that cause urine to become more acid include ammonium chloride, methenamine mandelate (Mandelamine), or sodium acid phosphate, and those that can cause urine to become alkaline include alkaline salts, such as sodium bicarbonate or potassium citrate.

In spite of the variables that influence urinary pH, most random urine samples show a pH of less than 6.6.

The nurse may be asked to perform urinary pH tests at the bedside for patients with a variety of metabolic disorders. Table 13-17 lists conditions in which urine is persistently acid or alkaline.

Several simple methods may be used by the nurse to measure urinary pH.

Table 13-17.   Clinical Conditions Associated With Persistently Acid or Alkaline Urine

Symptom	Imbalance Indicated by Symptom
Acid Urine	Metabolic acidosis: Daibetic acidosis, Ketosis of starvation, Severe diarrhea. Respiratory acidosis: Emphysema, Asthma. Metabolic alkalosis accompanied by severe potassium deficit
Alkaline Urine	Metabolic alkalosis: Excessive ingestion of alkalis, Severe vomiting. Respiratory alkalosis: Oxygen lack, Fever with its hyperpnea. Primary hyperaldosteronism. Acidosis accompanied by the following clinical conditions: *Chronic renal infection,* in which the infecting organism converts urea in newly-formed urine to ammonia. *Milkman's syndrome,* a severe chronic acidosis apparently secondary to renal tubular dysfunction. *Fanconi's syndrome,* a form of chronic acidosis secondary to renal tubular dysfunction. *Sulfanilamide intoxication* secondary to renal tubular dysfunction. *Pharmacologic alkalinuria* produced by a carbonic anhydrase inhibitor [such as acetazolamide (Diamox) or chlorothiazide (Diuril)]. *Persistent acidosis* secondary to renal tubular dysfunction in infants

Squibb Nitrazine Paper   Nitrazine Paper consists of a chemical (sodium dinitrophenolazonaphthol disulfonate) impregnated in cellulose. When Nitrazine Paper is dipped into urine, a chemical change takes place that causes the paper to change color. The color can vary from yellow to blue and is matched against the scale on the paper dispenser. The color changes correspond to specific pH levels ranging from 4.5 to 7.5 (Fig. 13-11). The nurse should keep the following points in mind while performing this test:

1. Only fresh urine should be used. (When urine is allowed to set for a time, urea breaks down into ammonia and the pH becomes more alkaline.)

2. The paper should be well moistened with urine but should not be left in the urine more than a few seconds—excessive fluid can wash away the chemicals from the paper.

3. After the paper has been dipped into the urine, the excess urine should be shaken off and the reading made immediately.

4. The color comparison between the Nitrazine Paper and the color scale on the dispenser should be made in a good light—avoid color comparison in pure fluorescent light.

Ames Combistix Dip Sticks   Combistix is a dip-and-read combination test for urine protein, glucose and pH. Barriers are impregnated in the dipstock to separate the three areas; otherwise, the chemicals from each portion would run together when moist-

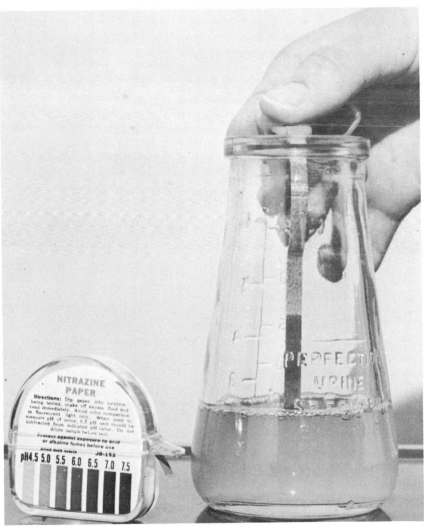

Figure 13-11.   Measuring urinary pH with Nitrazine Paper.

ened. The pH portion of the reagent strip is impregnated with methyl red and bromthymol blue. When dipped into urine, a color change takes place. The color varies from orange to blue and represents a pH range of from 5 to 9. The nurse should keep the following points in mind while performing this test:

1. Only fresh urine should be used.
2. Care should be taken to prevent excessive urine from washing chemicals from the other portions of the reagent strip onto the pH portion.

Regardless of the type of test used, it is important that the nurse read the manufacturer's directions carefully. Accurate results can be expected only when instructions are followed as directed.

CHANGES IN URINARY VOLUME Generally speaking, urinary output can safely range from 25 to 500 ml. per hour. The nurse should report hourly output below 25 ml. or above 500 ml., also an output of less than 500 ml. in a 24-hour period. Expected urinary volume can range from 1000 to 2000 ml./24 hr. (40 to 80 mg./hr.) in patients in a basal state; it may decrease temporarily to 750 to 1200 ml./24 hr. (30 to 50 ml./hr.) following physical stress. The expected urinary volume varies with each patient and is influenced by many factors. Urine volume is dependent on:

1. The amount of fluid intake
2. Water needs of the lungs, skin, and gastrointestinal tract
3. The amount of waste products to be excreted by the kidneys
4. The ability of the kidneys to concentrate urine
5. Blood volume
6. Hormonal influences
7. Age

Fluid Intake

1. In health, urinary volume is approximately equal to the volume of liquids taken into the body—this rule does not hold true in illness. (See Table 13-18.)
2. A large intake of liquids causes a large uri-

Table 13-18. 24-Hour Average Intake and Output of Water in an Adult

Intake		Output	
Oral liquids	1300 ml.	Urine	1500 ml.
Water in food	1000 ml.	Stool	200 ml.
Water of oxidation	300 ml.	Insensible:	
		Lungs	300 ml.
		Skin	600 ml.
Total	2600 ml.	Total	2600 ml.

Reprinted from Bland, J.: Clinical Metabolism of Body Water and Electrolytes. Philadelphia: W. B. Saunders Co., 1963, p. 48, with permission.

nary output; a small intake causes a small urinary output.

3. Adults usually pass between 1000 to 1500 ml. of urine in 24 hours. (Most persons void five to ten times during the waking hours; each voiding is usually between 100 to 300 ml.)

Water Needs of the Lungs, Skin, and Gastrointestinal Tract

1. Water is available for urine formation only after the needs of the skin, the lungs, and the gastrointestinal tract have been met.
2. Excessive sweating causes a decreased urinary volume—daily urinary volume is several hundred ml. less in the summer.
3. Increased water loss from the lungs occurs with hyperpnea—this loss can cause a reduction in the urinary volume.
4. Excessive losses of fluid in vomiting and diarrhea can also cause a decreased urinary volume.

Amount of Waste Products to Be Excreted

1. Under most circumstances, urine volume varies directly with the urinary solute load—a solute excess causes an increased need for water excretion.
2. Excessive fluid loss may occur as the result of increased solute loads found in diabetes mellitus, thyrotoxicosis, fever, and response to stress.
3. A decreased solute load causes a decreased urinary volume.

Ability of the Kidneys to Concentrate Urine

1. Kidneys able to concentrate urine normally have less need for water than damaged kidneys—a normal individual with a urinary specific gravity of 1.029 to 1.032 requires 15 ml. of water to excrete 1 Gm. of solute, whereas an individual with nephritis and a urinary specific gravity of 1.010 to 1.015 requires 40 ml. of water to excrete 1 Gm. of solute.
2. Low concentrating ability of the kidneys results in large urinary output.
3. Provided renal concentration is normal, the least amount of urine needed for excretion of daily metabolic wastes is 400 to 500 ml.
4. An acutely ill patient, or one with poor kidney function, may need to excrete as much as 3000 ml. of urine daily to rid the body of waste products.

Blood Volume

1. A decreased blood volume causes decreased urinary output primarily due to changes in arterial pressure and pressure in the glomeruli. (This phenomenon explains the oliguria or anuria of profound shock.)
2. An increased blood volume causes increased urinary output, again primarily due to changes in arterial pressure and pressure in the glomeruli.

Hormonal Influences

1. An increased secretion of antidiuretic hormone occurs when the blood volume is decreased—the kidneys increase water reabsorption, and the urinary volume is decreased.
2. An increased secretion of aldosterone occurs when the blood volume is decreased—the kidneys increase sodium reabsorption, and the urine volume is decreased.
3. A decreased secretion of antidiuretic hormone occurs when the blood volume is increased—the kidneys decrease water reabsorption, and the urinary volume is increased.

4. A decreased secretion of aldosterone occurs when the blood volume is increased—the kidneys excrete more sodium and the urinary volume is increased.

Age

1. Data presented by Behnke indicate that the aged have a smaller urinary output (0.8 ml./min.) than do younger adults (1.0 ml./min.).
2. The decreased urinary volume in the aged is related to a decreased renal blood flow, secondary to vascular changes—the narrowed vessels decrease plasma filtration and cause less urine to be formed.
3. The decreased urinary volume in the aged may also be related to diet—most aged persons consume much more carbohydrate than protein. (Carbohydrate presents less of a solute load than the nitrogenous end products of protein.)
4. The aged tend to drink less than younger adults.
5. The aged have a decreased concentrating power. It is important for the nurse to remember that when an increased solute load is presented to such patients, a large urinary volume will result. Such patients require a larger water intake when the renal solute load is high. (See Table 13-19 for conditions associated with urinary volume changes.)

Table 13-19. Significance of Urinary Volume Changes

Symptom	Imbalance Indicated by Symptom
Oliguria	Fluid volume deficit
	Sodium deficit
	Potassium excess
	Severe sodium excess
	Renal calcification due to calcium excess
	Shock
	Renal insufficiency (late in disease)
Polyuria	Interstitial fluid-to-plasma shift
	Diabetes insipidus
	Increased renal solute load:
	Diabetes mellitus
	Infection
	Calcium excess
	Hyperthyroidism
	Renal insufficiency (early)
	"Salt-losing" nephritis

Measuring and Recording Fluid Intake and Output

INTAKE-OUTPUT RECORDS A workable intake-output record has appropriate columns for all types of fluid gains and losses. The volumes and types of fluid taken into the body are entered on the left side of the record, and the volumes and types of fluids lost from the body are entered on the right. The intake side of most records provides a column for oral intake and another column for parenteral fluids or other avenues of fluid gain. The output side usually provides a column for urine output and another column for gastrointestinal fluid losses or other routes of fluid loss. The record should be sufficiently simple so that the method of its use is self-evident, and necessary instructions should be incorporated in the record.

It is easy to become confused by intake-output records because they vary from hospital to hospital and even within the same hospital. For example, a burn unit requires a different intake-output record from that required in a general surgical unit.

The type of intake-output record used often depends on the patient's condition. A patient with a severe fluid balance problem may require an hourly summary of his fluid gains and losses, so that the physician can plan treatment according to immediate needs. Figure 13-12 depicts a bedside record suitable for an hourly fluid gain and loss summary. Many patients require only 8-hour summaries of their fluid gains and losses. Figure 13-13 depicts a bedside record suitable for this purpose. Both of these records provide for a 24-hour total. Some hospitals use a small intake-output slip at the bedside; at the end of each shift, the total is transferred to a summary sheet on the patient's chart. Completed intake-output records are attached to the patient's chart and kept as permanent records.

The use of the bedside intake-output record is facilitated when it is kept on a clipboard with an attached pen.

INDICATIONS FOR INTAKE-OUTPUT MEASURE-MENT Physicians often indicate which patients are to have records kept of their daily fluid intake and output. However, the failure of the physician to request intake-output measurement is no reason to omit it when the patient has a real or potential water and electrolyte balance problem. Many physicians assume that the nurse will initiate intake-output meas-

urement when necessary, without a written order. Patients with the following conditions should automatically be placed on the fluid intake-output measurement list:

Following major surgery
Thermal burns or other serious injuries (especially head and facial bone injuries)
Suspected or known electrolyte imbalance
Acute renal failure
Oliguria
Congestive heart failure
Abnormal losses of body fluids
Lower nephron nephrosis
Diuretic therapy
Corticoid therapy
Inadequate food and fluid intake
Coma

NEED FOR ACCURATE INTAKE-OUTPUT RECORDS Most discrepancies between gains and losses of body fluids can be detected when an accurate record is kept of the total fluid intake-output. The content of the gained and lost fluids is as important as their volume and, because the electrolyte content of the individual body fluids varies widely, the amount of each fluid lost should be designated on the intake-output record. The amounts and kinds of fluids taken into the body should also be recorded.

Ideally, the physician should be able to use the nursing intake-output records as a major tool in diagnosis as well as in the formulation of fluid replacement therapy. However, most physicians regard the usual intake-output record with the proverbial grain of salt. They are justified in complaining that an accurate account of a patient's intake-output is extremely difficult to obtain in the average hospital.

CAUSES OF INACCURATE INTAKE-OUTPUT RECORDS Neglect in keeping accurate nursing intake-output records is widespread and causative factors are extremely difficult to pinpoint. However, the difficulty seems to be related to a combination of the following factors:

Failure to comprehend the value of accurate intake-output records
Understaffed patient-care units
Lethargic and improperly motivated personnel
Lax supervision

LIQUID INTAKE AND OUTPUT RECORD

Patient's Last Name	First Name

History Number

Location	Service	Date

Time A.M. or P.M.	INTAKE (in cc.)					OUTPUT (Measured or estimated in cc.)					
	Oral or tube		Parenteral		Running Total	Sweat + to ++++	Urine	Other (feces, vomitus, etc.)			Running Total
	Type	Amount	Composition	Amount				Type	Amount		

Figure 13-12. Liquid intake and output record suitable for hourly measurement. (From Bland, J.: Clinical Metabolism of Body Water and Electrolytes. Philadelphia: W. B. Saunders Co., 1963, p. 215. Used with permission)

Decatur Memorial Hospital
24-HOUR INTAKE AND OUTPUT RECORD
11 P.M.–11 P.M.   **Record Output**
Time: Check

LIQUID MEASUREMENTS (Average) 1 oz. 30cc
Jello ....120cc   Fruit Juice Glass 100cc
Ice Cream ..120cc   Reg. Drinking Glass 240cc
Cup ....150cc   Squat Tray Glass 200cc
Soup Bowl ..120cc   Bedside Water Pitcher .900cc
Coffee Pot ..240cc   Paper Cup & Glass 180cc

Directions: Enter amount ON LINE in square. When time of act is significant, write time in top corner of square and circle it. When recording a series, center time in top square only. A new form must be put at bedside when 24 Hour Record is removed for totalling.

ORAL INTAKE (Include Tube Feedings)

	11–7	7–3	3–11

8-Hour Oral Totals ....

PARENTERAL FLUID INTAKE
(Blood, Plasma, I.V., Sub. Fluids)
Record Time Started)

	11–7	7–3	3–11

8-Hour Parenteral Totals ....

8-Hour Total Intake 11–7 _____ + 7–3 _____ + 3–11 _____ = Total 24-Hour Intake

NOTE: Record amount of Parenteral Fluid started. Make entry and minus sign if not taken. Subtract when totalling.

URINE OUTPUT (Record Urethral Catheter—C; Ureteral—U)

Describe urine if significant	11–7	7–3	3–11

8-Hour Urine Output Totals ....

ALL OTHER OUTPUT   (Emesis, Gastric Suction, Bile, Liquid Stool)

Record	11–7	7–3	3–11

Diaphoresis M–moderate P–profuse

8-Hour Output (All except Urine) Totals ....

8-Hour Total Output 11–7 _____ + 7–3 _____ + 3–11 _____ = Total 24-Hour Output

Form No. 9314 Rev. 7/76

Figure 13-13. Twenty-four hour intake-output record. (Courtesy of Decatur Memorial Hospital, Decatur, Illinois)

Unqualified personnel giving direct care to seriously ill patients

Inadequate in-service education programs for all levels of personnel

Failure to devise or implement a workable intake-output record

ACHIEVING ACCURATE INTAKE-OUTPUT RECORDS   It is not technically difficult to measure fluid intake and output or to record the measurements. Yet, persistent effort is required if one is to achieve an accurate account of gains and losses of fluids.

There are innumerable possibilities for error in the measurement and recording of fluid gains and losses; however, some errors occur much more frequently than others. Common errors and suggestions on overcoming them are shown in Table 13-20.

Table 13-20.   Overcoming Common Errors

Common Errors	Suggestions
Errors Involving Both Intake and Output:	
1. Failure to communicate to the entire staff which patients require intake-output measurement (Body fluids are often discarded without being measured, and oral fluids are not recorded, merely because staff members are not aware of the patients on intake-output)	a. A "measure intake-output" sign should be attached to the patient's bed to serve as a reminder. b. A list of all patients requiring intake-output measurement should be posted in a convenient work area for quick reference. c. Also for quick reference, the cardex should contain a list of all patients requiring intake-output measurement. d. An adequate patient report should be given to all personnel.
2. Failure to explain intake output to the patient and his family (Most patients will cooperate if they know what is expected of them)	a. Both the patient and his family should receive a simple explanation of why intake-output measurement is necessary. b. Careful instructions are necessary to acquaint the patient and his family with their role in helping to achieve an accurate intake-output record.
3. Well meaning intentions to record a drink of water or an emptied urinal at a later, more convenient time are often forgotten	Measurements should be recorded at the time they are obtained.
4. Failure to measure fluids that can be directly measured because it takes less time to guess at their amounts	Measure *all* fluids amenable to direct measurement—guesses should be reserved for fluids that cannot be measured directly.
Errors Related to Intake:	
5. Failure to designate the specific volume of glasses, cups, bowls, and other fluid containers used in the hospital (Each person may ascribe a different volume to the same glass of water)	The bedside record should list the volumes of glasses, cups, bowls, and other fluid containers used in the hospital (see Fig. 13-13).
6. Failure to obtain an adequate measuring device for small amounts of oral fluids (Patients frequently drink small quantities of fluids; the amounts must be estimated unless a calibrated cup is available—frequent estimates increase the margin of error)	Small calibrated paper cups should be kept at the bedside for such a purpose.
7. The amount of fluid taken as ice chips is frequently under-estimated	The nurse should consider that a full glass of ice chips is approximately half a glass of water when melted; for example: a 200 ml. glass filled with ice chips will contain approximately 100 ml. of water after the ice is melted (Fig. 13-14).

Table 13-20. (Continued)

Common Errors	Suggestions
8. Failure to consider the volume of fluid displaced by ice in iced drinks frequently causes an overstatement of ingested oral fluids	Only small amounts of ice should be used for iced drinks so that the accurate amount of fluid ingested can be recorded.
9. Assuming that the contents of empty containers were drunk by the patient (Patients sometimes give their coffee or juice to a visiting relative or other patients in the room; they may forget to tell the person checking the tray)	The patient should be asked what fluids he drank.
10. Failure to detect that a patient has exaggerated his fluid intake, perhaps to avoid unwanted oral fluids or a parenteral infusion	Patients who frequently try to convey the idea that they will drink fluids after the nurse has left the room should be suspected.
11. Failure to accurately record the amount of parenteral fluid administered on each shift	a. The actual amount of parenteral fluid run in on each shift should be recorded. b. The amount of solution left in the bottle at the end of a shift should be noted, in pencil, on the bedside record—this makes it easier for the next shift to determine the amount run in on their time.
12. Failure to note inadequate intake of solid foods (It is frequently forgotten that solid foods are mainly water, and failure to eat solids causes an increased need for liquids)	Notations concerning inadequate food intake should be made in the appropriate place on the patient's chart.

Errors Related to Output:

Common Errors	Suggestions
13. Failure to estimate fluid lost as perspiration (Many nurses fail to recognize perspiration as a major source of fluid loss)	a. An attempt should be made to describe the amount of clothing and bed linen saturated with perspiration—it has been estimated that one necessary bed change represents at least 1 L. of lost fluid. b. Some intake-output records require the nurse to estimate perspiration as +, ++, +++, or ++++ (+ represents sweating that is just visible, and ++++ represents profuse sweating).
14. Failure to estimate "uncaught" vomitus (Frequently, "uncaught" emesis is recorded merely as a lost specimen)	The amount of fluid lost as vomitus should be estimated, and recorded as an estimate—it is better to make a guess than to give no indication at all as to the amount.
15. Failure to estimate the amount of incontinent urine (Intake-output records often indicate the number of incontinent voidings but give no indication of the amounts; obviously, such records are of little value)	The amount of incontinent urine should be estimated—it is helpful to note the amount of clothing and bed linen saturated with urine.
16. Failure to estimate fluid lost as liquid feces	a. The patient should be encouraged to use the bedpan rather than the toilet so that the fluid loss can be directly measured. b. The amount of fluid lost in incontinent liquid stools should be estimated.
17. Failure to estimate fluid lost as wound exudate	a. The amount of drainage on a dressing should be measured and charted—this can be done by measuring the width of the stained area and determining the thickness of the dressing. b. If extreme measures are necessary, the dressing can be weighed before application and again when removed.

Table 13-20.   (Continued)

Common Errors	Suggestions
18. Failure to check a urinary catheter for patency when there is decreased drainage of urine (It is sometimes too quickly assumed that decreased drainage from a catheter is due to decreased urine formation)	Decreased drainage from a urinary catheter is an indication to irrigate it and check for patency before charting the absence of, or decrease in, urinary output.
19. Failure to obtain an adequate measuring device for hourly or more frequent checks on urinary output (An error of even 10 ml. could be significant when dealing with small amounts of urine)	A handy device for frequent volume checks on urinary output is the Davol Uri-meter (Fig. 13-15). This device is calibrated to measure small amounts of urine—after the hourly amount has been measured, the petcock can be opened and the urine drained into a collecting bag.
20. Failure to record the amount of solution used to irrigate tubes and the amount of fluid withdrawn during the irrigation	a. One method for dealing with this problem is to add the amount of irrigating solution to the intake column, and to add the amount of fluid withdrawn to the output column. b. Another method is to compare the amount of irrigating solution used and the amount of fluid withdrawn during the irrigation—if more fluid was put in than was taken out, the excess is added to the intake column; if more fluid was taken out than was put in, the excess is added to the output column.

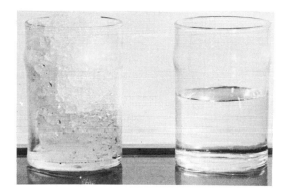

Figure 13-14.   Liquid volume of a glass of ice chips.

Body Weight

The daily weighing of patients with potential or actual fluid balance problems is of great clinical value because (1) accurate body weight measurements are much easier to obtain than accurate intake-output measurements and (2) rapid variations in weight closely reflect changes in fluid volume. A loss of body weight will occur when the total fluid intake is less than the total fluid output; conversely, a gain in body weight will occur when the total fluid intake is greater than the total fluid output (Table 13-21). For instance, a gain or loss of 1 kg. (2.2 lb.) of body

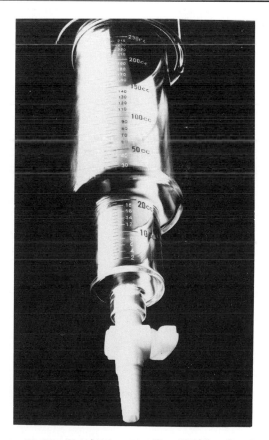

Figure 13-15.   Davol Uri-meter. (Davol Rubber Co., Providence, Rhode Island)

Table 13-21.   Significance of Weight Changes

Symptom	Imbalance Indicated by Symptom
Rapid loss of 2% total body weight	Mild fluid volume deficit
Rapid loss of 5% total body weight	Moderate fluid volume deficit
Rapid loss of 8% total body weight	Severe fluid volume deficit
Rapid gain of 2% total body weight	Mild fluid volume excess
Rapid gain of 5% total body weight	Moderate fluid volume excess
Rapid gain of 8% total body weight	Severe fluid volume excess
Chronic weight loss	Protein deficit

weight is approximately equivalent to the gain or loss of 1 L. of fluid.

The nurse should recall that fluids can be lost to the body in the pooling that occurs, for example, with intestinal obstruction. Such losses, which can cause a serious fluid volume deficit, are not reflected by weight changes.

Daily weight measurement may be indicated in the same conditions listed earlier as indications for fluid intake-output measurement. At the minimum, all patients should be weighed on admittance, so that a baseline can be established for later comparison.

It is important that the same scale be used for repeated measurements, since any two portable scales seldom give the same reading. The daily variations in weight should reflect true body weight changes rather than variations between scales.

Ambulatory patients may be weighed on small portable scales. Seriously ill patients confined to bed can be weighed with a bed scale (Fig. 13-16).

The weighing procedure with a bed scale can be performed with a minimum of effort for both the patient and the nurse. The patient is turned on one side, making room for the scale board on the mattress. The scale is rolled under the bed, automatically positioning the weighing board over the mattress. The board is lowered until it rests on the mattress. The patient is turned onto the scale board with his body weight evenly distributed; the arms should be folded over the chest, if possible, or placed at the patient's side on the board in order to prevent them from hanging off the side of the board. The board is raised hy-

draulically a few inches above the mattress, the patient is weighed, and the board is lowered to the mattress; the patient is moved off the board and the scale is removed. The In-Bed scale is particularly safe, since the patient remains within the confines of the bed during the entire process.

It is useless to weigh the patient daily if the procedure is not performed the same way each day. The nurse should strive for accurate weight measurements, because the physician often bases the administration of fluids and diuretics on the recorded weight changes. The following practices should be followed:

The same scales should be used each time.
The weight should be measured in the morning before breakfast.
The patient should empty his bladder before each weight measurement.
The same or similar clothing should be worn each time (the clothing should be dry).
The patient may be weighed wearing his glasses and wristwatch if desired—if so, they should be worn during each weight measurement.
A summary of all of the above points should be written on the cardex or the nursing care plan, so that a uniform weighing procedure is followed.

Frequency and Character of Stools

The nurse should record bowel movements and any significant facts related to them, on the chart. The consistency of the stool (solid or liquid) and the frequency of evacuation should be noted.

Abnormal fecal losses and their causal relationship to fluid imbalances are discussed earlier in this chapter. Table 13-22 lists some of the fluid imbalances accompanied by changes in the character and the frequency of bowel movements.

Table 13-22.   Significance of Stool Changes

Symptom	Imbalance Indicated by Symptom
Hard fecal mass	Fluid volume deficit
Intestinal colic with diarrhea	Sodium deficit Potassium excess
Ileus, abdominal distention (little or no stool or flatus passed) Diminished bowel sounds	Potassium deficit

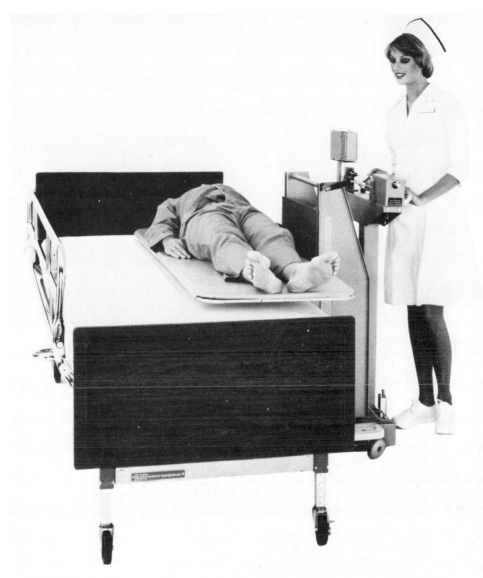

Figure 13-16. In-Bed[R] Scale. (Courtesy of Acme Scale, Co., Oakland, California, of which In-Bed is a registered trademark)

Blood Gases

Clinically, blood gas quantities may be roughly assessed by observing various signs in the patient. For example, insufficient oxygenation of blood may result in cyanosis. A decrease in the pulse rate and respiratory rate after a few minutes of oxygen administration demonstrates that hypoxemia was present. Elevation of the arterial pCO_2 concentration (up to 9 per cent) causes increased respirations, as does an increased hydrogen ion concentration. However, despite the help obtained from these observations, it is necessary to do blood gas analyses in seriously ill patients.

While caring for certain acutely ill patients, the nurse may be required to observe blood gas changes and take appropriate actions (within the treatment regimen prescribed by the physician). The changing blood gas values must be compared to each other and to previous readings and should be evaluated in relation to the patient's clinical appearance and medical history.

Some physicians leave an order to take samples for blood gas studies P.R.N. This requires the nurse to understand factors affecting blood gases and to recognize symptoms indicating a need to take a sample; such symptoms may include changes in respirations, color, level of consciousness, and restlessness. The nurse should recognize significant blood gas values and report them to the physician, because blood gas variations are early clues to changes in the patient's condition.

Blood gas analysis includes measurement of hydrogen, oxygen, and carbon dioxide tensions in arterial blood and expressed, respectively, as pH, pO_2, and pCO_2. These arterial blood gas values are:

pH—7.38 to 7.42
pCO_2—38 to 43 mm. Hg
pO_2—95 to 100 mm. Hg

Arterial blood specimens may be obtained from arterial punches or, less commonly, from indwelling arterial catheters. Common sites for arterial punch include the radial and brachial arteries. Nursing responsibilities in obtaining arterial blood samples for blood gas analysis are discussed in Chapter 24.

The nurse must understand the relationship between pH and pCO_2:

1. A fall in pH and a rise in pCO_2 indicates respiratory acidosis, often present in hypoventilation. Among the possible causes are emphysema, excessive secretions blocking the respiratory tract, heavy sedation, splinting caused by pain in the chest area, tight dressings, and improperly regulated mechanical respirators (causing respirations to be too slow or shallow).
2. A low pH occurring with a low pCO_2 indicates metabolic acidosis. The pH is low because the body is deficient in base bicarbonate, and the pCO_2 becomes low when the lungs attempt to compensate by eliminating more CO_2 (hyperventilation).
3. A high pH and a low pCO_2 indicates respiratory alkalosis, the primary problem of which is hyperventilation. Possible causes include anxiety, fever, hypoxia and improperly regulated mechanical respirators (causing respirations to be too fast or deep). If the hyperventilation is due to pain and anxiety, an appropriate analgesic should be administered.

4. A high pH and a high pCO_2 indicates metabolic alkalosis, of which the primary problem is an excess of base bicarbonate. The lungs attempt to compensate by retaining more carbon dioxide and, thus, elevate the carbonic acid level.

Arterial pO_2 is naturally much higher than venous pO_2 because arteries carry oxygenated blood.

Hypoventilation results in a decreased pO_2 and an elevated pCO_2, a situation that indicates the nurse should try to improve pulmonary ventilation. Such actions may include (depending on the circumstance):

Turning the patient from side to side at frequent intervals to allow for gravitational drainage of mucus from the various lung segments
Placing the patient in Fowler's or semi-Fowler's position to allow for greater chest expansion
Suctioning the patient as necessary to rid the respiratory tract of excessive secretions
Increasing activity, as outlined by the physician, to promote ventilatory and circulatory improvement
Performing other functions as prescribed by the physician, such as postural drainage, chest tapping, and intermittent positive pressure breathing treatments

A low pO_2 with a normal pCO_2 is an indication to administer oxygen in a concentration and by a route prescribed by a physician.

A postoperative patient with a low pO_2 and a low central venous pressure probably has a blood volume deficit and requires replacement therapy.

A patient with poor tissue perfusion will also have a low pO_2. Such a patient displays poor color and a lower-than-normal body temperature. In this instance, the nurse should provide warmth with extra blankets.

(The reader is encouraged to see Chapter 24 for a more thorough discussion of arterial blood gas studies.)

CONCLUSION

The preceding discussion of planned nursing observations has been quite general. The reader is encouraged to further explore and assimilate pertinent and detailed nursing observations (in context with appropriate nursing actions) in the chapters dealing with specific conditions (Chapters 17 through 27).

BIBLIOGRAPHY

Beland, I., and **Passos, J.:** Clinical Nursing, ed. 3. New York: Macmillan Publishing Co., 1975.

Berk, J., et al.: Handbook of Critical Care. New York: Little, Brown & Co., 1976.

Boedeker, E., and **Dauber, J.** (eds.): Manual of Medical Therapeutics, ed. 21. New York: Little, Brown and Co., 1974.

Condon, R., and **Nyhus, L.** (eds.): Manual of Surgical Therapeutics, ed. 3. New York: Little, Brown & Co., 1975.

Given, G., and **Simmons, S.:** Gastroenterology in Clinical Nursing, ed. 2. C. V. Mosby, 1975.

Luckman, J., and **Sorensen, K.:** Medical-Surgical Nursing: A Psychophysiological Approach. Philadelphia: W. B. Saunders Co., 1974.

Macleod, J. (ed.): Davidson's Principles and Practice of Medicine, ed. 11. London: Churchill Livingstone, 1975.

Maxwell, M., and **Kleeman, C.:** Clinical Disorders of Fluid & Electrolyte Metabolism, ed. 2. New York: McGraw-Hill Book Co., 1972.

Stroot, V., et al.: Fluids and Electrolytes: A Practical Approach, ed. 2. F. A. Davis Co., 1977.

— 14 —

The Nurse's Role in Preventing Imbalances of Water, Electrolytes, and Other Nutrients

"He who does not prevent a crime when he can, encourages it." Seneca

It is better to prevent disturbances of water, electrolytes, and other nutrients than to have to treat them after they have developed. Any patient can develop a serious nutritional disturbance if his needs for nutrients are not considered and met; consequently, the practical application of the principles of nutrition is as much a part of nursing as is the administration of medications. Examples of common clinical events that can lead to nutritional disturbances include:

1. Inadequate intake
2. Excessive losses from such conditions as
   a. Fever
   b. Excessive perspiration
   c. Vomiting
   d. Gastric or intestinal suction
   e. Diarrhea

3. Medical therapy, such as the prolonged use of diuretics, laxatives, enemas, or steroids
4. Catabolic effects, such as those induced by
   a. Immobilization
   b. Draining dedubitus ulcers
   c. Surgical operations (hemorrhage, toxic destruction of protein)
   d. Trauma

When one considers how frequently the nurse encounters situations such as these in her daily practice, the need for a carefully considered plan of action on her part becomes evident. *Such a plan must include meticulous observation of the patient.*

Compared to other healing disciplines, the profession of nursing is unique in that its ministrations are applied continuously to the hospitalized patient. The nursing staff is responsible for the intelligent execution of orders for solid foods and liquids during the entire 24-hour period. Far more is required than a rote performance of duties. Initiative is mandatory on the part of the nurse if the prescribed therapy is to produce optimal results.

In assuring the patient's nutritional welfare, the nurse functions in the framework formulated by the physician. Nevertheless, much is left to her discretion. For example, the order "diet as tolerated" is frequently written on surgical services, and the physician assumes that the nursing staff understands the patient's condition so as to execute properly such a diet order. Indeed, it would be impossible for the physician to detail step-by-step exactly what should be done for every patient, even when the diet order is relatively specific. When the nurse knows the general purpose and scope of the diet, she can exercise her judgment in accordance with the individual patient's needs.

The nurse should constantly be aware of the problems that may be posed by medication. Suppose a thiazide diuretic has been ordered. Since the nurse knows that this medication will, in all probability, increase the patient's need for potassium, she can encourage the ingestion of high potassium foods and, in addition, alert the physician to the possible need for a potassium supplement.

In instances such as those cited above, the nurse can often institute action to meet the new situation and, on other occasions, she must report her findings to the physician and seek his direction. Among the valuable resource personnel available to the nurse for consultation is the dietitian, who can frequently provide helpful suggestions if she is given background information based on careful nursing observations. The wise nurse consults other members of the health team when confronted by problems that tax her knowledge. Obviously, the patient benefits from such coordination.

The busy physician can easily miss notations in the nursing notes concerning a patient's inadequate intake of food and liquids. Sometimes such notations are not made because of laxity in checking the patient's tray after meals, or in recording the findings on the patient's chart, which should always contain a meaningful summary of the patient's food and fluid intake by the members of the nursing staff.

The importance of accurate nursing observations is revealed in questions commonly asked by physi-

cians when they evaluate the state of the patient's water and electrolytes balance:

1. Has the patient been eating and drinking normally? If not, for how long?
2. Have abnormal losses of body fluids occurred, as perspiration, vomiting, gastric or intestinal suction, drainage from enterostomy, colostomy, or fistulas, liquid stools, wound, or burn exudate?
3. Has there been an acute weight loss or an acute weight gain?
4. Have therapeutic fluids been given by tube or parenterally (if patient has been under treatment by another physician)?
5. Has the patient been on a restrictive diet (if patient has been under treatment by another physician)?
6. Has the patient been given medications that might cause body fluid disturbances?

Obviously, conditions that cause disturbances of water and electrolytes can also cause deficits of other nutrients, such as protein, carbohydrate, fat, or vitamins.

INADEQUATE INTAKE

Intake Via the Gastrointestinal Route

With respect to the intake of water, electrolytes, vitamins, and other nutrients, the oral route has long been preferred for the prevention of deficits and the correction of mild deficits already present. It offers several advantages:

1. Because it allows gradual absorption, the oral route provides far greater efficiency in the utilization of administered nutrients.
2. Large quantities of water, electrolytes, and other nutrients can be ingested over a short period without upsetting water and electrolyte balance.
3. The oral route is far less expensive.
4. The oral route appeals to the patient as being more natural.

(Naturally, the gastrointestinal tract must be functional if the oral route is to be used.)

The ingestion of nutrients is so commonplace that its significance is frequently overlooked, possibly because the oral route lacks the dramatic impact of parenteral or nasogastric feedings. Yet, oral administration can frequently prevent serious disturbances of the body fluids.

Since the oral route is the normal way to obtain nutrients, it possesses a distinct psychologic appeal. Frequently a patient feels he is quite ill simply because he is denied food by the oral route.

NURSING MEASURES TO PROMOTE EATING

Illness or imposed dietary restrictions may greatly decrease the desire to eat, and offering an adequate diet does not guarantee that the patient will accept it. The real test of nursing skill is not to order and serve a diet; rather, it lies in getting the patient to eat it. The nurse should keep the following points in mind:

- Review the patient's eating habits, his food likes and dislikes, and the cultural and religious beliefs that influence his eating habits.
- Permit the patient to make dietary choices when possible, since this will increase the acceptability of the diet.
- Display a sincere interest in the patient and avoid a forceful, goading approach to encourage eating.
- Eliminate unpleasant sights and odors at mealtime (e.g., change soiled dressings, empty ileostomy bags, remove from sight such items as bedpans, urinals, dead flowers).
- Minimize strong emotions near mealtime, when possible, since they affect both appetite and digestive processes adversely. (Incidents that irritate the patient should be noted on the nursing care plan and avoided, if possible, in the future.)
- Avoid unpleasant procedures in the vicinity at mealtime.
- See that the patient is clean before eating (change soiled linens, wash face and hands).
- Provide comfort measures as needed before meals (e.g., the patient with a distended bladder may need to be catheterized; the patient in pain may require a p.r.n. medication).
- Position the patient in high Fowler's, if permitted, to facilitate ease of swallowing.

- Situate the tray so that it is easy for the patient to reach.
- Help the patient prepare the tray if this is necessary (open milk cartons, pour coffee, cut up food). Remember that a weak patient, or one with an I.V. tube in his hand, cannot easily perform these activities.
- Serve food portions appropriate to the patient's appetite (remember that a patient with a small appetite can be repelled by large portions of food).
- Avoid unnecessary interruptions during meals (the not-too-eager appetite can be easily discouraged by the poor planning of nursing activities).
- Be sure that patients with dentures have them in place before serving the meal. Patients with ill-fitting dentures or few teeth may require soft or liquid foods to provide adequate nourishment. Dietary departments will usually grind hard to chew foods for such patients if requested.
- Serve trays last to patients who must be fed. (It is frustrating for patients to wait for someone to return to feed them.)
- Feed patients in a friendly, unhurried manner, allowing sufficient time to chew and swallow comfortably. Offer liquids and solids alternately in manageable amounts.
- Allow the patient's family to bring him favorite foods from home, if permitted, under nursing supervision.
- Encourage the patient to be as physically active as allowed to stimulate his appetite.

Every effort should be made to prevent nausea and vomiting after meals; therefore, the patient should not be turned quickly or subjected to excessive physical activity. On the other hand, mild exercise should not be condemned, for it may aid digestion. If nausea should occur, appropriate medication may be given in accord with medical orders. In the absence of a p.r.n. order for nausea, the nurse might seek a medical order. The cause of the nausea should be sought and noted on the chart.

Although the points just enumerated are well-known to most nurses, *we are convinced that they cannot be overemphasized.* One does well to remember that any program of diet therapy is worthless if the patient does not eat! Conversely, any measure capable of promoting food and liquid intake contributes to the patient's welfare. The nurse should impress the importance of these facts on the auxiliary staff members, who are frequently charged with important responsibilities associated with feeding the patients.

ELEMENTAL DIETS Elemental diets* are powdered mixtures of basic nutrients (eight essential amino acids plus a number of nonessential amino acids, simple sugars, electrolytes, minerals, trace elements, and essential fatty acids). When mixed with water the powdered mixture forms a stable solution, similar in content to those used for parenteral hyperalimentation. Elemental diets are frequently used to maintain caloric and nitrogen balance over long periods of time when the patient is unable to eat conventional foods. These diets are low in bulk and require only minimal digestive effort before total absorption in the small intestine. Biliary, pancreatic, and gut secretions are decreased with the use of elemental diets, making them useful in such conditions as pancreatitis, fistulas, and inflammatory bowel disease. Some elemental diets are available with low sodium content for patients requiring low sodium intake. Points to consider in the use of elemental diets include the following:

1. Elemental diets are hyperosmolar, causing them to draw fluid into the stomach if consumed too rapidly, thus resulting in gastric distention, nausea, vomiting, cramping, and diarrhea. Some diets have added flavorings to mask their metallic taste; these flavorings further increase the osmolarity of the feeding.

2. To prevent these untoward gastrointestinal symptoms, the patient should be instructed to sip a glass of the solution slowly over a period of an hour. *The mixture should never be drunk all at once* (although patients may try to do so to avoid prolonging the unpleasant flavor). If given by tube feeding, the solution should be administered slowly.

3. Chilling improves the palatability of most flavors; however, patients with swallowing problems should take the liquid at room temperature.

4. *After the elemental diet is reconstituted, it becomes perishable and must be refrigerated.* It is best

to prepare no more than is needed in a 24-hour period.

5. Intake and output records should be kept and extra water should be provided to maintain an adequate urinary output. Periodic measurement of urinary glucose, acetone, and pH may be ordered. Because of the diet's high carbohydrate content, some depleted patients may develop hyperglycemia, requiring insulin for regulation.

6. Because elemental diets are hypertonic, they should be used cautiously in patients sensitive to hyperosmolarity (such as diabetics).

7. Remember that stool bulk is greatly diminished when elemental diets are the sole source of intake. (These diets were originally designed for astronauts with the purpose of producing minimal fecal waste while providing adequate nutrition.)

8. Daily weights should be recorded at first, then at least biweekly. After positive nitrogen balance has been achieved, the patient will begin gaining weight.

9. It is wise to monitor the blood urea nitrogen, glucose, serum electrolytes, and proteins at least weekly for patients receiving elemental diets.

Tube Feedings

INDICATIONS FOR TUBE FEEDINGS Oral intake might be impossible, even though adequate gastrointestinal function is present, in such situations as:

1. Semiconsciousness or unconsciousness
2. Oral surgery
3. Extreme anorexia
4. Swallowing problems
5. Weakness caused by chronic debilitating conditions
6. Disorientation
7. Serious mental diseases, such as major psychoses

The nurse must be aware of these conditions and report inadequate intake when any of them are present. The patient should not be permitted to develop malnutrition before another route for intake of nutrients is adopted. One solution to the problems posed by such patients is the use of tube feedings. Tube feedings have many advantages, especially when the problems requiring them are likely to be of long duration.

When oral intake is inadequate, tube feedings are

* Vivonex (Eaton Laboratories); Flexical (Mead Johnson & Co.); Precision LR (Doyle Pharmaceutical Co.).

used to administer the protein and calories necessary for tissue healing in such conditions as fractures, decubitus ulcers, and burns. An intake of at least 1600 to 2000 calories must be provided if the protein is to be used for tissue repair; otherwise, it will be used to meet energy needs.

Disorders of the gastrointestinal tract, such as biliary or pancreatic fistulas, or delayed emptying of the stomach, may necessitate passing a feeding tube beyond the affected area in order to administer nutrients. One of the few contraindications for tube feedings is the complete obstruction of the lower gastrointestinal tract.

Even if the underlying disease process cannot be corrected, the patient can live more comfortably during the weeks and months remaining if he is adequately nourished. The incidence of trophic ulcers, wasting, and debilitation is decreased by adequate nourishment.

Anorexia and malnutrition create a vicious cycle: anorexia leads to malnutrition; malnutrition promotes anorexia. The use of tube feedings for several weeks improves the patient's nutrition, as well as his appetite, thus interrupting the cycle. Visual evidence of the general improvement brought about by tube feedings is presented in Figure 14-1.

ROUTES FOR TUBE FEEDINGS Routes of administration for tube feedings include nasogastric intubation, gastrostomy, jejunostomy, and cervical pharyngostomy.[1] Nasogastric tube feeding is easily accomplished but has the disadvantage of nasal discomfort when the tube is in place for more than a few days. When a tube cannot be passed through the esophagus, a tube may be surgically introduced directly into the stomach (gastrostomy) or jejunum (jejunostomy). Jejunostomy feedings are preferred for patients with weak gag reflexes who are likely to aspirate vomitus. Cervical pharyngostomy is sometimes used for long-term feeding. It consists of introducing a feeding tube into the hypopharynx through a stab wound in the side of the neck. The distal end of the tube is then advanced through the esophagus into the stomach; a suture is used to hold the proximal end of the tube in place.

TUBE FEEDING MIXTURES Any tube feeding mixture should provide all the required solid nutrients—protein, carbohydrate, fat, minerals, and vitamins—and should incorporate generous quantities of

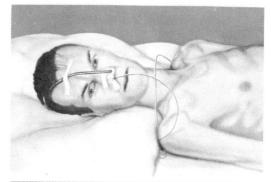
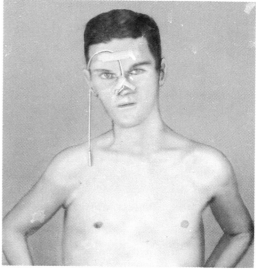

Figure 14-1. Improvement in nutritional status as a result of tube feedings. (From Barron, J.: Tube feeding of postoperative patients. Surg. Clin. N. Am. 39:1489, 1959, with permission from W. B. Saunders Co., Philadelphia)

water. Additional water, however, must be supplied if the daily requirement is to be met. It is especially necessary to provide adequate water for the elderly, confused, lethargic, and comatose, since these patients frequently do not experience or express normal thirst. The physician should prescribe the contents of the tube feeding and should designate the quantity and the times when it should be given.

Whole foods can be liquefied in a blender and administered by means of a tube, providing the ingredients of a natural diet with all known and unknown dietary essentials, relatively inexpensively. They sometimes cause less diarrhea and other untoward symptoms than commercial preparations. The content of such mixtures is readily varied if diarrhea should occur. Commercial strained baby foods can be administered as tube feedings. (See Table 14-1.)

Table 14-1. Composition and Nutritive Value of Blenderized Tube Feeding Mixture

	Unit	2000 ml.*	1000 ml.
Strained peas	Jars	1	½
Strained carrots	Jars	1	½
Strained beets	Jars	1	½
Strained applesauce	Jars	1	½
Strained beef	Jars	3	1½
Strained liver	Jars	1	½
Eggs	(Number)	2	1
Strained orange juice	ml.	200	100
18% cream	ml.	180	90
Milk.	ml.	700	350
Glucose	Gm.	60	30
Salt	Gm.	5	2

Reprinted from Artz, C., and Hardy, J.: Complications in Surgery and Their Management. Philadelphia: W. B. Saunders Co., 1961, p. 352, with permission.
* 2000 ml. contain approximately 1977 calories, 11 Gm. of sodium chloride, 120 Gm. protein, 89 Gm. fat and 174 Gm. of carbohydrate. Each 500 ml. would contain about 495 calories and 30 Gm. of protein.

Numerous convenient ready-to-use feeding mixtures* are available commercially and are widely used although they are more costly than blenderized feedings. Also used for tube feeding is a blenderized mixture of whole milk, powdered milk, egg yolks, orange juice, cream, yeast, and salt (Table 14-2).

Low bulk diets, described earlier in the chapter, may be used for tube feedings. Because they are hyperosmotic, they should be administered slowly by gravity drip or by a feeding pump.

TUBE FEEDING METHODS Every nurse should thoroughly understand both the role and the method of tube feedings, which can be administered by gravity flow or by mechanical pump. Many variations have been devised for administering tube feedings by gravity flow.

1. An *Asepto syringe* can serve as a funnel; it is frequently used to administer the feeding mixture (Fig. 14-2). The syringe attaches directly to the nasogastric tube, and flow rate is regulated by the height at which the nurse holds the syringe. Although the equipment is simple and easy to use, this method has sev-

---

* Meritene (Doyle Pharmaceutical Co.); Compleat-B (Doyle Pharmaceutical Co.); Ensure (Ross Laboratories); Isocal (Mead Johnson Laboratories); Sustacal (Mead Johnson Laboratories); Sustagen (Mead Johnson Laboratories); Portagen (Mead Johnson Laboratories); Nutri-1000 (Syntex Laboratories).

Table 14-2. Milk-base Tube Feeding Mixture

Contents	Approximate Amounts
Homogenized milk	4 cups
Instant nonfat dry milk	6 ounces
Egg yolks	4 yolks
Orange juice	7 ounces
Cream	1 cup
Brewer's yeast	3 tablespoons
Salt	1 teaspoon
Water	as needed

eral disadvantages. The tube feeding mixture is often administered too rapidly because the nurse lacks sufficient time to remain at the bedside for a slow delivery of the feeding. Also, the flow rate can be only crudely adjusted by raising or lowering the syringe.

2. *Disposable gravity-flow gastric feeding units* are available commercially and are desirable because the flow rate of the feeding mixture can be adjusted in drops and the constant attendance of the nurse is not required. One kind of disposable bag is the Davol Gastric Feeding Unit (Fig. 14-3). It consists of a graduated polyethylene bag, drip chamber, petcock shut-off for measurement of flow, wide plastic tubing, and a Sims connector for at-

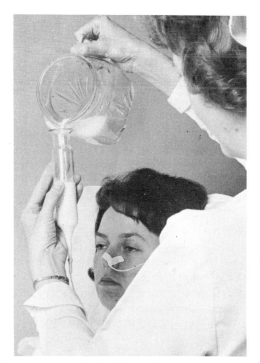

Figure 14-2. Tube feeding with an asepto syringe.

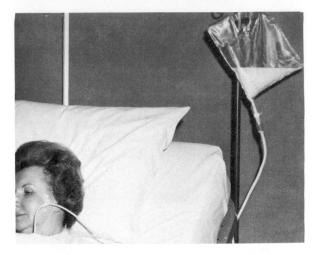

Figure 14-3. Tube feeding with Davol Gastric Feeding Unit. (Davol Rubber Co., Providence, Rhode Island)

tachment to the feeding tube. Another type of disposable feeding unit is the Kangaroo Tube Feeding Set (Fig. 14-4). This bag has a pouch to insert ice cubes to cool the feeding or warm water to heat the mixture, as indicated.

3. The *mechanical pump method* is more dependable than the gravity drip method for slow constant delivery of tube feedings. Factors that may cause an uneven flow rate in the gravity drip method include:

A. A change in the patient's position after the flow rate has been adjusted; almost invariably the patient will desire to change his position during the feeding, especially when the mixture is given slowly.

B. Failure to adjust the flow rate as frequently as necessary; frequent checks are indicated to assure maintenance of the desired flow rate.

C. A viscous mixture may clog the tube, especially when the flow has been disrupted by a position change.

A food pump, on the other hand, assures a constant flow rate regardless of the patient's position. A thick feeding may necessitate periodic rinsing of the tubing. An example of a commercial food pump is the Barron food pump* (Fig. 14-5). The pump can be used to deliver intermittent or continuous feedings.

The equipment includes the pump mechanism, the food container, an outer insulated container for ice, and the latex tubing (Fig. 14-6).

To prevent spoilage, the feeding solution is cooled by placing the food bottle in the non-drip insulated ice container.

The speed of the feeding, determined by the physician, is controlled by a pulley on the underside of the pump. (See Figure 14-7). There are four speeds for delivery of the solution:

1. First speed (low)— 43 ml./hr.
2. Second speed — 65 ml./hr.
3. Third speed —113 ml./hr.
4. Fourth speed —200 ml./hr.

* Randolph Surgical Supply Co., Ferndale, Michigan.

Figure 14-4. Kangaroo tube-feeding set keeps food solutions warm or cold as long as desired. The 1000-ml. feeding bag is of clear plastic and shows both volume issued and consumed. Clear polyvinyl drip chamber permits visual check on flow rate. Feeding chamber may be filled and sealed by dietitian thus eliminating need for intermediate containers. This is a sterile disposable product. (Courtesy of Chesebrough-Pond's, Inc. From Brunner, L., and Suddarth, D.: The Lippincott Manual of Nursing Practice, ed. 2, Philadelphia: J. B. Lippincott, Co., 1978, p. 505. Used with permission)

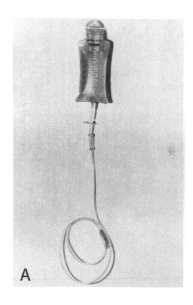

A

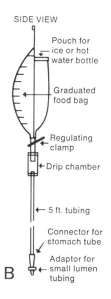

B

SIDE VIEW

- Pouch for ice or hot water bottle
- Graduated food bag
- Regulating clamp
- Drip chamber
- 5 ft. tubing
- Connector for stomach tube
- Adaptor for small lumen tubing

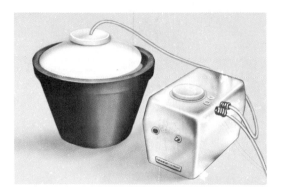

Figure 14-5. Barron Food Pump. (Manufactured by Randolph Surgical Supply Co., Ferndale, Michigan. From Friedrich, H.: Oral feeding by food pump. Am. J. Nurs. 62:63, 1962, with permission)

Selection of the Feeding Method When the tube feedings are ordered, the physician may indicate a specific method for administering the feeding solution. If he has no preference, the nurse may decide which method is best for the patient.

Factors to be considered in determining the best method to use include (1) the patient's condition, (2) the viscosity of the feeding mixture, and (3) the type of equipment available.

The patient's condition is an important factor. For example, comatose patients must have a slow delivery of solution to prevent gastric distention and vomiting, with possible tracheal aspiration. A food pump set at a slow speed or a gravity drip method suitable for slow delivery of the mixture should be

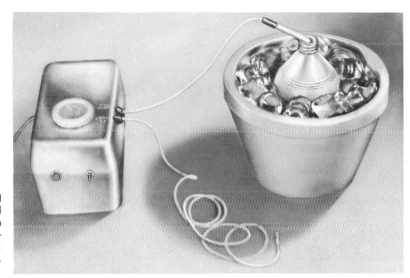

Figure 14-6. Pump mechanism, food container, insulated ice container, and tubing of the Barron Food Pump. (From Barron, J.: Tube feeding of postoperative patients. Surg. Clin. N. Am. 39: 1488, 1959, with permission from W. B. Saunders Co., Philadelphia)

Usually the slowest speed is necessary when the patient is first started on tube feedings, to minimize nausea, vomiting, cramping and diarrhea; the speed is gradually increased to the desired rate. To prevent distention, the end of the tubing should be kept below the level of the feeding solution so that air is not pumped into the stomach.

When used properly, food pumps conserve the nurse's time. The instructions accompanying the pump should be carefully studied before the feedings are started; otherwise the results will not be satisfactory.

Some intravenous infusion pumps may also be used to administer gastrointestinal feedings (such as the Ivac 530* or the Sigmamotor Volume†).

* Ivac Corporation, San Diego, California.
† Sigmamotor, Inc., Middleport, New York.

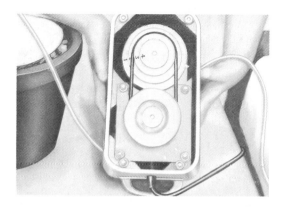

Figure 14-7. Pulley for regulating speed of Barron Food Pump. (From Friedrich, H.: Oral feeding by food pump. Am. J. Nurs. 62:63, 1962, with permission)

used. Patients receiving duodenal or upper jejunal feedings require a slow, constant feeding rate; best results are obtained with a mechanical food pump set at a low speed. All patients, however, do not require a constant, slow delivery of the feeding mixture. Many alert patients, free of gastrointestinal problems, can tolerate fairly rapid feedings if the amount given each time is small; any of the feeding methods described earlier can be adapted for their needs.

Failure to consider the viscosity of the feeding mixture can result in clogging the apparatus. A thick mixture is best given with a mechanical food pump or with a gravity drip apparatus having wide diameter tubing.

The type of equipment available greatly influences the method chosen; most hospitals have their own routine set-ups for tube feedings.

PREVENTION OF TUBE FEEDING COMPLICATIONS Although tube feedings have proved to be of immense value, they can cause trouble if given incorrectly. Complications of tube feedings include:

1. Diarrhea
2. Nausea
3. Vomiting
4. Aspiration pneumonia
5. Inadequate provision for water requirements
6. Metabolic alkalosis (primary base bicarbonate excess)

In order to avoid untoward reactions from tube feedings, the nurse should keep the following in mind:

1. The patient should be in a sitting position when receiving tube feedings. If this is not permitted, the head of the bed should be elevated to a 45 degree angle. The head of the bed should remain elevated for from 30 minutes to one hour following the feeding. This precaution is taken to prevent the aspiration of gastric contents if vomiting or regurgitation occurs; aspiration of the feeding mixture can cause pneumonia or strangulation. If the patient has a cuffed tracheostomy or endotracheal tube, the cuff should not be deflated during the feeding nor within an hour afterwards to prevent possible aspiration.

2. Check the position of the nasogastric tube prior to introducing the feeding mixture:

a. The nurse can ask the patient to speak—if the tube is in the trachea, he will be unable to do so.

b. The proximal end of the tube can be placed in a glass of water and if many bubbles appear as the patient exhales, the tube is in the respiratory tract. Remember that the absence of bubbles establishes that the tube is not in the breathing passage; it does not prove that the tube is in the stomach. Also remember that trapped air in the stomach can produce occasional bubbles.

c. Another method involves listening with a stethoscope placed over the stomach while introducing 5 to 10 ml. of air through the tube. If the tube is properly positioned, air will be heard entering the stomach. Belching will occur immediately if the tip of the tube is in the esophagus.

d. A common check used to determine if the feeding tube is in the stomach is the withdrawal of a small quantity of gastric juice prior to each feeding. (It may be necessary to turn the patient or slightly withdraw or advance the tube to situate the tip below the gastric fluid level.)

3. It is wise to check for gastric retention by aspirating the tube with an asepto or piston syringe prior to each feeding. The presence of a sizable volume of the previous feeding is an indication to withhold further feedings until the situation is reported to the physician. (Sometimes clear liquid feedings are given initially when the ability of the stomach to empty is in question.) Gastric distention predisposes to regurgitation and aspiration of stomach contents.

4. Avoid bacterial contamination of the tube feeding mixture and administration apparatus. Do not prepare more than a 24-hour volume of the mixture at one time and keep it refrigerated until ready for use (unless, of course, the mixture is in a ready to use unopened can). Administration equipment should be *rinsed thoroughly* after each use.

5. The tube feeding mixture should be neither too hot nor too cold, since such temperature extremes cause nausea and discomfort, especially if the feeding is given quickly. Refrigerated feedings should be warmed to room or body temperature by placing the container in a basin of hot water. The mixture should

not be overheated since this can curdle the protein in some feedings and clog the tubing.

6. It is wise to administer a small amount of water prior to giving the feeding mixture to assure patency of the tube and to moisten it (prevents feeding mixture from adhering to the wall of the tubing).[2]

7. The tube feeding mixture should be given slowly and in small amounts in order to avoid distention, nausea, and excessive peristalsis. When the intermittent method is used, the amount given at each feeding is determined by dividing the total 24-hour dose by the number of feedings. Frequently, 2000 ml. is given over a 24-hour period. Divided feedings may be given at intervals of 2, 3, or 4 hours. Individual feedings frequently vary between 150 and 250 ml., requiring approximately 30 minutes to administer. A single feeding should not exceed 300 ml. unless it is to be given very slowly.

8. From 20 to 50 ml. of lukewarm water should be administered through the tube after each feeding when the intermittent method is used (sometimes more than this amount is required to adequately clear the tubing and prevent clogging). Afterwards, the tube should be clamped and secured to the patient's clothing.

9. Additional water should be given as necessary to maintain a satisfactory urinary output (remember, the greater the protein intake, the greater the need for water). Extra water is particularly necessary when the patient has fever, decreased renal concentrating ability, or extensive tissue breakdown. Malfunctioning kidneys require more water to excrete a given amount of solute than do normal kidneys, and because aged patients frequently have impaired renal function, they require more water than do the young. Hypernatremia and an elevated blood urea nitrogen may develop after administration of an excessive solute load and inadequate water. Usually, 2000 to 2500 ml. of fluid daily (tube feeding volume plus extra water) will provide enough water if the feeding mixture contains less than 100 Gm. protein, 10 Gm. salt, and 2500 calories.[3] Early in protein overloading, the urine volume is large even though the water intake is inadequate; this can easily lead the staff to think that the water intake is adequate. In such instances, however, output actually exceeds intake. By the accurate recording of careful observations, the nurse can unmask the true situation. Confused or unconscious patients should be observed carefully for inadequate water intake, since they are not aware of thirst.

10. The amount of feeding taken should be recorded, as should the amount of water added before, between, and after feedings.

11. Urine output should be recorded and, unless abnormal fluid losses are occurring, the amount of water taken by mouth should roughly equal the urinary output.

12. If nausea should occur, the feeding should be stopped and the patient given a rest period until further medical orders are received. A p.r.n. medication for nausea may be necessary. It may be helpful to dilute the mixture and administer it more slowly; other times a change in the content of the feeding mixture may be required.

13. If diarrhea occurs, the feeding should be discontinued until further medical orders are received. Medication, such as Kaopectate or paregoric, may be ordered and given through the tube. Sometimes a modification is made in the feeding, such as decreasing its carbohydrate content.

14. The esthetic factors for patients taking food by mouth also apply to patients receiving tube feedings. Unpleasant stimuli inhibit the flow of juices needed for food digestion.

15. Even though the patient is not taking nourishment orally, one should respect his need for a clean mouth. Regurgitation can occur in patients receiving tube feedings, and when it does, the patient should be given a mouthwash. Even semi-alert patients can taste tube feedings. The nares should be cleaned and lubricated often to minimize discomfort caused by the tube.

16. Constipation may sometimes be a problem when liquefied natural foods are administered very slowly into the stomach. The nurse should observe the frequency and character of bowel movements so that constipation can be detected before a fecal impaction occurs. Sometimes laxatives are added through the feeding tube to correct constipation; other times, a change in the content of the feeding mixture may be needed.

Intake Via the Parenteral Route

The nurse's role in administering parenteral nutrients is discussed in Chapter 16.

CONDITIONS THAT CAUSE EXCESSIVE LOSSES

Fever

An increased metabolic rate accompanies fever. Each degree Fahrenheit the temperature is elevated causes a 7 per cent increase in metabolic rate, whereas each degree of Centigrade (Celsius) elevation causes a 13 per cent increase. Prolonged fever, particularly if it is high, can easily lead to body fluid disturbances, especially when the body's requirements for water and electrolytes are neglected. Fever causes an increased loss of water and electrolytes from lungs, skin, and kidneys. The increased metabolism that accompanies fever depletes the body stores of glycogen and causes an increased catabolism of protein. The increased solute load resulting from protein breakdown places an extra burden on the kidneys and losses of sodium, chloride, and potassium are increased.

The patient suffering from prolonged fever needs to have his intake of all nutrients augmented, and yet the feverish patient usually has anorexia. Moreover, there appears to be decreased intestinal motility and subnormal absorption of nutrients during fever. Catabolism of body tissues can easily lead to metabolic acidosis (primary base bicarbonate deficit).

The patient with prolonged fever requires increased water. The amount of additional water required depends on the degree of temperature elevation. For example, a temperature between 101 and 103°F. increases the 24-hour fluid requirement by at least 500 ml. and a temperature above 103°F. increases it by at least 1000 ml.[4]

The patient's intake of the bulk nutrients—protein, fat, and carbohydrate—should be increased; so should his intake of the water soluble vitamins, including members of the B complex and C. Adequate electrolytes, too, should be provided, particularly sodium and potassium. The effort to increase the patient's nutritional intake should not, of course, overtax his ability to ingest and digest food. Small, frequent servings will help avoid overtaxing the gastrointestinal tract. If the patient is unable to ingest adequate nutrients by mouth, then feedings by nasogastric tube or by the parenteral route should be considered.

Sweet concentrated liquids can cause abdominal distention and loss of appetite. Carbonated beverages, on the other hand, are usually well tolerated, as are fruit juices, tea, coffee, and water. The fat of fluid whole milk tends to slow down the emptying time of the stomach; skim milk is probably preferable for most patients.

Often a liquid diet is indicated for the acutely ill patient, providing 800 to 1200 calories, and providing water and calories needed to prevent severe depletion. The patient should be returned to a full diet as soon as he is able to ingest it.

If possible, the daily intake of protein for the febrile patient should be 60 to 100 Gm. or more. High protein drinks, such as powdered or liquid commercial protein concentrates, or eggnog, frequently are useful. Fats are an excellent source of calories and can be given in the form of egg yolk, milk, cream, ice cream, margarine and butter, provided they are tolerated, but when fats are not tolerated, carbohydrates can be used to provide generous quantities of calories.

While the patient is convalescing from a febrile illness, a diet generous in all essentials should be administered in order to repair deficits.

Excessive Perspiration

Sensible perspiration, or sweat, is a hypotonic liquid containing sodium, potassium, chloride, and small amounts of magnesium, ammonia, and urea. Insensible perspiration consists of water only and is lost through evaporation from body surfaces, including the skin and the lungs.

High environmental temperatures can cause the loss of large quantities of body water and electrolytes. In hot surroundings some workmen have been found to lose 8 to 10 L. of sweat a day.

Perspiration losses can be recorded both on the intake-output sheet and on the nurse's notes. The saturation of pajamas and bed linen should be recorded, as should the number of times it has been necessary to change them. Because it is difficult to estimate the amount of perspiration, some persons tend to ignore it altogether. Moderate intermittent sweating increases the 24-hour fluid need by 500 ml., moderate continuous sweating by 1000 ml., and profuse continuous sweating by 2000 ml. or more.[5]

Insensible loss equals approximately 1000 ml./m² of body surface/day in the hospitalized patient but, when respiration is hyperactive or fever is present, this loss may be greatly increased. Sweat losses (sensible perspiration) depend chiefly upon temperature, humidity, metabolic rate, and fever and, in disease, may equal 1000 or more ml./m.^{2} of body surface/day. Sweat losses can be roughly measured by weight changes if one considers other gains and losses of fluids.

Liquids should be given freely to the heavily perspiring patient and should contain both water and electrolytes. If sweat losses are replaced by water alone, sodium deficit (low sodium syndrome, hyponatremia, heat exhaustion) can easily occur. Among the sources of salt are the salt content of foods, salty broths, salt added at the table, and commercial salt tablets. Naturally, one should guard against producing a sodium excess caused by the administration of excessive quantities of sodium chloride. The patient on a low sodium diet often develops excellent sodium conservation. This applies only to patients not receiving diuretics, since diuretics counteract the body's sodium conserving action.

When the heavily perspiring patient is unable to take fluids by mouth, parenteral fluid orders should be requested from the physician.

Vomiting

One should know when to advise against oral intake, as well as when to encourage it. For example, the patient who is vomiting persistently should not drink water, since vomited water will carry with it gastric electrolytes.

Since persistent vomiting calls for parenteral administration of fluids, the nurse should report its presence to the physician. Untreated vomiting can lead to metabolic alkalosis if gastric fluid alone is lost or metabolic acidosis if proportionately more duodenal fluid is lost than gastric juice. Ketosis may result if caloric intake is inadequate.

When vomiting ceases or decreases in frequency, the patient can be given bland foods in small amounts. Toast, crackers, ginger ale and, in some instances, milk—especially skim milk—are tolerated well, but orange juice tends to increase peristalsis.

Recall that vomitus consists of water, hydrogen, chloride, sodium, potassium, and other chemicals, and as much as 6 L. of gastric secretion can be lost in a 24-hour period.

The reinstitution of a normal diet can repair mild deficits, particularly if the diet is supplemented with between-meal feedings of potassium-rich foods such as meats, fruits, vegetables, milk and fruit juices. Excellent commercial potassium supplements are available and have the advantage that they can be given in doses containing known quantities of potassium. Examples are K-Lor, Kaon, and K-Lyte.

Gastrointestinal Suction

The patient receiving gastrointestinal suction should never be given large amounts of water or ice chips by mouth, since water washes electrolytes from the stomach, causing metabolic alkalosis. Statland cited a patient who was receiving suction and was permitted to ingest 21 L. of water. The water was drawn back from the suction tube, leaving the patient in profound alkalosis, which proved fatal.

Sometimes the order is given to permit ice chips sparingly; the term "sparingly" can readily be stretched by well-meaning but ill-advised persons to the point where the intake of plain ice is excessive. Some physicians allow approximately an ounce of plain ice chips per hour to relieve oral dryness.

Diarrhea

Diarrhea results in the loss of water, electrolytes, and partially digested nutrients. Prolonged diarrhea frequently results in potassium deficit, as well as in metabolic acidosis, and prolonged watery diarrhea can result in sodium excess, since water is lost in excess of electrolytes. During the acute stage of diarrhea, the gastrointestinal tract is usually put at rest through parenteral alimentation. Food is given by mouth as soon as it can be tolerated, and some physicians institute oral feedings by the use of oral electrolyte solutions; others use skim milk. Some doctors employ tea and toast.

Liberal fluid intake should be encouraged with frequent, high caloric feedings. Such foods as puddings, custards, and milk supply calories and protein and are well tolerated, provided the patient does not have a special sensitivity to them. The diet is gradually changed to normal.

MEDICAL THERAPY THAT CAUSES NUTRITIONAL DISTURBANCES

Diuresis

The primary purpose of diuretics is to promote the excretion of sodium and water from the body (Fig.

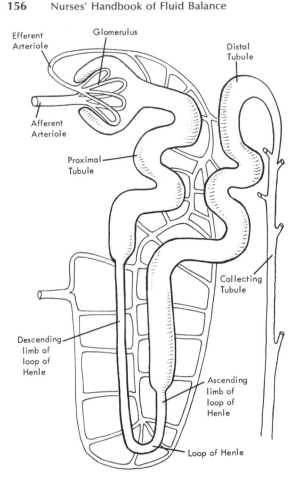

Figure 14-8. The nephron—the functional unit of the kidney. Secretion and absorption of water, electrolytes and other solutes in the proximal and the distal tubule can be influenced by drugs of many types. (From Rodman, M., and Smith, D.: Clinical Pharmacology in Nursing, Philadelphia: L. B. Lippincott Co., 1974, p. 330)

14-8). In varying degrees, most diuretics tend also to promote the excretion of potassium. Diuretics associated with hypokalemia include the thiazides, the mercurials, furosemide (Lasix), and ethacrynic acid (Edecrin) (Table 14-3).

Although the usual diet provides potassium in amounts ranging from 75 to 125 mEq. per day, losses of potassium by patients receiving any of the above diuretics can amount to several times this amount. Failure to eat well should be reported to the physician, because potassium deficit is even more apt to occur when the dietary intake is inadequate or when there are other abnormal losses of potassium from the body. Unfortunately, the body apparently has no adequate mechanism for the conservation of potassium, and, the patient dying of a potassium deficit may lose

Table 14-3. Diuretic Drugs

Nonproprietary Name	Trade Name	Daily Dosage Range	Comments
Thiazide-Type Diuretics			
Bendroflumethiazide N.F.	Naturetin	2.5 to 20 mg.	Mild, general purpose oral diuretics
Benzthiazide N.F.	Exna; Aquatag	25 to 200 mg.	Thiazides act by inhibiting Na$^+$ reabsorption in the ascending loop of Henle
Chlorothiazide N.F.	Diuril	500 to 100 mg.	
Cyclothiazide N.F.	Anhydron	1 to 2 mg.	
Hydroflumethiazide N.F.	Saluron	25 to 200 mg.	May cause hypokalemia, hyperglycemia, hyperuricemia, and hypochloremic alkalosis
Hydrochlorothiazide U.S.P.	Esidrix; HydroDiuril; Oretic	25 to 200 mg.	K$^+$ supplements or extra dietary K$^+$ are often necessary when thiazides are used routinely
Methyclothiazide N.F.	Enduron	2.5 to 10 mg.	
Polythiazide N.F.	Renese	1 to 4 mg.	Observe for arrhythmias and other symptoms of digitalis toxicity in digitalized heart patients (recall that hypokalemia intensifies the action of digitalis)
Trichlormethiazide N.F.	Naqua; Metahydrin	2 to 4 mg.	
			Thiazides cause lengthy lithium retention and thus patients taking lithium may require lower dosages of lithium carbonate

Table 14-3. Diuretic Drugs (Continued)

Nonproprietary Name	Trade Name	Daily Dosage Range	Comments
Other Diuretics			
Ethacrynic acid U.S.P.	Edecrin	25 to 200 mg. orally	These are *potent* diuretics—indicated for refractory edema of congestive heart failure, cirrhosis, and nephrosis
Sodium ethacrynate U.S.P.	Sodium Edecrin	0.5 to 1.0 mg. per kg. body weight, I.V.	Both drugs block reabsorption of Na^+ from the ascending loop of Henle
Furosemide U.S.P.	Lasix	40 to 80 mg. orally 20 to 40 mg. I.V. or I.M.	May be given by I.V. push for rapid action in emergencies
			Prone to cause hypokalemia (action not inhibited by alkalosis)
			Potassium supplements often needed
			Observe for arrhythmias in digitalized patients; drug-induced hypokalemia can cause fatal arrhythmias
			Daily weights are indicated to detect excessive diuresis; excessive and rapid weight loss may cause an acute hypotensive episode
			Ethacrynic acid and furosemide may be ototoxic
Potassium-Conserving Diuretics			
Spironolactone U.S.P.	Aldactone	25 mg. orally, 2 to 4 times daily	Triamterene acts on the distal renal tubule to depress the exchange of Na^+
Triamterene U.S.P.	Dyrenium	100 to 200 mg. orally	Spironolactone inhibits action of aldosterone (recall that aldosterone causes Na^+ retention and K^+ excretion)
			Both drugs tend to reduce K^+ excretion and may lead to hyperkalemia, thus, *K^+ supplements are contraindicated*
			Often combined with thiazides for effective diuresis—in this case, the hypokalemic tendency of the thiazides may offset the hyperkalemic tendency of triamterene and spironolactone (examples of such combinations are Dyazide and Aldactazide)
Mercurial Diuretics			
Mercaptomerin sodium U.S.P.	Thiomerin	0.2 to 2 ml. I.M.	Not used extensively—have largely been replaced by thiazides, which are safer and easier to administer
Merethoxylline procaine	Dicurin; Procaine	0.5 to 2 ml. I.M.	May cause hypochloremic alkalosis and hypokalemia; alklaosis inhibits effectiveness of diuretic action.

Adapted from Rodman, M., and Smith, D.: Clinical Pharmacology in Nursing. Philadelphia: J. B. Lippincott Co., 1974, pp. 333–334.

30 to 40 or more mEq. a day in the urine in spite of his dire need.

Determination of the daily urinary excretion of potassium through analysis of the potassium content of the 24-hour urine specimen helps guide potassium replacement. A useful rule of thumb suggests that the patient receive a daily quota of potassium equal to his daily urinary excretion plus 10 per cent. Thus, if a patient was found to be excreting 160 mEq. of potassium in the urine each day, the total potassium intake for prevention of a deficit would be 176 mEq. daily. If the dietary intake of potassium was estimated at 75 mEq.—a frequent average intake—then one would administer about 100 mEq. of potassium as a supplement. This quantity of potassium can be readily administered by use of one of the available pharmaceutical potassium supplements. The concentrations of potassium are variable, so read the labels carefully. The need for potassium supplementation of the diet of patients receiving potassium-losing diuretics becomes more pronounced when the diuretic has been taken for a long period.

Potassium supplements should be diluted as indicated by the manufacturers to avoid gastrointestinal irritation and a saline laxative effect. Remember that hyperkalemia may result from overdosage of potassium or from maintenance or therapeutic doses in patients with severe renal impairment. Potassium supplements should not be used in patients receiving potassium-sparing diuretics (spironolactone and triamterene).

When possible, diuretics should be administered intermittently rather than daily, allowing the patient to partially restore his potassium supply by dietary means. Regardless of the methods used to reduce the possibility of potassium deficit, the patient should be observed closely for undue fatigue, weakness, anorexia, flaccid muscles, and gaseous abdominal distention, and all patients receiving diuretics associated with potassium loss should have occasional plasma potassium determinations.

The patient should be encouraged to consume adequate quantities of potassium rich foods, such as:

- bananas
- oranges
- grapefruit
- dried fruits
- cantaloupe
- avocados

- fruit juices (such as prune, orange, and grapefruit)
- meats (avoid high-sodium varieties such as bacon, sausage, ham, and luncheon meats)
- fresh tomatoes
- milk (intake may be limited if more than mild sodium restriction is necessary)

An excellent source of the potassium content of foods, as well as other dietary values, is *Bowes and Church's Food Values of Portions Commonly Used*, J. B. Lippincott Co., Philadelphia, 1975. This book is particularly helpful to the nurse because food contents are expressed in terms of common servings rather than in portions of 100 Gm. (Table 14-4).

Potassium-conserving diuretics include spironolactone (Aldactone) and triamterene (Dyrenium). Aldactone is an aldosterone blocking agent and, thus, promotes sodium loss and potassium retention, whereas Dyrenium has a unique mode of action, interfering with the exchange of sodium ions for potassium and hydrogen ions. Hyperkalemia can occur when potassium-conserving diuretics are used in patients with renal insufficiency since such patients already have a tendency for potassium retention. Symptoms to be alert for include paresthesias of the extremities, nausea, weakness, and intestinal cramping with diarrhea. If hyperkalemia is severe, cardiac arrest can occur. Only patients with adequate renal reserve should receive potassium-conserving agents. Periodic plasma potassium determinations should be obtained. Diuretics that allow retention of potassium are often used in conjunction with diuretics that cause potassium loss, as their combined use reduces the possibility of hyperkalemia.

Frequently, the sodium intake of patients receiving diuretics is restricted, reducing the need for large doses of potentially harmful diuretics. Usually, sodium restriction will not involve less than 1000 mg. of sodium a day, because the use of low sodium diets containing lower levels of sodium in patients receiving diuretics can cause acute sodium deficit.

Low sodium diets and diuretics may be used to treat a variety of conditions, such as congestive heart failure, nephrosis, hepatic cirrhosis and toxemia of pregnancy. Because low sodium diets are commonly used, the nurse should know what constitutes such diets and be able to instruct patients in their use.

An average daily diet not restricted in sodium contains 6 to 15 Gm. of salt, whereas low sodium

Table 14-4. Potassium Content of Various Foods in Common Portions

Food, Amount	mEq. of K
Beverages:	
Whole Milk, 240 ml.	9.11
Non-Fat or Skim Milk, 240 ml.	5.11
Instant Coffee, Folgers (2 Gm. in 240 ml. water)	6.14
Prune juice (½ cup)	6.14
Tomato Juice, ½ cup (canned)	7.29
Orange Juice, ½ cup (fresh)	5.68
Grapefruit Juice, ½ cup (canned)	4.41
Grape Juice, bottled, ½ cup	3.84
Apple Juice, ½ cup	3.20
Coca-Cola, 180 ml.	2.25
Pepsi-Cola, 240 ml.	0.18
Ginger-Ale, 240 ml.	0.03
Fruits:	
Banana, raw, 1 medium	16.12
Figs, dried, 7 small	19.96
Grapefruit, raw, ½ medium	10.24
Orange, 1 medium	9.21
Peaches, dried, uncooked, ½ cup	28.16
Raisins, dried seedless, 2 tbsp.	3.68
Apricots, raw, 2–3 medium	7.06
Cereals:	
Oatmeal, cooked, 1 cup	3.32
Corn Flakes, 1 cup	1.02
Meats and Meat Substitutes:	
Canadian Bacon, cooked, 1 slice	2.32
Frankfurther, cooked, 1 average	2.72
Ham, cooked, 2 slices	13.31
Hamburger, cooked, 1 patty	9.77
Rib Steak, cooked, 1 serving (½ lb. raw)	9.93
Pink Salmon, ½ cup (canned)	7.42
Cheese, American Cheddar, 1 piece (2 x 2 x 1)	2.96
Egg, whole, 1 medium	1.23
Others:	
Brazil Nuts, shelled, ⅓ cup	17.15
Bre'r Rabbit Syrup, 1 tbsp.	6.91
Bar Candy, chocolate covered, 2½ oz.	14.84

Adapted from Church, C. F., and Church, H. N. (eds.): Bowes & Church's Food Values of Portions Commonly Used, ed. 12. Philadelphia: J. B. Lippincott Co., 1975.

diets can range from a mild restriction to as low as 200 mg. of sodium a day, depending on the patient's needs. The American Heart Association has prepared booklets describing mild, moderate, and strict sodium-restricted diets. The moderate sodium-restricted diet allows 1000 mg. of sodium daily; the strict diet allows only 500 mg. of sodium daily. The booklets are available to patients on request of their physicians.

Patients requiring only a mild sodium restriction have a great deal of freedom in planning their meals and may salt most foods lightly (about half as much as usual) during preparation. Because most canned and processed foods are already salted, no additional salt should be added. Salt should not be used at the table. (One level teaspoon of salt contains about 2300 mg. of sodium.) Foods high in sodium content should be avoided. Examples of such foods include:

Sauerkraut and other vegetables prepared in brine	Salt pork
	Sardines
	Processed cheese
Bacon	Bouillon cubes
Luncheon meats	Peanut butter
Frankfurters	Catsup
Ham	Mustard
Kosher meats	Olives
Sausage	Pickles
Meat tenderizers	Worcestershire sauce
Relish	Potato chips
Horseradish	Pretzels

Patients on a low sodium diet must limit their intake of commercially processed foods which contain sodium benzoate, monosodium glutamate, and baking powder. Baking soda (sodium bicarbonate) should not be used as an antacid, since one level teaspoon of baking soda contains 1000 mg. of sodium. Baking soda used in excessive amounts can produce metabolic alkalosis, particularly in the aged.

Tooth pastes, tooth powders, and mouth washes may be high in sodium content; therefore, patients on sodium restricted diets should be instructed not to swallow these products and to rinse their mouths well with water after their use. Medicines not prescribed by the physician should be avoided, as some medicines contain enough sodium to interfere with the desired intake. Among these are certain laxatives, pain relievers, sedatives, cough syrups, and antibiotics. Chewing tobacco and snuff are high in sodium.

Salt substitutes are sometimes used to make low sodium diets more palatable. Commercial salt substitutes include Co-Salt (potassium chloride, ammonium chloride, choline, and lactose) and Neocurtasol (potassium chloride, potassium iodide, potassium glutamate, glutamic acid, calcium silicate, and tricalcium phosphate). Note that these preparations contain potassium and should be used cautiously in patients with a tendency toward hyperkalemia (such as those with renal disease or Addison's disease).

Prolonged Use of Laxatives and Enemas

The abuse of laxatives and enemas in our society is appalling. One reason for their widespread use is misunderstanding of the term constipation, which really refers to a hard, dry stool, difficult to evacuate. Even though the patient may not have a bowel movement for several days, *he is not constipated unless his stools are hard, dry and difficult to evacuate.* Some persons normally have bowel movements every day; others may have them every 3, 4, or 5 days. If the latter individuals have soft stools, they are not regarded as constipated.

It is the compulsion to have a daily evacuation that has led to the frequent use of laxatives and enemas. Many patients feel they must be "cleaned out" daily or their health will be impaired, a misconception which should be corrected by the nurse at every opportunity; otherwise, patients will continue to use laxatives and enemas unnecessarily. Reliance on laxatives and enemas decreases the natural reflex activity of the colon; hence, *stronger* laxatives and *more* enemas are required.

The repeated administration of plain water enemas causes electrolytes to be drawn into the bowel, since the body always tries to make any collection of fluid isotonic with extracellular fluid. Therefore, when the enema is evacuated, it carries not only water, but electrolytes with it. Sodium deficit, potassium deficit, or both can be produced by repeated water enemas.

Should the patient actually be constipated, he should be provided a diet with these characteristics:

1. Generous quantities of fruits, vegetables, and bran cereals
2. Increased water intake
3. Regular meal hours

Stool softeners, such as Colace (dioctyl sodium sulfosuccinate) are useful physiologic tools for increasing the softness of the stools, and a glass of warm water or hot coffee first thing in the morning can stimulate the evacuation reflex.

Adrenocorticosteroids

Administration of adrenocorticosteriods may cause sodium and water retention and excretion of potassium, particularly when prolonged high doses are employed. For patients on such doses, the potassium intake should be increased and the sodium intake restricted, because, if potassium loss is not replaced, metabolic alkalosis and potassium deficit may result. Edema and hypokalemia are particularly dangerous to digitalized congestive heart failure patients. Individuals taking corticosteroids and potassium-losing diuretics concomitantly should receive potassium-supplements.

The nurse should be alert for signs of fluid volume excess, such as weight gain, edema, and increased blood pressure and should also observe for signs of potassium deficit, such as weakness, fatigue, anorexia, flaccid muscles, and gaseous abdominal distention. The newer synthetic steroids, such as triamcinolone (Aristocort or Kenacort), do not have a strong influence on electrolytes and, thus, are associated with fewer fluid balance problems. A token rise in blood pressure may occur within a few weeks of regular corticosteroid therapy; it is of no consequence to normotensive individuals but may necessitate sodium restriction and adjustment of antihypertensive drug dosage for those with existing hypertension.

Prolonged administration of cortisone encourages negative nitrogen balance, and dietary treatment includes a generous intake of protein, a potassium supplement, and an adequate caloric intake to prevent weight loss. The use of cortisone can also cause decreased tolerance to carbohydrates, with hyperglycemia and glycosuria. Corticosteroids sometimes induce reversible Cushingoid changes (moon facies, acne, and hirsutism). These symptoms may occur in patients taking 25 mg. or more of prednisone (or its equivalent) daily for longer than 2 weeks.

The hydrochloric acid and pepsin contents of the stomach are increased, a fact which may be related to the occurrence of ulcers in patients on steroid therapy. Patients are sometimes advised to take an antacid just before, and between, doses of corticosteroids.

Wounds heal more slowly in patients taking systemic corticosteroids because these medications retard formation of granulation tissue. Postoperative patients on steroids usually have their sutures in place longer than others because they are more likely to suffer wound dishiscence. High doses of vitamins (particularly vitamin C) are needed in postoperative patients to promote wound healing. Supplemental vitamin C also helps counter the bruises frequently evident in patients taking systemic corticosteroids.

Normally, the adrenal cortex produces about 25 mg. of hydrocortisone a day; during stressful periods it can secrete as much as 300 mg. a day.[6] When corticosteroids are supplied medically and then withdrawn, the adrenal cortex needs time to assume its normal function (it may take from 3 to 9 months for it to be able to secrete normal daily needs). It may require up to two years before the adrenal cortex is able to produce amounts needed during stress.[7] Patients being withdrawn from corticosteroids should wear a special alert tag or bracelet indicating a need for extra hydrocortisone during periods of stress. Early symptoms of acute adrenal insufficiency may include weakness, nausea, fainting, loss of appetite, and fever.

CATABOLIC EFFECTS THAT CAUSE NUTRITIONAL DISTURBANCES

Immobilization

CALCULI   All patients subjected to long periods of bedrest develop metabolic disturbances, one of which is the increased excretion of calcium. As pointed out by Kottke and Blanchard:

> The long bones of the lower extremities are designed to bear weight, and as long as weight is being borne by them, the calcium is maintained in the matrix of the bones. When the stresses of weight bearing have been removed, the calcium is very soon mobilized and enters the blood stream with the resulting increased concentration of circulating calcium in the blood. This increased calcium is filtered out through the kidneys, where it is deposited as calcium salts to form kidney and bladder stones.[8]

Disuse osteoporosis can cause the urinary calcium level to triple after only two weeks of bedrest; calculi develop in 15 to 30 per cent of patients immobilized for more than a few weeks.[9] Other causes of renal

calculi are excessive calcium excretion caused by hyperparathyroidism and by excessive ingestion of milk, alkali, and vitamin D; increased urinary excretion of uric acid, as in gout; renal infection with formation of stones containing pus and blood; and increased urinary excretion of cystine (an inborn error of metabolism).

Measures to prevent calculi include:

- Preventing urinary stasis by turning the patient frequently, elevating the head of the bed, and having the patient sit up if allowed
- Scheduling frequent active and passive exercises—encouraging weight bearing and ambulation as soon as possible
- Forcing fluids to 3000 to 4000 ml./24 hr, unless contraindicated, to increase urinary volume to 3000 ml./24 hr. (small crystals have less tendency to accumulate mass when urine flow is great and continuous)
- Lowering urinary pH for patients with the following kinds of urinary calculi may be indicated to increase their solubility:

Calcium carbonate ⎫
Calcium phosphate ⎬ (90% of all stones)
Calcium oxalate ⎭

The physician may prescribe acidifying drugs such as sodium acid phosphate or methenamine mandelate. Calcium stones will not form in urine with a pH below 6.6. Food and fluids yielding an acid-ash may be prescribed and are listed in Table 14-5. To keep the urine acid, intake should emphasize high-grade protein (especially meat), cranberries, plums, prunes, and cranberry juice. Patients tending to form calcium phosphate stones are sometimes given aluminum hydroxide gel to retard the absorption of phosphate from the gut.

- Elevating urinary pH to the alkaline level for patients with the following kinds of urinary calculi may be indicated to increase their solubility:

Uric acid (5 to 8 per cent of all stones)
Cystine (1 to 3 per cent of all stones)

The physician may prescribe alkalinizing drugs such as potassium citrate, sodium citrate, and citric acid. Foods and fluids yielding an alkaline-ash may be prescribed and are listed in Table 14-5. To alkalinize urine, dietary emphasis should be on citrus fruits, milk, and most vegetables (especially legumes). A low purine diet may be indicated for patients tending to form uric acid stones; allopurinol (Zyloprim) may be used to block uric acid formation.

Pathologic fractures can occur as a result of bone rarefaction. Increased calcium excretion begins in the first week of immobilization and continues for a period of 4 to 8 weeks. After this period, the calcium drops back to normal or subnormal levels.

Some authorities feel that when calcium is being lost from the body, the intake should be increased over normal, and others believe that only the amount of calcium required for maintenance of body stores should be permitted. When calcium is restricted, the patient is permitted only one pint of milk a day; of course, other foods high in calcium, such as cheese and salmon, should be excluded from the diet.

NEGATIVE NITROGEN BALANCE Nitrogen balance is a measure of protein metabolism, indicating that the rate of protein synthesis in the body equals that of protein degradation. Negative nitrogen balance refers to a state in which nitrogen loss exceeds intake; it indicates that protein catabolism exceeds protein anabolism. (Recall that approximately 1 Gm. of nitrogen is contained in about 6.25 Gm. of protein.) The immobilized patient develops a state of negative nitrogen balance after approximately four days of

bedrest. By the tenth day of immobilization, the state of negative nitrogen balance reaches its peak and gradually returns toward normal. It is important to encourage the intake of foods high in protein (meat, eggs, fish, milk) to compensate for the increased loss of protein. Commercial high protein products are also available for complete dietary intake or supplemental feedings. (See discussion of elemental diets and high protein tube feedings in this chapter.)

Clinically, negative nitrogen balance is manifested by the following symptoms:

- anorexia
- muscle weakness and wasting
- weight loss
- decreased state of awareness
- hypoalbuminemia with associated edema
- anemia

Decubitus Ulcers

A draining decubitus ulcer can quadruple the body's need for protein, as the ulcer exudate is high in protein content. The fact that most patients with decubiti are immobilized further contributes to the increased protein need.

It is often difficult for the patient to consume sufficient protein, since his appetite is usually poor. The nurse must use all her ingenuity to find foods rich in protein but acceptable to the patient. Usual food sources of protein can be supplemented by commercial high protein supplements or by skim milk powder. Both can be added to food without changing

Table 14-5. Acid-Base Reaction of Foods

Potentially Acid or Acid Ash Foods	Potentially Basic or Alkaline Ash Foods
Breads, all types	Fruits, all types (except cranberries, plums, and prunes)
Cakes and cookies, plain	Jams and jellies, honey
Cereals and crackers	Milk, cream, and buttermilk
Cheese, all types	Molasses
Eggs	Nuts: almonds, coconut, chestnuts
Fish and shellfish	Vegetables, all types except corn and lentils
Fruits: cranberries, plums, and prunes	
Macaroni, spaghetti, noodles	
Meats and poultry	
Nuts: Brazil, filberts, peanuts, walnuts	
Vegetables: corn and lentils	

Neutral Foods

Butter or margarine	Cooking fats and oils	Starches, corn and arrowroot
Candy, plain	Syrups	Sugars

Reprinted from Cooper, L., et al.: Nutrition in Health and Disease, ed. 14. Philadelphia: J. B. Lippincott Co., 1963, p. 542, with permission.

the bulk or flavor appreciably. Two tablespoons of dry skim milk powder supplies 6 Gm. of protein and can be added to cereal, scrambled eggs, pudding, soup, hamburger, and other foods.

The increased protein need must be considered as important as turning the patient often and keeping the skin clean and dry.

Hemorrhage

The well-nourished person usually can regenerate red blood cells following one episode of hemorrhage. Chronic blood loss, however, depletes the red cell stores and results in anemia. The body compensates for the decrease in circulating blood volume that accompanies hemorrhage by drawing fluid from the tissue spaces into the vascular compartment—an interstitial fluid-to-plasma shift of water and electrolytes. The total extracellular fluid volume is unchanged; only the distribution of the fluid is affected.

The patient who has suffered chronic hemorrhage should be provided a diet rich in protein, iron, and vitamin C. Up to 1000 Gm. of protein a day should be given; excellent sources of protein are meat, eggs, cheese, and fish. Protein supplements can also be employed between meals, at bedtime, or both. Iron can be supplied as meat, liver, prunes, apples, grapes, spinach, beans, enriched cereals, and eggs. In addition, it is well to give an additional source of iron, preferably ferrous sulfate, by mouth. Vitamin C intake can be increased by generous servings of citrus fruits. Lastly, the fluid intake should be generous.

Trauma

Trauma, such as burns, fractures, wounds, and crushing injuries, causes loss of protein through direct destruction of tissues. It contributes further to the loss through the so-called toxic destruction of protein, an increased catabolism brought on mysteriously by the trauma. It also promotes the accumulation of protein-rich fluid at the site of the injury, which contributes further to possible protein depletion. Immobilization made necessary by the injury also causes losses of protein and, in addition, of electrolytes.

Because of these losses and because of the requirements for optimal healing, the protein, electrolyte, and vitamin C intake of the injured patient should be increased; as much as 150 Gm. of protein daily is frequently administered. (Of course, high

potassium foods should be withheld until adequate renal function has been established, since cellular breakdown releases large amounts of potassium into the bloodstream.) The diet should be high in calories to prevent ingested protein from being consumed for energy purposes. The use of "oral" hyperalimentation with elemental diets has been effective in producing positive nitrogen balance in traumatized patients.

REFERENCES

1. **Noone, R.,** and **Grahan, W.:** Cervical pharyngostomy for tube feeding. J.A.M.A. 216:314, 1971.

2. **Given, B.,** and **Simmons, S.:** Gastroenterology in Clinical Nursing, ed. 2. St. Louis: C. V. Mosby, 1975, p. 20.

3. **Boedeker, E.,** and **Dauber, J.** (eds.): Manual of Medical Therapeutics, 2 ed. Boston: Little, Brown & Co., 1974, p. 4.

4. **Condon, R.,** and **Nyhus, L.** (eds.): Manual of Surgical Therapeutics, ed. 3. Boston: Little, Brown, & Co., 1975, p. 203.

5. Ibid., p. 204.

6. **Newton, D., Nichols, A.,** and **Newton, M.:** You can minimize the hazards of corticosteroids. Nursing 77, June, pp. 30–31, 1977.

7. Ibid.

8. **Kottke, F.,** and **Blanchard, R.:** Bedrest begets bedrest. Nursing Forum 3: 71, 1964.

9. **Luckman, J.,** and **Sorensen, K.:** Medical-Surgical Nursing—A Psychophysiologic Approach. Philadelphia: W. B. Saunders Co., 1974, p. 307.

BIBLIOGRAPHY

Blackburn, G.: Intake: Perspectives in Clinical Nutrition, 5. Adaptation to Starvation. Eaton Laboratories, Norwich, N.Y. 1973.

Browse, N.: The Physiology and Pathology of Bedrest. Springfield, Ill.: Charles C Thomas, 1965.

Brunner, L., and **Suddarth, D.:** Textbook of Medical-Surgical Nursing, ed. 3. Philadelphia: J. B. Lippincott Co., 1975.

Burton, B.: Human Nutrition, ed. 3. Published for H. J. Heinz Co., Pittsburgh. New York: McGraw-Hill Book Co., 1976.

Diet Manual—Massachusetts General Hospital Dietary Department. Boston: Little, Brown and Co., 1976.

Houghey, E., and **Sica, F.:** Diuretics: How safe can you make them? Nursing 77, Feb., pp. 34–39.

Manzi, C.: Edema: how to tell if it's a danger signal. Nursing 77, April, pp. 66–77.

Pearson, E., et al.: Intake: Perspectives in Clinical Nutrition. 1. Metabolism—The Balance of Life. Eaton Laboratories, Norwich, N.Y., 1973.

Robinson, C.: Basic Nutrition and Diet Therapy, ed. 3. Macmillan, 1975.

Rodman, M., and **Smith, D.:** Clinical Pharmacology in Nursing. Philadelphia: J. B. Lippincott Co., 1974.

Trunkey, D., et al.: Intake: Perspectives in Clinical Nutrition. 6. Nutrition and trauma. Eaton Laboratories, Norwich, N.Y., 1973.

— 15 —

The Treatment of Body Fluid Disturbances

"Rational therapy of patients with disturbances in their
body fluids requires a working clinical diagnosis
which is founded on a mental image of the nature,
and a reasonably accurate estimate of the
magnitude of the disturbances present."
Michael James Sweeney

PRELIMINARY TESTING

In planning therapy for the patient with an actual or potential disturbance of the body fluids, the first step is to determine the status of the kidneys. Various types of solutions, particularly those containing potassium, can be hazardous if renal function is not adequate. The presence of any one of the following criteria indicates suppressed kidney function:

1. Specific gravity of urine above 1.030
2. Less than three voidings in 24 hours
3. No urine in the bladder

Renal depression almost invariably occurs in patients who have suffered massive acute losses of extracellular fluid, and so many patients with fluid imbalances have oliguria or even anuria. Before administering fluid therapy, it is necessary to determine if the suppression of urination is due simply to an extracellular fluid volume deficit or whether it is due to serious renal impairment. If urinary suppression is caused simply by volume deficit, the therapeutic test will reveal that fact by reestablishing urinary flow, making it safe to proceed with the fluid therapy program, including the administration of potassium-containing solutions.

The therapeutic test consists of administration of a special solution, frequently called an initial hydrating solution or a pump-priming solution. Such a solution often provides sodium, 51 mEq./L., chloride, 51 mEq./L., and glucose, 50 Gm./L. It actually represents a solution containing one part of isotonic solution of sodium chloride in 5 per cent glucose, and two parts of 5 per cent glucose in water. The solution is administered at the rate of 8 ml./m.^{2} of body surface/minute for 45 minutes. When the kidneys begin to function, as shown by the restoration of the flow of urine, then the initial hydrating solution is discontinued and therapy is started with other types of solutions. If the urinary flow is not restored, the infusion rate is reduced to 2 ml./m.^{2} body surface/minute and continued for another hour. If urination has not occurred at the end of this period, the physician assumes he is dealing with renal impairment rather than functional depression, thus demanding a battery of laboratory tests plus careful management by nephrologists or similarly qualified specialists.

THE GOALS OF FLUID THERAPY

In planning day-to-day therapy for the individual patient, including what type of solution is needed in what amount, the physician considers the three goals of therapy:

1. Any preexisting deficits of water and electrolytes must be repaired.
2. Water and electrolytes must be provided to meet the patient's maintenance requirements.
3. Continuing abnormal losses of water and electrolytes through such routes as vomiting, diarrhea, tubal drainage, wound drainage, burn drainage, diuresis, and the like, must be replaced.

There are various, widely different methods for achieving these goals. Rather than describe several methods, we will present one simple method that has worked out well in practice, that will help give the nurse a basic understanding of the principles involved in fluid therapy. From the standpoint of clinical results, this method is no better than other methods of fluid therapy and certainly has its drawbacks and limitations—we have chosen it for pedagogical reasons. The method that we shall describe briefly is that developed by Butler and his coworkers at the Massachusetts General Hospital, and which has, since that time, been used with great success in many parts of the world.

ADMINISTERING FLUID THERAPY

In perhaps 90 per cent of patients with fluid imbalances, a single solution of the type such as that devised by Butler can be used to provide water and electrolytes for maintenance and repair. Such a solution is so designed that *when used to meet the patient's fluid volume requirement, it supplies electrolytes in quantities balanced between the minimal needs and the maximal tolerances of the patient.* The Butler-type solution is actually one third to one half as concentrated as plasma, providing free water for urinary formation and metabolic activities and, in addition, both cellular and extracellular electrolytes. It incorporates 5 or 10 per cent of carbohydrate to minimize tissue destruction, reduce ketosis and spare protein. The Butler-type solution utilizes the body homeostatic mechanisms, which select the electrolytes that are required and reject those that are not needed. Butler-type solutions, when used properly, have a great margin of safety and are enormously useful in managing body fluid disturbances that result from acute differences between intake and output of water and electrolytes not controllable by the body homeostatic mechanisms. Probably 90 per cent of all body fluid disturbances are of this nature and include extracellular fluid volume deficit, sodium excess, potassium deficit, and the four acid-base disturbances. In the text, when we refer to *balanced solution,* we mean the type of hypotonic, multiple-electrolyte solution (containing both extracellular and cellular electrolytes) as recommended by Butler, Lowe, and others. (See Table 16-5.)

EXTRACELLULAR FLUID VOLUME DEFICIT The goal of therapy in this imbalance is to provide both cellular and extracellular electrolytes to compensate for losses without altering the composition of the extracellular fluid. While a treatment solution containing water and electrolytes in the proportions present in extracellular fluid may appear to be the logical choice, it is not, since such a solution would not provide the water needed for urinary excretion and for replacement of plain water lost from the skin and lungs. A balanced solution provides the body homeostatic mechanisms not only with free water for these purposes, but also with the materials they need to restore volume and at the same time maintain the normal composition of the extracellular fluid.

SODIUM EXCESS OF EXTRACELLULAR FLUID In sodium excess, which is often accompanied by volume deficit, the goal of therapy is to provide water to dilute the concentration of electrolytes both in the extracellular fluid and in the cellular fluid while supplying maintenance amounts of electrolytes to reestablish the normal composition of the body fluid. The free water in balanced solutions dilutes the electrolyte concentration excess, and the body homeostatic mechanisms are also supplied with the electrolytes they may need to reestablish the normal water-to-electrolyte ratio.

POTASSIUM DEFICIT OF EXTRACELLULAR FLUID The purpose of therapy in potassium deficit is to repair the deficit while providing adequate amounts of potassium for maintenance needs. Balanced solutions contain sufficient potassium to repair both cellular and extracellular deficits and at the same time provide potassium and other electrolytes for maintenance.

PRIMARY BASE BICARBONATE DEFICIT OF EXTRACELLULAR FLUID (METABOLIC ACIDOSIS) In this imbalance, one needs to provide bicarbonate ions to replace acid ions, to promote excretion of nonbicarbonate anions, and to counteract the processes responsible for producing ketosis. Balanced solutions contain at least 20 mEq. of lactate/L., which the liver converts into base bicarbonate, to be broken down by the kidneys into bicarbonate ions, which are conserved, and acid ions, which are excreted. Balanced solutions also contain free water to promote urinary excretion, thus speeding up the washing out of acid ions, and carbohydrate to reduce ketosis by providing the body with a nonfat energy source, thus decreasing the burning of body fat. Since metabolic acidosis usually causes a loss of water and electrolytes—especially sodium, potassium, and chloride—culminating in fluid volume deficit, a balanced solution also supplies the water and electrolytes needed to maintain fluid volume and to prevent secondary electrolyte deficits from developing.

Some authorities have emphasized that since lactic acid acidosis can well occur in a variety of clinical situations, it appears illogical to administer lactate in order to correct acidosis. They advocate the forthright intravenous administration of sodium bicarbonate, maintaining that if the patient's compensation for bicarbonate deficit (metabolic acidosis) is inadequate, then sodium bicarbonate should be administered. In doing so, one should endeavor to raise the bicarbonate toward normal, but not all the way to normal. Thus, a small amount of bicarbonate is given, then the patient is reassessed and more is given if

needed. In calculating the amount of bicarbonate required, recall that this anion is present not only in the extracellular fluid, but also in the cellular fluid. Considering both locations, one can regard bicarbonate as present in 40 per cent of the body weight. Therefore, 40 per cent of the patient's body weight ideally should have a bicarbonate concentration of approximately 24 mEq./L. Example: a 70 kg. person has a bicarbonate of 10 mEq./L., and we want to raise it, in our stepwise approach to correcting it, to 20 mEq./L. Forty per cent of his total body weight of 70 kg. = 28 kg., which represents 28 L. of body fluid that should have a bicarbonate concentration of 24 mEq./L. So, in raising the bicarbonate concentration from 10 to 20 mEq./L., we multiple $10 \times 28 = 280$ mEq. of bicarbonate. (We would give this amount, note the patient's response, then give more if the bicarbonate did not reach 20 mEq./L. Later, we could give additional bicarbonate until the level was at 24 mEq./L., in accordance with the need.)

PRIMARY BASE BICARBONATE EXCESS OF EXTRACELLULAR FLUID (METABOLIC ALKALOSIS) The goal of therapy in this imbalance is to provide nonbicarbonate anions, such as chloride, to replace bicarbonate ions. Because metabolic alkalosis is almost always accompanied by potassium deficit and will not respond to therapy unless potassium is also supplied, balanced solutions must contain adequate amounts of both chloride and potassium. When such a solution is administered, the body homeostatic mechanisms will selectively retain the chloride ions to replace bicarbonate ions, as well as potassium to correct the potassium deficit.

PRIMARY CARBONIC ACID DEFICIT OF EXTRACELLULAR FLUID (RESPIRATORY ALKALOSIS) Parenteral therapy is of secondary importance in this imbalance, since the chief effort should be directed toward managing the condition that initially caused hyperventilation. The function of fluid therapy in this disturbance is to complement the efforts of the kidneys as they attempt to compensate, by excreting bicarbonate and retaining acid. Therefore, the object of fluid therapy in respiratory alkalosis is to provide chloride ions that can be used to replace bicarbonate ions and at the same time provide free water to replace water lost through the lungs in overbreathing. Balanced solutions contain adequate amounts of both chloride and free water, so they are useful for supportive therapy. Caution must always be observed in correcting carbonic acid deficit too rapidly, especially when the imbalance has existed for several days.

PRIMARY CARBONIC ACID EXCESS OF EXTRA-CELLULAR FLUID (RESPIRATORY ACIDOSIS)

Fluid therapy is also of secondary importance in managing this disturbance, because the function of parenteral fluids in respiratory acidosis is to support the corrective efforts of the homeostatic mechanisms by supplying them with ions such as lactate or acetate that can be converted into bicarbonate. Balanced solutions are useful here since they contain lactate ions.

In all the imbalances just described, balanced solutions can be used both for repair and for maintenance. Dosage is relatively simple and is based primarily on the patient's fluid volume, which is assessed mainly by acute changes in body weight. A moderate fluid volume deficit is indicated by weight loss up to 5 per cent in a child or adult, up to 10 per cent in an infant, and by symptoms moderate in degree, whereas a severe fluid volume deficit is indicated by an acute weight loss of over 5 per cent in a child or adult, and over 10 per cent in an infant, with symptoms and laboratory findings severe in degree.

In the patient whose fluid volume is normal at the time therapy is started, his maintenance requirements can be met by the administration of 1500 ml. of a Butler-type solution/m.² body surface/day. In the patient who has a moderate preexisting deficit, 2400 ml./m.² body surface/day will both correct this deficit and meet maintenance needs. If the patient has a severe preexisting deficit, then one can correct the deficit and provide maintenance by giving 3000 ml. of a Butler-type solution/m.² body surface/day.

The Butler-type solution is given intravenously, by mouth, or by nasogastric tube, but *not subcutaneously*. The dose should be calculated carefully, regardless of what route is used. In giving the solution intravenously, the usual rate of administration is 3 ml./m.² of body surface/minute.

Various modifications of the Butler-type solution are made available by manufacturers of parenteral solutions. The usual solution for older children and adults contains 75 mEq. of total cation (and hence of total anion), and that used for infants and small children contains 48 mEq. of total cation (and hence of total anion). Manufacturers gladly provide informa-

tion concerning available solutions and their proper use.

For replacing continuing abnormal losses (concurrent losses) from vomiting, drainage from an intestinal tube or fistula, severe diarrhea, and so on, replacement solutions with a composition resembling the body fluid lost are added to the daily fluid ration. Thus, to replace gastric juice, one administers a gastric replacement solution intravenously and to replace intestinal or duodenal juices, he uses an intestinal replacement solution intravenously. For replacing concurrent losses of hypotonic fluids, such as perspiration and watery diarrheal fluids, additional amounts of balanced solution are added to the amount the patient is already receiving for repair and maintenance. Concurrent losses are replaced on a volume for volume basis at a flow rate of 3 ml./m.² body surface/minute. Caution must always be exercised in correcting carbonic acid excess too rapidly, especially if the imbalance has existed for several days.

CALCULATING DOSAGE

Among the most beautiful passages in the medical literature are these from the clinical reports of early physicians who used parenteral fluid therapy. Latta, of Leith, Scotland, thus described the effect of an intravenous solution administered to a patient suffering from cholera in 1832:

> . . . Like the effects of magic, instead of the pallid aspect of one whom death had sealed as his own, the vital tide was restored and life and vivacity returned . . .

Cantini, who practiced in Naples, Italy, and died in 1893, wrote as follows:

> The cold, cyanotic, dehydrated, comatose patients, lying pulseless and almost lifeless, became animated after the subcutaneous infusion of warm salt water. Remarkably their pulse and voice often returned in a few minutes and they are even able to sit alone in bed . . .

Neither Dr. Latta nor Dr. Cantini felt much need for precise knowledge of parenteral fluid dosage, nor was a great need experienced for many decades to come, for as long as it remained an emergency measure, to be performed only as a last resort, the clinical response of the patient—if respond he did—was regarded as gauge enough for proper dosage. Now, with striking advances in the knowledge of clinical fluid disturbances during the past four decades, there has been a great extension in the use of parenteral fluids. The medical profession has, therefore, felt a mounting need for simple, widely applicable dosage gauges suitable for assisting the physician in determining the volume and the rate of administration of parenteral fluids.

The gauges for dosage most frequently used have been body surface area and body weight related to age; caloric requirement has been employed to a lesser extent. Some authorities feel that body weight related to age possesses an important shortcoming: requirements for water and electrolytes determined on the basis of body weight are different for patients of different ages. However, when using body surface area, expressed in terms of square meters of body surface per day, requirements for water and electrolytes are approximately the same for patients of all age groups, as shown in Figure 15-1 for approximate water requirement and approximate sodium requirement.

Body surface area is proportional to many essential physiologic processes, including heat loss, blood volume, glomerular filtration rate, organ size, respiration, blood pressure, and nitrogen requirements. Alan Butler and his coworkers at the Massachusetts General Hospital were the first to emphasize that the basic water and electrolyte requirements are also proportional to body surface area, regardless of the age or size of the patient. They pointed out that since body surface area provides a quantitative index of our total metabolic activity, it also provides us with a remarkably useful gauge for determining doses and proper rate for parenteral administration of water and electrolytes in fluid therapy. In addition, body surface area can provide nurses with a simple, rapid method of checking the correctness of parenteral fluid orders, especially in regard to volume and rate of administration, and in particular to determine if orders for sodium and potassium in parenteral solutions are within the realm of safety.

There are various methods of measuring body surface area, including the covering method, geometric method, skinning method, and other investigational methods. Clinicians employ simple nomograms that enable one to rapidly estimate body surface area from height and body weight. Actually, one can quickly obtain the approximate surface area from weight alone, as shown in Table 15-1.

The table is simple to use: an infant weighing 10 lb. would have an approximate surface area of 0.27 m.²; a child weighing 50 lb. would have an approximate surface area of 0.87 m.²; an adult weighing 150 lb. would have an approximate surface area of 1.75 m.².

The body surface areas arrived at by use of the weight chart are approximate only, and apply to individuals of average body build. In general, obese or stocky individuals have less surface area than tall

APPROXIMATE WATER REQUIREMENT   **APPROXIMATE SODIUM REQUIREMENT**

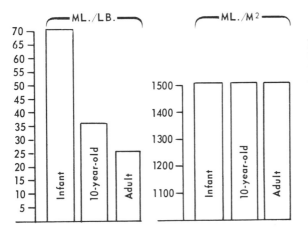
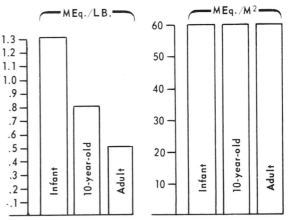

Figure 15-1.   We can use the same values for water and sodium requirements for persons of all ages if we use body surface area, rather than weight, as the dosage criterion.

Table 15-1.   Chart for Converting Weight to Surface Area

(Figures are approximate and apply only to individuals of average build.)

Pounds	Surface Area in Square Meters
4	.15
6	.20
10	.27
15	.36
20	.45
30	.60
40	.72
50	.87
60	.97
70	1.10
80	1.21
90	1.33
100	1.4
125	1.6
150	1.75
175	2.0
200	2.2
250	2.7

lanky persons of the same weight (just as a long, low one-story ranch house has more external surface than a two- or three-story house of equal floor space). For example, our 10-lb. infant would have a surface area of 0.2 m.² if he were only 16 inches tall, but he would have 0.3 m.² of surface area if he were 28 inches in height. Our 50-lb. child would have 0.68 m.² of surface area if he were 2 feet, 10 inches tall and 0.84 m.² if his height were 3 feet, 10 inches. Our 150-lb. adult would have 1.47 m.² of surface area if he were only 4 feet, 4 inches tall and 1.86 m.² if he had a height of 6 feet.

The body surface area gauge for dosage is especially useful for checking the correctness of water and electrolytes ordered for patients with body fluid disturbances. Remember the following rules:

1. For maintenance, administer 1500 ml./m.² body surface/day.
2. For correction of a moderate deficit in extracellular fluid volume plus maintenance, administer 2400 ml./m.² body surface/day.
3. For correction of a severe deficit in extracellular fluid volume plus maintenance, administer 3000 ml./m.² body surface/day.
4. Concurrent losses are replaced with an appro-

priate replacement solution on a volume for volume basis.

5. Except when giving initial hydrating solutions (as described above), the recommended rate is 3 ml./m.² body surface/minute. Slower rates of infusion may be used when the daily parenteral fluid ration is given over a 24-hr. period, as for infants and small children because of technical difficulties involved in repeated venipuncture.

By applying these rules, the nurse can quickly check the correctness of an order for fluid therapy. Let us suppose that the physician has written an order for a liter of solution to be given over a 24-hour period to an infant weighing 20 lb. with a moderate fluid volume deficit. A quick check of the conversion chart shows that a 20-lb. baby would have 0.45 m.² of body surface; the volume of fluid for correction of a moderate fluid volume deficit in such a baby should be 0.45 times 2400 ml., or about 1080 ml.

Let us suppose, on the other hand, that a large man with a severe fluid volume deficit is to receive 3 L. of solution for the first 24 hours. Reference to the conversion chart shows that a 175-lb. man would have a body surface area of 2.0 m.²; 2.0 times 3000 ml., the requirement per m.² of body surface per day for a severe fluid volume deficit, is 6 L., or 6000 ml.; 3 L., therefore is grossly inadequate.

Suppose that a 12-year-old boy with no fluid imbalance is to be given water and electrolytes for maintenance for a few days following abdominal surgery. The physician orders 3 L. of his favorite maintenance solution. The boy's body surface area is 1.33 m.² and maintenance should call for 1500 ml. times 1.33, or 1995 ml., approximately 2 L. of fluid. The extra liter ordered might embarrass the boy's homeostatic mechanisms, and the physician should appreciate having the order questioned. Of course, in the presence of fever or heavy sweating, the extra fluid might well be entirely proper.

Using the above information, the rate of administration for the infant with 0.45 m.² of body surface would be 0.45 × 3 × 60 = 81 ml./hr.; for the 2.0 m.² man, 2 × 3 × 60 = 360 ml./hr.; for the 1.33 m.² boy, 1.33 × 3 × 60 = 240 ml./hr. This applies, of course, when the total infusion is to be given within a period shorter than 24 hours.

The quantity of sodium or potassium being administered parenterally can quickly be checked by recalling that the average daily maintenance requirement for sodium is 50 to 70 mEq./m.^{2} of body surface/day, also valid for potassium. The minimal need for each of these cations is 10 mEq./m.^{2} of body surface/day, and the maximal tolerances, 250 mEq./m.^{2} of body surface/day.

IMBALANCES REQUIRING SPECIFIC TYPES OF THERAPY

The simple plan of therapy described above is not suitable for treating the remainder of our 16 basic imbalances, including extracellular fluid volume excess, sodium deficit, potassium excess, calcium deficit, calcium excess, magnesium deficit, protein deficit, and the two shifts involving the water and electrolytes of plasma and interstitial fluid. These imbalances require specific therapy.

In extracellular fluid volume excess, calcium excess, and potassium excess, the object of therapy is to remove from the extracellular fluid excesses of a single electrolyte or of a combination of water and electrolytes.

EXTRACELLULAR FLUID VOLUME EXCESS
Fluid therapy usually is not indicated in this imbalance; rather, therapy is directed toward the causative factors. Symptomatic treatment consists of restriction of fluids, administration of diuretics, or both. When the excess has resulted from excessive administration of isotonic solutions, discontinuing the infusion may be all that is required in the patient with functional homeostatic mechanisms. Administration of a balanced solution at the rate of 1 ml./m.^{2} body surface/minute will provide free water to aid in excretion of excess electrolytes and at the same time will provide potassium and other electrolytes that may be deficient. If the excess has developed over a long period of time, as may occur in the patient with chronic kidney disease, chronic liver disease, or congestive heart failure, withholding of fluids is not indicated. The homeostatic mechanisms do not function normally in patients with these conditions and treatment is directed toward the underlying condition. The volume excess may also be corrected by use of a low sodium diet. Finally, the patient with chronic malnutrition may develop a volume excess, largely because of plasma protein deficit; in this case, treatment is directed toward improving the patient's nutritional status.

CALCIUM EXCESS OF EXTRACELLULAR FLUID
This imbalance is always secondary to a metabolic disease, so primary treatment is directed toward correcting the underlying cause. The patient should be placed on a low calcium diet, and those requiring therapy for other imbalances should be given only calcium-free solutions. Hypercalcemic crisis is the most critical syndrome of calcium excess and it represents an emergency situation requiring urgent therapy lest the patient die of cardiac arrest. Unfortunately, medical management of hypercalcemic crisis has generally been unsatisfactory, and none of the regimens tried has been consistently successful because of slow action or inherent toxicity. Inorganic phosphate appears to be effective in rapidly lowering serum calcium levels, beginning within 3 minutes of the start of the infusion, with return to normal calcium values within 24 hours. Despite their effectiveness, phosphate solutions produce several undesirable side effects; nevertheless, the urgency of the situation appears to justify their use. Sulfate solutions are also effective and do not produce the widespread side effects associated with phosphate solutions, but they take longer to act and tend to produce magnesium deficit; consequently, magnesium supplements should be available when a sulfate solution is being used.

POTASSIUM EXCESS OF EXTRACELLULAR FLUID
The method used to treat this imbalance depends upon the status of the patient's homeostatic mechanisms. An uncomplicated potassium excess can be corrected simply by avoiding additional potassium intake, either orally or parenterally. If the homeostatic mechanisms are functioning normally, a 5 per cent solution of sodium bicarbonate is the preferred solution in treatment of severe potassium excess, since the kidneys retain sodium in preference to potassium, which causes increased urinary excretion of potassium. In patients whose homeostatic mechanisms are impaired, insulin and dextrose are useful in forcing potassium from extracellular fluid back into the cells, the most satisfactory method of producing a temporary fall in the extracellular fluid potassium level. Carbonic anhydrase inhibitors and ion exchange resins can also be used in treating this imbal-

ance, but they tend to produce metabolic acidosis, an undesirable side effect. When potassium excess is accompanied by severe kidney disease, peritoneal dialysis or hemodialysis may be necessary.

Patients suffering from severe disruptions in electrolyte concentration or composition of the extracellular fluid often need immediate replacement therapy. The patient may have functional homeostatic mechanisms, but the magnitude of the deficit is so severe, or the deficit has developed so rapidly, that balanced solutions cannot provide adequate electrolytes to correct the imbalance. Therefore, specific repair solutions are required for sodium deficit, calcium deficit, and magnesium deficit.

SODIUM DEFICIT OF EXTRACELLULAR FLUID
In treating this imbalance, one must administer sodium chloride in such concentration as to return the sodium level to normal without subsequently producing a fluid volume excess. If fluid volume is normal or excessive, a 3 or 5 per cent solution of sodium chloride is used, dosage being based on the deficit of sodium in the plasma. Hypertonic solutions of sodium chloride should be administered only intravenously; they are given at a rate of 1 ml./m.^{2} body surface/minute. When the sodium deficit is accompanied by extracellular fluid volume deficit, an isotonic solution of sodium chloride, or normal saline, is used to correct the sodium deficit and, when the sodium deficit has been repaired, the volume deficit can be corrected with a balanced solution. Isotonic solution of sodium chloride is administered intravenously at a flow rate of 3 ml./m.^{2} body surface/minute.

CALCIUM DEFICIT OF EXTRACELLULAR FLUID
The accepted mode of therapy for this disturbance is administration of a 10 per cent solution of calcium gluconate combined with an isotonic solution of sodium chloride, particularly important if severe muscle spasms or convulsions have occurred. The recommended dose for children is 1 ml. of the 10 per cent solution of calcium gluconate/kg. body weight, diluted with two volumes of isotonic solution of sodium chloride administered over a 10-minute period; the total dose of 10 per cent calcium gluconate solution should not exceed 10 ml. in any one infusion. Older children and adults can be given a dose of 10 ml. of 10 per cent calcium gluconate solution diluted with two volumes of isotonic solution of

sodium chloride. If the disease process that originally caused the hypocalcemia cannot be immediately controlled, it may be necessary to repeat the infusion. In the patient with hypoparathyroidism, administration of a phosphorus-free balanced solution promotes absorption of calcium and, thus, helps maintain the normal levels of calcium and phosphorus in the plasma.

MAGNESIUM DEFICIT OF EXTRACELLULAR FLUID
Magnesium sulfate either by mouth or intravenously is the treatment of choice in magnesium deficit. Parenteral treatment includes intravenous administration of a 10 ml. ampule of 50 per cent magnesium sulfate solution combined with 1 L. of a balanced solution containing no calcium or phosphorus. This is necessary because the symptoms of magnesium deficit are exaggerated by high intakes of calcium and, particularly, of phosphorus. Flow rate should be no faster than 6 ml./m.^{2} body surface/minute. Response is usually comparatively rapid, and tetanic symptoms often disappear within a matter of hours. However, since a significant percentage of the administered magnesium will be lost in the urine, supplemental doses may be necessary. It is important to keep in mind that tetany caused by magnesium deficit cannot be corrected by administration of calcium, and vice versa.

MAGNESIUM EXCESS OF EXTRACELLULAR FLUID
Magnesium excess occurs so infrequently as not to deserve a place in our basic classification. However, when it is present, administration of magnesium-containing products should be discontinued promptly; extracellular fluid volume deficit, if present, should be corrected; and calcium gluconate can be administered intravenously. If respiratory failure occurs, artificial respiration will be necessary. *Magnesium salts should never be given to patients with acute or chronic renal disease.*

PROTEIN DEFICIT OF EXTRACELLULAR FLUID
The goal of therapy in protein deficit is to help prevent the vicious circle of nutritional deficiency, which goes from anorexia to malnutrition to still further anorexia. The only way to break the circle is to provide protein and adequate calories to prevent amino acids from being used for energy purposes, plus potassium and magnesium for effective utilization of protein. The most desirable therapy is high-protein foods or supplements orally or by nasogastric

tube but, if the patient cannot tolerate such therapy or if his condition contraindicates such feedings, administration of protein hydrolysate solutions containing essential amino acids, adequate calories in the form of dextrose or alcohol or both, and electrolytes for maintenance requirements will prevent further development of protein deficit in most patients.

PLASMA-TO-INTERSTITIAL FLUID SHIFT Therapy of this imbalance is directed toward limiting the shift, if possible; maintaining plasma volume; treating vascular collapse and heart failure if they occur; and preparing for the possibility of a secondary interstitial fluid-to-plasma shift. Unfortunately, massive plasma-to-interstitial fluid shifts often cannot be restricted except by correcting the primary cause. For localized shifts, a tight binder around the affected part may effect relief; if a massive shift involves loss of plasma, plasma volume can be restored or maintained by administering plasma or a plasma expander, such as dextran, intravenously. An electrolyte replacement solution with a composition resembling extracellular fluid should be used if the shift involves only water and electrolytes. A gastrointestinal replacement solution or lactated Ringer's solution is ideal if the kidneys are functioning normally but, if kidney function is depressed, isotonic solution of sodium chloride may be given. The amount of plasma, dextran, or electrolyte solution needed varies with the weight of the patient and the magnitude of the shift. Vascular collapse and heart failure are usually fatal complications following prolonged lack of oxygen during shock; treatment includes administration of oxygen and stimulants such as caffeine, nikethamide (Coramine), epinephrine, and norepinephrine. Lastly, to help limit the severity of the secondary interstitial fluid-to-plasma shift that occurs with remobilization of edema fluid, unnecessary administration of fluids during the plasma-to-interstitial fluid shift should be avoided.

INTERSTITIAL FLUID-TO-PLASMA SHIFT The rapid interstitial fluid-to-plasma shift that occurs with remobilization of edema fluid following the reverse shift or following excessive intravenous administration of hypertonic solutions is unpreventable and may be so severe as to overload the renocardiovascular system. When this occurs, the goal of therapy is to reduce the amount of fluid returning to the heart, accomplished by placing tourniquets around the extremities in such a way that they block venous return but do not interfere with arterial circulation. Phlebotomy may be necessary. If the shift occurs as a compensatory measure following internal or external loss of whole blood, it can be halted by transfusion of whole blood.

WHOLE BLOOD DEFICIT A whole blood deficit should be repaired by giving whole blood but, if the extracellular fluid volume is excessive, red cells should be given alone.

COMPLEX COMBINED IMBALANCES The severe burn is an excellent example of a complex combination of body fluid imbalances. Therapy of this condition requires knowledge of the hazardous aftermaths of the burn, which include losses of body fluid, shock, renal depression, and remobilization of edema fluid. Carefully controlled therapy must be directed at the correction of the imbalances secondary to these aftermaths.

Types of Solutions

Solutions vary greatly from hospital to hospital. The nurse is urged to become familiar with the solutions employed in the hospital in which she works. This information can be gained by talking with the hospital pharmacist or with knowledgeable physicians and by carefully reading the excellent literature provided by the pharmaceutical company that supplies the parenteral solutions for the hospital. Certainly among the valuable resource personnel, we should emphasize the local pharmaceutical company representative and the medical departments of their respective companies.

BIBLIOGRAPHY

Bennett, W., Singer, I., and **Coggins, C.:**   A guide to drug therapy in renal failure. J.A.M.A. 230:1544–1553, 1974.

Chatton, M.:   Handbook of Medical Treatment, ed. 13. Los Altos, Calif.: Lange Medical Publications, 1972.

Kempe, C., Silver, H., and **O'Brien, D.:**   Current Pediatric Diagnosis and Treatment, ed. 4. Los Altos, Calif.: Lange Medical Publications, 1976.

Knochel, J.:   Dog days and diriasis, how to kill a football player. J.A.M.A. 233:513–515, 1975.

Schneider, H., Anderson, C., and **Coursin, D.** (eds.):   Nutritional Support of Medical Practice. New York: Harper & Row, 1977.

— 16 —

Parenteral Fluid Administration— Nursing Implications

"I injected one hundred and twenty ounces, when like the effects of magic, instead of the pallid aspect of one whom death had sealed as his own, the vital tide was restored, and life and vivacity returned!" Thomas Latta, 1831

Intravenous therapy is a major component of patient care; millions of patients in hospitals receive this treatment each year. The nurse plays a major role in the administration of parenteral fluids. Her exact responsibilities are not uniformly defined and vary with geographical areas and individual hospitals. Many hospitals have wisely organized intravenous therapy teams to start, and assist in maintaining, infusions. Nevertheless, regardless of who starts the fluids, the nurse shares in the responsibility of assuring their safe and therapeutic administration. To ably assume this responsibility, she must understand basic principles of safe fluid administration and become familiar with parenteral fluids. If intelligent observations are to be made during their infusion, the purposes, contraindications, and complications associated with their use must be known.

ROUTES AND TECHNIQUES OF PARENTERAL FLUID ADMINISTRATION

Intravenous

INDICATIONS FOR USE   Veins provide an excellent route for the quick administration of water, electrolytes, and other nutrients. Fluids administered intravenously at the proper rate and in the proper dose pass directly into the extracellular fluid. They are rapidly acted upon by the body homeostatic mechanisms and, hence, in proper doses, do not produce abnormal changes in volume or electrolyte concentration of extracellular fluid. The intravenous route is essential when nutrients are needed in a hurry, such as glucose in severe hypoglycemia, 5 per cent sodium chloride in severe sodium deficit, or calcium gluconate in acute calcium deficit. Relatively large volumes of fluids can be given by the intravenous route, provided due care is exercised.

GENERAL PSYCHOLOGIC CONSIDERATIONS

Few persons are without some fear or dread of a needle being introduced into their veins. Normal fears are exaggerated in illness, since many patients associate intravenous fluids with critical illnesses and are disturbed when such therapy is employed. It is the nurse's responsibility to explain away as much of the fear as possible and point out that I.V. fluids are commonly used until oral intake is again possible.

Because all patients are individuals, the nurse must plan her approach on an individual basis. The nurse must always remember that although I.V. therapy is commonplace to her, it is far from routine to the patient. A detailed explanation of why and how the fluids are given is indicated for some; others want only a brief account. In any event, the patient should *never* be approached with no explanation at all; the fear of not knowing what is to happen can be worse than the most painful venipuncture.

Only persons capable of skillful venipuncture should start fluids on anxious patients; just one traumatic experience may make I.V. therapy totally unacceptable to them. The nurse who starts fluids must always appear confident—patients sense insecurity and are understandably upset by it. An I.V. therapy department with competent therapists provides many advantages, one of which is the skill developed by such therapists in performing venipuncture.

SELECTION OF SITE

Suitable Superficial Veins   A number of superficial veins are available for venipuncture. Those most commonly used include:

Veins in and around the cubital fossa (antecubital, basilic, and cephalic veins)
Veins in the forearm (basilic and cephalic veins)
Veins in the radial area of the wrist
Veins in the hand (metacarpal and dorsal venous plexus)
Scalp veins in infants

Criteria for Selection   Selection of a vein depends upon a number of factors:

Availability of sites (depends upon condition of veins)
Size of needle to be used
Type of fluids to be infused
Volume, rate and length of infusion
Degree of mobility desired
Skill of operator

Hand Veins   The early use of hand veins (Fig. 16-1) is important if parenteral therapy is to be prolonged. This allows each successive venipuncture to be made above the previous site, eliminating pain and inflammation caused by irritating fluids passing through a vein injured by previous venipuncture. Because of their small diameter, hand veins do not accommodate large needles—a small gauge scalp vein needle is sometimes used for venipuncture in the hand.

Small veins cannot accept hypertonic or otherwise irritating fluids because less blood is present in small veins to dilute such solutions. These peripheral veins collapse sooner in the presence of shock than do more centrally located veins. And, finally, extravasation of blood may occur in venipuncture in this area, particularly when there is thin skin and inadequate connective tissue.

Forearm Veins   The cephalic vein flows upward along the radial border of the forearm and is an excellent site for venipuncture (Fig. 16-2). Also, the size of the vein will accommodate a large needle. The accessory cephalic vein joins the cephalic vein below the elbow, and it too is a good site for venipuncture. Both veins are frequently used for blood administration. When prominent, the median antebrachial vein can be used for venipuncture. The location of superficial veins of the forearm is somewhat variable and not always well-defined.

Venipuncture in a forearm vein allows the patient some arm movement without the risk of puncturing the posterior venous wall.

Elbow Veins   The median cephalic and median basilic veins are found in the antecubital fossa; both veins are readily accessible to venipuncture because they are large and superficially located. In addition,

Sections of this chapter concerned with starting and maintaining intravenous infusions were prepared with the assistance of Darnell Roth, R.N., I.V. Therapist, Alexian Brothers Hospital, St. Louis, Missouri.

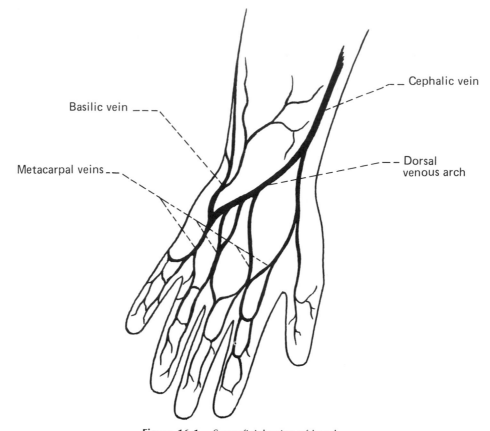

Figure 16-1. Superficial veins of hand.

they are kept from rolling and sliding by surrounding tissues. They will accommodate large needles, large volumes of fluids, and all but the most irritating intravenous fluids.

Because arteries in the antecubital area, though usually more deeply located, lie in close proximity to veins, it is easy to mistake an artery for a vein in this area. Aberrant arteries are not uncommon in the cubital fossa. (These arteries, more superficially located than usual, are found in one out of ten persons.) Injection of fluids into an artery usually causes the patient to complain of sudden severe pain in the arm and hand, caused by arteriospasm. This is an indication to stop the infusion immediately.

When frequent blood specimens are necessary, it is wise to save the veins in the antecubital area for this purpose; large quantities of blood can be obtained from them. These veins can be used many times without damage if good technique is used. (It is extremely difficult to get sufficient blood from small veins.)

A disadvantage in using veins in the antecubital area is the restriction of elbow flexion during the infusion. Therefore, when long-term infusions are anticipated or the patient is uncooperative, it is best to use the veins in the forearm, because the patient can be moved and ambulated with less danger of dislodging the needle. The nurse should remember that damage to veins in the antecubital area can limit the use of sites below.

A right-handed person has more freedom if the infusion is given in the left arm; however, the need for multiple venipunctures is an indication to employ alternate sites in both arms.

Lower Extremity Veins Usually, lower extremity veins are not recommended for venipuncture since their use can result in dangerous complications. Thrombus formation at the venipuncture site occurs to some degree in all venipunctures, but when ankle veins are used, the thrombus can extend to deep veins and may result in pulmonary embolism.

Venipuncture should not be performed on a varicose vein or at a site below a varicosity, as such veins do not readily transport fluids into the general circulation, and they may cause a pooling of fluid in veins around the injection site. Pooling of infused medications can cause an untoward reaction when a toxic concentration reaches the general circulation. Varicose veins are easily traumatized, and moreover, they are difficult to enter because they tend to roll; moreover, the blood flow in them is frequently reversed.

GENERAL CONSIDERATIONS

1. When feasible, it is best to use veins in the upper part of the body.
2. When multiple punctures are anticipated, it is best to make the first venipuncture distally and work proximally with subsequent punctures.
3. Avoid venipuncture in the affected arm of patients with axillary dissection, as in radical mastectomy (embarrassed circulation affects the flow of the infusion, causing increased edema).
4. Avoid checking the blood pressure on the arm receiving an infusion because the cuff interferes with fluid flow, forces blood back into the needle, and may cause a clot to form.
5. When the patient is on his side, the upper arm should be used for venipuncture. The lower arm has increased venous pressure which interferes with fluid flow and may cause clot formation in the needle.

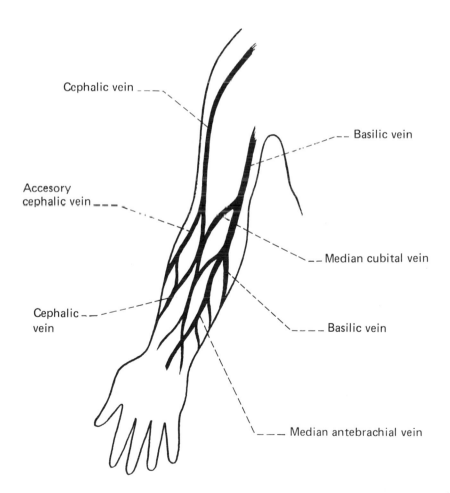

Figure 16-2. Superficial veins of forearm.

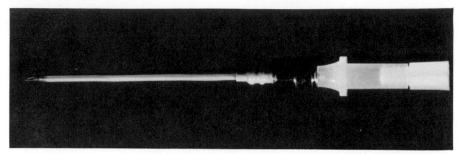

Figure 16-3.   Jelco Cathlon I.V. Placement Unit. Note that the catheter is *over* a needle. (Jelco Laboratories, Raritan, New Jersey)

6. Restraints should not be placed on or above the infusion site. (When the involved extremity must be immobilized, the restraint should be applied to the arm board only; *never* over the injection site since it would act as a tourniquet and obstruct flow.)

7. An armboard should be used when the venipuncture site is over an area of flexion (such as the wrist or elbow).

8. Hold the infusion bottle sufficiently high during ambulation of the patient and transport via wheelchair or stretcher to maintain a constant flow rate. When the patient is ambulating, the arm receiving the infusion should be placed across the abdomen to immobilize it and the I.V. pole should be rolled with the other hand.

9. Instruct the patient with a venipuncture in the hand or arm to avoid such movements as combing hair, brushing teeth, or cutting up food, with the affected arm whenever possible.

METHODS FOR VENOUS ENTRY   Fluids may be introduced into a vein by means of:

A metal needle

A plastic needle (catheter mounted on a needle) (See Figure 16-3)

A plastic catheter threaded through a metal needle (See Figure 16-4)

A plastic catheter introduced by means of a cutdown (minor surgical procedure)

SELECTION OF METHODS   Short-term infusions are usually given through metal needles—either a regular straight needle or, most often, a scalp vein needle. The scalp vein needle is approximately three-fourths of an inch long and has attached plastic wings, used for holding the needle during venipuncture (Fig. 16-5). This needle has a thin wall and provides a larger lumen with a smaller needle diameter and because the bevel is short, there is less danger of accidentally puncturing the posterior wall of the vein.

Scalp vein needles are available in two types:

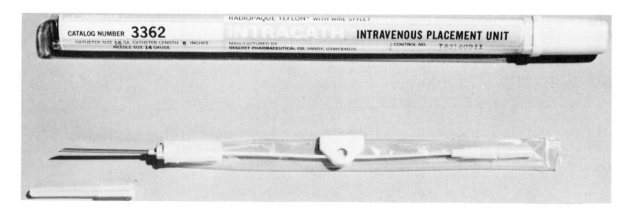

Figure 16-4.   *A,* Deseret Intracath. (Courtesy of Deseret Pharmaceutical Co., Sandy, Utah) *B,* (on facing page), note that the catheter is extended *through* the needle.

→

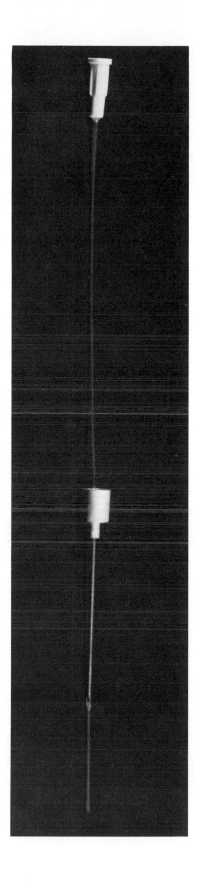

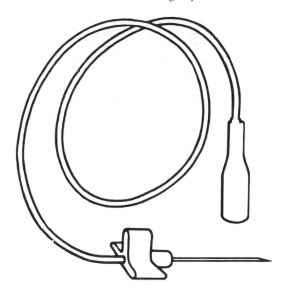

Figure 16-5. Pediatric Scalp Vein Infusion Set. (Courtesy of Cutter Laboratories, Berkeley, California)

one with a variable length of plastic tubing attached to an adaptor that accommodates an administration set and the other with a short length of tubing ending in a resealable injection site (sometimes referred to as a "heparin lock" or an "intermittent infusion set"). The resealable injection site allows intermittent injection of medications or parenteral fluids without repeated venipunctures (Fig. 16-6). Patency of the needle is maintained by periodically flushing the needle with a dilute solution of heparin. Each time medication is injected into the resealable site, it is important to cleanse the area thoroughly with a sterile alcohol wipe. Prior to injecting the medication, it is imperative to confirm that the needle is still in the vein. (*Never* automatically inject medication without first verifying proper positioning of the needle.)

Another device available for intermittent infusions is pictured in Figure 16-7. A stylet is inserted into the lumen of the catheter when I.V. fluids are not needed; it is removed when infusions are to be resumed. Such a device reduces the need for "keep-open" infusions and allows the patient more freedom of movement. A *new* sterile stylet is inserted into the catheter after each intermittent injection of medication (using scrupulous aseptic technique).

The size of the needle to be used depends on the vein as well as on the type of solution. Scalp vein needles range in size from a 25 gauge to a 16 gauge. (The smaller the gauge number, the larger the inter-

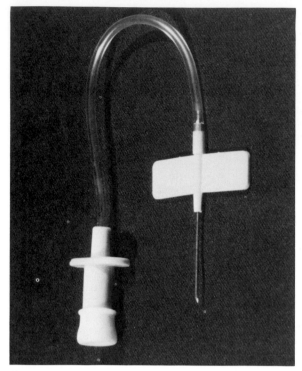

Figure 16-6. Bard Intermittent Infusion Set. Note the resealable injection site. (C. R. Bard, Inc., Murray Hill, New Jersey)

nal diameter of the needle.) If possible, the gauge of the needle should be appreciably smaller than the lumen of the vein to be entered, as when a large needle occludes the flow of blood, irritating solutions may produce chemical phlebitis. If a small needle is used, irritating fluids can mix readily with blood, decreasing the chance of phlebitis. A large gauge needle is required for high viscosity fluids, such as blood. (Blood usually is administered through an 18- or 19-gauge needle.)

A plastic needle is a catheter mounted on a metal needle. When the venipuncture is made, the catheter is slipped off the needle into the vein and the metal needle is removed. Plastic needles do not infiltrate as easily as metal needles because of their pliability. Most plastic catheters are Teflon coated for ease of insertion. It is recommended that plastic catheters be radiopaque (so that they can be more readily located in the event of catheter emboli.)

An intracatheter is a catheter inserted through a metal needle and used when a longer catheter is desired. Often it is used to administer drugs or irritating solutions that may cause tissue necrosis if infiltration occurs.

A cut-down may be performed when veins become exhausted from prolonged therapy and when peripheral veins have collapsed from shock. The necessity of signing a surgical permission form for the cut-down procedure is determined by individual hospital policy. The advent of plastic intracatheters introduced through a needle has reduced the need for surgical cut-downs.

TECHNIQUES OF INSERTION

Venipuncture with a Metal Needle After a suitable site has been located, the next step is to distend the vein, usually accomplished by a tourniquet; it also helps to steady the vein when the tourniquet is placed no higher than 2 inches above the site of injection. It should be tight enough to impede venous flow while arterial flow is maintained, but never too tight —a common error.

Occasionally, it may be necessary to distend the vein by placing it in a dependent position for several

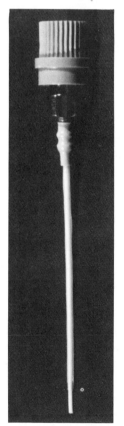
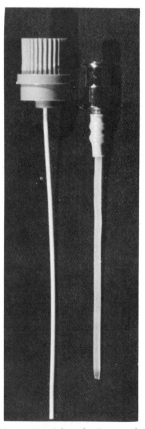

Figure 16-7. Jelco Cathlon I.V. set: *A*, with stylet inserted; *B*, with stylet removed. (Jelco Laboratories, Raritan, New Jersey)

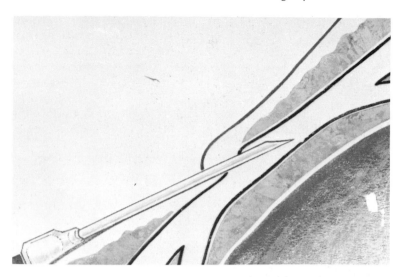

Figure 16-8. Needle bevel position for venipuncture. (Courtesy of Pfizer Laboratories, New York)

minutes. Sometimes a light slap or tap with the therapist's fingers over the proposed site of venipuncture helps; so does exercising the muscles distal to the site of puncture. However, exercising should not be done when blood is being drawn for determination of serum electrolytes, since a false reading may result.

A large gauge needle always causes pain; its insertion may be preceded by locally injecting a small amount of 1 per cent procaine. This should be done only by order of the physician; in addition, the patient should be questioned about allergy to procaine. The injection of procaine should be done intradermally, in only extremely small amounts. Sometimes it is advantageous to insert the procaine above the proposed site for venipuncture since distal anesthesia occurs after a short wait. Frequently, the operator does not wait a sufficient time for the full anesthetic effect of the procaine, which results in a tendency to use larger amounts of procaine than are necessary.

Seventy percent alcohol is frequently used to prepare the injection site; it is most effective if the skin is scrubbed with friction for a full minute with a "clean to dirty" circular motion. Unfortunately, skin preparation most often consists of a quick light wipe with the sponge, failing to significantly reduce the bacteria count. Povidone-iodine solution is highly desirable for cleansing the injection site because it provides effective bactericidal, fungicidal, and sporicidal activity. (Because of occasional allergy to iodine, the patient should be questioned about this before its use.) Aqueous benzalkonium chloride and other quarternary ammonium compounds are not effective skin antiseptics and should not be used for

this purpose. Scientific evidence does not substantiate the need to shave hair from the injection site to reduce bacterial flora; in fact, the nicks incurred from shaving may actually predispose to infection. Shaving does, however, facilitate removal of tape from a very hairy site.

Generally, the bevel of the needle should be facing upward during insertion (Fig. 16-8). However, the introduction of a large needle into a small vein may require the bevel to face downward; otherwise, the needle would pierce the posterior wall of the vein when the tourniquet is removed.

With the tourniquet in place, the needle should pierce the skin to one side of, and approximately one half to one inch below, the point where the needle will enter the vein. As the needle enters the skin it should be at about a 45 degree angle; after the skin is entered, the needle angle is decreased. Although it seems more logical to enter the vein from above with one quick thrust, there seems to be less flattening of the vein when a lateral approach is used. The free hand is used to palpate the vein while the needle is being introduced. An experienced operator can feel a snap as the needle enters the vein; after this, less resistance is offered to the needle. At this point, one should proceed very slowly with the insertion of the needle, threading it into the lumen approximately one half to three fourths of an inch. The tourniquet is then released. Frequently a thin stream of blood is seen in the tubing when the needle enters the vein. If in doubt, pinch the tubing just above the needle and release it; usually this will cause a flashback of blood into the tubing.

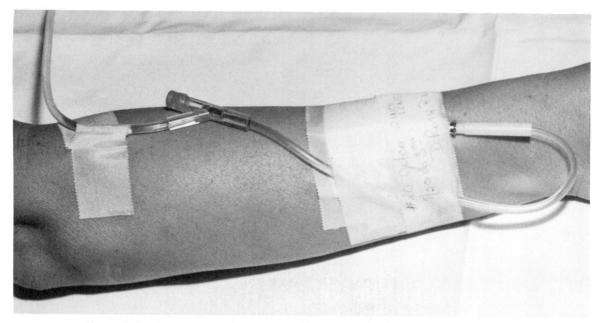

Figure 16-9. Venipuncture dressing. (See Figure 16-10 for close-up view of labeling.)

Fluid should be allowed to run in, and the area should be observed for swelling. The presence of swelling indicates that the needle is not in the vein and fluid is entering the subcutaneous area. The infusion should be discontinued immediately when swelling is noted or if the venipuncture attempt was unsuccessful; a venipuncture must then be made in another area. A tourniquet should not be reapplied immediately to the same extremity; if applied too soon, a hematoma will develop and the patient will experience unnecessary pain and discomfort.

After successful venipuncture, the next step involves anchoring the needle comfortably and safely. A piece of tape should be diagonally wrapped around the needle hub to prevent "to and fro" motion of the needle, which predisposes to phlebitis; then, a piece of tape should be applied over the hub to further stabilize it. A sterile 2 × 2 inch gauze pad should cover the entry site. (Some hospitals use povidone-iodine sponges or antibiotic ointment on the dressing.) Tape should be applied in such a way that the tubing may be changed easily. A loop of tubing should be secured with tape independently of the needle so that an accidental tug on the tubing will not dislodge the needle or catheter. The date and time of insertion should be written on the tape to alert personnel to the need to remove the device within a safe period of time. Also, the gauge and length of the device used

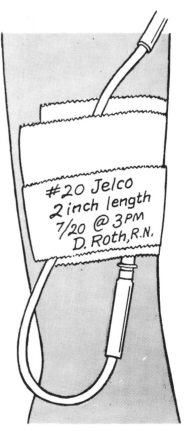

Figure 16-10. Close-up view of venipuncture dressing labeling.

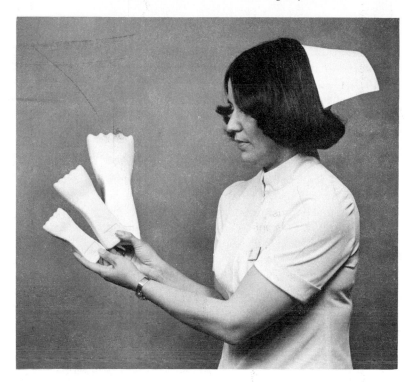

Figure 16-11. Various sizes of arm supports are available to suit individual needs. (Courtesy of The Master Medical Corporation, Phoenix, Arizona)

for venipuncture should be noted, as well as the name or initials of the person performing the venipuncture (Figs. 16-9 and 16-10). (It is important that the gauge of the venipuncture device be noted on the tape. Should an emergency situation arise, it is readily apparent to those responding whether or not the device in place will accommodate viscous fluids.)

An armboard may be necessary at times to immobilize the involved extremity and decrease the likelihood of infiltration (Fig. 16-11). It should be applied in such a way as to allow normal anatomic flexion of the fingers (Fig. 16-12). At no time should the fingers be flattened out on the armboard.

Plastic Catheter Mounted Over a Needle A venipuncture is performed in the usual manner, with the needle inserted far enough to ensure entry of the catheter into the vein. After the catheter is slid into the vein to the desired length, the needle is carefully removed. If the venipuncture is not successful, withdraw the catheter completely from the puncture site

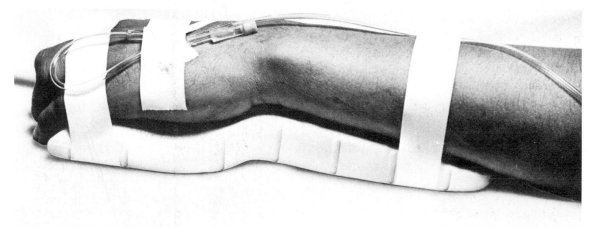

Figure 16-12. Master I.V. Arm Support allows normal flexion of fingers. (Courtesy of The Master Medical Corporation, Phoenix, Arizona)

before reinserting the needle; reinsertion of the needle with the catheter in place could sever the catheter, resulting in catheter embolism. (The manufacturer's directions should be followed closely.) A small sterile dressing should be applied to the puncture site after the catheter is anchored securely with tape.

Plastic Catheter Inserted Through a Needle After performance of a normal venipuncture, the catheter is inserted into the vein through the needle. If venipuncture is not successful, pull out the needle and catheter together. The catheter should not be pulled out first because the sharp edges of the needle could sever it as it is being withdrawn, resulting in catheter embolism. (The manufacturer's directions should be followed closely.)

Only an experienced operator should attempt venipuncture by this method because of the higher incidence of complications associated with its use (such as tissue trauma, infection, and severed catheter emboli.) When removing a catheter from a vein, do not use scissors to remove tape as it is possible to cut the catheter accidentally. Always *check the length* of the catheter when it is removed.

Some feel that plastic catheters are about twice as prone to produce venous complications as metal needles. It has been suggested that because metal needles infiltrate more quickly than plastic devices they are changed more frequently. It is known that the longer the intravenous device remains in place, the higher the rate of positive cultures. Plastic catheters should not remain in place longer than 72 hours (some recommend changing them every 48 hours). This time limit is difficult to enforce when the patient's veins are exhausted, particularly when the hospital is not equipped with an I.V. therapy team.

An antibiotic ointment is sometimes applied to minimize the occurrence of catheter sepsis. The catheter should be anchored securely with tape and a sterile dressing should cover the area; the dressing should be changed daily to inspect the site and apply more ointment. The date of insertion, and the gauge, length, and type of catheter used should be noted.

Hypodermoclysis

Hypodermoclysis, the administration of a solution subcutaneously, compares unfavorably with the intravenous route and is used less and less because of its many problems and associated discomfort to the patient.

The types of fluids that can be given subcutaneously are few, since they must closely resemble the electrolyte content and tonicity of extracellular fluid if they are to be absorbed. Some of the fluids generally considered reasonably safe for subcutaneous administration include:

Isotonic saline (0.9%)
Half-isotonic saline (0.45%) with 2½% dextrose
Ringer's solution
Half-strength Ringer's with 2½% dextrose
Lactated Ringer's solution
Half-strength lactated Ringer's with 2½% dextrose

Fluids that are contraindicated for subcutaneous administration include electrolyte-free solutions, hypertonic solutions, alcohol, amino acids, solutions of high molecular weight such as albumin, and those whose pH differs significantly from body pH (such as gastric replacement solution). Orders for the subcutaneous administration of any of these solutions should be questioned.

The subcutaneous administration of a 5 per cent dextrose in water solution attracts electrolytes from the surrounding tissues and from the plasma, which enter the pool created at the infusion site. (This electrolyte movement occurs to make the solution absorbable.) Often the pool remains at the infusion site for some time before it is absorbed, and the subsequent decreased plasma sodium level can cause hypotension and even shock. If the patient is already suffering from sodium deficit, the ultimate result can be death. Aged hospitalized patients may already have low plasma sodium levels secondary to extracellular fluid losses and, since such patients develop sodium deficit more readily than younger adults, they should certainly not receive electrolyte-free solutions subcutaneously.

Probably the only advantage hypodermoclysis has over the intravenous route is that it is easier to start. It is most often used for obese patients, infants, and the aged, for all of whom intravenous fluids are difficult to start. Suitable sites include the subcutaneous tissues on the lateral aspect of the thigh or abdomen, fatty tissue of the subscapular region, and loose fatty tissue at the base of the breasts. Infections into the tissues at the injection site. If an order for Wydase is not included with the fluid order, a call to the physician could be advantageous. The patient must be checked often when this route is used; a large amount of swelling can develop unless the flow rate is adjusted carefully. A small sterile gauze pad should be placed under the needle hub and another should cover the injection site. Following the removal of the needle, a light sterile dressing should be applied, as edematous injection sites are fertile fields for infections.

COMMENT   Much discomfort is usually associated with hypodermoclysis. This route is undependable, especially when large amounts of fluids are needed in a hurry. Fluids are not absorbed well from the subcutaneous tissue when blood volume is severely reduced because of accompanying peripheral collapse. The fluids that can be given safely are quite limited and, ironically, the patients for which hypodermoclysis is most often used (infants, the aged, and the obese) are the ones most prone to be harmed by them. Most authorities feel that a cut-down carries less risk than does hypodermoclysis.

GENERAL CONSIDERATIONS IN FLUID ADMINISTRATION

Determining Flow Rate

PHYSICIAN'S ORDERS   The physician should order the type of solution and, ideally, its rate of flow. In turn, the nurse is responsible for initiating most infusions and maintaining the proper rate of flow. Nurses must be aware of the composition of the prescribed solution, its desired effect, its usual rate of administration and complications that may be associated with its use.

FACTORS INFLUENCING THE DESIRED RATE OF ADMINISTRATION   Factors considered in determining the best flow rate for the infusion include:

Type of fluid
Need for fluids
Cardiac and renal status
Body size
Age

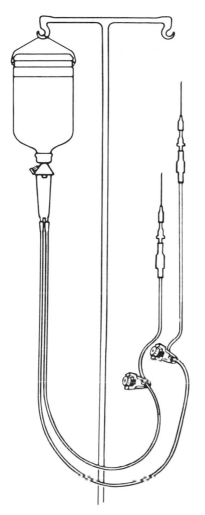

Figure 16-13. Hypodermoclysis Setup (Safticlysis™ Long-leg Setup). (Courtesy of Cutter Laboratories, Berkeley, California)

are not uncommon with hypodermoclysis and are usually proportionate to the distention that occurs (because of tissue ischemia) and to the length of time required for the infusion.

Most often, two needles are used and the fluid is infused into two sites at once; the inverted Y-tubing from the solution bottle separates and goes to two sites (Fig. 16-13). The rate of infusion depends upon how well the fluid is absorbed from the injection site. When the fluid is absorbed well, 250 to 500 ml. can be given at one site in one hour to an adult but, after a short while, the fluid is not this readily absorbed and the tissues become hard and swollen. To hasten absorption, hyaluronidase (Wydase), may be injected

Patient's reaction during the infusion
Size of the vein

The desired rate for the infusion varies with the type of fluids used. For example, isotonic solutions can usually be given more rapidly than very hypertonic solutions. Although the other variables must also be considered, it is helpful for the nurse to know the usual infusion rates for various solutions. They are given in the descriptions of parenteral fluids in the next section of this chapter.

The patient's need for fluids influences the desired rate of administration; for example, a patient in hypovolemic shock needs fluids in a hurry. The infusion in this instance is much faster than usual. The presence of cardiac or renal damage can greatly alter the desired infusion rate, because the heart and kidneys both play a major role in the utilization of fluids introduced intravenously. If the pumping action of the heart is inadequate, a rapid infusion of fluids could cause a dangerous fluid excess. The failure of the kidneys to excrete unneeded water and electrolytes can also result in excessive amounts of these substances in the body.

Body surface area is an important criterion for fluid infusion rate. As mentioned in Chapter 15, the flow rate is 3 ml./m.^{2} of body surface/minute. This rate does not apply to all types of fluids and must at times be altered. Generally speaking, however, it is logical that a large individual can tolerate a greater amount of fluid per minute than a smaller individual, if other factors are equal.

Aged patients almost always have some degree of cardiac and renal impairment; therefore, fluids are administered more slowly to them than to younger adults.

One of the best guides to safe flow rate is the patient's reaction to the infusion; the fact that individuals respond differently to parenteral fluid infusions, just as they do to other medications, must never be forgotten. For this reason, the patient should be checked at least every 30 minutes during an infusion. The nurse should be aware of symptoms associated with the improper administration of various solutions so that she can know what to look for. Reactions associated with different parenteral fluids are described later in the chapter.

VARIATIONS OF DROP SIZE WITH DIFFERENT COMMERCIAL SETS   Most nurses think in terms of

Table 16-1. Variation in Size of Drop in Commercial Administration Sets— Approximate No. of Drops to Deliver 1 ml.

Company	"Regular" Set	"Special" Sets
Abbott Lab.	15	60 (Microdrip) 10 (Blood Set)
Travenol Lab.	10	50 (M-50 Minimeter) 60 (Metal Drip System)
Cutter Lab.	20	60 (Saftiset Sixty Set)
McGaw Lab.	15	60

Adapted from Weisberg, H.: Water, Electrolyte and Acid-Base Balance, ed. 2. Baltimore: Williams & Wilkins, 1972, p. 286.

"drops per minute" when considering rate of fluid flow. It must be remembered that commercial parenteral administration sets vary in the number of drops delivering 1 ml. (Table 16-1). Unless one knows which administration set is to be used, it is more practical to consider the number of milliliters to be infused in 1 minute. From this figure, the number of drops per minute can be computed when the drop size of the administration set is learned.

Formula:
Drop Factor × ml./min. = drops/min.

For example, to deliver 3 ml./minute using a set with 10 drops to 1 ml., a flow rate of 30 drops/minute would be necessary. To administer the same amount using a set with 15 drops to 1 ml., a flow rate of 45 drops/minute would be necessary. Drop size can vary somewhat according to the viscosity of the fluid being infused. Other factors affecting drop size include room temperature and height of the bottle; however, for practical purposes, the calibration of the I.V. set (gtts/min) should be accepted as valid. (Manufacturers list the drop factors on the administration set packages.)

CALCULATION OF FLOW RATE   If the nurse knows the amount of fluid to be given in a prescribed time interval, plus the drop factor of the administration set to be used, she can easily compute the desired number of drops/minute. The following formula is used:

Drops/min. =

$$\frac{\text{Total volume infused (ml)} \times \text{Drop factor (drops/ml.)}}{\text{Total time of infusion in minutes}}$$

Sample Problem:

Infuse 1000 ml. of 5% D/W in 2 hours (Assume an administration set with 10 drops to 1 ml. is to be used)

Total volume = 1000 ml.
Drops/ml. = 10
Total time of infusion in minutes = 120

$$\frac{1000 \times 10}{120} = \text{approximately 80 drops/min.}$$

To save the nurse's time, some handy calculators* have been devised by manufacturers of parenteral fluids to determine the desired flow rate when the above factors are known, directions for which are included with the calculators.

A tape which indicates the hourly fluid rate should be placed on the bottle for convenient checking (Fig. 16-14).

MECHANICAL FACTORS INFLUENCING GRAVITY FLOW RATE

After the desired flow rate has been regulated, there are several mechanical factors that may alter it:

1. Change in needle position: A change in the needle position may push the bevel against or away from the venous wall. An adequate flow rate becomes diminished when the needle is pushed against the vein, whereas it is increased when the needle moves away from the venous wall. Care must be taken to prevent speed shock by making sure the solution is flowing freely before adjusting the rate.
2. Height of the solution bottle: Because infusions flow in by gravity, a change in the height of the infusion bottle or bed can increase or decrease the rate—the greater the

---

* Abbott Laboratories (Normosol Calculator); Travenol Laboratories (Minislide Calculator); McGaw Laboratories (Solution-Administration Set Conversion Chart).

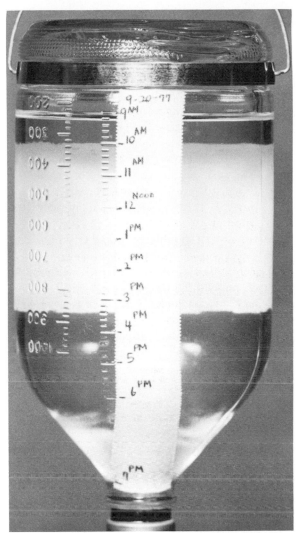

Figure 16-14. Tape on the I.V. container indicates where the fluid level should be each hour.

distance between the patient and the bottle, the faster the rate.

3. Patency of the needle: A small clot may occlude the needle lumen and decrease or stop the flow rate—when released, the rate increases. Clot formation may occur when an increase in venous pressure in the infusion arm forces blood back into the needle, causes of which can include lying on the infusion arm or constriction with a blood pressure cuff. A plugged needle should never be irrigated since the dislodged clot could cause an infarction; if infected, it could cause spread of the infection to another part of the body. (To check for a plugged needle, kink the tubing a

few inches above the injection site; then, pinch the tubing immediately above the needle. If resistance is met, and if there is no flashback of blood, the needle is probably plugged and should be removed.) Attempting to remove the clot by aspirating with a syringe may collapse the vein around the needle, possibly traumatizing the venous wall.[1]

4. Venous spasm: A cold or irritating solution may retard flow rate by producing venous spasm. A warm pack placed proximal to the infusion site will relieve this condition.

5. Plugged air vent: A plugged air vent can cause an infusion to stop. Thus, patency of the air vent should be checked when no other cause is apparent for the stopped infusion.

6. Condition of final filter: Final filters can cause decreased flow rates should particulate matter block the filtering surface or if an air lock develops.

7. Crying in infants: This problem raises venous pressure and, thus, slows the rate of flow.

PARENTERAL FLUIDS— SPECIAL CONSIDERATIONS

Parenteral Nutrition

Parenteral nutrition frequently is lifesaving. As Doctor Elman said, "Parenteral alimentation does not compete with oral alimentation; it competes only with death." Substances that can be given intravenously include:

Carbohydrates
Proteins
Fat emulsions
Alcohol
Vitamins
Water
Electrolytes

Provision of nutrients intravenously is indicated when it is desired to put the gastrointestinal tract at relative rest, as in the presence of nausea, vomiting, diarrhea, peritonitis, ileus, or fistula. Intravenous nutrition is also indicated when the patient cannot take nutrients by an enteral route. In considering the nutritional needs of the patient exclusively on paren-

teral feedings, it should be borne in mind that the recommended energy need of an adult at bedrest is 1600 calories; this is a basal figure and does not allow for fever, high environmental temperatures, or other causes of increased metabolism.

It is difficult to restore the nutritionally depleted patient by the intravenous route using routine fluids; however, it is possible to maintain the state of nutrition fairly well with their use for a short period of time. The advent of hyperalimentation has made it possible to support life and maintain growth and development for prolonged periods. (See the discussion of parenteral hyperalimentation.)

The goal of parenteral nutrition is chiefly to pinch-hit until the patient can again take nutrients by mouth. Every effort should be made to restore a patient receiving parenteral feedings to the oral or tube route as soon as possible. The nurse can contribute to this restoration by reporting signs of improvement, such as the absence of nausea and vomiting, and by encouraging the patient to take materials by mouth as soon as permissible.

Carbohydrates   Included in the carbohydrates that can be administered and absorbed intravenously are glucose, fructose, and invert sugar. These are all monosaccharides and, therefore, ready for utilization by the body cells. Disaccharides and polysaccharides cannot be utilized when given by the intravenous route. Table 16-2 presents an analysis of various parenteral carbohydrate solutions.

To provide the patient with sufficient calories through the administration of carbohydrate alone would necessitate giving a large quantity of a dilute solution, or a smaller quantity of a concentrated solu-

Table 16-2.   Parenteral Carbohydrate Solutions

Types of Solutions	Calories/L.	Tonicity
Dextrose		
2½% Dextrose	85	Hypotonic
5% Dextrose	170	Isotonic
10% Dextrose	340	Hypertonic
20% Dextorse	680	Hypertonic
50% Dextrose	1,700	Hypertonic
Fructose		
5% Fructose	187.5	Isotonic
10% Fructose	375	Hypertonic
Invert Sugar		
5% Invert sugar	187.5	Isotonic
10% Invert sugar	375	Hypertonic

tion. To supply 1600 calories with a 5 per cent dextrose solution would require 9 L., a volume exceeding the tolerance level of most patients. Mixtures of carbohydrate and alcohol are useful because of their rich caloric contribution and limited bulk.

Concentrated solutions, such as 20 per cent or 50 per cent dextrose, are useful for supplying calories for individuals with renal insufficiency or who for other reasons are unable to tolerate large volumes. In order that the glucose be utilized, concentrated solutions must be administered slowly. When administered rapidly, such solutions act as a diuretic and pull interstitial fluid into the plasma for subsequent renal excretion. Such hypertonic solutions damage veins in direct proportion to their tonicity, and when used, they should be injected into large functioning veins so that they will be diluted by the relatively large blood volume.

Carbohydrate is often administered parenterally to minimize the ketosis of starvation, since, when ingestion of carbohydrate and fats is inadequate, the body burns its own fats to supply caloric needs. As a result of this process, ketone bodies are formed and, since these are acids, they neutralize bicarbonate and produce metabolic acidosis (primary base bicarbonate deficit). Ketones require water for renal excretion and, thus, cause an increased demand for renal water expenditure.

One advantage of carbohydrate as a source of calories lies in the fact that, following its utilization, there remains only water and carbon dioxide to be used by the body or excreted. Nevertheless, when solutions of carbohydrate are administered too rapidly, the body cannot utilize all the carbohydrate and part of it is excreted in the urine. The body receives no benefit from the excreted glucose, and further, the glucose may carry with it other important nutrients. If a hypertonic carbohydrate solution is infused too rapidly, hyperinsulinism may occur, because the pancreas secretes extra insulin to metabolize the infused carbohydrate; discontinuance of the administration may leave an excess of insulin in the body. Symptoms of excess insulin include nervousness, sweating, and weakness. It is not uncommon for small amounts of isotonic carbohydrate solution to be given after hypertonic solutions to "cover" for the extra insulin and allow the return to normal secretion.

Rates of Administration The maximal speed for administration of glucose to normal adults without producing glycosuria is approximately 0.5 Gm./kg./hr. At this rate, it would take 3 hours for the injection of 1 L. of 10 per cent dextrose. Some maintain that fructose can be administered more rapidly than glucose and that invert sugar's optimal rate of administration lies somewhat between the two. Whether fructose and invert sugar offer real advantages from the standpoint of rate of administration appears open to question.

PROTEINS Protein is necessary for cellular repair, wound healing, growth, and for the synthesis of certain enzymes, hormones, and vitamins; proteins are available commercially as either protein hydrolysates* or crystalline amino acids.† Protein hydrolysates are derived from either casein or fibrin and are a mixture of essential and nonessential amino acids bonded together as polypeptides. Crystalline amino acids also contain essential and nonessential amino acids; however, they lack the polypeptide bonding and are thought of as a purer source of protein. (Peptides have been shown to cause nausea and vomiting.) Metabolism of crystalline amino acids results in less nitrogen waste than does metabolism of protein hydrolysates.

Recall that nitrogen balance is the accepted measure for protein balance. A patient is in nitrogen balance if the rate of protein synthesis equals that of protein degradation; he is in negative nitrogen balance if protein catabolism exceeds protein anabolism. Patients may be kept in positive nitrogen balance when protein preparations are administered intravenously with sufficient calories to prevent breakdown of the protein for energy purposes. A healthy adult requires approximately 1 Gm. of protein per kg. of body weight daily to replace normal protein losses; healthy growing infants and children require 1.4 to 2.2 Gm. of protein per kg. of body weight.

The initial rate of infusion of protein hydrolysates should be slow (not more than 2 ml. per minute) to permit careful observation for adverse effects. Excessively rapid infusion may cause nausea, vomiting, fever, and chills. Other untoward effects may include vasodilatation, urticaria, and abdominal pain. The

---

* Aminosol (Abbott Laboratories); Hyprotigen (McGaw Laboratories); Amigen (Travenol Laboratories); C.P.H. (Cutter Laboratories).
† Aminosyn (Abbott Laboratories); FreAmine II (McGaw Laboratories); Travasol (Travenol Laboratories).

infusion should be stopped if any of the above symptoms occur.

Protein solutions have a high NH_4^+ level and should be administered with especial care to patients with hepatic insufficiency or emaciation; a rate slower than that used for other I.V. solutions should be employed. Seriously impaired renal function constitutes a contraindication to the administration of either protein hydrolysates or crystalline amino acid solutions, since the seriously impaired kidney cannot normally excrete nitrogenous wastes.

Supplemental medications should not be added to the solution or injected into the administration tubing without first checking their compatability with the pharmacist. All protein solutions should be examined carefully before they are infused; either particulate matter or cloudiness should call for discarding the solution. Solutions should be used immediately after being opened since they are subject to spoilage.

Crystalline Amino Acids Used in Peripheral Veins to Promote Positive Nitrogen Balance A new concept in the use of parenteral nutrients to promote positive nitrogen balance is being investigated; it employs the administration of isotonic solutions of crystalline amino acids, in the absence of carbohydrates, into a peripheral vein (Table 16-3). This method provides few calories, reduces insulin formation, and mobilizes the body's own fat to meet energy needs. Fat mobilization and ketogenesis are efficient and desirable mechanisms in the reduction of bodily protein wasting.[2] This method can work only with those patients having adequate fat stores (usually present even in appreciably emaciated individuals.) It is sometimes recommended for seriously malnourished patients requiring only short-term therapy (several weeks) for undernutrition. The preservation of body cell mass can be attained by peripheral amino acid infusion; restoration of depleted body cell mass can be attained only by hyperalimentation. Patients requiring long-term parenteral nutrition or those with severe undernutrition should receive hyperalimentation fluids via a central vein (even though this method is associated with greater technical, septic, and metabolic complications).

During the first few days of therapy, the patient should receive 1 or 2 liters of isotonic amino acids a day; this amount is gradually increased to 3 to 4 liters a day if the blood urea nitrogen (BUN) doesn't exceed 30 to 40 mg. per cent, if the blood sugar falls toward

Table 16-3. Parenteral Amino Acid Solutions

Type of Solution	Calories/L.	Tonicity
5% Amino Acids	175	Isotonic
5% Amino Acids 5% Dextrose	345	Hypertonic

100 mg. per cent and if ketones appear in the urine. Patients receiving solely isotonic amino acid solutions develop ketosis of starvation within two or three days; ketonuria should remain positive as a sign of adequate adaptation to a state of starvation. A significant rise in the BUN level for three consecutive days is an indication to discontinue the amino acid infusions; protein solutions must be used cautiously in patients with hepatic or renal failure. If adequate oral feedings cannot be resumed in two or three weeks, and particularly if the patient continues to display negative nitrogen balance, the patient may need to progress to hyperalimentation.

PARENTERAL HYPERALIMENTATION The infusion of large amounts of basic nutrients sufficient to achieve tissue synthesis and growth is known as parenteral hyperalimentation. Commercial sets are available for mixing varying quantities of protein hydrolysates* or crystalline amino acids[+] and hypertonic dextrose solutions. Sufficient calories must be supplied to spare the protein for protein synthesis. Hyperalimentation solutions are highly concentrated; a typical adult solution consists of approximately 25 per cent dextrose and 3 to 4 per cent protein, supplying close to 1000 calories per liter. The hyperalimentation solution must be infused through an indwelling catheter into a large vein, such as the superior vena cava. Initially in adults, 1 or 2 liters is administered daily; this is gradually increased according to the patient's tolerance to a maximum of 4 or 5 liters daily. Caloric needs vary widely; for example, severe catabolic states may increase caloric need to as much as 10,000 calories daily. (An immobilized patient can rarely eat more than 3000 calories a day; it would be difficult to consume more than 5000 calories a day without causing vomiting and diarrhea.)

Because the solution is hypertonic, it must be

---

* Amigen (Travenol Laboratories); Aminosol (Abbott Laboratories); Hyprotigen (McGaw Laboratories).
+ Aminosyn (Abbott Laboratories); FreAmine II (McGaw Laboratories); Travasol (Travenol Laboratories).

administered slowly and constantly over the 24-hour period. *Too rapid administration may cause osmotic diuresis which, untreated, can lead to dehydration, convulsions, and death.* Patients particularly sensitive to hyperosmolarity, such as overt or latent diabetics, should be watched especially closely during hyperalimentation. All patients should be observed at least every 30 minutes; the use of a second clamp on the administration set acts as a safeguard should the first clamp fail. A more accurate and safe flow rate is assured when the hyperalimentation solution is administered with a mechanical infusion pump. (Infusion pumps are described later in this chapter.) If the administration of the hyperalimentation solution should fall behind schedule, no attempt should be made to "catch up" by speeding up the infusion; a severe hyperosmotic reaction could result.

Parenteral hyperalimentation requires frequent clinical evaluation of hepatic and renal function as well as daily laboratory determinations of blood sugar, serum osmolarity, and electrolyte levels (Na^+, Mg^{++}, K^+, HCO_3^-) for the first week and then as indicated. Hyperammonemia can be a problem in patients with severe hepatic damage and in pediatric patients; amino acids can contribute to a rising BUN in patients with renal disease. Urine should be tested for sugar and acetone every six hours; an attempt is made to keep the blood sugar below 200 mg. per cent and the urine sugar below 2+. Some patients require the administration of regular insulin during hyperalimentation to control hyperglycemia and glycosuria, particularly during the first week of therapy. Allergic reactions should be watched for when protein solutions are used in patients sensitive to amino acids.

Because potassium is needed for the transport of glucose and amino acids across the cell membrane, as much as 180 mEq. of potassium may be given with 4000 calories. Magnesium, calcium, sodium, and phosphorus are included as indicated. Some commercial preparations are available with electrolytes already added. Electrolyte disorders that may accompany parenteral hyperalimentation include:

- hypomagnesemia (may be due to insufficient Mg in the hyperalimentation solution)
- hypophosphatemia (usually due to inadequate amount of phosphate in hyperalimentation solution)
- hypokalemia (may be due to excessive loss of

K with inadequate replacement)
- hyperammonemia (may be due to hepatic dysfunction)
- hyperchloremic acidosis (may be due to excess Cl content in solution)

Symptoms of hypomagnesemia may include weakness, vertigo, positive Chvostek sign, and convulsive seizures. Hypophosphatemia may be manifested by confusion, paresthesias, and hyperventilation. Hypokalemia typically produces muscular weakness and cardiac arrhythmias. Hyperammonemia can cause lethargy, seizures, and coma.

In addition to electrolytes, water soluble vitamins are supplied daily; fat soluble vitamins may be supplied weekly.

Sterile dressing changes should be done every 48 hours, more frequently if necessary, only by nurses skilled in this procedure. (Danger of infection and air embolism are greater when a large central vein is cannulated.) During the tubing change, when the catheter is open to air, the patient should perform the Valsalva maneuver to increase positive pressure and, thus, decrease the chance of air being drawn into the vena cava (recall that venous pressure in the central vessels is low). The Valsalva maneuver is accomplished by having the patient bear down with his mouth closed (forced expiration against a closed glottis). A final membrane filter usually is used to trap particulate matter, air, or bacteria inadvertently present in the hyperalimentation solution. (Final filters are described later in the chapter.) Recall that only clear solutions are suitable for administration. An unexplained temperature elevation is an indication to halt hyperalimentation until the source of the fever is found (or, at least, to start all over with a new catheter, tubing, and solution). The possibility of catheter-induced septicemia must be considered. Accurate daily weights and intake-output measurements are mandatory during hyperalimentation.

Mixing of hyperalimentation solutions should ideally be done under a laminar hood by personnel skilled in aseptic additive procedures; the solution should never be prepared more than 24 hours in advance. Hyperalimentation solution should be used promptly after mixing; if the solution is not used immediately, it should be refrigerated in the interim (never longer than 24 hours). Each unit should hang at room temperature preferably no longer than 8 hours.

It is advisable that the hyperalimentation catheter not be used to obtain blood samples or to administer other fluids. Hyperalimentation fluids should be discontinued *gradually*; sudden cessation of the administration of hypertonic dextrose can result in hyperinsulinism (caused by continued endogenous insulin production).

FAT EMULSIONS   Fats supply more than twice the calories of proteins or carbohydrates since 1 Gm. of fat yields 9 calories, while a gram of carbohydrate or a gram of protein yields only 4 calories. Fat emulsions for intravenous use have been in and out of vogue in the United States for a number of years. The presently available fat emulsion in this country (Intralipid 10%)* is prepared from soybean oil 10 per cent (neutral triglycerides of predominantly unsaturated fatty acids), egg yolk phospholipids 1.2 per cent, glycerine 2.25 per cent, and water for injection. The emulsified fat particles are approximately 0.5 microns in size. Emulsions of fat are used in conjunction with carbohydrates and amino acids to provide total parenteral nutrition for patients requiring parenteral feedings for extended periods. No more than 60 per cent of the total caloric intake of the patient should be made up of fats; carbohydrates and amino acids should comprise the remaining 40 per cent or more of the caloric intake. When fat emulsions are used to correct a fatty acid deficiency, 8 to 10 per cent of the caloric intake should be supplied by fats.

Intralipid 10% provides 1.1 calories per ml. in an isotonic solution that is suitable for peripheral and central vein infusion. It is supplied in a 500 ml. container with a special administration set.

Fat emulsions are contraindicated in patients with a disturbance of fat metabolism such as pathological hyperlipemia, lipoid nephrosis, and acute pancreatitis if accompanied by hyperlipemia. Fat emulsions should be administered with caution in patients with severe liver damage, pulmonary disease, anemia or blood coagulation disorders, or when there is danger of fat embolism.

General precautions to keep in mind when administering intravenous fat emulsions include:

Do not mix fat emulsions with electrolyte or other nutrient solutions

Do not place additives in the fat emulsion container

* Manufactured in Sweden by Vitrum for Cutter Laboratories, Inc.

Do not use any bottle in which there appears to be an "oiling out" of the emulsion

Do not use filters with fat emulsions

Do not store the remaining contents of a partly used bottle for later use

Give slowly and increase the rate as the patient's response allows. The initial rate of infusion in adults should be 1 ml./min. for the first 15 to 30 minutes of infusion; if no untoward reactions occur, the rate can be increased so that 500 ml. will be infused over a period of 4 hours. In pediatric patients, the initial rate of infusion should be 0.1 ml./min. for the first 10 to 15 minutes; if no untoward reactions occur, the rate can be increased to permit infusion of 1 Gm./kg./4 hr.

Store Intralipid 10% under refrigeration at 4 to 8° C.

Monitor liver function frequently; if tests indicate that liver function is impaired, the infusion of the fat emulsion should be discontinued

Monitor the patient's ability to eliminate the infused fat from the circulation (the lipemia should clear between daily infusions)

Observe carefully for adverse reactions that may occur with intravenous fat emulsion administration:[3]

- dyspnea and cyanosis
- allergic reactions
- hyperlipemia
- hypercoagulability
- nausea and vomiting
- headache
- flushing
- increase in temperature
- sweating
- back or chest pain
- dizziness
- hepatomegaly and splenomegaly
- leukopenia
- deposition of a brown pigment in the reticuloendothelial system
- overloading syndrome (focal seizures, fever, leukocytosis, and shock)

ALCOHOL SOLUTIONS   One Gm. of absolute ethyl alcohol yields 6 to 8 calories. Obviously an excellent source of calories, alcohol has been combined with carbohydrates to provide a high calorie repair solution. When alcohol is infused with carbohydrate, it is apparently burned preferentially, thus permitting the glucose to be stored as glycogen. Alcohol spares body protein by providing readily accessible calories, and its sedating effect is highly desirable for patients with pain. *Sedation can be achieved in the average adult without symptoms of intoxication by giving 200 to 300 ml. of a 5 per cent solution per hour.*

The nurse should be aware of the physiologic and psychologic effects of alcohol parenterally administered; these include dulling of memory, loss of ability to concentrate, an improved sense of well-being, increased respiration and pulse, and vasodilation. Alcohol solutions should *not* be employed in shock, impending shock, epilepsy, severe liver disease, or in patients with coronary thrombosis. Nausea and vomiting do not occur as frequently when alcohol is given parenterally as when a comparable amount is taken orally. However, whenever the rate of administration of alcohol given parenterally exceeds its metabolic destruction by the body, restlessness, inebriation, and coma can occur.

The parenteral administration of alcohol, particularly of hypertonic solutions, can cause phlebitis. Tissue necrosis can occur if the needle accidentally leaves the vein and permits solution to perfuse the surrounding tissue spaces. Care should be taken to see that the needle is carefully anchored in the vein and that the site is inspected frequently to detect infiltration.

Table 16-4 shows the caloric values and the tonicity of various solutions of alcohol.

PARENTERAL VITAMINS Vitamins should be administered parenterally when there is inadequate oral intake or when parenteral fluid therapy is necessary for longer than two or three days. Although not food in themselves, vitamins are essential for the utilization of other nutrients. The need for vitamins is increased during periods of stress such as acute illness, infection, surgery, burns, injury, and convalescence. Some parenteral fluids have vitamins incorporated, and special vitamin preparations designed for injection with parenteral fluids are also available.

The vitamins most frequently needed in parenteral alimentation are vitamin C and members of the B complex, all of which are water soluble and stored by the body only in small amounts; they serve as coenzymes in the essential metabolic processes of the cells. Vitamin deficiency has been observed after only one week of parenteral administration of glucose and water alone. However, since most patients

Table 16-4. Parenteral Alcohol Solutions

Type of Solution	Calories/L.	Tonicity
Alcohol 5% Dextrose 5%	450	Hypertonic
Alcohol 10% Dextrose 5%	730	Hypertonic
Alcohol * Dextrose Fructose	960	Hypertonic

* Polyonic M 900 (Cutter Laboratories)

are on parenteral therapy for only limited periods, they do not require the fat soluble vitamins A and D since they are better retained by the body. If I.V. therapy is prolonged, fat-soluble vitamins should be supplied weekly.

Because there is some waste of parenterally infused vitamins through urinary excretion, it is necessary to administer generous amounts to assure an adequate intake. Hence, the patient who is on exclusive parenteral alimentation is usually given more than the daily vitamin requirement—sometimes as much as ten times the minimal requirement. A basic formula of parenteral vitamins is as follows:

Thiamine .... 10 mg.
Riboflavin .... 5 mg.
Niacinamide .... 50 mg.
Calcium pantothenate .... 20 mg.
Pyridoxine hydrochloride .... 20 mg.
Folic Acid .... 5 mg.
Vitamin B_{12} .... 15 μg.
Vitamin C .... up to 1 Gm.
                                     as indicated

Vitamin C is particularly important in surgical patients to promote wound healing, whereas the B complex vitamins provide factors to aid carbohydrate metabolism and the maintenance of normal gastrointestinal function. (An occasional patient may show extreme sensitivity to the B complex vitamins.) Sometimes vitamin K is given; flushing, sweating, and a constricted feeling in the chest may follow the intravenous injection of vitamin K.

WATER The patient on parenteral fluids exclusively can be provided with water by means of solutions of carbohydrates, the most common of which is 5 per cent dextrose in water. Also useful are the various hypotonic electrolyte solutions, such as 0.45 per cent sodium chloride or half-strength Ringer's. Isotonic electrolyte solutions provide no free water at all—they merely expand the extracellular fluid volume, ignoring the patient's need for water for renal excretion, insensible loss, and metabolic purposes; consequently, they should never be used to supply free water.

It should always be remembered that one should *never give water alone by a parenteral route.* If pure water were injected directly into the bloodstream, the red blood cells would absorb water, swell, and burst with resultant damage to the kidneys and hemoglobinuria.

ELECTROLYTE SOLUTIONS   A wide variety of electrolyte solutions are available for parenteral administration. Some of the more common solutions are listed in Table 16-5 for quick reference. Included in the table are the following:

> Electrolyte content
> Trademarks (brand names)
> Precautions for administration
> Usual rate of administration

Electrolyte solutions are considered isotonic if the total electrolyte content (anions + cations) approximates 310 mEq./L.; they are considered hypotonic if the total electrolyte content (anions + cations) is below 250 mEq./L.; and they are considered hypertonic if the total electrolyte content (anions + cations) exceeds 375 mEq./L.

Administration of Potassium Solutions   Potassium may be given in the form of commercially prepared electrolyte solutions, or a potassium salt may be added as a supplement to an intravenous fluid, such as 5 or 10 per cent dextrose in water. (Extreme care required in measuring.)

The nurse should keep the following facts in mind when potassium-containing solutions are administered (see Table 16-5):

1. Usually a liter of solution containing 20 to 40 mEq. of potassium is infused over an 8 to 12 hour period. At no time should the rate of infusion exceed 20 mEq. of potassium (suitably diluted) per hour for normal adults. Older adults should receive potassium solutions at an even slower rate, preferably no faster than 20 to 30 mEq. over a 3 to 4 hour period.
2. Potassium solutions should never be allowed to run with the flow valve wide open or be given under pressure; high concentrations of potassium in the bloodstream can result in cardiac arrest.
3. Small ampules containing concentrated solutions of potassium salts for addition to I.V. fluids are meant to be mixed with at least 1 L. of solution. They should never be directly administered in concentrated form by I.V. push because of the danger of cardiac arrest. When adding KCl to the fluid container, it is important to first fill the I.V. tubing with the plain fluid; then the KCl can be added and vigorously agitated to ensure its proper dispersion in the container.
4. It is wise to limit the potassium concentration in 1 L. of fluid to 20 to 40 mEq., never more than 60 mEq., since an accidental rapid infusion rate is less dangerous when potassium content is moderate. (Note that some dextrose solutions are available commercially with varying concentrations of KCl, usually 10 to 40 mEq./L., already added.)
5. Solutions containing potassium should be conspicuously labeled so that other personnel can readily note its presence (Figs. 16-15 and 16-16).
6. When potassium chloride is added to an I.V. solution, it should be thoroughly mixed by shaking the bag or bottle to prevent accidental infusion of a large bolus of the drug. (It is important to squeeze the medicine ports of plastic bags while they are in the upright position and then to mix the solution thoroughly.)
7. In the treatment of severe hypokalemia, it may be necessary to administer potassium in nondextrose solutions since the dextrose may cause a further fall in plasma potassium with ensuing cardiac arrhythmias.
8. Potassium should be administered only after adequate urine flow has been established. A decrease in urine volume to less than 20 ml./hr. for two consecutive hours is an indication to stop potassium infusion until the situation is evaluated. Urinary suppression may be due either to inadequate fluid intake or renal impairment; the rapid infusion of a hydrating solution (such as 5 per cent D/W or a hypotonic electrolyte solution) should cause an increase in urine output if the problem is fluid

Table 16-5. Electrolyte Solutions

Solution*	Tonicity	Na+	K+	Ca++	Mg++	NH4+	Cl-	Lactate	HCO3-	Acetate	Gluconate	HPO4	Citrate	Brand Names	Reasons for Use	Comments
Sodium Chloride 0.45% (One-half isotonic saline)	Hypotonic	77					77								Supply daily salt requirements; Supply water for excretory purposes	Available commercially with varying concentrations of carbohydrates
Sodium Chloride 0.9%	Isotonic	154					154								Replace Na+ and Cl-; Expands extracellular fluid volume; Correct mild metabolic alkalosis	Widely used as a routine electrolyte replacement solution even though it supplies only Na+ and Cl- (Many feel its routine use should be replaced by a solution that more closely resembles extracellular fluid, such as Lactated Ringer's); Does not supply free water for excretory purposes; Cl- is supplied in excess of normal plasma Cl- level—excessive use of isotonic saline can cause Cl- to replace part of the body HCO3- (metabolic acidosis); Sometimes erroneously referred to as "normal saline" or "physiologic saline"
Sodium Chloride 3%	Hypertonic	513					513								Rapid correction of severe low-salt syndrome	Available commercially with varying concentrations of carbohydrates; Contraindicated unless severe salt depletion is present
Sodium Chloride 5%	Hypertonic	855					855									Use with caution in edematous patients; Administer a small volume at a slow rate (such as 200 ml. over a minimum of 4 hr.)

mEq./L.

* K-containing solutions should be infused with caution and are contraindicated when these conditions are present: oliguria, potassium excess, renal disease, Addison's disease. (see section on K-solutions)

Table 16-5. (Continued)

Solution*	Tonicity	mEq./L.												Brand Names	Reasons for Use	Comments
		Na^+	K^+	Ca^{++}	Mg^{++}	NH_4^+	Cl^-	Lactate	HCO_3^-	Acetate	Gluconate	HPO_4^{--}	Citrate			
Ringer's	Isotonic	147	4	5			156								Replaces K^+ and Ca^{++} in addition to Na^+ and Cl^-	Contains an excess of Cl^- in relation to normal plasma Cl^- level Available commercially with carbohydrates
Lactated Ringer's (Hartmann's)	Isotonic	130	4	3			109	28							Routine electrolyte maintenance solution Correct metabolic acidosis Replace fluid lost as bile, diarrhea, and in burns	Electrolyte concentration closely resembles extracellular fluid Same precautions as for any K-containing solution* (It is permissible to use Lactated Ringer's in burns since the amount of K^+ is so small as to be inconsequential) (May at times be administered cautiously in the presence of decreased urinary output) Available commercially with carbohydrates
Acetated Ringer's	Isotonic	130	4	3			109			28					Replace extracellular fluid losses	Acetated Ringer's Solution is identical to Lactated Ringer's with the exception that it contains acetate instead of lactate as its HCO_3^- precursor Acetate is metabolized largely by muscle and other peripheral tissues rather than by the liver May be preferred to Lactated Ringer's in metabolic acidosis associated with liver dysfunction, hypothermia, circulatory insufficiency and extracorporeal circulation It requires less oxygen for metabolism than does Lactated Ringer's (particu-

Solution	Tonicity	Composition (values as printed)						Commercial products	Uses	Remarks
										larly important in shock with its tissue hypoxia)
										Same precautions as for any K-containing solution*
										(May at times be administered cautiously in the presence of decreased urinary output)
										Available commercially with carbohydrate
Gastric (Cooke and Crowley)	Isotonic	63	17			70	150	Electrolyte No. 3 Cutter Lab. Travenol Lab.; Isolyte G McGaw Lab.; Ionosol G Abbott Lab.	Replace gastric fluid lost in vomiting and gastric suction	Should not be used as a routine maintenance solution. pH of solution is acid (3.3–3.7), similar to that of gastric juice. Contraindicated in hepatic insufficiency. The ammonium ions are converted by the liver to urea and hydrogen ions, thereby replacing the H^+ deficit resulting from gastric juice loss. Same precautions as for any K-containing solution*. Available commercially with carbohydrates
Duodenal	Isotonic	138	12	5	3	108	53	Ionosol C-CM Abbott Lab.	Replace duodenal fluid loss. Correct mild acidosis	Same precautions as for any K-containing solution*. Available commercially with carbohydrates
Duodenal (modified)	Hypotonic	79.5	36	4.5	3	63	60	Electrolyte No. 1 Cutter Lab. McGaw Lab. Travenol Lab.; Ionosol D Abbott Lab.	Replace pancreatic and duodenal fluid losses. Supply water for excretory needs. Correct deficits of K^+, Ca^{++}, Mg^{++}, Na^+ and HCO_3^-. Correct acidosis	Same precautions as for any K-containing solution (Note that the K^+ content is high)*. Available commercially with carbohydrates

* K-containing solutions should be infused with caution and are contraindicated when these conditions are present: oliguria, potassium excess, renal disease, Addison's disease. (see section on K-solutions)

Table 16-5. (Continued)

Solution*	Tonicity	mEq./L.												Brand Names	Reasons for Use	Comments
		Na^+	K^+	Ca^{++}	Mg^{++}	NH_4^+	Cl^-	Lactate	HCO_3^-	Acetate	Gluconate	HPO_4^{--}	Citrate			
Sodium Lactate 1/6 M (Alkalinizing Solution)	Isotonic	167						167							Correct severe metabolic acidosis	Contraindicated in liver disease, shock, and right-sided heart failure (lactate ions are improperly metabolized in these conditions) Contraindicated in alkalosis
Sodium Bicarbonate 1.4%	Isotonic	167							167						Correct severe metabolic acidosis	Contraindicated in metabolic and respiratory alkalosis
Sodium Bicarbonate 5% (Alkalinizing Solution)	Hypertonic	595							595						Alkalinize urine (as in hemolytic reactions requiring rapid alkalinization of urine to reduce nephrotoxicity of blood pigments)	Contraindicated when hypocalcemia is present; alkalinization of plasma may produce signs of tetany Administer a small volume at a slow rate (such as 100 ml. of a 5% solution over 2 hr.) Administer with extreme caution to salt-retaining patients with cardiac, renal or liver damage (Severe acidosis in edematous patients should be treated with 5% bicarbonate solution in small volumes)
Ammonium Chloride 0.9% (Acidifying Solution)	Isotonic					168	168								Correct severe metabolic alkalosis in children	Contraindicated in disturbed hepatic function, renal failure or any condition with a high NH_4^+ level
Ammonium Chloride 2.14% (Acidifying Solution)	Hypertonic					400	400								Correct severe metabolic alkalosis in adults	Contraindicated in disturbed hepatic function, renal failure or any condition with a high NH_4^+ level Excessive amounts of this solution can cause metabolic acidosis with: drowsiness hyperpnea nausea and vomiting

Solution	Tonicity	Na	K	Ca	Mg	Cl	HCO₃/lactate	(misc)	Commercial Preparations	Uses	Precautions
Balanced electrolyte (*Fox*)	Isotonic	140	10	5	3	103	47 55 47	8	Isolyte E — McGaw Lab. Polysal — Cutter Lab. Plasma-Lyte — Travenol Lab.	Replaces gastrointestinal losses of: small intestinal juice, bile, diarrhea. Burn treatment. Postoperative fluid replacement. Correct Na⁺ deficit	Electrolyte content similar to plasma except that it has twice as much K⁺ (K⁺ content is similar to that of intestinal juice). Same precautions as for any K-containing solution*. Available commercially with carbohydrates
Butler (*Electrolyte No. 88*)	Hypotonic	57	25		5–6	45	25–31	13	Electrolyte No. 2 — McGaw Lab. Travenol Lab. Cutter Lab. Ionosol B — Abbott Lab.	Supply water. Supply maintenance needs of Na⁺, Mg⁺⁺, K⁺, and Cl⁻. Replace fluid loss from the large intestine	Same precautions as for any K-containing solution*. Available commercially with carbohydrate
Modified Butler (*Electrolyte No. 48*)	Hypotonic	25	20		3	22	23	3	Electrolyte No. 48 — Travenol Lab. Cutter Lab. Ionosol MB — Abbott Lab. Isolyte P — McGaw Lab.	Supply water. Used in pediatrics to treat dehydration of acidosis, diarrhea and burns	Same precautions as for any K-containing solution*. Available commercially with carbohydrates
Balanced Hypotonic Solution	Hypotonic	40	13		3	40	16		Normosol-M — Abbott Lab. Polyonic M-56 — Cutter Lab. Plasma-Lyte 56 — Travenol Lab. Isolyte H — McGaw Lab.	Supply water. Supply electrolytes for older children and adults	Same precautions as for any K-containing solution*. Available commercially with carbohydrates
Balanced Isotonic Solution	Isotonic	140	5		3	98	27	23	Isolyte S — McGaw Lab. Normosol-R — Abbott Lab.	Extracellular fluid replacement solution. Recommended	Same precautions as for any K-containing solution*. Available commercially with carbohydrates

* K-containing solutions should be infused with caution and are contraindicated when these conditions are present: oliguria, potassium excess, renal disease, Addison's disease. (see section on K-solutions)

Table 16-5. (Continued)

Solution*	Tonicity	mEq./L.												Brand Names	Reasons for Use	Comments
		Na^+	K^+	Ca^{++}	Mg^{++}	NH_4^+	Cl^-	Lactate	HCO_3^-	Acetate	Gluconate	HPO_4^{--}	Citrate			
														Plasma-Lyte 148 Travenol Lab.	substitute for isotonic saline	Contains no calcium; therefore can be administered simultaneously with blood
														Polyonic R 148 Cutter Lab.	Correct mild acidosis	
Electrolyte No. 75 (Talbot)	Hypotonic	40	35				40		20			15		Electrolyte No. 75 Travenol Lab.	Supply water	Same precautions as for any K-containing solution*
		40	35				20					15		Ionosol T Abbott Lab.	Supply maintenance electrolyte needs	Contains more K+ than most maintenance solutions
		40	35				40		20		15			Isolyte M McGaw Lab.	Correct K+ deficit	Available commercially with carbohydrates
Maintenance electrolyte solution	Hypotonic	40	16	5	3		40			12				Polysal M Cutter Lab.	Supply water	Same precautions as for any K-containing solution*
		40	16	5	3		40		12					Plasma-Lyte M Travenol Lab.	Supply maintenance electrolyte needs—contains Ca++ and Mg++ in addition to Na+ and K+	Available commercially with carbohydrates
		40	16	5	3		40			24				Isolyte R McGaw Lab.		

* K-containing solutions should be infused with caution and are contraindicated when these conditions are present: oliguria, potassium excess, renal disease, Addison's disease. (see section on K-solutions)

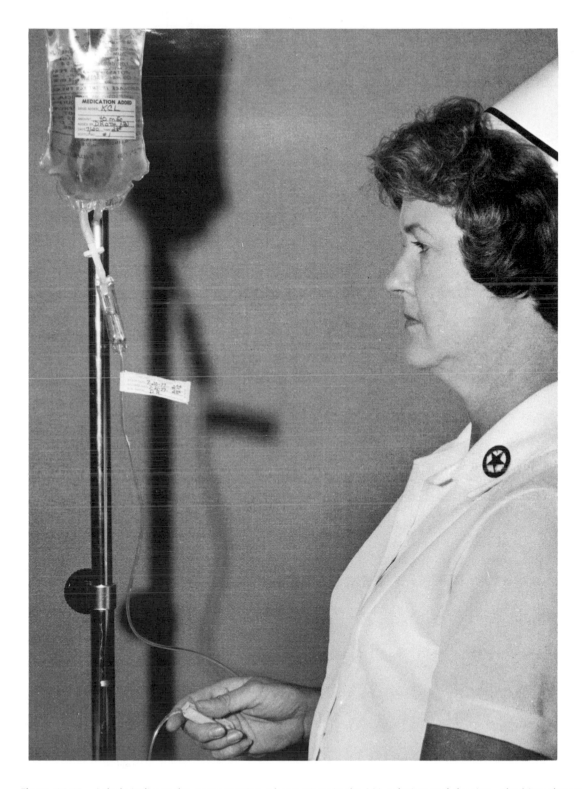

Figure 16-15. Labels indicate the concentration of potassium in the I.V. solution and the time of tubing change.

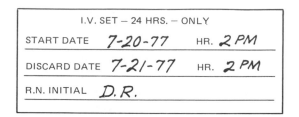

MEDICATION ADDED		
DRUG ADDED	*KCl*	
AMOUNT	*40 m. Eq.*	
ADDED BY	*D. Roth, R.N.*	
DATE	*7/20*	TIME *2 PM*
BOTTLE NO.	*# 1*	

I.V. SET — 24 HRS. — ONLY		
START DATE	*7-20-77*	HR. *2 PM*
DISCARD DATE	*7-21-77*	HR. *2 PM*
R.N. INITIAL	*D. R.*	

Figure 16-16. *Left,* Close-up view of additive label; *Above,* Close-up view of tubing change label.

volume deficit. Once urinary output is adequate, potassium infusion may be resumed. However, failure of the hydrating solution to increase urinary output indicates renal impairment and is an indication to withhold potassium. Recall that potassium is mainly excreted by way of the kidneys; when the kidneys are nonfunctional, a high potassium level builds up in the bloodstream (hyperkalemia).

9. A solution containing sizable amounts of potassium (30 to 40 mEq./L.) is sometimes associated with pain in the vein it is entering, especially if infused into a vein where a previous venipuncture has been performed. Slowing the rate usually relieves this sensation. Because administration of a potassium solution into the subcutaneous tissues is painful, it is rarely administered by means of hypodermoclysis; when it is, the concentration should be no higher than 10 mEq./L. to avoid local pain and tissue damage. Care should be taken to avoid accidental subcutaneous infiltration of more concentrated potassium solutions since *severe* tissue damage may result.

Administration of Calcium Solutions

1. Calcium salts should not be added to I.V. solutions containing sodium bicarbonate since the precipitate calcium carbonate will form.
2. Calcium should not be added to I.V. solutions containing phosphate since calcium phosphate may be precipitated.

3. Solutions containing calcium may cause tissue sloughing if they are allowed to infiltrate into the subcutaneous tissues; thus, patients receiving calcium solutions should be observed frequently to prevent this complication.
4. Intravenous calcium administration usually is contraindicated in digitalized patients since calcium ions exert an effect similar to that of digitalis and can cause digitalis toxicity with adverse cardiac effects.
5. Excessive or too rapid administration of calcium intravenously can cause cardiac arrest, preceded by bradycardia. Recall that hypercalcemia may cause the heart to go into spastic contraction.

Administration of Magnesium Solutions

1. Question the use of magnesium solutions in patients with oliguria (recall that 99 per cent of parenterally administered magnesium is excreted via the kidneys).
2. Avoid rapid administration of magnesium solutions since they may cause uncomfortable sensations of heat; more importantly, they may cause coma, respiratory depression, and cardiac arrest.
3. Observe the patient's respirations and deep tendon reflexes. A respiratory rate below 12 to 14 per minute should be reported to the physician, as should poor to absent deep tendon reflexes (such as the knee jerk).
4. Have calcium gluconate immediately available to counteract serious symptoms of hypermagnesemia, should they occur.

Incompatible Combinations of Additives and Parenteral Fluids

The nurse is frequently required to add medications to parenteral fluids. There is a fast-growing number of medications and types of parenteral fluids on the market; thus, the number of possible combinations is astronomical. It is impossible, without help, for the nurse to know which medications can be safely mixed with certain intravenous fluids and such assistance must come from several sources:

pharmacist
manufacturer's directions
publication of new admixture information

The nurse should keep the following points in mind when adding medications to parenteral fluids:

1. Thoroughly review the literature provided by the manufacturers of the I.V. fluid; most companies have prepared charts noting the compatability of various medications with their solutions. Also, review the literature provided by the manufacturers of the additive.

2. When possible, it is best to add only one medication to each solution bottle, as the complex interaction between two additives may render the solution incompatible.

3. When in doubt, the nurse should check with the pharmacist because he is best qualified to predict incompatabilities. (Some hospitals have wisely added pharmacy-centralized intravenous additive programs in an attempt to provide safer admixture preparation.)

4. Use freshly prepared solutions whenever possible and monitor infusing fluids periodically for physical changes. Some incompatabilities do not become apparent until the solution has been mixed for awhile. A physical incompatability may be manifested by a haze, color change, or effervescence. Chemical incompatabilities are more difficult to detect because they do not always produce a visible change.

5. The formation of a precipitate when a medication is added to an intravenous fluid is an indication to discard the solution unless the directions accompanying the medication state otherwise. The intravenous administra-

tion of a solution containing insoluble matter may result in embolism or other damage to the heart, liver, and kidneys.

6. An administration set with a final filter should be used whenever possible to trap undetected precipitates.

7. The degree of solubility of an additive varies with the pH, as most incompatibilities are related to changes in pH. Solutions of a high pH seem to be incompatible with solutions of a low pH. (A chart listing the pH of certain drugs and parenteral solutions can help the nurse predict potential incompatibilities.)

8. Sodium bicarbonate and calcium salts should never be mixed since they form an insoluble precipitate (calcium carbonate).

9. Dilantin and Valium should not be mixed with any intravenous solution since they precipitate out. They are both incompatible with any other drug in syringe or solution.

10. It is best not to mix multiple vitamin complexes with potassium penicillin G or ampicillin since the acidic ascorbic acid lowers the pH and causes degradation of the antibiotic.[4]

11. It is best not to mix heparin with antibiotics since heparin may affect the stability of certain antibiotics.[5]

12. Hydrocortisone should not be mixed with tetracycline or cephalothin since a precipitate will form.[6]

13. It is best not to administer sodium bicarbonate and epinephrine jointly since sodium bicarbonate tends to neutralize epinephrine; they may be administered intermittently through the same tubing if it is flushed first.[7]

14. Although the current literature is conflicting, it has been suggested that the anticoagulant activity of heparin is decreased in the presence of dextrose.[8] It may be desirable, then, to use an electrolyte solution (such as isotonic saline) as a diluent for heparin infusions. If dextrose is desired, an increased dose of heparin may be needed to achieve the desired anticoagulant effect.[9]

If, after researching the literature, the nurse finds that an order for an additive is incorrect, she should contact the physician for a change in orders.

SPECIAL EQUIPMENT FOR INFUSIONS

DROP SIZE REDUCTION   When potent medications are added to intravenous solutions, extreme precautions must be taken to prevent too rapid administration.

Manufacturers of intravenous equipment provide administration sets delivering from 50 to 60 drops/ml. These microdrip sets allow for greater control of fluid flow rate.

VOLUME CONTROL SETS   There are several commercial sets designed to administer limited amounts of solution in precise volume, all of which are extremely useful in the infusion of potent medications. They are also valuable in pediatric intravenous therapy.

Abbott Laboratories has designed a rigid plastic cylinder (Soluset) that is available in 100 ml. or 250

ml. capacities; the maximum amount of solution that can be infused is limited to the amount in the cylinder. Amounts larger than capacity may be given by refilling the chamber. The Soluset-100 is fitted with a Microdrip orifice, which provides approximately 60 drops/ml., whereas the Soluset-250 provides approximately 15 drops/ml.

Travenol Laboratories has designed the pliable plastic Pedatrol set, divided into 5 aliquots of 10 ml. each (Fig. 16-17). By simply moving a hemostat's position on the set, the maximum amount of solution to be infused can be limited to 10, 20, 30, 40 or 50 ml.; when empty, the set can easily be refilled from the solution bottle above. Travenol Laboratories also has the In-Line Buretrol set, especially designed for use in pediatrics for metered intravenous administration of blood or solutions; it has a capacity of 150 ml., with markings at 1 ml. intervals.

McGaw Laboratories has developed the Metriset,

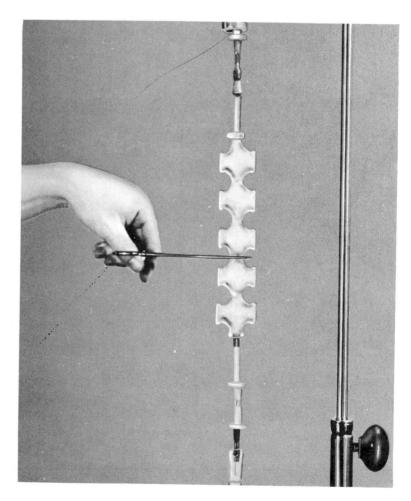

Figure 16-17.   Pedatrol Administration Set. (Courtesy of Travenol Laboratories, Deerfield, Illinois)

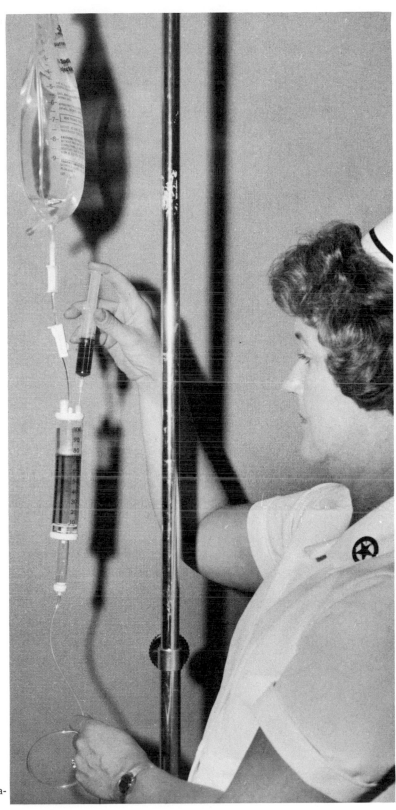

Figure 16-18. Metriset. (McGaw Laboratories, Santa Ana, California)

a calibrated chamber that controls the volume to 100 ml., wherein medications may be added directly into the set through a medication plug (Fig. 16-18). Cutter Laboratories has a pediatric measuring apparatus (Volu-Trole Set) consisting of a regular I.V. infusion set plus a flexible transparent plastic metering chamber graduated in 10 ml. divisions (approximately 60 drops/ml.).

BOTTLE ARRANGEMENTS   A series hookup may be used to add more fluid or to change fluids while an infusion continues (Fig. 16-19). The two bottles are connected by plastic tubing, with the airvent closed in the primary bottle and the secondary bottle vented—the secondary bottle will empty first. If the specific gravity is higher in the secondary bottle, there will be no mixing of solutions; there will be mixing if the specific gravity is higher in the primary bottle.

A parallel hookup may be used to administer two solutions alternately or simultaneously (Fig. 16-20). This type of hookup is more dangerous than a series hookup, because if either of the bottles empties completely and its clamp closure is not complete, large quantities of air will leak in by way of the empty bottle and form air bubbles in the infusion tubing. The nurse must exercise great care when using a Y-type set; complete clamp closure should be made when

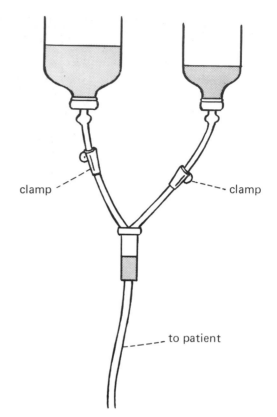

Figure 16-20.   Bottles connected in parallel (Y-type) setup.

there is still a little fluid in the bottle. Well meant intentions to administer every drop in the bottle are not warranted.

PLASTIC CONTAINERS   Flexible I.V. containers are available from Travenol Laboratories (Fig. 16-21), Abbott Laboratories (Fig. 16-22), and McGaw Laboratories. Plastic bags reduce the potential for air emboli since they are not vented; also, the possibility of contamination by way of an air filter is eliminated. They are lighter, easier to handle, and more easily stored and discarded than glass bottles. In addition, they are less likely to injure patients or nursing personnel if accidentally dropped during administration.

INTRAVENOUS PIGGYBACK SETUPS   Intermittent infusion of an intravenous medication into an established I.V. line is referred to as a "piggyback" and is a widely used procedure. This method has several advantages over the direct introduction of a concentrated medication into the vein via a syringe (I.V. push):

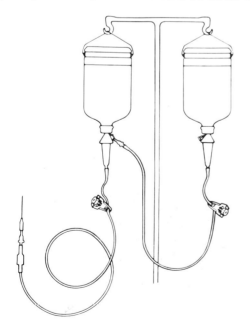

Figure 16-19.   I.V. Tandem Setup (Saftiset™ Tandem Set). (Courtesy of Cutter Laboratories, Berkeley, California)

- the medication can be diluted in a larger volume of diluent, thus reducing the possibility of chemical phlebitis
- the nurse does not have to be constantly present during administration of piggyback infusions (this is a definite advantage over the I.V. push method which frequently requires the nurse to spend 10 minutes or more at the bedside for safe injection of the medication)
- the diluted medication can be delivered more

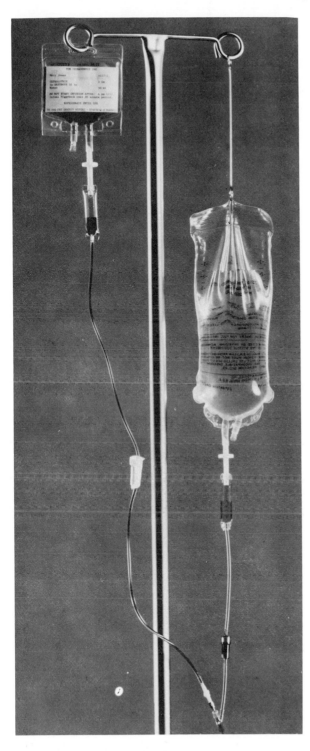

Figure 16-21. Viaflex™ primary container with Mini-Bag™ (piggyback setup). (Courtesy of Travenol Laboratories, Deerfield, Illinois)

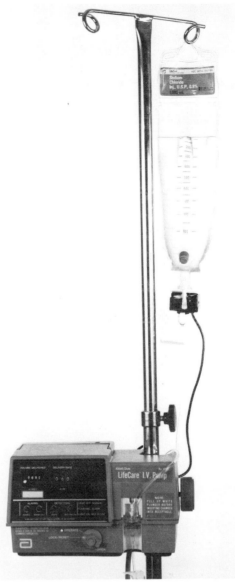

Figure 16-22. LifeCare™ I.V. pump with LifeCare™ solution in flexible plastic container. (Courtesy of Abbott Laboratories, North Chicago, Illinois)

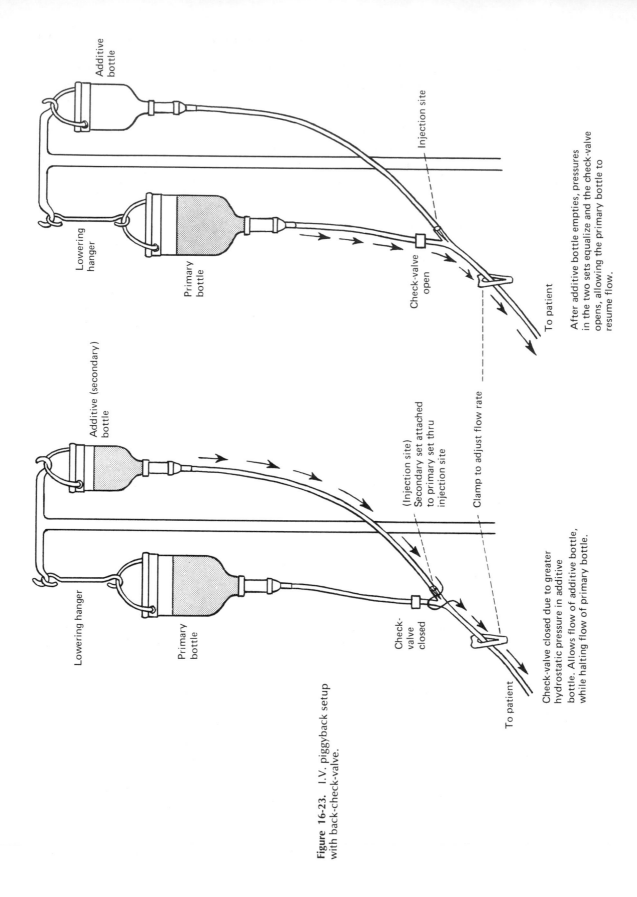

Figure 16-23. I.V. piggyback setup with back-check-valve.

Additive bottle

Lowering hanger

Primary bottle

Check-valve open

To patient

Injection site

After additive bottle empties, pressures in the two sets equalize and the check-valve opens, allowing the primary bottle to resume flow.

Additive (secondary) bottle

Lowering hanger

Primary bottle

Check-valve closed

To patient

(Injection site)
Secondary set attached to primary set thru injection site

Clamp to adjust flow rate

Check-valve closed due to greater hydrostatic pressure in additive bottle. Allows flow of additive bottle, while halting flow of primary bottle.

slowly, allowing time for observation for adverse reactions before the entire dose is given

To perform a piggyback infusion, the primary bottle is lowered by means of a hook below the secondary (additive) bottle. The secondary setup is attached by means of a 1-inch 20-gauge needle into the injection site of the primary set after first thoroughly scrubbing the site with an alcohol sponge. Remember that the injection site at the distal end of the tubing may be exposed to drainage and excreta. The needle should be securely taped in place to avoid accidental dislodgement. A smaller gauge needle may break and enter the administration set; a longer needle can more easily puncture the tubing and allow the entrance of air and contaminants. When the clamp on the additive bottle is fully opened, its fluid will flow in owing to its greater hydrostatic pressure. (The rate of flow is determined by the clamp on the primary set.)

A convenient and safe method for piggybacking makes use of sets with check-valves* to prevent air from entering the vein when the additive bottle empties and to prevent or minimize mixing of the primary and additive fluids. The valve automatically occludes flow from the primary bottle while the additive bottle is infusing and then shuts off the additive bottle when it empties, allowing the primary bottle to automatically resume flow (Fig. 16-23). The latter is of great value because the vein is kept open by the uninterrupted fluid infusion. (Some piggyback setups require the nurse to be present to switch the flow to the primary bottle; if not performed quickly, the needle clogs.) Rate of flow for both bottles is the same (unless readjusted) since both are controlled by the clamp on the primary set.

Remember that there is danger of air embolism when two vented containers are allowed to infuse simultaneously. This danger can be avoided by allowing only one bottle to flow at a time. If two vented solutions must run simultaneously through the same needle, care must be taken to assure that the first container to drain is tightly clamped off before it completely empties. An unclamped empty container in a Y-type setup allows air bubbles to enter the bloodstream.

---

* Continu-Flo Set and Add-A-Line Secondary Set (Travenol Laboratories); Additiv® Set for Piggyback Hookups (McGaw Laboratories); Abbott Automatic Piggyback System (Abbott Laboratories).

FINAL IN-LINE FILTERS   It has been recommended that intravenous fluids be administered through in-line final filters (Fig. 16-24) to remove particulate matter (undissolved substances unintentionally present in parenteral fluids). This foreign matter may consist of particles of glass, rubber, metal, molds, bacteria, or drug precipitates. A number of filter devices are available commercially for this purpose.

Final filters are available as membrane filters or depth filters. The former are screen-type devices that are calibrated in pore size (such as 0.22 micron, 0.45 micron, or 5 microns); the latter are made of pressed fragmented material of nonuniform pore size. Depth filters are assigned a nominal rating according to the particle size that will be trapped 98 per cent of the time. Membrane filters will block the passage of air (under normal pressure) when wet, depth filters will not. Both the 0.45 and 0.22 micron filters will block bacteria. A 0.45 micron filter will retain all particles larger than 0.45 micron; the 0.22 micron filter blocks all particles larger than 0.22 micron (absolute sterilization). An in-line membrane filter with a self-venting mechanism to vent air that has entered the administration set has been developed (Fig. 16-25).

It is imperative that the nurse read and follow the manufacturer's directions carefully to avoid plugging or rupturing the filter. The latter is particularly dangerous since it may allow fragments of the filter to enter the administration set; also, the air blocking ability of the filter is lost when it is ruptured. Filters should be changed within 24 hours, or more often as indicated.

FILTER ASPIRATION NEEDLE   A filter aspiration needle (Fig. 16-26) is a device attached to the syringe used to draw the intravenous medication from its container (either a rubber-topped vial or a glass ampule). The filter needle traps particles 5 microns in size and larger (such as glass, rubber, or metal) and, thus, allows the use of a more particulate-free fluid. A new needle is applied before the medication is injected into the I.V. container (use of the filter needle for this purpose would allow the trapped particles to be injected into the intravenous fluid).

INFUSION PUMPS   A number of infusion pumps are available commercially and are being used in many patient care areas (neonatal, pediatric, and adult intensive care units; labor and delivery; x-ray, surgery, and increasingly on general medical-surgi-

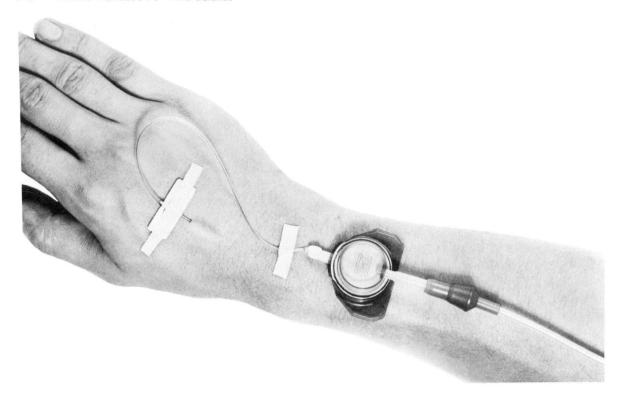

Figure 16-24.   Final filter. (Courtesy of Travenol Laboratories, Deerfield, Illinois)

cal units). They are used to allow more accurate administration of fluids and critical drugs than is possible with routine gravity flow setups. Their precise rate of flow is particularly desirable in the administration of hyperalimentation fluids, chemotherapy, and other potent medications (such as dopamine, heparin, lidocaine, nitroprusside, oxytocin, pitressin, and aramine). Pumping mechanisms may be classified as linear peristaltic, rotary peristaltic, and piston and cylinder. Peristaltic pumps move fluid by compressing the I.V. tubing; piston and cylinder pumps apply pressure to the fluid rather than to the tubing, much like a plunger pushes fluid through the barrel of a syringe.

Pumps that have flow rates calibrated in terms of ml./hr. rather than in drops/min. are called volumetric pumps. These pumps provide greater accuracy than those measuring drops since many factors can affect drop size (such as fluid viscosity and drop rate formation). Most pumps require individualized special administration sets, although a few use standard I.V. sets.

Circulatory overload is less apt to occur when infusion pumps are used to control the flow rate; also,

needles are less apt to clog with the use of infusion pumps since the pressure generated by the pumps exceeds maximum venous pressure. Many infusion pumps may be used to administer fluids intraarterially; some infusion pumps are occasionally used to administer slow gastrointestinal tube feedings.

The Harvard Syringe Infusion Pump—Model 2620 (Fig. 16-27) is an example of a syringe pump (designed to administer an accurate small dosage of medication or fluid). It uses either B-D 50 ml. or Monoject 60 ml. disposable syringes and is capable of infusing 0.1 to 99 ml./hr. This device can increase the infusion rate in 0.1 ml./hr. increments, making it particularly valuable in the administration of very potent drugs. (Most other infusion pumps increase in 1 ml. increments.) Alarms indicate when only 5 ml. are left in the syringe and when it is empty. The pump stops when the syringe empties. This pump is not intended for the infusion of large volumes of fluids.

The Ivac 530 Pump (Fig. 16-28) is a peristaltic pump that acts directly on the I.V. tubing; it can be adjusted to deliver between 1 to 99 drops per minute and uses any normal adult or pediatric administration set. (It is wise to move the tubing up or back a few inches every 8 hours to avoid damage to the section of the tubing manipulated by the pumping mechanism.) This pump can become portable with the use of available rechargeable batteries. It has alarms that are activated by an empty container, occluded tubing, or discharged batteries, at which point pumping action stops.

The Ivac 600 Pump (Fig. 16-29) is a volumetric pump capable of infusing from 1 to 999 ml./hr. It can become portable with the use of available rechargeable batteries. Alarms are activated by an empty container, occluded tubing, or discharged batteries, at which point pumping action stops.

The Sigmamotor Volumet (Fig. 16-30) is a volumetric pump using a peristaltic pumping action. It can be set to infuse from 1 to 499 ml./hr. An indicator shows the total volume of fluid infused up to any given point in 1 ml. increments. A battery is available to allow for patient mobility. A low battery signals an alarm; when the alarm goes off, the flow rate is switched over to a "keep-open" rate. The pump has an "air-detect" alarm that signals when the container has run dry or when there is a leak in the I.V. set. It then switches to a keep-open rate of 1 ml./hr. (there is sufficient fluid in the tubing to keep the vein open for 5 hours).

The Imed 922 Volumetric Infusion Pump (Fig. 16-31) is a volumetric cassette infusion pump that can be set to infuse from 1 to 299 ml./hr. (It is also marketed by McGaw Laboratories as the McGaw VIP Volumetric Infusion Pump). A rechargeable battery capable of operating without recharging for a number of hours allows for patient ambulation or transfer. Once the desired volume has been infused, an alarm is triggered and the pump maintains a keep-open rate of 1 ml./hr. Alarms also sound when air enters the tubing (pump shuts down) and when the tubing is occluded.

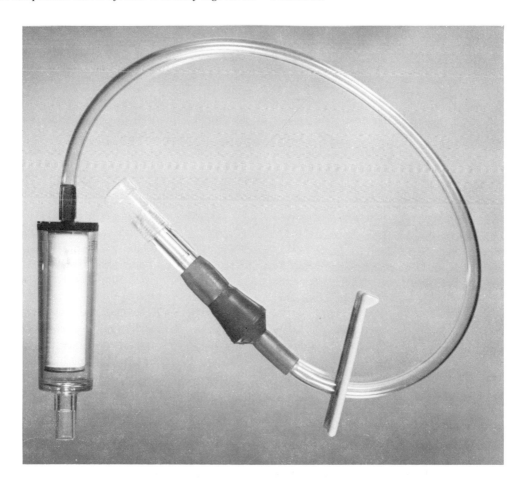

Figure 16-25. Ivex-2 micrometer filter set. (Courtesy of Abbott Laboratories, North Chicago, Illinois)

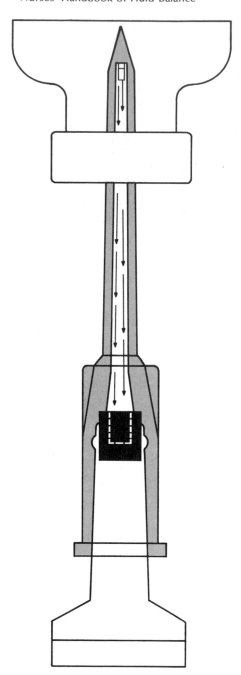

Figure 16-26. Monojet filter aspiration needle, manufactured by Sherwood Medical Industries, St. Louis, Missouri. (Drawn from a brochure.)

The Abbott/Shaw LifeCare I.V. Pump (see Fig. 16-22) is a volumetric pump capable of infusing 1 to 999 ml./hr. It has an infiltration detector that consists of a flat rubber pad with temperature sensors applied to the venipuncture site; infiltration of cool I.V. fluid

into the tissues activates the alarm and stops fluid delivery. If air is introduced into the pump chamber, the system shuts off and activates an alarm. The volume of fluid administered is displayed on the "volume administered" dial. Emptying of the container causes an alarm to signal and the pump to switch to a keep-open rate of 4 ml./hr. (There is sufficient fluid in the tubing to keep the vein open for over an hour.)

The Extracorporeal 2100 Infusion Pump (Fig. 16-32) is a volumetric pump capable of infusing from 1 to 999 ml./hr. The flow rate and infusion time (in hours) can be read on digital readouts. When the infusion time (up to 9 hours) is completed, the pump slows to a keep-open rate of 3 ml./hr. and activates a visual alarm. Rechargeable batteries allow patient mobility; a low battery will signal an alarm. The pump automatically switches to battery operation if hospital power fails. An empty bottle detector minimizes the danger of air embolism caused by an empty container; the pump will stop and activate alarms when air is detected.

Nursing considerations in the use of infusion pumps include the following:

1. *Read the manufacturer's directions carefully prior to using any infusion pump since there are many variations in available models.* (Instruction manuals should be readily available on all units using infusion pumps). It is best to learn how to safely operate each type of infusion pump under the direction of someone knowledgeable in its use (such as an inservice program presented by a representative of the manufacturer). It is particularly important to read the manufacturer's recommendations before administering blood with an infusion pump since some models damage red cells and cause hemolysis.
2. Remember that some types of final filters may be damaged by the high pressures exerted by infusion pumps; thus, it is important to read directions furnished by manufacturers of specific filters prior to using them with infusion pumps. Some filters may cause rate inaccuracies.
3. Check the venipuncture site for infiltration since most pressure pumps keep infusing fluid even though the tissue may be greatly distended, unlike the markedly diminished flow rate accompanying infiltration of a gravity-flow solution.

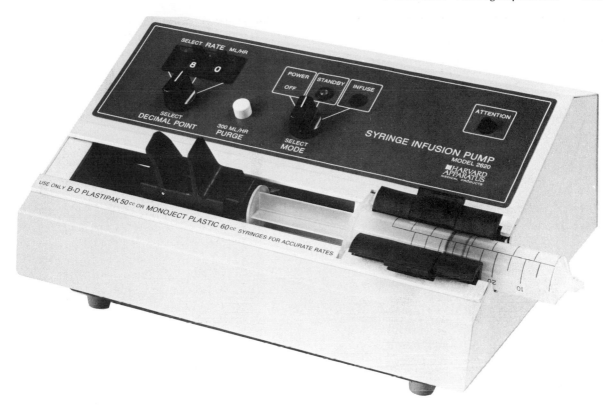

Figure 16-27. Harvard Syringe Infusion Pump—Model 2620. (Courtesy of Harvard Apparatus, Millis, Massachusetts)

4. Check infusion rates closely when batteries are the power source since low batteries may greatly alter the flow rate.

5. Closely monitor the fluid level in the container and adjust the pump as indicated to keep the infusion at the desired rate. Remember that all infusion pumps have some degree of inaccuracy. Also, remember that meters indicating the total volume infused may be misleading if there is a leak or if the tube is blocked, since meters count pump cycles rather than measuring the amount of fluid.[10]

6. Check the function of occlusion detectors (present on a number of pumps) by periodically pinching the tubing shut several times each shift. Recall that an occlusion detector senses increased back pressure due to pinched tubing, clogged final filter, clogged bottle airway, or an unopened tubing clamp.

7. Remember that any machine is subject to malfunction and, thus, it is necessary to continue to check the venipuncture site, flow rate, and amount of fluid in the container. Patients sometimes change the settings on the pump, making it necessary to check these at regular intervals also. Although most pumps are equipped with alarms to signal trouble, it is unwise to rely too heavily on any mechanical device.

8. When using drop sensitive pumps, always check the sensor eye to be sure it is clean and dry. The sensor eye should be cleansed only with water (detergents can cause a film that leads to malfunctioning of the sensor device).

COMPLICATIONS OF INTRAVENOUS FLUID ADMINISTRATION

Patients receiving parenteral fluids should be observed often to detect the early appearance of complications. The nurse should periodically check the rate of flow, the amount of solution in the bottle, the appearance of the injection site and the patient's general response to the infusion.

Complications sometimes occurring with intravenous infusions include:

Pyrogenic reactions

Local infiltration
Circulatory overload
Thrombophlebitis
Air embolism
Speed shock

PYROGENIC REACTIONS   The presence of pyrogenic substances in either the infusion solution or the administration setup can induce a febrile reaction.

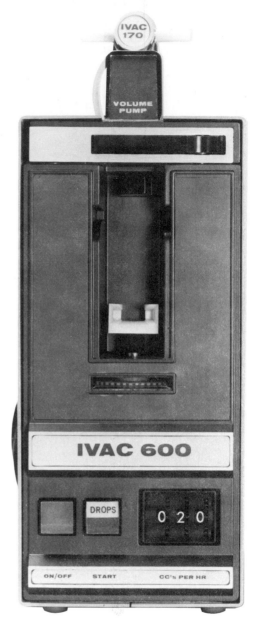

Figure 16-29.   Ivac 600 Pump. (Courtesy of Ivac Corporation, San Diego, California)

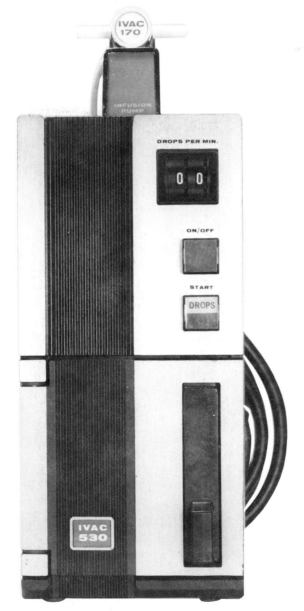

Figure 16-28.   Ivac 530 Pump. (Courtesy of Ivac Corporation, San Diego, California)

(Pyrogens are foreign proteins capable of producing fever.) Such a reaction is characterized by:

An abrupt temperature elevation (from 100 to 106° F.) accompanied by severe chills (the reaction usually begins about 30 minutes after the start of the infusion)
Backache

Headache

General malaise

Nausea and vomiting

Vascular collapse with hypotension and cyanosis, which may occur when the reaction is severe

The severity of the reaction depends upon the amount of pyrogens infused, the rate of flow, and the patient's susceptibility. Patients having fever or liver disease are more susceptible than others.

If these symptoms occur, the nurse should stop the infusion at once, check the vital signs, and notify the physician. The solution should be saved so that it can be cultured if necessary.

The wide use of commercially prepared solutions and administration sets has dramatically decreased the number of pyrogenic reactions. It must be remembered, however, that contaminants can enter the solution flask after the seal is broken. It is, there-

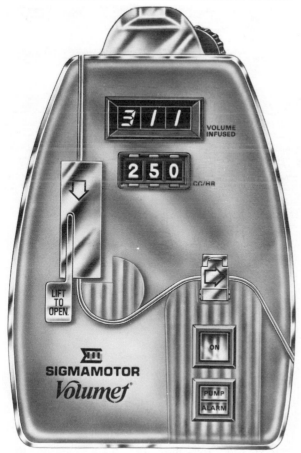

Figure 16-30. Sigmamotor Volumet. (Courtesy of Sigmamotor, Inc., Middleport, New York)

fore, a wise practice to indicate on the bottle the date and time that the seal was broken; electrolyte and dextrose solutions should be in use no longer than 24 hours. This is important to remember when patients are on slow "keep-open" infusions.

For very slow infusions, it is wise to use 250 ml. bottles to assure change of the containers within a safe period of time. Administration sets should be changed at least every 24 hours, and any evidence of cloudiness or other particulate matter in a normally clear solution is an indication to discard it. The administration set should be changed after the administration of blood or other protein-containing solutions since these substances become a growth medium for bacteria.

Prior to initiating an infusion, the nurse should squeeze plastic containers to detect leaks and inspect glass containers against light for cracks or bright reflections that penetrate into the wall of the bottle; if either are present, the solution is no longer sterile and must be discarded. Administration sets should also be routinely inspected for cracks or discolorations prior to use.

Unless the nurse uses the most careful technique, contaminants can be introduced when medications are added to the infusion fluid (Fig. 16-33).

Because traffic generates airborne contamination, medications should be added in an isolated area. Some hospitals are equipped with Laminar Flow Clean Air Work Stations; these stations provide a filtered air screen to reduce contamination of intravenous fluids during handling (Fig. 16-34).

A final filter is another safety device to prevent the infusion of bacteria and particulate matter. The filter is situated between the infusion tubing and the needle, allowing for final sterilization filtration immediately before the solution enters the bloodstream. It also prevents air from entering the circulatory system during mechanical infusion. (Changing the filter set every 24 hours prevents a potential buildup of material.)

LOCAL INFILTRATION   The dislodging of a needle and the local infiltration of solution into the subcutaneous tissues is not uncommon, especially when a small, thin-walled vein is used and the patient is active. Infiltration is characterized by:

1. Edema at the site of injection: compare the infusion area with the identical area in the

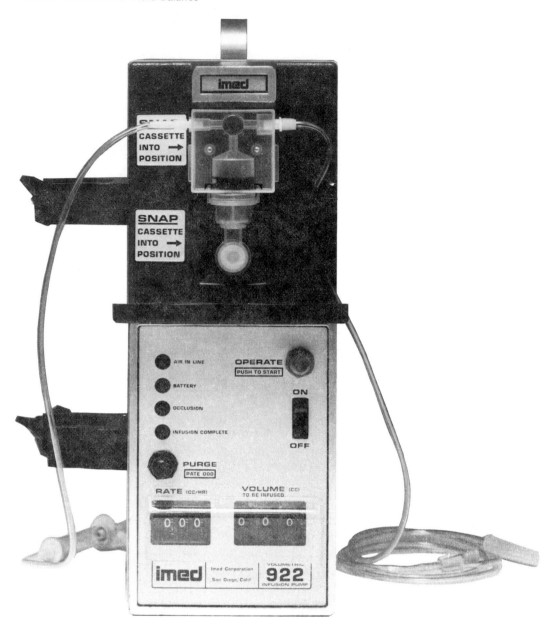

Figure 16-31. Imed 922 Volumetric Infusion Pump. (Courtesy of Imed Corporation, La Jolla, California)

opposite extremity; otherwise swelling may not be readily noticeable. Temperature of the skin around the insertion site is cooler than the rest of the skin because the I.V. fluid is cooler than the body.

2. Discomfort in the area of the injection (the degree of discomfort depends on the type of solution)

3. Significant decrease in the rate of infusion, or a complete stop in the flow of the fluid

4. Failure to get blood return into tubing when the bottle is lowered below the needle (this method is not always foolproof—sometimes the needle lumen is partially in the vein with its tip in the subcutaneous tissue)

Hypertonic carbohydrate solutions, potassium solutions, and solutions with a pH varying greatly from that of the body (such as protein hydrolysates, sixth molar sodium lactate, or ammonium chloride)

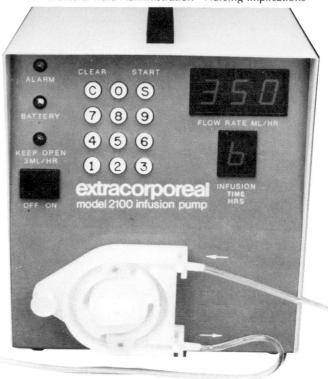

Figure 16-32. Extracorporeal Model 2100 Infusion Pump. (Courtesy of Extracorporeal Medical Specialties, King of Prussia, Pennsylvania)

often cause great pain if they infiltrate into the subcutaneous tissues. Tissue slough may result from the local irritation, especially when norepinephrine (Levophed) is the offending solution.

The infusion should be discontinued immediately when infiltration is apparent. When in doubt, an infiltration can be confirmed by applying a tourniquet (or applying pressure with the fingers) to restrict venous flow proximal to the injection site; if the flow continues, regardless of the venous obstruction, the needle is obviously not in the vein.

Close observation with early detection of infiltration will greatly reduce the severity of this all too common complication. A summary of frequently occurring contributing factors to infiltration include:

Hyperactive patient
Improperly taped venipuncture device
Improper technique of person initiating therapy (such as pushing bevel of needle through the posterior wall of the vein)
Poor selection of venipuncture site (such as over an area of flexion)
Improper handling of extremity and/or equipment during transportation

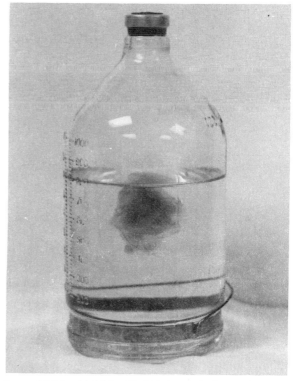

Figure 16-33. Mold in this I.V. bottle indicates break in aseptic technique.

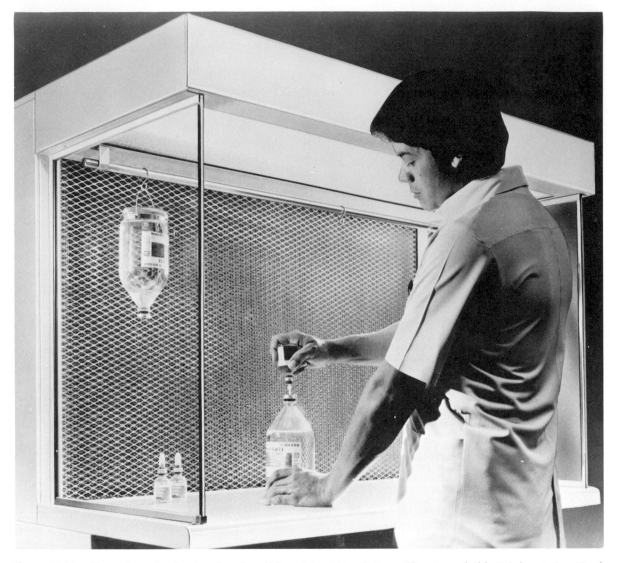

Figure 16-34. Clean air center (laminar-flow hood) for mixing I.V. solutions. (Courtesy of Abbott Laboratories, North Chicago, Illinois)

CIRCULATORY OVERLOAD Overloading the circulatory system with excessive intravenous fluids may cause the following symptoms:

Increased venous pressure
Venous distention (engorged neck veins)
Increased blood pressure
Coughing
Shortness of breath, increased respiratory rate
Pulmonary edema with severe dyspnea and cyanosis

The nurse should be particularly alert for circu-latory overload in patients with cardiac decompensation. If the above symptoms occur, the infusion should be stopped and the physician notified immediately. If necessary, the patient can be raised to a sitting position to facilitate breathing. Patients prone to circulatory overload may require central venous pressure monitoring during infusions.

THROMBOPHLEBITIS The condition associated with clot formation in an inflamed vein is known as thrombophlebitis. Although some degree of venous irritation accompanies all intravenous infusions, it is usually of significance only in infusions kept going in the same site for more than 12 hours. Thrombophlebitis at an infusion site may be manifested by:

Pain along the course of the vein

Redness and edema at the injection site

If severe, systemic reactions to the infection (tachycardia, fever, and general malaise)

Mechanical factors can produce thrombophlebitis. Needle movement can cause venous irritation when the infusion site is near a joint; careless technique in venipuncture, or in removing an infusion needle, can seriously traumatize the vein.

Irritating solutions, such as alcohol, can be instrumental in causing thrombophlebitis. Hypertonic solutions are often associated with venous irritation; carbohydrate solutions in excess of 10 per cent almost always produce this reaction. Solutions with an alkaline or acid pH are more frequently associated with thrombophlebitis than are the solutions that approximate body pH.

Dextrose solutions are irritating to veins because of their low pH. (The U.S.P. specification for pH of dextrose solutions ranges between 3.5 and 6.5.) Five per cent dextrose in water has a pH ranging between 4.0 and 5.0, a low pH necessary to prevent caramelization of the dextrose during sterilization and to preserve the solution's stability during storage. Studies have shown a significant decrease in thrombophlebitis when buffered dextrose solutions have been used. For example, Abbott Laboratories provides a sodium bicarbonate 1% additive solution (Neut) to increase the pH of intravenous solutions to a less irritating level. This small amount of basic solution will not alter the patient's plasma pH. However, increasing the pH of solutions containing additives can produce incompatibility problems, since some additives are only stable at a low pH.

Once thrombophlebitis is detected, the infusion is stopped and restarted in another site to allow the traumatized vein to heal. Usually, cold compresses are applied to the thrombophlebitic site, after which warm moist compresses can be employed to relieve discomfort and promote healing.

AIR EMBOLISM The danger of air embolism is present in all intravenous infusions, even though it does not occur frequently. The widespread use of plastic blood bags has decreased the occurrence of air emboli when blood is pumped in under pressure. According to Rogers,[11] a normal adult can tolerate as much as 200 ml. of air intravenously, but as little as 10 ml. may be fatal to seriously ill patients.

The nurse should take the following measures to prevent the occurrence of air embolism.

1. The disposable tubing should be inspected for cracks or defects.
2. The needle and any other attachments in the setup should be tightly fitted to the infusion tubing to prevent the entrance of air.
3. An infusion should be discontinued before the bottle and tubing are completely emptied; otherwise, air from the bottle will enter the bloodstream if there is a negative pressure in the vein receiving the infusion. (If the vein has a positive pressure, the fluid will stay at this level; normally venous pressure is 4 to 11 cm. above the level of the heart.)
4. The extremity receiving the infusion should not be elevated above the level of the heart since this results in venous collapse and negative venous pressure. Negative pressure in the vein receiving the infusion draws in air if there are any defects in the apparatus or if the solution flask is emptied.
5. The clamp used to regulate the fluid flow rate should be kept at a low level—preferably no higher than the level of the heart, certainly no higher than 4 to 11 cm. above the heart. If the flow regulating clamp is placed above this height, a negative pressure will develop in the tubing below. The negative pressure can be great enough to draw in sizable amounts of air should a loose connection or defect exist between the needle and the clamp. The chance of defects occurring between the needle and the clamp is much greater when the clamp is positioned high on the tubing.
6. Permitting the infusion tubing to drop below the level of the extremity may help prevent air from entering the vein if the infusion flask empties unobserved. There is nothing wrong with enlisting the patient's help in observing the infusion bottle and notifying the nurse when the infusion is about to run out. A tape can be placed on the side of the infusion flask showing the level at which the patient should buzz the nurse.

7. The first bottle to empty in a Y-type set (parallel hookup) should be completely clamped off; otherwise, air will be drawn into the vein from the empty bottle. The potential danger of air emboli exists when fluids from two vented containers run simultaneously through the same needle. The use of administration sets with check-valves for piggybacking fluids prevents this problem (see discussion of piggybacking earlier in this chapter).
8. Great care should be taken when solutions in vented containers are given under pressure since air may be accidentally forced into the bloodstream when the container empties.
9. Some types of electric infusion pumps can pump air into the vein if the infusion bottle is allowed to empty. Be sure to read and follow the manufacturers' directions for safe use of pumps.
10. Air emboli are more apt to occur when the infusion is given via a central vein. Recall that there is a low pressure in the central veins that can pull air in during tubing changes or when connections in the administration apparatus are not airtight. To prevent this complication during tubing change, it is recommended that the patient perform the Valsalva maneuver (forced expiration with the mouth closed) when the tubing is disconnected from the catheter. All connections in the administration setup should be tightly secured to prevent air from being drawn in. If a stopcock is part of the I.V. setup, the outlets not in use should be completely shut off.

The presence of an air embolism is manifested by sudden vascular collapse, with the following symptoms:

Cyanosis
Hypotension
Weak rapid pulse
Venous pressure rise
Loss of consciousness

The occurrence of these symptoms in the patient receiving an infusion should lead one to suspect air embolism.

If an air embolism occurs, administration tubing should be promptly clamped. Some physicians place the patient on his left side with his head down and the lower extremities elevated, on the theory that this allows the air to rise into the right atrium and away from the pulmonary outflow tract.

BLOOD EMBOLISM   A blood embolism may result from the unwise irrigation of a plugged needle or catheter. Irrigation may dislodge the clot into the circulation, possibly resulting in an infarction. Also, the irrigating fluid may embolize small infected needle thrombi, resulting in septicemia. *Plugged needles should be removed—not irrigated.*

SPEED SHOCK   Speed shock may be defined as the systemic reaction that occurs when a substance foreign to the body is rapidly infused into the bloodstream. Too rapid administration of intravenous fluids can cause sensations of chest constriction or throbbing headache. Too rapid administration of fluids containing drugs can flood the bloodstream with the drug and cause toxic concentrations in organs having a rich blood supply (such as the heart and brain). Syncope and shock may occur. The nurse should check the flow rate often and reduce it if untoward symptoms develop.

ADMINISTRATION OF BLOOD, PLASMA, AND DEXTRAN

Blood

Whole blood can be preserved with a solution of sodium citrate, citric acid, and glucose. Sodium citrate acts as an anticoagulant by combining with ionized calcium and, thus, interrupting the clotting mechanism, whereas citric acid and glucose prolong the viability of red blood cells. Blood preserved with acid-citrate-dextrose (A.C.D.) solution can be kept safe for use up to 21 days after collection from the donor, if stored at 4°C. (39°F.). Whole blood can also be preserved with citrate phosphate dextrose solution (C.P.D.) for up to 21 days. Blood preserved in C.P.D. anticoagulant has a higher pH while containing less acid than A.C.D. blood; therefore, it imposes less acid load. This is particularly important if a large volume of blood is infused.

PACKED RED BLOOD CELLS Sometimes it is necessary to administer packed red blood cells, obtained by centrifuging whole blood and drawing off approximately 200 to 225 ml. of plasma. This is the case when a patient with congestive heart failure or fluid volume excess requires blood. Advantages of packed cells, besides reduced volume, include reduced chemical content and reduced agglutinins. Potassium, sodium, and citrate content is substantially reduced, decreasing the danger of hyperkalemia, sodium overload, and citrate toxicity. Because most of the plasma is removed, the amount of anti-A and anti-B agglutinins is also reduced. Packed cells with a hematocrit of 70 per cent can be infused with little difficulty.

BLOOD TRANSFUSION REACTIONS Whole blood transfusions often are indicated in the presence of a significantly decreased blood volume. Blood replacement therapy is often lifesaving, but, without careful attention to its hazards, it may also be lethal. Because the nurse shares a large responsibility in assuring safe blood administration, she should be familiar with complications associated with its use.

Stored Blood and Potassium Excess Continual destruction of red blood cells occurs when blood is stored; at the end of 21 days only 70 to 80 per cent of the original number of cells remain. The longer the blood ages, the higher its plasma potassium level becomes. One day old blood has a plasma potassium content of approximately 7 mEq./L.; blood stored for 21 days has a plasma potassium content of approximately 23 mEq./L. Not only is potassium released from the destroyed red blood cells but there is also a transfer of potassium from the intact cells into the surrounding plasma.

Aged blood should not be given to patients with oliguria or anuria since there is danger of causing potassium excess. Potassium excess may be recognized by the following symptoms:

Gastrointestinal hyperactivity (nausea, intestinal colic, and diarrhea)
Vague muscular weakness, first in the extremities, later extending to the trunk
Paresthesia of hands, feet, tongue, and face
Flaccid paralysis (involving respiratory muscles last)
Apprehension
Slowed pulse rate (may also be irregular)

Cardiac arrest and death when plasma potassium level reaches 10 to 15 mEq./L. (due to marked dilation and flaccidity of the heart)

The incidence of cardiac arrest during surgery is correlated with the rapid infusion of large quantities of aged blood.

Citrated Blood and Hypocalcemia Rarely, symptoms of calcium deficit can be caused by the rapid administration of large volumes of citrated blood. It should be recalled that A.C.D. and C.P.D. preserved bank blood contain citrate in excess of that needed to combine with the calcium in the blood collected. Under certain circumstances, the excess citrate, when infused into the bloodstream, can combine with ionized plasma calcium and cause tetany. The excess citrate normally causes no difficulty since the liver can remove it from the blood within a few minutes; also, binding of ionized calcium by citrate causes rapid mobilization of calcium from the bones. Therefore, when blood transfusions are given at slow rates (less than 1 L./hr.) there is usually no danger of citrate toxicity.[12] (One source states that an adult ordinarily can tolerate the administration of the amount of excess citrate in a unit of blood every 10 minutes without undue symptoms.[13]) However, patients with severe liver disease cannot tolerate usual administration rates since the liver is unable to remove citrate from the blood quickly enough to prevent a reaction. Also, patients with inadequate bone stores of calcium (such as young children and osteoporotic adults) are more susceptible to citrate toxicity during massive transfusions. (It may occur in infants receiving exchange transfusions with citrated blood.)

Citrate-induced ionized calcium deficit may cause the following symptoms:

Tingling of the fingers and circumoral region
Hyperactive muscular reflexes
Muscle spasms (respiratory muscle spasm can kill the patient within a few minutes[14])
Bradycardia, arrhythmias, and hypotension

If citrate toxicity is anticipated or suspected, the patient is given calcium gluconate or calcium chloride to correct the deficit of ionized calcium. (The physician injects the calcium preparation into a vein remote from the transfusion site.)

Circulatory Overload Discussed earlier in the chapter as a possible complication of all intravenous infusions, circulatory overload is particularly likely to occur in massive blood replacement for hypovolemia or when blood is given to a patient with normal blood volume. In addition to inducing pulmonary edema, the increased blood volume may cause hemorrhage into the lungs and the gastrointestinal tract.

To guard against the occurrence of circulatory overload, many physicians order the monitoring of venous pressure during the rapid replacement of large volumes of blood. (The procedure is discussed in the last section of this chapter.) Aged patients and patients with cardiac damage should be closely observed for circulatory overload even when small volumes of blood are given; venous pressure monitoring is frequently used to protect such patients from overload. Administration of packed cells decreases the likelihood of fluid overload.

Allergic Reactions   Allergic reactions to blood are reported to occur in 1 to 4 per cent of all transfusions. Symptoms may include flushing, chills, pruritus, and urticaria; rarely do bronchospasm, angioneurotic edema, and vascular collapse occur. (Urticaria occurs only in allergic blood reactions, not in the other types of transfusion reactions.) The allergic reaction results from transfer of donor antigen to a sensitive recipient; frequently the donor has just ingested the antigen prior to donating blood. Reactions are much more apt to occur in patients with a history of asthma, hay fever, or atopy; it has been suggested that such patients be transfused with washed packed plasma-free red blood cells to decrease the likelihood of an allergic reaction. Symptoms usually do not occur until 250 ml. of whole blood or 125 ml. of packed red blood cells have been transfused;[15] they may not occur until the transfusion has been completed. Blood administration is often slowed if a minor reaction occurs; it is stopped immediately if severe symptoms are present. Antihistamines usually relieve mild symptoms; but the rarer, more severe reactions require epinephrine or steroids. Sometimes antihistamines are used prophylactically when an allergic reaction is considered likely.

Serum Homologous Hepatitis   Associated with blood transfusion is the risk of transmitting serum hepatitis, and, therefore, persons known to have had hepatitis are not allowed to give blood. Nonetheless, not all persons with hepatitis have had the condition diagnosed; thus, the danger always exists. There is no way to eliminate this risk completely but, recently, researchers have found an agent (Australian antigen)

that is linked with serum hepatitis. More importantly, tests have been devised to detect the agent and to allow blood banks and hospitals to screen blood for serum hepatitis. Unfortunately, the accuracy of the tests is estimated at only about 25 per cent.

The incidence of Australian antigen in voluntary donors is about 1:11,000. Statistics indicate that paid donors cause up to five times as many cases of serum hepatitis as unpaid donors. (Drug addicts often sell blood to raise money for more drugs, with serum hepatitis fast spreading among them, because most use unsterile equipment for intravenous injections.) It is regrettable that in many cities, as much as half the blood comes from commercial sources.

The incubation period for serum hepatitis is from 6 weeks to 6 months; symptoms include malaise, anorexia, vomiting, abdominal discomfort, enlarged liver with tenderness, diarrhea, headache, fever, and jaundice. Serum hepatitis is particularly serious in the elderly and in patients already debilitated by serious illness or injury.

The incidence of serum hepatitis is lessened with the use of frozen red blood cells and washed packed cells; it is assumed that freezing and washing the cells decrease the concentration of virus in the plasma.

Hypothermia   Cold solutions are quickly warmed as they mix with circulating blood during usual administration rates. Rapid massive replacement of cold blood has caused cardiac arrest, and one study in a new York hospital showed a significant decrease in cardiac arrest (from 58.3 to 6.8 per cent) when cold blood was warmed to body temperature during rapid massive infusion (6 pints or more per hour). In addition to cardiac arrest, cold blood can cause hypothermia and peripheral vasoconstriction. When it is deemed necessary to warm blood, an automatic blood warmer may be used.

Blood temperature should not exceed 110° F. (43.3° C) since temperatures above this level cause increased hemolysis of red cells. (Usually blood warmers automatically shut off when the blood temperature reaches 100° F.)

Febrile Reactions   Minor febrile reactions occur in 2 per cent of all recipients of blood transfusions and are characterized by fever (rarely exceeding 103° F. [39.5° C.]), flushing, chills, and headache. Usually they are due to sensitivity to donor white cells; less frequently they are caused by sensitivity to platelets and plasma proteins in patients who have received numerous transfusions in the past. Symptoms do not usually occur until more than 250 ml. of blood has infused. It may be necessary to administer blood that has had the white cells and platelets removed for patients with a history of severe reactions. Febrile reactions may also result from contamination of the administration setup. The patient does not appear toxic and is usually treated with aspirin to relieve the fever; therapy is essentially symptomatic.

Such a reaction is sometimes confused with an incompatible blood reaction and so it should be noted that febrile reactions tend to occur toward the end of the transfusion or even after it is completed (an acute hemolytic reaction usually occurs during the infusion of the first 100 ml. of incompatible blood). Also, the back pain so characteristic of a hemolytic reaction is often absent in a febrile reaction.

Bacterial Contamination Before blood is used it should be inspected for bacterial growth signs, such as discoloration or gas bubbles. If these are present the blood should be discarded. If blood used for transfusion is grossly contaminated with gram-negative organisms, the recipient usually develops a high fever, intense flushing, vomiting, diarrhea, headache, and symptoms of shock which may prove fatal. As little as 50 ml. of contaminated blood can precipitate this reaction. Blood samples should be drawn and cultured; the patient is usually treated with appropriate antibiotics, steroids, and fresh uncontaminated blood. (It has been reported that approximately 0.1 per cent of all units of whole blood are contaminated with cold-growing organisms.[16])

Acute Hemolytic Reaction The most dreaded reaction to blood transfusion is that caused by the administration of grossly incompatible whole blood or packed cells. (It is reported to occur in 1 out of every 3000 transfusions.[17]) A transfusion of incompatible blood causes rapid cell agglutination in the recipient and eventual intravascular hemolysis. The incompatible transfusion is most often caused by the careless administration of the wrong blood; it can also be the result of inadequate crossmatching. Some hemolytic reactions are caused by the administration of blood accidentally hemolyzed from improper handling. Symptoms of an acute hemolytic reaction usually occur during the transfusion of the first 100 ml. (sometimes as little as 5 to 10 ml.) of blood and may include:

Lumbar and flank pain (flank pain caused by hemoglobin precipitation in the renal tubules)

Tachypnea and tachycardia
Feeling of constriction in the chest or precordial pain
Urge to defecate or urinate
Fever and severe shaking chills (a hemolytic reaction may cause considerable fever and general toxicity; these effects, in the absence of renal shutdown, are rarely fatal)
Jaundice (usually does not occur unless more than 3000 ml. of blood is hemolyzed in less than a day)
Later hemoglobinuria and acute renal tubular necrosis may occur
The only signs of serious transfusion reaction in an anesthetized or otherwise unconscious patient may be increasing tachycardia, shock, and oozing of blood at the site of operation (bleeding may follow disseminated intravascular coagulation, which presumably follows the release of erythrocytic thromboplastic substances)

Because an acute hemolytic reaction becomes evident during transfusion of the first 20 to 100 ml. of blood, it is highly desirable that the patient be carefully observed during this part of the infusion. If the transfusion is stopped early, acute renal tubular necrosis and death rarely occur; if more than several hundred ml. are infused, renal shutdown and death are common. Renal shutdown is due to blockage of the tubules with hemoglobin and to the powerful vasoconstriction caused by toxic substances released from the hemolyzed blood.

The blood transfusion should be discontinued immediately when a hemolytic reaction is evident. The blood bottle and set should be refrigerated so that further compatibility tests may be made. All urine should be saved and observed for discoloration; urine is sent to the laboratory for evaluation of hemoglobin content. The onset of a hemolytic reaction may be delayed when factors of less moment than those involving the ABO system are present. For example, a patient who has received multiple transfusions in the past may have become sensitized to Rh or to the minor factors, and his hemolytic reaction might have a delayed onset. The slow developing type of hemolytic reaction may be characterized by jaundice appearing hours or days after the transfusion.

Hemolytic reactions are more prone to occur in patients who have had past transfusions and tend to be proportionate to the number of such transfusions, regardless of when given.

Treatment of an incompatible blood reaction usually consists of rapid administration of dilute fluids to promote diuresis. Alkaline fluids, such as sixth molar sodium lactate, increase the solubility of hemoglobin and aid in its excretion. An osmotic diuretic (usually mannitol) may be given intravenously to promote fluid excretion by the tubules and to overcome renal vasoconstriction; further treatment is dependent upon the amount of renal damage present. It is impossible to overstress the need to check and recheck all labels for both donor and patient, as errors in labeling still constitute a frequent cause of reaction.

SAFE BLOOD ADMINISTRATION   To help assure that blood transfusions be as safe as possible, the nurse should keep the following points in mind:

1. Be aware of the complications associated with blood administration; keep their descriptions in mind while observing the patient.
2. *Give the right blood to the right patient.*
   a. Read the labels identifying the blood and check them carefully with the patient's full name, obtained from the wrist identification band. The bed card should not be relied on solely to identify the patient; these cards are often not up to date.
   b. The patient should be called by name and his response observed; this practice in itself is not foolproof because some patients respond to any name.
   c. Location of the patient should not be relied upon as the sole means of identification; patients are moved frequently in most hospitals.
   d. Particular precautions are necessary when the patient has a common name; many errors have been made by not checking further than the last name and first initial. This is not to imply that two patients with the same uncommon name cannot be confused; it *has* happened. Most importantly, the label on the container should be matched with the patient's wrist identification band; the name and number on both should be identical.

3. Blood sent to nursing divisions should be started within 30 minutes, because *rapid deterioration of red blood cells occurs after blood has been exposed to room temperature for more than two hours.* Ward refrigeration is inadequate for storing blood because it is not controlled and has no alarm to signal fluctuation of temperature. (Accidental freezing of blood renders it unsuitable for use.)
4. The patient's temperature should be taken before the transfusion to serve as a baseline for later temperature comparisons. An elevated temperature during a transfusion may indicate either a pyrogenic or an incompatible blood reaction and, for this reason, the temperature should be checked hourly during the blood administration and for several hours afterwards.
5. The blood should be inspected before use for discoloration or gas bubbles; if these are present, the blood is probably contaminated and must be discarded.
6. Blood should always be given through a filter to remove the particulate matter formed during storage. Stored bank blood contains cellular degradation debris that can cause a condition known as post-transfusion lung syndrome when multiple units have been transfused through a standard (170 micron) mesh filter. A micropore filter (40 microns and under) should be used when more than 4 units of whole blood are to be transfused in one day.[18]
7. Do not start whole blood with 5 per cent dextrose in water or hook whole blood in series or parallel with it. Isotonic saline is compatible with blood and is often used to start blood. "Balanced electrolyte" solutions are available without calcium and are also used to start blood.
8. Do not use a calcium-containing solution (such as lactated Ringers) to start citrated blood or hook it in series or parallel with citrated blood, as calcium ions may cause the blood to clot and clog the infusion apparatus.
9. If it is necessary to warm blood before administration, a blood warmer can be used, as described earlier. Hot water should never

be used to heat blood because excess heat destroys red blood cells.

10. The first 50 ml. of blood should be delivered slowly while the patient is observed closely. If no adverse reactions occur, the rate may be increased as ordered. Frequent observations should continue during the transfusion.

11. Unless the patient has severe hypovolemia, blood transfusions should be given no faster than 500 ml. every 30 minutes. The presence of factors such as cardiac, renal, or liver damage may necessitate much slower rates. A patient with normal blood volume should receive blood at a slow rate to prevent circulatory overload. Usually a unit of blood can be given in less than a 2-hour period. Remember that blood cells deteriorate rapidly after exposure to room temperature for more than 2 hours.

Blood can be given under pressure by applying a pressure sleeve to the plastic blood container (Fig. 16-35). Air, forced into the sleeve by means of a pressure bulb, exerts force on the flexible container and increases the flow rate.

Plasma

Plasma is the liquid component left after blood has been centrifuged and the red blood cells removed. It is prepared commercially and dispensed as liquid, frozen, or dried plasma.

Storage of plasma presents less of a problem than blood storage; therefore, it is more readily available than blood. For this reason, plasma is sometimes used in emergency situations to restore blood volume until whole blood can be obtained. Plasma is indicated for the replacement of volume when there is little or no deficit of red blood cells, as in severe crushing injuries or burns. The use of fresh frozen plasma provides coagulation factors for patients with clotting abnormalities.

There is risk of hepatitis transmission with plasma. Less chance of hepatitis transmission exists when single donor plasma is used; consequently, the use of pooled plasma (derived from the blood of many donors) is to be discouraged.

Serum albumin is the chief protein of plasma. A 5 per cent solution can be used in the emergency treatment of hypovolemic shock; a 25 per cent solution can be used to treat the hypoproteinemia of

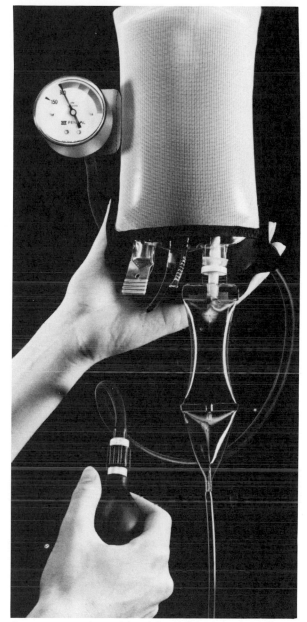

Figure 16-35. Plastic blood bag with pressure infusor. (Courtesy of Fenwal Laboratories, Morton Grove, Illinois)

nephrotic and cirrhotic edema. There is no hepatitis hazard associated with the use of albumin. There is also no hepatitis risk with the use of plasma protein fraction (such as Plasmanate*). Plasma protein fraction is the fraction of plasma left after the fibrinogen and much of the globulin have been removed. It is often used as a plasma expander in the treatment of hypovolemia.

* Plasmanate (Cutter Laboratories).

Dextran

Dextran is a polymer of glucose having a large molecular weight. It is sometimes used for emergency treatment of hypovolemic shock.

When infused into the bloodstream, the large dextran molecules increase intravascular osmotic pressure and draw in interstitial fluid to restore blood volume. When blood loss is not severe, dextran may serve as the total replacement fluid. If blood loss is severe, dextran should be followed by whole blood when available.

Dextran does not require special storage. Because it is prepared synthetically rather than from blood, there is no danger of serum homologous hepatitis.

Dextran 70* has a molecular weight close to that of serum albumin—about 70,000. Dextran 70 6% is available in isotonic saline or in nonelectrolyte solutions (such as 5% D/W or 10% invert sugar in water). The latter is used for patients requiring a low sodium intake. Dextran is for intravenous use only, and the usual dose is 500 ml. More than this amount can be given but is not recommended, since dextran is not broken down rapidly and will expand the intravascular space for some time. By so doing, it limits the rapidity of red blood cell replacement.

Dextran may act as an allergen and occasionally causes reactions of varying degrees of severity. Symptoms of a severe allergic reaction may include:

Generalized urticaria
Chest tightness
Wheezing
Nausea and vomiting
Dyspnea
Hypotension

The patient should be observed closely for anaphylaxis during the first 30 minutes of the infusion. (Allergic symptoms have been known to appear after the administration of as little as 10 ml. of dextran.) If any of these symptoms appear, the infusion should be stopped immediately; Adrenalin may be necessary to control a severe reaction. In mild reactions, withdrawal of the dextran will usually suffice.

Particular caution is necessary when dextran is administered to patients with heart disease or renal disease, because of the danger of congestive heart failure and pulmonary edema. Careful monitoring of venous pressure during rapid dextran administration is sometimes indicated to guard against circulatory overload. (A precipitous rise in venous pressure is an indication to stop the infusion immediately.) If venous pressure is not monitored, the infusion must be given more slowly and the patient observed carefully for signs of circulatory overload. The physician should indicate the desired flow rate.

A transient increase in bleeding time is sometimes seen several hours following the administration of dextran (particularly if more than 1000 ml. has been given). For this reason, patients should be observed for any bleeding tendencies. Dextran should be used with caution in patients with thrombocytopenia and severe bleeding disorders.

A dextran of lower molecular weight—about 40,000—has been developed; it is referred to as dextran 40.* Ten per cent dextran 40 is available in 5% D/W and in 0.9% sodium chloride. Like dextran 70, it expands the plasma volume and is used in the treatment of shock; however, because of its smaller molecular weight, it has a shorter action period and is more readily excreted.

Studies have shown that capillary blood flow is often decreased or stopped in shock, probably owing to blockage of these small vessels with red blood cells. Dextran 40 enhances blood flow, particularly in the small vessels, by increasing blood volume, decreasing blood viscosity, and by reducing the aggregation of red blood cells in the capillaries.

Blood samples for typing, crossmatching, and other tests should be obtained before the dextran infusion is started (dextran can interfere with the accuracy of some laboratory tests).

Poorly hydrated patients receiving dextran are in danger of becoming more dehydrated. (Recall that dextran acts by pulling water from the extravascular space.) Other parenteral fluids should be administered as necessary to prevent extravascular dehydration and to maintain an adequate urinary output.

---

* Gentran 75 (Travenol Laboratories); Macrodex (Pharmacia Laboratories); Dextran 70 (Cutter Laboratories); Dextran (Abbott Laboratories).

* Gentran 40 (Travenol Laboratories); LMD (Abbott Laboratories); Rheomacrodex (Pharmacia Laboratories); Dextran 40 (Cutter Laboratories).

CENTRAL VENOUS PRESSURE MEASUREMENT

Central venous pressure refers to the pressure in the right atrium or vena cava and provides information about the following parameters:

Blood volume
Effectiveness of the heart's pumping action
Vascular tone

Pressure in the right atrium is usually 0 to 4 cm. of water; pressure in the vena cava is approximately 4 to 11 cm. of water.

Venous pressure can also be measured in peripheral veins (as in the arm). Peripheral venous pressure reflects central pressure fairly well if the limb in which it is measured is not acutely compressed between the manometer and the heart. When accuracy is of utmost importance, however, venous pressure should be measured in a central vein.

A low central venous pressure may indicate decreased blood volume or drug-induced vasodilatation (causing pooling of blood in peripheral areas). A high

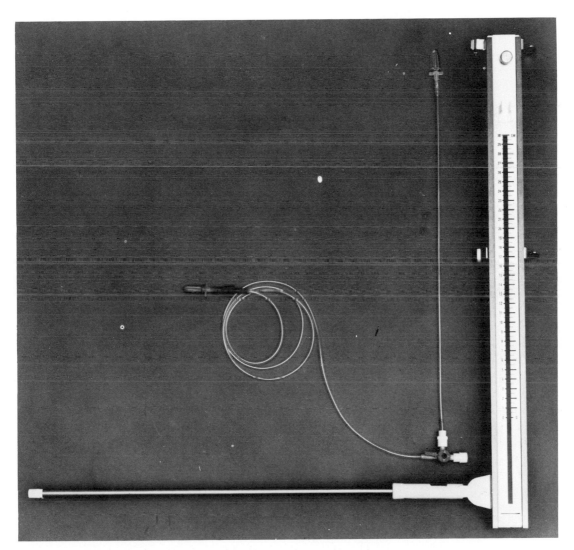

Figure 16-36. Apparatus for measuring central venous pressure: B-P Manometer Stand and Venous Pressure Manometer Set. (Courtesy of Bard-Parker, Division of Becton, Dickenson, & Co., Rutherford, New Jersey)

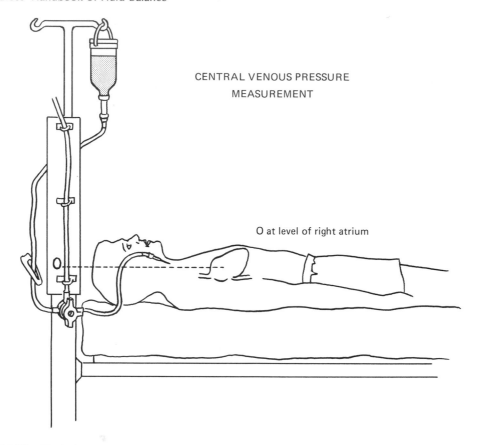

CENTRAL VENOUS PRESSURE
MEASUREMENT

O at level of right atrium

Figure 16-37. Central venous pressure measurement with zero-point of manometer at level of right atrium.

central venous pressure may indicate increased blood volume, heart failure, or vasoconstriction produced by vasopressors (causing the vascular bed to become smaller). More important than absolute values are the upward or downward trends in central venous pressure; these trends are determined by taking frequent readings (often every 30 to 60 minutes). It is always important to evaluate central venous pressure in reference to other available clinical data such as blood pressure, pulse, respirations, breath and heart sounds, fluid intake, and urinary output. For example: a rise in central venous pressure paralleling that of systolic blood pressure is an indication of adequate fluid volume replacement; or, a low central venous pressure persisting after fluid volume replacement may be a sign of continued occult bleeding. Sometimes the rate of an intravenous infusion is titrated according to the patient's central venous pressure; when this is necessary, the physician should designate the desired limits so that the nurse can adjust the flow rate accordingly.

Equipment used to measure central venous pressure is relatively simple, consisting of a CVP catheter, water manometer, three-way stopcock, and a routine I.V. setup (Fig. 16-36). After the physician has threaded the CVP catheter into the vena cava, the catheter is connected by way of the stopcock to the manometer and the infusion apparatus. The manometer is attached to an I.V. pole with the zero point at the level of the patient's right atrium (mid-axillary line) (Fig. 16-37).

Readings should be made, if possible, with the patient flat in bed; if not, they should be made with the patient in the same position each time (the position should be indicated when charting the pressure). When the catheter is properly positioned in the vena cava, the fluid should fluctuate 3 to 5 cm. in the manometer with respirations. If the patient is being ventilated on a respirator, it should be disconnected temporarily for the brief period it takes to read the CVP, since a respirator will cause a false high reading. If the respirator cannot be discontinued, it should be noted that readings were made with it in operation (a trend can still be noted although the absolute readings are not accurate). Sometimes methylene blue or vitamin B complex is added to color the I.V. solution and facilitate reading the fluid level in the manometer. In order to read venous pressure, it is necessary to:

1. Turn the stopcock so that the solution will flow from the container to the manometer, allowing it to reach a level of 30 cm. (See system 2 in Fig. 16-38).
2. Then, turn the stopcock to direct manometer flow to the patient (see system 3 in Fig. 16-38). The fluid level should drop, reaching a reading level in about 15 seconds.
3. The reading should be made at the upper level of the respiratory fluctuation of fluid in the manometer (fluid falls slightly on inspiration and rises slightly on expiration).
4. Turn the stopcock to allow resumption of the infusion to keep the catheter patent and to supply needed fluids (See system 1 in Fig. 16-38).

Meticulous aseptic technique should be used for dressing changes, catheter care, and tubing changes.

Check frequently for signs of redness, swelling, and infection at the insertion site. The connections should be checked frequently to be sure they are secure (to prevent the occurrence of air embolism). Remember that air embolism is more likely to occur when a catheter is placed in the central veins where pressure is low.

REFERENCES

1. **Plumer, A.:** Principles and Practices of Intravenous Therapy, ed. 2. Boston: Little, Brown & Co., 1975, p. 71.
2. **Blackburn, G.** and **Flatt, J.:** Metabolic response to illness: protein-sparing effect. Comprehensive Ther. Vol. I, No. 5, 1975.
3. **Cutter Solutions.** Cutter Laboratories, Berkeley, Calif., 1977.
4. **Frenier, E.:** Problems of I.V. incompatabilities. Am. J. I.V. Ther. Vol. 3, 1976, p. 23.
5. Ibid.
6. Ibid., p. 22.
7. Ibid.
8. Ibid.
9. Ibid.
10. **Beaumond, E.:** The new infusion pumps. Nursing 77, July 1977, p. 33.

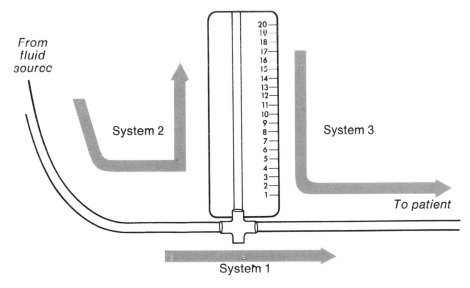

System 1 allows flow from the container to the patient (routine infusion)
System 2 allows flow from the container to the manometer (allows manometer to fill)
System 3 allows flow from the manometer to the patient (allows reading of CVP)

Figure 16-38. Fluid flow systems in central venous pressure measurement. (Hudak, C., et al.: Critical Care Nursing, ed. 2. Philadelphia: J. B. Lippincott, Co., 1977, p. 187)

11. **Boedeker, E.,** and **Dauber, J.** (eds.): Manual of Medical Therapeutics, ed. 21. Boston: Little, Brown & Co., 1974, p. 287.

12. **Guyton, A.:** Textbook of Medical Physiology, ed. 5. Philadelphia: W. B. Saunders Co., 1976, p. 96.

13. **Condon, R.,** and **Nyhus, L.** (eds.): Manual of Surgical Therapeutics, ed. 3. Boston: Little, Brown & Co., 1975, p. 298.

14. **Guyton:** Textbook of Medical Physiology, p. 96.

15. **Condon** and **Nyhus:** Manual of Surgical Therapeutics, p. 294.

16. Ibid., p. 295.

17. Ibid.

18. Ibid., p. 300.

BIBLIOGRAPHY

Berk, J., et al.: Handbook of Critical Care. Boston: Little, Brown & Co., 1976.

Dudrick, S., et al.: Long-term parenteral nutrition: its current status. Hospital Practice 10:47–58, 1975.

Goldman, D.: Improving infection control in I.V. therapy. Am. J. I.V. Ther. March 1977.

Goldman, D., et al.: Guidelines for infection control in intravenous ther. Ann. Intern. Med. Vol. 79, 1973.

Hudak, C., et al.: Critical Care Nursing, ed. 2, Philadelphia: J. B. Lippincott Co., 1977.

Klotz, R.: The team approach to fluid and electrolyte therapy. Am. J. I.V. Ther. Sept/Oct. 1974.

Kurdi, W.: Refining your I.V. therapy techniques. Nursing 75, Vol. 5, 1975.

Lee, D., and **Kleeman, C.:** Phosphorus depletion in man. Medical Monographs. McGraw Laboratories, Santa Ana, Calif., 1976.

Recommended Guide to Parenteral Nutrition. Travenol Laboratories, Deerfield, Ill., 1976.

Robinson, L., and **Vanderveen, T.:** Pharmacy-based infusion pump program. Am. J. Hosp. Pharm. 34:697–705, 1977.

Schulte, W., et al.: Positive nitrogen balance using isotonic crystalline amino acid solution. Arch. Surg., Vol. 110, 1975.

Sheldon, G., and **Grzyb, S.:** Phosphate depletion and repletion: relation to parenteral nutrition and oxygen transport. Ann. Surg. 182:683–689, 1975.

Turco, S.: Inaccuracies in I.V. flow rates. Am. J. I.V. Ther. June/July, 1976.

— 17 —

Fluid Balance in the Surgical Patient

THE BODY'S RESPONSE TO SURGICAL TRAUMA

Although a surgical procedure may be lifesaving, the body responds to it as trauma. Postoperative responses bear a direct relationship to nursing care.

Endocrine Response (Stress Reaction)

PERIOD OF FLUID RETENTION AND CATABOLISM The stress reaction described by Selye, representing a response to surgical trauma, is present for the first two to five days. The intensity of changes depends on the severity and duration of the trauma.

A scale of 10 has been proposed to grade the severity of trauma. An appendectomy or a simple herniorrhaphy is rated low on the scale, around 1 or 2, whereas severe trauma, such as deep burns or pelvic evisceration, rates high on the scale. In the middle of the scale are abdominal surgical procedures such as subtotal gastrectomy or colectomy. Postoperative apprehension and pain enhance the stress reaction, and extreme preoperative apprehension can initiate the stress reaction before surgery. Anesthesia also constitutes a form of stress.

The endocrine responses may be briefly outlined as follows (see Fig. 17-1):

1. Increased ACTH (adrenocorticotrophic hormone) secretion from the anterior pituitary
2. Increased mineralocorticoid and glucocorti-

coid secretion from the adrenal cortex (in response to stimulation by ACTH)
   a. Mineralocorticoids (desoxycorticosterone [DOCA] and aldosterone) cause:
      (1) Na^+ retention
      (2) Cl^- retention
      (3) K^+ excretion
   b. Glucocorticoids (mainly hydrocortisone) cause:
      (1) Na^+ retention
      (2) Cl^- retention
      (3) K^+ excretion
      (4) Catabolism
         (a) protein breakdown
         (b) gluconeogenesis and elevated blood sugar
      (5) Fat mobilization
      (6) Drop in eosinophil count
3. Increased ADH (antidiuretic hormone) secretion from posterior pituitary, causing decreased urinary output
4. Vasopressor substances (epinephrine and norepinephrine) secreted from the adrenal medulla to help maintain blood pressure, a response stimulated by fear, pain, hypoxia and hemorrhage

The body's response to stress appears purposeful. For example, sodium retention, chloride retention, potassium loss, and increased ADH secretion help to maintain blood volume. Sodium and chloride

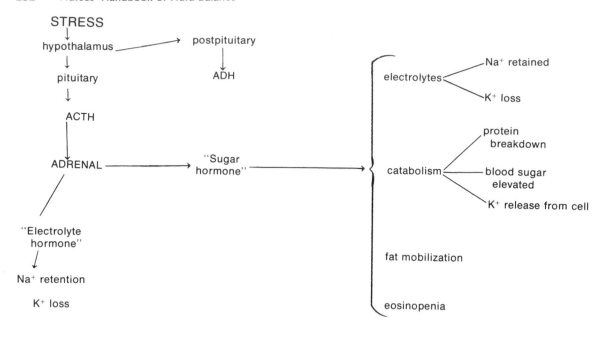

Figure 17-1. Effect of stress on electrolyte excretion. (Adapted from Statland, H.: Fluids and Electrolytes in Practice, ed. 3. Philadelphia: J. B. Lippincott Co., 1963, p. 45)

retention cause water retention, cellular potassium loss releases cellular water into the extracellular space, and ADH secretion causes decreased fluid excretion by way of the kidneys. Glucocorticoids cause protein breakdown, make amino acids available for healing at the site of trauma, and cause conversion of protein and fat to glucose (gluconeogenesis), creating a ready supply of glucose for use during the stress period. (The elevated blood sugar may be mistaken for diabetes mellitus.)

As a result of stress, the early postoperative patient loses more urinary nitrogen than normal, even though his protein intake is low or absent. Because the body nitrogen losses exceed intake, the patient is said to be in negative nitrogen balance. Laboratory findings during the stress period include reduced eosinophil count and elevated level of serum 17-hydroxycorticosteroid hormones; both indicate increased adrenal activity.

The changes described here are *normal* responses to trauma and do not require corrective measures.

PERIODS OF DIURESIS AND ANABOLISM   After the second to fifth postoperative days, adrenal activity is decreased and a mild water and sodium diuresis

occurs. The body also begins to retain potassium. Following an uncomplicated abdominal operation, it is not uncommon for a normal adult male to lose from 4 to 9 lb. during the first postoperative days.

Anabolism, the building up of body protein, usually begins by the seventh to the tenth postoperative day. At this time the urinary nitrogen losses are decreased even though the patient is consuming protein foods. Thus, the renal excretion of nitrogen no longer exceeds the nitrogen intake from protein foods, and the patient begins to gain weight, provided oral intake is adequate.

Tissue Injury

Trauma results in the formation of edema in and about the operative site for the first few days after surgery. The fluid closely resembles plasma; its volume is roughly proportionate to the amount of tissue trauma. Traumatic edema is functionally sequestered as a "third-space" and cannot be readily mobilized to meet body needs. While the amount of fluid lost in edema is not in itself significant, it may enhance the extracellular fluid volume deficit created by peritonitis, hemorrhage, or other complications. The edema fluid is reabsorbed and excreted during the diuretic phase of the stress reaction.

Immobilization

Despite the emphasis on early ambulation, postoperative patients are much less physically active than normal. Immobilization favors increased renal nitrogen and calcium excretion and negative nitrogen balance, with muscle atrophy occurring from disuse. However, except for weight loss and temporary weakness, immobilization for a few days does not significantly affect metabolism.

Starvation Effect

Most patients eat inadequately, or not at all, during the first few postoperative days; thus, a starvation effect is induced. Accompanying starvation is a daily weight loss of about ½ lb., reflecting a decrease in lean and fatty tissue mass. Renal nitrogen excretion is increased as a result of lean tissue catabolism.

The weight loss following surgery is generally constant as revealed by accurate weighing procedures and recording the findings on a weight chart. A weight gain, in the face of starvation, indicates fluid retention. Usually the patient will regain his normal weight in two or three months if preoperative nutrition was good, operative trauma was of only moderate severity, and there was prompt return of gastrointestinal function.

PREVENTION OF POSTOPERATIVE COMPLICATIONS BY CAREFUL PREOPERATIVE PREPARATION

Nutrition

A patient in good nutritional condition preoperatively withstands postoperative negative nitrogen balance and early starvation without serious effects. On the other hand, the nutritionally depleted patient goes to surgery under a serious handicap—a poor tolerance for operative stress. Increased susceptibility to infection results from a diminished ability to form antibodies and from the superficial atrophy in the mucous membrane linings of the respiratory and gastrointestinal tracts that often accompanies malnutrition. Hypoproteinemia follows prolonged negative nitrogen balance and increases susceptibility to shock from hemorrhage. The body gives top priority for nutrients to the incision site, and good wound healing is seen in some nutritionally depleted patients; in others, wounds fail to heal. Diminished supplies of protein and vitamin C retard wound healing.

When surgery is elective, the patient with a real or potential fluid balance problem is hospitalized early for preoperative evaluation and buildup. Weisberg advocates baseline electrolyte studies for all infants, adults over 50, and any patient subjected to an exploratory laparotomy or gastrointestinal surgery. During this time the patient is given a well-balanced diet to provide the body with substances to make its own repairs and to help the patient weather the impending surgical trauma. Specific oral or parenteral medications may be deemed necessary after evaluation of clinical and laboratory findings.

A primary nursing responsibility in the preoperative period is getting the patient to eat—sometimes difficult, especially when the patient's illness is such that his appetite is diminished. Fear and depression, common before surgery, may also deter the patient's desire to eat. (For nursing measures to promote eating see Chapter 14.) The benefits of activity are sometimes overlooked in the preoperative period; activity stimulates appetite and sleep, as well as general well-being.

Another important nursing responsibility is reporting inadequate oral intake, as when all efforts fail to promote eating. Nasogastric tube or parenteral feedings may then have to be given. (For nursing responsibilities in administering tube feedings see Chapter 14.) Anorexia accompanies malnutrition; correction of malnutrition with tube feedings often restores the patient's appetite. (For nursing responsibilities in parenteral nutrition see Chapter 16.)

Emotional Response

Emotional stimuli may produce changes in electrolyte metabolism, which are mediated through the hypothalamus and anterior pituitary gland with the adrenal cortex as the target organ. The patient's attitudes toward surgery may, thus, significantly affect his postoperative course. Some fear of surgery is natural; undue fear and apprehension, however, may initiate the adrenocortical stress reaction. Discomfort resulting from venipuncture or insertion of a gastric tube, as part of the preoperative preparation, may contribute to the stress reaction. Most nurses can recall more than one postponement of surgery because the patient was not emotionally ready for the experience.

The nurse has an ideal opportunity to observe the patient's behavior and to detect signs of apprehension or severe depression that may be missed by the surgeon. Patients display fear in different ways: some refuse to discuss the oncoming surgical event; others can talk of nothing else. (Significant behavior observations should be discussed with the physician.)

No nursing function is more important than providing emotional support for the surgical patient. The most effective support comes from persons who have a sincere interest in the patient's welfare and a respect for his feelings. Thoughtful explanations before new procedures and experiences do much to relieve fear. Inspiring confidence by performing all nursing functions with skill and confidence is also a form of emotional support. Willingness to listen when the patient feels like talking helps; many patients find it easier to verbalize fears to an understanding nurse than to a relative or close friend. This is understandable when one considers the patient's desire to spare his loved ones additional worry. (Some patients regard fear of surgery as a weakness and prefer to hide such fears from those close to them.)

Body Weight

All surgical patients should have an admission weight recorded on the chart. The preoperative body weight serves as a baseline for comparison with subsequent body weight measurements. Obtaining the weight of an ambulatory patient presents no problem; the patient confined to bed can be weighed on a bed scale. (For procedures in weighing the patient see Chapter 13.)

Intake-Output Measurements

Patients requiring preoperative electrolyte studies are placed on the nursing intake-output measurement list. An accurate record of fluids gained and lost from the body is of great importance in detecting inadequate intake and abnormalities in renal function and fluid balance. (For nursing responsibilities in measurement of fluid intake and output see Chapter 13.)

Medications

STEROIDS   The adrenals normally produce about 25 mg. of hydrocortisone a day; under stress, however, they may need to increase their output up to ten times above this amount. A patient's ability to withstand surgical stress depends upon his adrenals' ability to secrete extra hydrocortisone. It is wise to routinely ask all surgical patients if they have taken cortisone or any other steroid preparation for more than one or two weeks within the past six to twelve months. When a patient is on steroid therapy there is less need for adrenal secretion and the glands tend to atrophy from disuse; after withdrawal of steroid therapy, the adrenals gradually resume their function. However, if steroids are suddenly withdrawn and the patient is subjected to massive trauma, such as a major surgical procedure, the atrophied adrenal glands may be unable to respond to the stress signal; adrenocortical failure may follow cessation of adrenocortical substitution therapy. Symptoms include hypotension, nausea and vomiting, thready pulse, subnormal temperature early with later hyperpyrexia, hallucinations, confusion, stupor, or coma. The reaction usually occurs in the first 24 hours.

Preoperative patients who have received steroid therapy should have their adrenal function checked by the ACTH infusion test. If this discloses decreased adrenocortical responsiveness, steroids must be given to cover the operative and postoperative periods.

Today, because of medical specialization, one patient may have two or three physicians prescribing medications at the same time. The fact that the patient may recently have received steroids is often overlooked, and, in fact, many patients do not know what medicines they have taken; if this is the case, the nurse can ask for a description of the medication and why it was given. Conditions for which steroid therapy is often used should be kept in mind (for example, rheumatoid arthritis, asthma, dermatitis, and ulcerative colitis). When in doubt, the physician should check with those who prescribed medications for the patient.

DRUG ALLERGIES OR IDIOSYNCRASIES   The physician or the nurse should always ask the prospective surgical patient if he knows of any drug allergies, sensitivities, or idiosyncrasies he may have. If the patient does not understand the question, typical symptoms of sensitivity, such as urticaria, asthma, and the like, can be mentioned. One can also ask the patient if a physician has ever cautioned him to avoid a specific medication because of an unusual reaction to it. In questioning the newly admitted patient, the nurse will do well to remember that he is often upset and may have difficulty remembering.

Some patients assume that their physician remembers any drug allergies from office interviews prior to hospital admission, and unless specifically asked, they may not volunteer information. Allergies must be discovered before the patient is sedated or anesthetized; it is too late to ask when he is unconscious or semireactive after surgery, since most medications are ordered in the immediate postoperative period. Failure to ascertain the presence of allergies may be disastrous. The most dreaded allergic reaction is anaphylactic shock; other less dangerous reactions include skin eruptions and asthma.

Idiosyncratic reactions to drugs deserve consideration. For example, a narcotic may cause more depression in one patient than in another of equal weight and age. A dose creating the desired effect in one patient may overwhelm the patient who is unusually reactive to the drug. The aged are particularly sensitive to narcotics and should be given much smaller doses than younger adults; this is particularly important in aged surgical patients.

Pulmonary Ventilation

Inadequate pulmonary ventilation is common after surgery and can lead to respiratory acidosis (primary carbonic acid excess) or atelectasis. During the preoperative period, the nurse should teach the patient how to deep-breathe and cough postoperatively, explaining that these activities are excellent preventives against lung complications. Once the patient is properly motivated and knows what is expected of him, the nurse will have greater success in carrying through the common postoperative order to "have the patient cough and deep-breathe every hour."

Intermittent positive pressure treatments are sometimes used preoperatively and postoperatively to improve pulmonary ventilation in patients with chronic pulmonary conditions, such as emphysema. Other conditions that may contribute to postoperative ventilation problems include asthma, chronic bronchitis, heavy cigarette smoking, obesity, advanced age, and chest wall deformities. If other deep breathing devices are to be successfully used postoperatively, the patient should be allowed to practice their use *preoperatively*.

Chronic Illnesses

Certain chronic illnesses greatly increase the hazard of postoperative water and electrolyte imbalances. Such illnesses include:

Diabetes mellitus
Addison's disease
Renal disorders
Cardiac disorders
Hepatic disorders
Thyroid disorders
Pulmonary disorders

The presence of any of the above conditions requires careful preoperative preparation so that postoperative disturbances can be kept at a minimum.

The physician does a careful history and physical examination before surgery to detect preexisting illness. However, the patient may forget an important item and mention it later to the nurse, in which case, the information should be brought immediately to the physician's attention. The nurse should also be alert for symptoms of chronic illness.

Special Considerations in the Aged

Conscientious preoperative preparation often means the difference between success or failure of surgery in the aged, since the decreased body homeostatic adaptability of these patients predisposes to difficulty when they are exposed to stress.

These facts apply to the aged:

1. Malnutrition is more common in the aged than in younger adults.
2. Thirst is not as accurate a gauge of fluid needs as it is in younger adults. Sodium excess occurs with relative frequency in the aged because the thirst stimulus is often not intact and water intake is inadequate. In fact, many aged patients fail to recognize thirst when they are confused, whereas elderly patients who are alert and have access to water are not apt to develop sodium excess. Conditions causing water loss, such as fever and hyperpnea, contribute to a rise in plasma sodium. Clinical signs include dry, sticky mucous membranes and excitement. The nurse should offer the patient adequate

water and, when in doubt, the intake and output should be recorded. (A urinary volume that greatly exceeds oral intake is a signal to increase fluid intake.)

3. The aged patient will develop sodium deficit faster than younger adults; thus the nurse should be particularly alert for sodium deficit when the patient is losing body fluids containing sodium. This is particularly apt to occur when there is a free intake of water —either orally or parenterally. Sometimes the elderly patient may drink too much water; thirst satisfaction may require excessive water.

4. Moderate fluid volume deficit and decreased circulating blood volume are not uncommon in the aged *before* operation.

5. The plasma pH tends to remain fixed on the low side of normal, largely because of decreased pulmonary and renal function.

6. Decreased pulmonary function is common in the aged. It has been demonstrated that vital capacity is reduced with an increased residual volume, as rigidity of the chest wall interferes with normal pulmonary excursions. Since diminished respiratory function interferes with carbon dioxide elimination, many aged patients are in a state of impending respiratory acidosis. Because of this decline in pulmonary function, the nurse must help the aged patient achieve maximal ventilation. This can be accomplished by keeping the respiratory tract free of excessive secretions, providing maximal allowed activity, turning the bedfast patient from side to side at regular intervals and avoiding restrictive clothing or tight chest restraints.

7. Because renal response to pH disturbances is not as efficient in the aged, imbalances occur faster. There is a tendency toward metabolic acidosis as a result of decreased renal function.

8. Changes in pH are less well tolerated in the aged. Anemia, with its decreased hemoglobin, depletes one of the major buffer systems; emphysema is not uncommon in the aged and disrupts pH control.

9. The volume and acidity of gastric juice decreases gradually with age. Hypochlorhydria or achlorhydria is present in about a third of patients over 60. The aged patient with decreased gastric acidity may not develop metabolic alkalosis with vomiting or gastric suction; the primary disturbance in such a patient may be sodium deficit or potassium deficit.

10. Hypoxia is not well tolerated in the aged; for this reason local or spinal anesthetics are preferable to inhalation anesthetics.

11. Hypotension is poorly tolerated by the aged and, unless corrected quickly, is frequently complicated by renal damage, stroke, or myocardial infarct. (Shock becomes irreversible earlier than in younger patients.)

Preoperative dietary management is particularly important. Optimal nutrition helps the aged patient withstand the electrolyte deficits and pH changes occurring after surgery. Electrolyte solutions may be given intravenously prior to surgery to supplement dietary intake, and deficits of potassium and sodium especially should be corrected.

Sometimes, small, frequent blood transfusions are used to restore blood volume and to correct anemia. Ambulation and activity improve appetite and sleep. An accurate account should be kept of the patient's urinary output. In addition, renal function tests and an ECG may be indicated. And, finally, a conservative dose of preoperative medication is used to help avoid respiratory depression and hypoxia.

Immediate Preoperative Preparation

ENEMAS   A cleansing enema may be ordered either the night before or on the morning of abdominal or rectal surgery. Occasionally one still sees an order for "tap water enemas until returned clear"; fortunately, it is seen less and less. As many as five to ten enemas may be needed before the solution is "returned clear"; large amounts of sodium and potassium may be lost with the enema return, thus depleting the patient of valuable electrolytes when he can ill afford to lose them. Many surgeons feel that one cleansing enema, properly given, suffices.

WITHHOLDING FLUIDS   Some physicians allow the patient nothing by mouth for at least eight hours prior to surgery to reduce the risk of vomiting and aspiration on induction of anesthesia. Usually the patient is allowed to have the evening meal and then nothing but liquids until bedtime, after which time all oral intake is stopped. Other physicians allow oral fluids up to six hours before surgery.

VITAL SIGNS   All vital signs should be checked before the preoperative medication is given. An elevated temperature should be reported immediately; postponement of surgery may be necessary until the source of the fever is disclosed. An unusually rapid pulse and respiratory rate may indicate undue apprehension and should be reported.

A more accurate appraisal of the patient's blood pressure may be obtained by checking it both the evening before and the morning of surgery, and after sedative medication has been given. Postoperative blood pressure findings must be compared with the patient's usual blood pressure if they are to be evaluated correctly. For example, some patients normally have a systolic pressure of 90; unless this reading is established as the patient's norm, it may be inaccurately interpreted as a symptom of early shock.

POSTOPERATIVE GAINS AND LOSSES OF WATER, ELECTROLYTES, AND OTHER NUTRIENTS

Need for Intake-Output Measurement

Surgery often brings into play abnormal routes of fluid loss, such as gastric or intestinal suction, vomiting, or drainage from an ileostomy or colostomy. Failure to measure the amounts and kinds of fluids lost makes adequate replacement therapy almost impossible, and, without an accurate account of gains and losses, the early discovery of water and electrolyte imbalances is unlikely. It behooves the nurse, then, to automatically place postoperative patients on the intake-output list and to make a conscientious effort to keep the intake-output record accurate.

The 8-hour and 24-hour totals are significant in assessing fluid balance in general; it is equally important to know the types and amounts of fluids making up the total. For example, to state that a patient has lost a total of 3000 ml. of fluid in 24 hours is not as revealing as an itemized analysis of the loss:

1000 ml. urine
800 ml. gastric suction
200 ml. bile from T-tube drainage
1000 ml. estimated perspiration

The aim of fluid replacement therapy is to restore to the body the quantities of water and electrolytes lost. Special parenteral fluids are available to replace losses of gastric juice, intestinal juice, bile, and others.

(Chapter 13 tabulates the electrolyte content of most of the body fluids of concern in postoperative care plus imbalances to be expected with large losses of each fluid. The reader is encouraged to review this section because of its importance for the formulation of intelligent postoperative care.) A summary of this information is presented in Table 17-1.

Urinary Output

In health, the daily urinary output is roughly equal to the volume of liquids taken into the body. However, during postoperative stress reaction, the urine volume may tend to be low regardless of the amount of fluids taken in. Additional secretion of aldosterone and ADH (antidiuretic hormone) during the early phase of stress causes a reduction in renal capacity to excrete excessive water and sodium loads. Following a major surgical procedure the 24-hour output may be only 750 to 1200 ml. for the first few postoperative days. During this period, overadministration of water solutions can cause water intoxication (hyponatremia) and overadministration of isotonic electrolyte solutions may cause fluid volume excess with pulmonary edema and increased local edema at the surgical site. In intestinal surgery the increased edema may be sufficient to cause partial or complete obstruction.

An hourly urinary output below 25 ml. should be investigated. It is important to differentiate between the decreased urinary output of stress reaction (healthy physiologic response to surgery) and pathologic developments. Factors contributing to decreased urinary volume in the postoperative patient may include:

1. hypovolemia resulting from fluid loss incurred in surgery
2. preoperative dehydration
3. subtle accumulation of fluid at the surgical site
4. disturbance in myocardial function, causing decreased blood flow to the kidneys and, thus, decreased urine formation
5. renal failure (a serious cause of postoperative oliguria)

Table 17-1. Electrolyte Content of Gastrointestinal Fluids

Fluid	pH	Content (mEq./L.)	Likely Imbalances with Significant Losses
Gastric juice (fasting)	1–3	Na⁺ 60 K⁺ 9 Cl⁻ 84	Metabolic alkalosis Potassium deficit Sodium deficit Fluid volume deficit
Small intestine (suction)	7.8–8.0	Na⁺ 111 K⁺ 5 Cl⁻ 104 HCO₃⁻ 31	Metabolic acidosis Potassium deficit Sodium deficit Fluid volume deficit
(ileostomy-recent)		Na⁺ 129 K⁺ 11 Cl⁻ 116	Potassium deficit Metabolic acidosis Sodium deficit Fluid volume deficit
(ileostomy-old)		Na⁺ 46 K⁺ 3 Cl⁻ 21.4	Above imbalances less likely— volume and electrolyte content of drainage markedly diminishes when ileostomy adapts
Bile (fistula)	7.8	Na⁺ 149 K⁺ 5 Cl⁻ 101 HCO₃⁻ 40	Metabolic acidosis Sodium deficit Fluid volume deficit
Pancreas (fistula)	8.0–8.3	Na⁺ 141 K⁺ 5 Cl⁻ 77 HCO₃⁻ 121	Metabolic acidosis Sodium deficit Fluid volume deficit

Reprinted from Metheny, N.: Water and electrolyte balance in the postoperative patient. Nurs. Clin. N. Am. 10:50, 1975, with permission.

Measurement of urinary specific gravity is a simple method of evaluating renal function. A low fixed urinary S.G. (1.010 to 1.012) in the presence of oliguria indicates acute renal failure; however, a high urinary S.G. (1.026 to 1.036) suggests water conservation by a healthy kidney (water retention owing to stress reaction or dehydration). The oliguria of renal failure does not respond to increased intravenous fluid administration or to diuretics. Also, the serum creatinine level rises rapidly in renal failure while the urinary creatinine level remains low (indicating a disturbance in excretion of body wastes).

Fluid Intake

The usual daily fluid intake during the stress reaction should be about 1500 to 2000 ml., varying with the patient's need for replacement.

PARENTERAL FLUIDS Nausea, postoperative ileus, and gastrointestinal suction contraindicate oral fluids; intravenous fluids must be relied on to furnish the body with needed substances. Negative nitrogen balance can be reduced by the administration of dextrose solutions, and they frequently are used for this purpose in the postoperative period. Hypotonic multiple electrolyte solutions are used for maintenance water and electrolyte needs; specific electrolyte replacement solutions are used as indicated by the patient's condition.

After adequate renal function has been established, potassium is given daily to prevent potassium deficit, if the patient is not yet eating. Forty mEq. per day suffices unless large volumes of gastrointestinal fluids, rich in potassium, are being lost by vomiting, suction, or fistulas. (Nursing responsibilities in administering potassium solutions are discussed in Chapter 16.)

After the fluid retention of stress has subsided, a larger amount of fluid is given. If oral intake is still prohibited, an attempt must be made to supply body needs solely with parenteral fluids. Magnesium replacement may be necessary when parenteral fluid administration is prolonged. Magnesium deficit is not as rare as was once thought; prolonged administration of magnesium-free fluids dilutes the plasma magnesium level and may produce symptoms of deficit, particularly when magnesium loss has resulted from gastric suction. Parenteral vitamin preparations of the B complex group and vitamin C should be given daily when parenteral therapy is necessary for more than two days.

As described earlier, protein catabolism is increased in the immediate postoperative period (particularly the day of surgery and the following day). During this early period it is generally not considered beneficial to administer amino acids intravenously; emphasis is on providing water and electrolytes for maintenance needs and replacing abnormal losses. Amino acids may be started, if deemed necessary, on the second or third postoperative day. (See Chapter 16 for a discussion of the use of amino acids in promoting positive nitrogen balance when administered alone in peripheral veins and when used in hyperalimentation solutions.)

Parenteral solutions containing alcohol may be used postoperatively to supply calories and reduce pain. (Nursing responsibilities in the administration of carbohydrate solutions, electrolyte solutions, alcohol, and proteins are discussed in Chapter 16.)

ORAL INTAKE. Many physicians prefer that patients undergoing gastrointestinal suction receive nothing by mouth; others allow "ice chips sparingly" to relieve thirst. The term "sparingly" is open to interpretation by the staff, and more ice chips may be given than was intended by the physician, because of a thirsty patient's constant plea for more ice.

Drinking plain water causes a movement of electrolytes into the stomach to make the solution isotonic; before the water and electrolytes can be absorbed they are removed by the suction apparatus. This process can deplete the body of valuable electrolytes, primarily sodium, chloride, and potassium. Profound states of metabolic alkalosis or of sodium deficit have been caused by the unwise practice of giving plain water to a patient undergoing gastric suction. *If ice chips are to be given, they should be limited carefully.* (Some physicians allow approximately an ounce of plain ice chips per hour to relieve oral dryness.)

When oral feedings are allowed, the nurse should encourage the patient to eat those foods most likely to replace his probable deficits. For example, a patient with an ileostomy should receive high potassium foods and a patient with a cholecystectomy and bile drainage should receive high sodium foods. Contraindications to high potassium intake (such as renal disease) and to high sodium intake (such as cardiac disease) should, of course, be considered. The patient should be returned to a full diet as early as possible, because good nutrition decreases both the duration and the complications of convalescence.

POSTOPERATIVE PROBLEMS IN WATER AND ELECTROLYTE BALANCE

Water Excess

Water excess (sodium deficit) is also referred to as water intoxication or hyponatremia, an imbalance most likely to occur in the first one or two postoperative days, while the water retention effect of stress is still present. Excessive administration of water-yielding fluids, such as 5 per cent glucose in water, predisposes to this condition. Symptoms of water excess (sodium deficit) include the following:

1. Behavior changes
   a. inattentiveness
   b. confusion
   c. hallucinations
   d. shouting and delirium
   e. drowsiness
2. Acute weight gain
3. Overbreathing
4. Normal or elevated blood pressure
5. Skin color normal or pinker than usual
6. Neuromuscular changes
   a. cramping of exercised muscles
   b. isolated muscle twitching
   c. weakness
   d. headache
   e. blurred vision
   f. incoordination
   g. elevated intracranial pressure may occur with hypertension, bradycardia, decreased respiration, projectile vomiting, and papilledema
   h. convulsions
   i. hemiplegia

Table 17-2. Intravenous Fluids Used for Maintenance Needs
and Correction of Imbalances*

Type of Fluid	Electrolyte Content mEq./L.	Comments
5% Dextrose in water	None	Supplies 170 calories and free water for excretory purposes
5% Dextrose in lactated Ringer's solution	Na$^+$ 130 K$^+$ 4 Ca$^+$ 3 Cl$^-$ 109 Lactate 28	Sometimes used as a routine maintenance solution; electrolyte content approximates that of plasma (does not supply Mg). Dextrose supplies 170 calories
Isotonic saline (0.9% Sodium Chloride)	Na$^+$ 154 Cl$^-$ 154	Used to supply sodium chloride—expands extracellular fluid volume (not a good routine maintenance solution). Sodium and chloride content exceeds that found in plasma; excessive Na can cause edema, and excessive Cl can cause metabolic acidosis
Balanced isotonic solution	Na$^+$ 140 K$^+$ 5 Mg$^+$ 3 Cl$^-$ 98 Acetate 27 Gluconate 23	Used as an extracellular fluid replacement solution. Manufactured commercially under a variety of trade names. Note that it contains no Ca;—can be given simultaneously with blood. Supplies Mg
Gastric replacement solution	Na$^+$ 63 K$^+$ 17 NH$_4^+$ 70 Cl$^-$ 150	Used to replace gastric fluid loss. Acid pH of 3.3 to 3.7 is irritating; should be administered in a large functional vein. Manufactured under a variety of trade names. Contraindicated in hepatic insufficiency
Duodenal replacement solution	Na$^+$ 138 K$^+$ 12 Ca$^+$ 5 Mg$^+$ 3 Cl$^-$ 108 Lactate 50	Given to replace duodenal fluid loss and to correct mild acidosis. Manufactured under a variety of trade names. Supplies Mg
Butler solution (electrolyte 88)	Na$^+$ 57 K$^+$ 25 Mg$^+$ 5–6 Cl$^-$ 49–50 Lactate 25 HPO$_4^-$ 13	Given to replace fluid lost from the large intestine. Hypotonic fluid, supplying electrolytes and free water for excretory purposes. Manufactured under several trade names. Supplies Mg

Reprinted from Metheny, N.: Water and electrolyte balance in the postoperative patient. Nurs. Clin. N. Am. 10:55, 1975, with permission.

* The reader is encouraged to see Table 16-5 for a more extensive tabulation of intravenous fluids

The nurse should suspect water excess (sodium deficit) when several of these symptoms occur in the early postoperative period. Behavior changes are usually noticed first. The aged and the very young are particularly susceptible to this imbalance.

Prevention of body fluid disturbances demands the study of daily accurate body weight measurements; a sudden weight gain in the early postoperative period is an indication to decrease fluid intake. Fluid intake during the water-retention of stress should not exceed body fluid losses; a reasonable 24-hour intake for most patients is about 1500 to 2000 ml. Here again, much depends upon how accurately the nurse performs body weight and intake-output measurements.

Mild water excess can be corrected by prohibiting further water intake; however, brain damage or death may supervene if the condition is allowed to go untreated.

Respiratory Acidosis

Normally, carbon dioxide is given off by the lungs during exhalation. Respiratory acidosis (primary carbonic acid excess) occurs when the lungs retain carbon dioxide, because of decreased respiration depth or blockage of oxygen-carbon dioxide exchange at the alveolar level. Breathing excessive amounts of carbon dioxide will also produce this imbalance. The surgical patient may develop respiratory acidosis for one or several reasons:

1. Depression of respiration by anesthesia
2. Blockage of oxygen-carbon dioxide exchange in the lungs owing to atelectasis, pneumonia, or bronchial obstruction
3. Depression of respiration with too frequent or too large doses of narcotics
4. Shallow respiration because of abdominal distention and crowding of the diaphragm
5. Excessive breathing of carbon dioxide during anesthesia
6. Shallow respiration as a result of pain in the operative site or large cumbersome dressings

A threat to postoperative ventilation is posed by surgical procedures involving the diaphragm, such as hiatus hernia repair. Also, patients having thoracic or high abdominal incisions are particularly prone to develop ventilatory problems. For example, vital capacity is decreased by 40 per cent of normal on the day after subtotal gastrectomy. However, this loss of reserve still allows for adequate oxygen and carbon dioxide exchange if preoperative ventilation was normal. In addition to causing respiratory acidosis, decreased ventilation interferes with the correction of metabolic acidosis. (Recall that the lungs attempt to compensate for metabolic acidosis by eliminating more carbon dioxide.)

Indiscriminate use of oxygen in the postoperative period increases the chance of overlooking respiratory acidosis. Cyanosis is usually the chief criterion for detecting inadequate ventilation; oxygen therapy may prevent cyanosis and keep the skin color pink even though respiratory acidosis is progressing.

The nurse can help prevent respiratory acidosis

by encouraging the patient to cough and breathe deeply at regular intervals, unless contraindicated by the type of surgery. Even when coughing is to be avoided in neurological or eye surgery the patient can be encouraged to breathe deeply. Administration of narcotics requires good nursing judgment, with enough medication given to make coughing tolerable, yet not enough to produce shallow respiration. The timely use of analgesics enables the patient to expand his thoracic cavity with less discomfort during deep breathing treatments. It is best to position the patient in high Fowler's to allow for better gas distribution throughout the lungs. The sitting position allows for greater lung expansion because gravity pulls the abdominal organs away from the diaphragm. The nurse should splint the patient's incision while he coughs; this causes him to be less fearful and less apt to splint himself by muscular contraction, which limits ventilation. Of course, the patient should be taught how to splint his own incision when assistance is not available.

Turning the patient at regular intervals helps prevent pneumonia and atelectasis and, thus, discourages respiratory acidosis. Early ambulation probably helps avoid this complication by increasing the patient's breathing efforts.

Some physicians order IPPB (intermittent positive pressure breathing) treatments to improve pulmonary ventilation; others may prefer the use of blow bottles or devices such as the Dale-Schwartz rebreathing tube or the Adler rebreather.

The nurse should remember that seemingly small doses of barbiturates or narcotics may produce respiratory depression and acidosis in the aged patient. If the ordered dose appears inadequate or produces adverse effects, the nurse should report her observations to the physician and seek new orders. Conscientious physicians welcome such nursing observations; they realize that what may be a therapeutic dose in one patient may be ineffective or harmful to another. Observations made by the nurse take on added weight because she spends more time with the patient than does the physician.

Ileus

Peristalsis is inhibited for two to four days after intra-abdominal manipulation and, for this reason, patients with abdominal surgery usually receive nothing by mouth until bowel sounds indicate the return of peristalsis. Gastric intubation is often employed early in the postoperative period to prevent the bowel from becoming greatly distended with swallowed air and gastrointestinal fluids.

If paralytic ileus persists longer than normal, the patient must be maintained on intravenous fluids and gastric suction until peristalsis returns (as evidenced by passage of flatus). Factors that may prolong the expected period of ileus postoperatively include bacterial and chemical peritonitis, excessive handling of the intestines during surgery, advanced age, or actual mechanical obstruction. Oral intake should be withheld in any postoperative patient who is vomiting; the nature of the vomitus, as well as the degree of abdominal distention, should be noted and reported to the surgeon.

Large amounts of water and electrolytes may be sequestered into the bowel. The amount of fluid "lost" in this manner is not revealed by body weight change. Clinical signs of fluid volume deficit, decreased urinary volume, and increased urinary specific gravity help indicate the amount of fluid trapped in the bowel. (See the discussion of bowel obstruction in Chapter 19.)

Use of Plain Water as Irrigating Fluid for Suction Tubes

Fluid used to irrigate gastrointestinal tubes should be isotonic saline rather than plain water since the latter promotes electrolyte loss from the gastrointestinal mucosa. (See Chapter 14 for a discussion of this subject.) Sometimes there are specific orders for the frequency of the irrigation and the amount of solution to be used; other times the order is general and leaves the frequency of the irrigation and the amount of fluid to the nurse's discretion. In either event, the amount of fluid instilled should be removed; any difference between the amount instilled and amount removed should be recorded on the intake-output record.

Some physicians prefer hourly irrigation of the tube with 30 to 50 ml. of air to prevent clogging; air does not interfere with electrolyte balance or with intake-output record keeping. However, when blood or thick secretions are occluding the tube it may be necessary to use isotonic saline.

Imbalances Associated with Specific Body Fluid Losses

Metabolic alkalosis is most commonly seen in surgical patients as a result of the loss of large amounts of gastric secretions, either through vomiting or gastric suction. It is closely associated with potassium deficit, produced by the excessive loss of potassium-rich intestinal secretions or by prolonged parenteral therapy without potassium replacement. Potassium deficit is enhanced by the stress reaction in the early postoperative period.

Metabolic acidosis (primary base bicarbonate deficit) follows excessive loss of alkaline intestinal secretions, bile, and pancreatic juice. (See Table 17-1.)

Hemorrhage and Shock

Severe hemorrhage and hypovolemic shock are dreaded complications of surgery. The nurse should be alert for, and report promptly, symptoms of hemorrhage and hypovolemic shock such as the following:

- collapse of neck veins (see discussion of this subject in Chapter 13)
- poor capillary refill time (may take several seconds) as noted by pressing over fingernails
- anxiety (owing to hyperactivity of the sympathetic nervous system)
- decreased pulse pressure—often less than 20 mm.Hg. (when blood pressure changes are due to blood loss, the systolic pressure falls more rapidly than the diastolic pressure)
- brief initial rise in systolic pressure may occur as a result of increased release of epinephrine
- respiratory alkalosis in early shock (caused by hyperventilation)
- decreased systolic blood pressure of 10 mm.Hg. or more when position changed from lying to standing or sitting (early sign)
- pulse rate increased by more than 20 per minute when position changed from lying to standing or sitting—later, pulse remains rapid and thready in all positions
- decreased urinary output (increased ADH and aldosterone secretion causes water and sodium retention by kidneys)

- pale, cool, moist skin (caused by peripheral vasoconstriction)
- eventually, blood pressure remains low even in flat position as the body's defense mechanisms are unable to cope with hypovolemia (systolic pressure generally does not fall significantly until a blood volume deficit of at least 15 to 25 per cent has been sustained)
- metabolic acidosis in late shock (resulting from lactic acid buildup caused by hypoxia)
- central venous pressure usually below normal (isolated CVP reading may mean relatively little—but, the change caused by fluid replacement is quite significant)

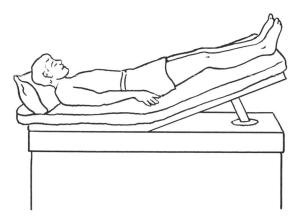

Figure 17-2. Elevation of legs during shock.

Prompt correction of the cause of hemorrhage and replacement of fluids are mandatory to prevent irreversible shock and death. Blood is the fluid of first choice, but electrolyte solutions or dextran usually are effective until blood is available. (Nursing responsiblities in the administration of blood, dextran, and electrolyte solutions are described in Chapter 16.) Treatment of shock is aimed at improving tissue perfusion rather than just elevating blood pressure. Vasopressors are not generally indicated in hypovolemic shock and may be quite dangerous in that they can cause arteriole occlusion. Success of therapy can be gauged partially by closely observing urinary output; a calibrated device for measuring small urine volumes must be used to detect significant hourly changes (see Fig. 13-7). An attempt is made to keep the hourly urine volume at 50 ml./hr.; an output of less than 25 ml./hr. should be promptly reported. (These volumes apply to adults.)

Central venous pressure may be monitored to evaluate vascular volume. Hypovolemia usually causes a low CVP; adequate fluid replacement should elevate the CVP toward normal. (See discussion of CVP monitoring in Chapter 16.)

Elevating the legs to a 45 degree angle (Fig. 17-2) temporarily releases about 500 ml. of blood and, thus, partially relieves the effect of moderate hypovolemia; in severe hypovolemia there may be insufficient blood in the extremities to be of value. Trendelenburg position is contraindicated in most instances since it allows the abdominal viscera to interfere with respirations by pressing against the diaphragm; also, the abdominal contents press against the vena cava, interfering with venous return.

Oxygen may be administered in shock to lessen hypoxia; an attempt is made to maintain an arterial pO_2 of at least 80 mm.Hg. Recall that hemoglobin is an important mechanism in oxygen transport; reduced hemoglobin content in the bloodstream results in decreased oxygenation of body tissues. Most acid-base problems in shock will improve spontaneously when tissue perfusion is improved; however, treatment with bicarbonate solutions may be necessary in some instances when severe acidosis is present.

The period of hypotension must be kept at a minimum because it results in decreased blood flow and damage to vital organs, primarily the brain, the heart, and the kidneys. Hypotension in a patient with arteriosclerosis is particularly dangerous because of the high incidence of thrombosis, resulting in either cerebral vascular accident or myocardial infarct. Acute renal insufficiency may follow prolonged hypotension, particularly in the aged.

Acute Renal Insufficiency

Acute renal insufficiency may complicate surgery. Usually it is secondary to reduction of renal blood flow (as in shock) or to a hemolytic blood transfusion reaction. The aged patient has a higher incidence of acute renal insufficiency.

The nurse can help prevent acute renal insufficiency by being alert to, and reporting, *early* symptoms of shock; prompt correction of shock prevents a pronounced reduction in renal blood flow. (Nursing responsibilities in preventing hemolytic blood transfusion reactions are discussed in Chapter 16. Acute renal failure is discussed in detail in Chapter 20.)

BIBLIOGRAPHY

Condon, R., and **Nyhus, L.** (eds.): Manual of Surgical Therapeutics, ed. 3. Boston: Little, Brown & Co., 1975.

Berk, J., et al.: Handbook of Critical Care. Boston: Little, Brown & Co., 1976.

Garrett, J.: Oliguria in postoperative patients. Nurs. Clin. N. Am. 10:59, 1975.

Given, B., and **Simmons, S.:** Gastroenterology in Clinical Nursing, ed. 2. St. Louis: C. V. Mosby, 1975.

Freeman, J., et al.: Metabolic effects of amino acids vs. dextrose infusion in surgical patients. Arch. Surg. 110:916, 1975.

Luckman, J., and **Sorenson, K.:** Medical-Surgical Nursing. Philadelphia: W. B. Saunders Co., 1974.

Metheny, N.: Water and electrolyte balance in the postoperative patient. Nurs. Clin. N. Am. 10:49, 1975.

Shock—its definition, classification, diagnosis, pathophysiology, monitoring, and treatment. From Wilson, R.: A Manual of Practices & Techniques in Critical Care Medicine. The Upjohn Co., June, 1976.

18

Fluid Balance in the Badly Burned Patient

Burns cause a series of major water and electrolyte changes. The purpose of this chapter is to explore these changes and their implications for nursing care. A background discussion of physiologic changes accompanying burns precedes the discussion of treatment and nursing care.

EVALUATION OF BURN SEVERITY

The severity of water and electrolyte changes is largely dependent on the *burn depth* and the *percentage of body surface* involved.

Burn Depth

Burns may be classified as first, second, or third degree, according to the depth of skin damage. (A more recent classification of burns is partial-thickness and full-thickness: deep partial-thickness burns extend into the dermis and full-thickness burns extend into the subcutaneous tissue or deeper.) Factors considered in determining burn depth (Table 18-1) include the following:

Amount of sensation remaining (pinprick test may be done to determine the degree of sensation)
Appearance of the burned surface

Nature of burning agent plus length of exposure to it

In a first-degree burn, vasodilation is the only important change, whereas a second-degree burn is characterized by damaged capillaries and the appearance of blebs containing fluid.

Third-degree (full-thickness) burns result in thrombosed capillaries and the formation of an eschar (dead tissue), and each per cent of a third-degree burn is about twice as severe as each per cent of a second-degree burn.

PERCENTAGE OF SURFACE INVOLVED

The "rule of nines" is commonly used to estimate the severity of burns in adults. It divides the body surface into areas of 9 per cent or its multiples:

Head	=	9%
Each arm	=	9%
Each leg	=	18%
Front of torso	=	18%
Back of torso	=	18%
Genitalia	=	1%

Unless used cautiously, this method can result in dangerously high estimates. A more detailed break-

Table 18-1. Diagnosis of Burn Depth

	Degree	Nature of Burn	Symptoms	Appearance	Course
Epidermal Burn (shallow partial-thickness)	First	Sunburn Low-intensity flash	Tingling Hyperesthesia Painful Soothed by cooling	Reddened; blanches with pressure Minimal or no edema	Complete recovery within a week Peeling
Intradermal Burn (deeper partial-thickness)	Second	Scalds Flash flame	Painful Hypesthesia Sensitive to cold air	Blistered, mottled red base, broken epidermis, weeping surface Edema	Recovery in 2 to 3 weeks Some scarring and depigmentation Infection may convert to third degree
Subdermal Burn (full-thickness)	Third	Fire	Painless Symptoms of shock Hematuria and hemolysis of blood likely	Dry; pale white or charred Leathery Broken skin with fat exposed Edema	Eschar sloughs Grafting necessary Scarring and loss of contour and function

Modified from Sako, Y.: Emergency management of the acutely burned patient. Hospital Medicine, p. 7, Wallace Laboratories, New York, October, 1964.

down is beneficial, since it contributes to a complete understanding of percentage of surface involved (Fig. 18-1).

After the percentage of partial-thickness and full-thickness burns is estimated, the therapeutic approach is planned. Burns are sometimes classified as minor, moderate, or major. Minor burns consist of partial thickness burns of less than 15 per cent of the body surface or full-thickness burns of less than 2 per cent of body surface. Moderate burns consist of partial-thickness burns of 15 to 30 per cent or full-thickness burns of less than 10 per cent. Major burns consist of partial-thickness burns of over 30 per cent or full-thickness burns of more than 10 per cent of the body surface.[1] Factors other than the percentage of burned body surface area can influence the severity of the burn. For example: burns are made more serious by the presence of prior renal, cardiac, or metabolic disorders; concurrent injuries; burns of the face, hands, or genitalia; respiratory burns; and extreme age variations (very young children and the elderly).

Chemical and electrical burns tend to require more attention than other types of burns.

WATER AND ELECTROLYTE CHANGES IN BURNS

Loss of Body Fluids in Burns

Body fluids are lost in severe burns as:

Plasma leaves the intravascular space and becomes trapped as edema fluid
Plasma and interstitial fluid are lost as exudate
Water vapor is lost from the denuded burn site
Blood leaks from the damaged capillaries

PLASMA-TO-INTERSTITIAL FLUID SHIFT Intravascular water, electrolytes, and protein are lost through damaged capillaries at the burn site. Clinically, the shift results in edema; the magnitude of this shift depends upon the burn depth and the percentage of surface area involved. Consider a specific example: an adult with a body surface of 1.75 m.² has about 10.5 L. of extracellular fluid. If he sustains a 50 per cent burn, the volume of edema fluid formed during the first day or two would approximate 5.25 L., a quantity exceeding the total plasma volume of the patient. Obviously all of the edema fluid is not derived from plasma; some of it comes from the body cells and some from administered fluids.

Proportionately greater amounts of water and electrolytes than of protein are lost from the plasma. (Protein molecules are larger and, thus, fewer escape through the damaged capillaries.) As a result, the circulating plasma protein becomes more concentrated, the increased osmotic pressure draws fluid from un-

damaged tissues in all parts of the body, and generalized tissue dehydration results. Sometimes it is difficult to visualize the presence of severe dehydration in a patient so obviously edematous; one must remember that the edema represents trapped fluids unavailable for body use.

BURN EXUDATE A protein-rich fluid is lost through the leakage of approximately equal parts of plasma and interstitial fluid from the burned surface. Visible fluid loss by way of the surface is mostly limited to second-degree burns, and the amount of fluid lost in this manner is proportional to the percentage of second-degree burns. Such losses do not increase appreciably in burns involving 50 per cent or more of the body. Burn exudate has approximately two thirds as much protein as plasma.

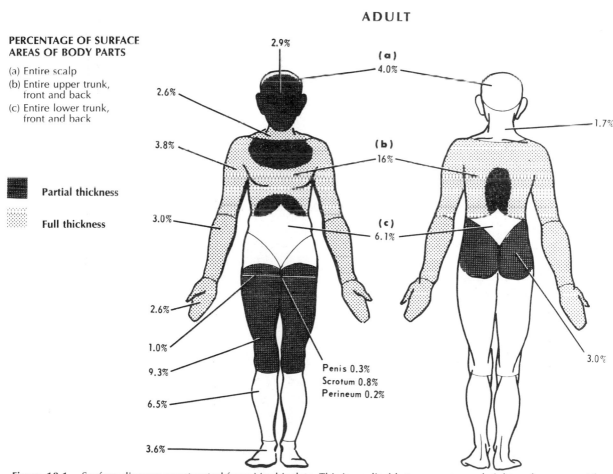

ADULT

PERCENTAGE OF SURFACE AREAS OF BODY PARTS

(a) Entire scalp
(b) Entire upper trunk, front and back
(c) Entire lower trunk, front and back

Partial thickness

Full thickness

Figure 18-1. Surface diagram constructed from Meeh's data. This is applicable to persons aged eight and up, except for the very obese. (From Moyer, C.: Treatment of large burns. Arch. Surg. 90:856, copyright 1965, American Medical Association, with permission)

WATER VAPOR AND HEAT LOSS   The intact skin serves as a barrier against the loss of water and heat. When skin is destroyed by a burn, increased water and heat loss result, and the larger the burned surface, the greater the loss of water vapor and heat. Burned infants are particularly vulnerable to heat loss.

The average water vapor loss from a major burn wound is thought to be from 2.5 to 4.0 L. per day. Maintenance of an environment saturated with water vapor decreases the transcutaneous water loss; for example, wounds covered with dressings of aqueous topical agents and dry covers lose only half the amount of water vapor lost through exposed wounds. Some physicians feel that early coverage of burn wounds with a temporary biological dressing (such as pig skin) decreases evaporative water and heat loss. Patients treated by exposure often shiver and complain of feeling cold; external heat sources should be provided for comfort. Ideally, the room temperature should be 82 to 84° F. (28 to 29° C.). Shivering increases the rate of metabolism, as does fever and infection (causing increased loss of water from the body).

WATER AND ELECTROLYTE CHANGES IN MAJOR BURN PHASES   The nurse should be aware of the water and electrolyte changes occurring in burns so that she can recognize significant changes in the patient. Observations are more meaningful when one has at least some idea of what to look for. An outline of expected water and electrolyte changes is presented in Table 18-2. (The reader is referred to earlier chapters for detailed descriptions of these imbalances. Planned nursing observations are discussed in Chapter 13.)

Physiologic Basis for Treatment and Nursing Care During the Fluid Accumulation Phase

The adequacy of early burn treatment largely depends upon the physician's and the nurse's understanding of physiologic derangements caused by burns, the organization of equipment, and the ability to act quickly and skillfully.

Need for Early Treatment

The shift of fluid from plasma to the interstitial space is rapid and well underway by the end of the first hour. The maximal speed of edema formation is reached by the end of the first eight to ten hours; the shift continues until the thirty-sixth to forty-eighth hour. (By this time, the capillaries have healed sufficiently to prevent further fluid loss.) The decreased plasma volume can lead to hypovolemic shock and renal depression (caused by decreased renal blood flow) unless quickly corrected by fluid replacement therapy. Oliguria or anuria are particularly threatening during this phase because of the excessive amounts of potassium flooding the extracellular fluid. (Remember that potassium is mainly excreted in urine; decreased urinary output causes a dangerous excess to build up in the bloodstream.) The sodium deficit requires prompt attention, as does the acidosis so frequently present.

Initial Patient Evaluation

Ideally a burn team made up of physicians and nurses skilled in the care of burn patients is on hand to treat burn emergencies. Unfortunately, the number of specialized burn units in the United States is inadequate and most burned patients must be cared for in general hospitals. When at all possible, patients should be transferred to a burn center for treatment. (Fortunately, burned patients withstand travel fairly well.)

Some hospital emergency rooms are staffed with at least one house physician. Unfortunately, however, *many* emergency rooms are staffed only with R.N.s and on-call physicians. While the nurse in this situation cannot initiate therapy without medical orders, she can obtain valuable information to expedite treatment when the physician arrives. Pertinent questions include:

1. When did the burn occur? (The degree of fluid shift is related to the length of time the burn has been present.)
2. What was the nature of the burning agent? (Notice in Table 18-1 that burns are classified in relation to burning agents frequently associated with them.)
3. What was the length of exposure to the burning agent? (Questions 2 and 3 are intended to help the physician establish the burn depth—appearance of the burns on admission is often misleading.)
4. Were any medications given prior to hospital admission? (Sometimes narcotics are given at the scene of the accident; it is im-

Table 18-2. Water and Electrolyte Changes in Different Burn Phases

Phase	Water and Electrolyte Changes	Comments
Fluid Accumulation Phase (Shock Phase)	Plasma-to-Interstitial Fluid Shift (edema at burn site)	Plasma leaks out through the damaged capillaries at the burn site—edema forms
First 48 hours	Generalized Dehydration	Undamaged tissues give up fluids to help increase plasma volume—part of it leaks through the damaged capillaries and helps form edema
	Contraction of Blood Volume	Loss of plasma causes a decreased circulatory volume
	Decreased Urinary Output	Secondary to:
		Decreased renal blood flow
		Increased secretion of ADH (antidiuretic hormone)
		Sodium and water retention caused by stress (increased adrenocortical activity)
		Severe burns may cause hemolysis of red blood cells; the ruptured cells release Hb. and it is excreted by the kidneys (hemoglobinuria can cause severe renal damage)
	Potassium Excess	Massive cellular trauma causes the release of K^+ into the extracellular fluid (recall that most of the body's K^+ is located *inside* the cells; only small amounts are tolerated in plasma)
	Sodium Deficit	Large amounts of Na^+ are lost in the trapped edema fluid and in the exudate (recall that Na^+ is the chief extracellular ion and large amounts are lost when extracellular fluid is lost)
		Research work done under the direction of C. A. Moyer indicates sodium deficit in unburned tissues is closely linked with burn shock (partial correction of Na^+ deficit relieved burn shock symptoms in some patients even though a substantially decreased blood volume persisted)
	Metabolic Acidosis (base bicarbonate deficit)	Develops within a few hours due to: Accumulation of fixed acids released from injured tissues Ineffective tissue perfusion
	Calcium Deficit	May occur after 12–24 hours in extensively burned patients—may be particularly marked in infants and children (presumably due to saponification of fat in the burned subcutaneous adipose tissue)
	Hemoconcentration (elevated hematocrit)	Relatively greater loss of liquid blood components in relation to blood cell loss
Fluid Remobilization Phase	Interstitial Fluid-to-Plasma Shift	Edema fluid shifts back into the intravascular compartments
(State of Diuresis) Starts 48 hours post-burn	Hemodilution (hematocrit decreased)	The blood cell concentration is diluted as fluid enters the vascular compartment and, in addition, at this time a decrease in the number of cells becomes evident (destruction of red blood cells at the burn site causes anemia —as much as 10% of the total number of RBCs may be destroyed)
	Increased Urinary Output	Fluid shift into the intravascular compartment, increases renal blood flow and causes increased urine formation

Table 18-2.   Water and Electrolyte Changes in Different Burn Phases (*Continued*)

Phase	Water and Electrolyte Changes	Comments
	Sodium Deficit	Sodium is lost with water when diuresis occurs
	Potassium Deficit (may occasionally occur in this phase)	Beginning about the fourth or fifth post-burn day, K⁺ shifts from the extracellular fluid into the cells
	Metabolic Acidosis	
Convalescent Phase	Calcium Deficit	Since calcium may be immobilized at the burn site in the slough and early granulation phase of burns, symptoms of calcium deficit may occur (recall that for some unknown reason calcium rushes to damaged tissues)
	Potassium Deficit	Extracellular K⁺ moves into the cells, leaving a deficit of K⁺ in the extracellular fluid
	Negative Nitrogen Balance (present for several weeks following burns)	Secondary to: Stress reaction; Immobilization; Inadequate protein intake; Protein losses in exudate; Direct destruction of protein at the burn site
	Sodium Deficit	

portant to avoid repeating drugs too soon, especially if respiratory tract burns or shock are present.)

5. Was the burn sustained in an enclosed area where heat and fumes were inhaled? (This question is highly significant in establishing the likelihood of respiratory burns.)
6. Are there any preexistent illnesses, such as cardiac or renal damage or diabetes, that will require therapy in addition to burn treatment? (Failure to ascertain the presence of such illnesses is not uncommon in the initial rush.)
7. What is the normal pre-burn weight? (The pre-burn weight is a baseline for comparison for later weight changes; the weight is also instrumental in determining drug doses.)
8. Is pain present? If so, how severe? (It should be remembered that severe pain can cause a drop in blood pressure and further complicate the patient's condition.)
9. Is the patient known to have any drug allergies?
10. What is the status of tetanus immunization? (All patients with severe burns should receive prophylaxis against tetanus.)
11. Are there any associated injuries requiring treatment? (For example: head injuries or fractures)

While asking these questions, the nurse can be busy with other activities, such as readying fluid equipment, removing loose clothing not stuck to the burns, and removing constrictive jewelry before edema becomes severe. The unit that is to receive the patient after initial treatment should be notified so that every necessary preparation can be made.

The physician will usually request that blood be drawn for determination of electrolytes, hemoglobin, hematocrit, glucose, and urea nitrogen. Arterial blood may be drawn for determination of pH, pCO₂, and pO₂.

Observing for Burn Shock

The nurse should be particularly alert for symptoms of burn shock:

Extreme thirst (caused by generalized cellular dehydration)
Increasing restlessness (persistent slight to moderate restlessness may be due to apprehension

and discomfort produced by the burn rather than to inadequate fluid resuscitation)

Sudden high pulse rate (heart beats faster to compensate for decreased blood volume)

Respiratory rate is often increased, but the character of breathing should be normal unless there are complicating factors

Blood pressure, when measurable, is either normal or low (the body may be too extensively burned to permit application of a blood pressure cuff) (the supine burned patient can often tolerate a large fluid volume deficit with little or no change in blood pressure; however, upon sitting or standing, hypotension and even syncope may occur—thus, the badly burned patient should be left supine for at least the first 48 to 72 hours)

Cool pale skin in unburned areas (indicative of cutaneous vasoconstriction—a compensatory mechanism that helps preserve normal blood flow)

Oliguria (owing to decreased renal blood flow and to increased levels of ADH and aldosterone)

Delirium or coma (presumably these symptoms are due to inadequate cerebral blood flow and are serious signs)

Seizures sometimes occur (may be the result of cerebral ischemia)

Fortunately, burn shock is slow in onset and can be prevented or corrected by the intravenous administration of fluids in sufficient volume to maintain an adequate urinary output.

Initial Urine Observations

An indwelling urinary catheter is usually inserted when burns involve 20 per cent or more of the body surface; the catheter should be connected to a device for hourly measurement of the urine flow. If the patient voids before the catheter is inserted, the urine should be measured and saved. The urine should be observed for discoloration resulting from blood; if present, the patient probably has severe third-degree burns. Hemolysis of red blood cells at the burn site (caused by trauma) causes the release of hemoglobin and, consequently, hemoglobinuria. Thermal trauma may also destroy muscle tissue, releasing myoglobin into the bloodstream to be filtered out by the kidneys.

Mannitol is given intravenously sometimes to promote diuresis and washing-out of the renal tubules.

Initial Observations of Respiratory Tract

The nurse should observe the patient closely for symptoms of respiratory burns. These include:

singed nasal hair
hoarseness
red painful throat
dry cough
moist rales and dyspnea
stridor
bronchospasm with prolonged wheezing

Such symptoms should be reported promptly. Burns about the face and neck can cause edema and pressure around the trachea; difficulty in breathing should, of course, be reported immediately.

Initial Wound Care

Dirt, debris, or loose skin should be removed by the physician with sterile instruments. Blisters that are not leaking should be left untouched since they act as sterile dressings. Many physicians favor gentle scrubbing of the burned area with soap and water or with antiseptics, whereas others feel this is unnecessary trauma in fresh major burns unless the wound is known to be contaminated by dirt or polluted water. In any event, all wounds should be cultured. As a rule, general anesthesia for debridement should be avoided during the shock phase of burns; adequate analgesia can usually be achieved by small intravenous doses of narcotics. (Fluid resuscitation should be underway before analgesics are administered.)

Intravenous Fluids

Intravenous fluids are life-saving in the treatment of moderate and severe burns. Burns involving 20 per cent or more of the body surface (less in the very young or the aged) usually require intravenous fluid therapy. The aim of early fluid therapy is to give the least amount of fluids necessary to maintain the desired urinary output and keep the patient relatively free of burn shock symptoms.

Physicians are of varied opinions about the kinds

of intravenous fluids used in burn treatment. Among those used initially are:

Lactated Ringer's solution
Isotonic saline
Plasma and plasma substitutes
Dextran
Blood
5% dextrose in water or saline
Alkalinizing solutions (1/6 M sodium lactate and
   1.2% sodium bicarbonate)
Hypertonic lactated saline

Lactated Ringer's solution is used to supply sodium and to help correct metabolic acidosis; 1 L. of this solution contains 130 mEq. of sodium and 28 mEq. of lactate, a bicarbonate precursor.

Isotonic saline (0.9% sodium chloride) can also be used to supply sodium, as 1 L. of isotonic saline contains 154 mEq. of sodium and 154 mEq. of chloride. It has the disadvantage of supplying an excessive amount of chloride ions which contribute to the acidosis rather than correcting it.

The use of plasma and plasma substitutes is advocated by some physicians, who reason that plasma or other colloids must be given to replace the plasma leaked through injured capillaries into the burn site. A frequently used colloid is Plasmanate, a plasma protein fraction that has good expansion properties without the disadvantage of possible viral hepatitis transmission (heat treated to destroy hepatitis virus). Some physicians prefer not to administer colloids until at least 36 hours post-burn (after the injured capillaries have healed sufficiently to retain the protein molecules). Others administer colloid preparations during early resuscitation. Twenty-five to fifty grams of albumin are sometimes added to each liter of Lactated Ringer's solution and administered during early burn resuscitation to help maintain intravenous osmotic pressure.

Plasma contains sodium (sometimes as much as 200 mEq./L.) and thus helps correct sodium deficit. However, it should be remembered that the use of plasma is associated with the risk of serum hepatitis. (See Chapter 16.) Some physicians favor the use of Dextran solutions as plasma volume expanders in the treatment of burns. Dextran solutions do not alter the pH of the blood and have no caloric value. (Nursing responsibilities in the administration of Dextran are

discussed in Chapter 16.) Some physicians feel that plasma and other colloids are unnecessary in burn therapy.

A few physicians still advocate the use of blood in early burn resuscitation; however, many feel that blood is contraindicated initially because the patient already suffers from hemoconcentration. Blood administration is associated with risks of hepatitis and transfusion reaction. (See Chapter 16.) In addition, blood is difficult to obtain and is expensive. (Blood transfusions are frequently required to correct burn anemia during the convalescent phase in severely burned patients. Burn anemia likely is due to poor nutrition, blood loss, infection, and decreased production of erythropoietin.)

A non-electrolyte solution, usually 5% dextrose in water, may be used to replace the normal insensible water loss and the increased transcutaneous water vapor loss. In addition, alkalinizing fluids, such as 1/6 M sodium lactate and 1.2% sodium bicarbonate are sometimes used to correct the metabolic acidosis associated with burns.

The use of a hypertonic lactated solution for fluid resuscitation in burned patients is advocated by Monafo to supply sodium in a minimal fluid load.[2] One liter of this solution contains 250 mEq. of sodium, 100 mEq. of lactate, and 150 mEq. of chloride.

Whenever intravenous fluids are given there is a danger of giving too much or not enough; both hazards are always present in burn therapy. To serve as a guide for the amount to be given early to burned patients, several formulas have been devised (Table 18-3). However, clinical assessment of urine output and vital signs are still mandatory in regulating fluid administration since these formulas are only meant to serve as guides. The goal of fluid therapy is to keep urinary output and central venous pressure within normal limits.

The nurse must be alert for symptoms of inadequate or excessive fluid administration. Inadequate fluid therapy in burned patients is indicated by:

decreased urinary output (Table 18-4)
elevated urinary specific gravity (provided renal
   function is normal)
decreased central venous pressure
thirst
restlessness and disorientation
hypotension and increased pulse rate

Table 18-3.   Formulas for Use of Intravenous Fluids in Burn Therapy

Formula	Adults	Children
	Brooke formula (Burns > 50% counted as 50%)	
	First 24 Hours	
a) Colloids (plasma, dextran or blood)	0.5 ml./kg./1% burn	Same as adults
b) Lactated Ringer's solution	1.5 ml./kg./1% burn	Same as adults
c) Electrolyte-free solution (5% D/W)	2000 ml.	According to age
	Second 24 Hours	
	Give: one-half the amount of a & b and all of c	
	Parkland Regimen	
	First 24 Hours	
	Lactated Ringer's solution is infused in the amount of 4 ml./Kg./% of burned body surface	

Circulatory overload is indicated by:

elevated central venous pressure
shortness of breath
moist rales
increased blood pressure

Central venous pressure measurement frequently is used to monitor the effects of intravenous fluid replacement therapy, particularly in infants, the aged, and patients with cardiac and renal disease. It is generally indicated when the burned surface is greater than 50 or 60 per cent. The margin for therapeutic error is small when the patient has deep extensive burns. Frequent checks of venous pressure allow more aggressive fluid replacement therapy without the risk of circulatory overload. Normal venous pressure is from 4 to 11 cm. of water, and a level of 15 to 20 cm. represents a significant elevation. When venous pressure becomes elevated above a point designated by the physician, the fluid infusion rate is curtailed.

If possible, the patient should be weighed daily for at least the first week, to get an indication of the amount of fluid retention present. Sudden weight gains indicate fluid retention; loss of weight accompanies the stage of diuresis and indicates loss of edema fluid. An in-bed scale may be used if the patient is immobilized. (See Chapter 13.)

Oral Electrolyte Solutions

Oral electrolyte solutions may be the sole source of fluids for the patient with minor burns and may be used in conjunction with intravenous fluids in moderately burned patients. Oral fluids should not, of course, be administered if the gastrointestinal tract is not functional. (Recall that paralytic ileus, gastric dilatation, and nausea are frequent complications of severe burns.) Some physicians prefer not to give fluids orally for the first day or two (or until bowel sounds are heard); fluids are offered slowly at first and increased as tolerated.

Thirst is an early symptom following burns. The patient permitted unlimited quantities of plain water is in danger of developing water intoxication (sodium deficit) because of simple dilution. It is characterized clinically by:

headache
depression
apprehension
tremors
muscle twitching
blurring of vision
vomiting
diarrhea
disorientation
excessive salivation

mania
generalized convulsions

The nurse must explain to the seriously burned patient that plain water (usually in the form of ice chips) should be taken in limited amounts, if at all. Physicians favoring the use of oral electrolyte fluids vary as to the exact contents and proportions of the solutions. One solution consists of 1 tsp. of sodium chloride and ½ tsp. of sodium bicarbonate in 1 L. of chilled water. Occasionally isotonic saline or sixth molar sodium lactate is used.

The solution should be prepared carefully; errors between teaspoons and tablespoons can be serious. Oral electrolyte solutions have a definite taste and some patients find them difficult to accept. Measures that help to make the solution more palatable include chilling it, making ice chips from it, flavoring it with lemon, or disguising it in juices (when allowed). Orange juice and other potassium-containing fluids should be withheld until renal function is established and the physician approves their use.

Oral solutions are not given in the presence of:

1. Acute gastric dilatation
2. Frequent vomiting
3. Peripheral vascular collapse
4. Mental confusion (there is danger of aspirating fluid into the lungs)

Observations of Urinary Output as a Basis for Therapy

Urinary output is the best single index of the adequacy of fluid replacement therapy; the nurse should take measures to assure its accurate measurement.

The output may be measured every half hour or hour as a guide to fluid replacement therapy. One commercial device available for measurement of small volumes of urine is the Davol Uri-Meter, described in Chapter 13. Any clear cylinder with small calibrations may be used. When dealing with small volumes any error can be significant.

Absent or decreased urinary output can be due to inadequate fluid replacement, gastric dilatation, or renal failure. Remember that a clogged catheter may falsely indicate oliguria. Patency of the catheter should be checked before assuming oliguria is present. Extreme care should be taken to record accurately the amount of fluid instilled as an irrigant and the amount of fluid removed.

If the urinary output has been inadequate for 3 hours or more, the physician may order a test to differentiate between the oliguria of inadequate fluid therapy and that of renal failure. One can carry out this test by infusing a solution composed of 5 per cent dextrose in 0.2 per cent sodium chloride or in 0.33 per cent sodium chloride over a period of 40 to 60 minutes. If the oliguria is due to inadequate fluid therapy, the urinary volume will increase; if it is due to renal failure, the output will remain small. In addition to oliguria, acute renal failure will manifest itself as a low urine osmolality. Fortunately, renal failure in burns is uncommon.

Gastric dilatation resulting from stress is not uncommon in burned patients. When it is present, fluids taken orally become trapped in the distended stomach. Thus, even though oral fluids are swallowed, they are not available for body use and urine formation. Gastric distention can be detected by effortless vomiting, nausea, epigastric distress, and grunting respiration. If vomiting occurs, a nasogastric tube is inserted to prevent aspiration of the vomitus. Additional parenteral fluids are needed to make up for the fluid lost in gastric suction. The severe stress imposed by a serious burn causes gastric hyperacidity that can lead to mucosal ulceration; an antacid is sometimes administered through the nasogastric tube every two hours on a clamp-and-release basis.

The physician usually indicates the desired urinary volume plus the variations in either direction to be reported. (See Table 18-4 for desired hourly urine volumes.)

The desired urinary volume should be realistic and approximate the minimum, not the maximum. Attempts to increase fluid input sufficiently to cause large urine volumes in the aged or the very young are dangerous. The kidneys will not excrete excessive fluids because of the body's reaction to stress (increased retention of sodium and water, plus increased secretion of the antidiuretic hormone).

Specific gravity tests are performed on urine, wherein a low reading indicates adequate hydration and a high reading indicates inadequate hydration. (See Chapter 13.)

An accurate intake-output record is a necessity.

Table 18-4.   Desired Urinary Output

Age Group	Desired Urine Flow (ml./hr.)
Adult:	
Male	30–50
Female	25–45
Child:	
1–10	10–25
1 or under	5–10

Adapted from Weisberg, H.: Water, Electrolyte and Acid-Base Balance, ed. 2. Baltimore: Williams & Wilkins, 1962, p. 386.

Treatment of Respiratory Tract Burns

Blood gases should be monitored closely when respiratory burns are present or suspected. Respiratory burns can cause dyspnea, stridor, and copious mucous secretions. Burns about the face and neck may produce sufficient edema to embarrass respiration. In these instances, an airway must be established. If possible, an endotracheal tube is inserted; if not, a tracheostomy is performed. Massive involvement of respiratory tissue nearly always is fatal, even when tracheostomy is performed.

The head of the bed should be elevated (unless contraindicated) and the patient should be encouraged to deep-breathe and cough every 20 minutes. It also is important that the patient be turned at least hourly. Fluid should be suctioned frequently from the respiratory tract to prevent its accumulation. In addition, humidifiers and bronchodilators are used to loosen secretions and improve ventilation; oxygen should be administered to decrease anoxia. Use of mechanical ventilation may be necessary.

Prophylactic antibiotics are given to prevent infection of the lungs and consequent increased edema. Some physicians prescribe intravenous corticosteroids to decrease the pulmonary inflammatory reaction. Lastly, parenteral fluids are administered cautiously to avoid overloading the circulatory system and causing pulmonary edema. (The desired urinary volume is slightly less when respiratory tract burns are present.)

Topical Antibacterial Agents

A number of agents may be applied locally to burn wounds to prevent or control infection. Among those in use are:

1. Silver sulfadiazine (Silvadene)
2. Cerium nitrate-silver sulfadiazine
3. Mafenide acetate (Sulfamylon) 10% cream
4. 0.5% aqueous silver nitrate solution
5. Gentamicin sulfate (Garamycin) 0.1% cream

While these local agents are often effective in controlling infection, they may, in varying degree, alter body electrolyte levels or cause other undesirable effects.

SILVER SULFADIAZINE   Silver sulfadiazine (Silvadene) is a soft, white, water-miscible cream containing silver sulfadiazine in micronized form. This substance is bacteriocidal for a number of gram-negative and gram-positive bacteria as well as yeast. Application to a depth of 1/16 inch is recommended once to twice daily; dressings may or may not be used. Since silver sulfadiazine is not a carbonic anhydrase inhibitor, cases of acidosis have not been reported (a problem that can occur with mafenide therapy—see discussion following). Silver sulfadiazine is somewhat better tolerated by patients than mafenide and is associated with less pain during dressing changes. Any of the adverse reactions associated with sulfonamides may possibly occur with the use of silver sulfadiazine (serum sulfa concentrations should be monitored). According to one source, the growth of gram-negative bacteria in patients with injuries covering 50 per cent or more of the skin surface is not reliably suppressed or prevented by silver sulfadiazine.

CERIUM NITRATE/SILVER SULFADIAZINE   A clinical trail conducted by Monafo and associates[3] was undertaken to study the effectiveness of a water-miscible cream containing both cerium nitrate and silver sulfadiazine on a group of 70 hospitalized burn patients. Simultaneous use of these two agents was prompted by the observed differences in the flora of silver- vs. cerium-treated wounds (the former being mostly gram-negative and the latter mostly gram-positive wounds). Studies indicate a possible synergistic antibacterial effect between these two agents. According to the researchers, even extensive burn wounds were consistently found to be free, or nearly free, of bacteria (particularly troublesome gram-negative strains). The cream was applied to the wounds and covered with cotton dressings once or twice daily and the wounds tended. It was found that absorption of topically applied cerium was minimal. The potential for methemoglobinemia exists with the use of cerium nitrate (as a result of the presence of nitrate ions); however, it was not observed in this study.

MAFENIDE Mafenide acetate (Sulfamylon) is a white, water-soluble cream that can diffuse through avascular burn tissue to help control infection. It is smeared on open burns with a gloved hand, or a sterile tongue blade, once or twice daily. The cream can be left on the wound uncovered or a light fine mesh gauze dressing can be used; dry cream and exudate must be removed before more cream is applied. Because it is water soluble, it can be washed off by tub bathing, shower, or bed bath. The antibacterial spectrum of mafenide includes the Clostridia and a variety of other gram-negative and gram-positive organisms commonly found in major burn wounds. However, the use of mafenide is associated with certain problems:

1. Metabolic acidosis. Mafenide is absorbed into the burn wound and is apparently eliminated principally in the urine. The drug is a potent carbonic anhydrase inhibitor; the tendency to metabolic acidosis apparently is due to carbonic anhydrase inhibition at the renal tubular level. Absorption of the drug causes urinary bicarbonate excretion to increase and the urine pH to become alkaline, which results in a plasma base bicarbonate deficit (metabolic acidosis). Most patients with adequate respiratory function tolerate mild acidosis fairly well; however, at times, the acidosis requires treatment with bicarbonate solutions or discontinuing the use of mafenide.
2. Hyperventilation. The respiratory system becomes the only functional method for maintaining body pH in the normal range because the renal buffering mechanism is impaired. Hyperventilation is a compensatory action to lighten the pCO_2 and raise the plasma pH. (Usually the acidosis is only partially compensated for by the respiratory system.) Hyperventilation is particularly evident in patients with burns of 50 per cent or more of

the body surface. After absorption, mafenide is metabolized into an acid, placing further demands on the lungs to maintain a normal pH. As a result, respiratory compensation may overshoot and cause a high arterial pH and a low pCO_2 (respiratory alkalosis).
3. Pain on application. Application of the cream causes most patients to complain of stinging, especially in the first few weeks. (The use of analgesics is sometimes necessary.)
4. Allergic reaction. This is mild in most cases but occasionally may require that the drug be discontinued.

AQUEOUS SILVER NITRATE SOLUTION The application of an aqueous 0.5% silver nitrate solution to burns is still used occasionally to combat infection. It is an effective antibacterial agent against organisms that regularly colonize burn wounds. The silver nitrate dressings are at least 1 inch thick, are held in place with stockinette, and are wet every two hours with warmed 0.5% silver nitrate solution. Dry sheets and a cotton blanket are used to cover the patient; the covers minimize convection currents and the rate of heat loss. Silver nitrate is associated with certain problems:

1. Leaching of electrolytes (Na, Cl, K, Ca, and Mg) and vitamins from the burn wound. This is due to the hypotonicity of the silver nitrate solution as well as to the ion-binding potential of the silver ion. 0.5% silver nitrate contains only 29.4 mEq./L. of $AgNO_3$, and the solute composition of the solution is much different from that of body fluids. *The patient's plasma electrolyte levels must be monitored closely so that adequate replacement therapy can be instituted; children should be monitored especially closely. Patients treated with topical 0.5% silver nitrate dressings should routinely receive supplementation of sodium chloride, potassium, calcium, and water solute vitamins, especially vitamin C.*
2. Staining. The staining property of silver nitrate is esthetically objectionable to the patient and to the staff. Silver nitrate stains everything it touches brown or black.
3. Pseudomonas superinfections.
4. Dressings must be re-wet every two hours

with warmed silver nitrate solution. Failure to keep the dressings wet results in an increased concentration of silver nitrate at the wound site (caused by evaporation of water from the dressings). Concentrations of silver nitrate greater than 1 or 2 per cent are caustic and damage tissue.

5. Methemoglobinemia may occur rarely. Bacterial reduction of nitrate ions to nitrite ions can result in systemic absorption of nitrite (presumably the cause of methemoglobinemia).

GENTAMICIN Gentamicin sulfate (Garamycin) may be applied topically and used systemically to treat burns. It is effective against a wide range of gram-negative and gram-positive organisms. Application of the cream is not associated with pain. The drug is not appreciably absorbed from the burn wound. Garamycin is primarily eliminated by the kidneys; it should be used systemically with caution on patients with impaired renal function. Nephrotoxicity and auditory or vestibular ototoxicity may occasionally occur when Garamycin is used systemically, particularly when renal function is impaired. Dizziness or vomiting should be reported immediately to the physician.

Systemic Antibacterial Agents

Because infection commonly occurs in burned patients, systemic antibiotics are commonly administered; the specific agent required is determined by culturing the source of the infection (such as wounds, urinary tract, or respiratory tract). Penicillin is often given as a prophylaxis against streptococcal or staphylococcal infections.

Control of Pain

The amount of pain present varies with the depth of the burn, the extent of surface area involved, and the patient's pain threshold. Third-degree (full-thickness) burns are painless because the nerve endings are destroyed; however, pain is experienced around the periphery of third-degree burns where first-degree and second-degree burns are present.

Burned patients complaining of severe pain may be given small doses of meperidine or morphine through the intravenous cannula put in place for fluid administration. The subcutaneous or intramuscular route should never be used to administer narcotics to a burned patient with circulatory collapse. Peripheral tissue perfusion is erratic when shock is present; thus, absorption of the drug may not occur or may be delayed. Failure to achieve the desired effect may prompt repeated doses by the same route. When peripheral circulation is improved after fluid resuscitation, there may be a rapid absorption and cumulative overdosage of the narcotic resulting in respiratory depression.

The administration of a large dose of an analgesic to an inadequately resuscitated patient in or near burn shock can be lethal.

An 18-year-old boy received superficial intradermal burns over 80% of his body in a flash fire and explosion at a motel that occurred at 8:00 a.m. He was initially alert and oriented when seen by a local physician who prescribed no treatment. He was taken 25 miles by automobile to his family physician; by this time 4 hours had elapsed since his accident. He was given 100 mg. of meperidine subcutaneously (but no intravenous fluids) and placed in an ambulance for transfer to St. John's Mercy Hospital—a distance of 75 miles. When he arrived, 8 hours after the accident, he was comatose and cyanotic, with infrequent, gasping shallow respirations. An endotracheal tube could not be inserted because of facial and cervical edema. Although tracheostomy and cannula phlebotomy were performed immediately, spontaneous breathing never resumed and the pupils remained fixed and dilated. There was persistent oliguria until his death in coma, 20 hours later. (*Comment: this patient had a potentially curable lesion; most of his burns were intradermal and shallow. Delayed resuscitation, together with an ill-advised dose of narcotic, led to his untimely and unnecessary death.*)[4]

It is important not to confuse the restlessness of burn shock with pain. A patient thrashing about in bed, without complaints of pain, may well be in burn shock. In this case, a narcotic is contraindicated; the physician usually orders an increased rate of parenteral fluid administration.

Adynamic Ileus with Gastric Dilatation

Adynamic ileus with gastric dilatation is common during the first day or two in patients with burns of 50 per cent or more of the body surface. Usual symptoms include nausea, effortless vomiting, hiccoughing, and abdominal distention. Oral intake should be withheld if vomiting is present, as the danger of tracheal aspiration of vomitus is great. The emesis should be measured and observed for blood. A naso-gastric tube may be inserted if symptoms persist; rarely is it necessary to leave the tube in longer than 24 hours. (Nasogastric tubes irritate the esophagus and stomach and may contribute to ulceration.)

The appearance of abdominal distention after the first few days postburn may indicate the presence of invasive wound sepsis, since ileus commonly occurs with this condition. Ileus may also be associated with gastroduodenal perforation. A routine observation of stools should be made for blood since ulcers of the gastrointestinal tract are not uncommon in burned patients.

Physiologic Basis for Treatment and Nursing Care During the Fluid Remobilization Phase

Remobilization of edema fluid represents an interstitial fluid-to-plasma shift which begins on the second or third day after the patient has been burned. Its usual duration is from 24 to 72 hours.

Observing Urinary Output

Reabsorption of edema fluid takes place about the second to fifth postburn day. The blood volume is greatly increased and large amounts of urine are excreted. The nurse should be alert for increasing urine volume and should report its presence to the physician.

If the expected diuresis does not occur, the possibility of renal damage must be considered.

Observing for Pulmonary Edema

Fatal pulmonary edema may occur because the reno-cardiovascular system is not capable of handling the volume of water and electrolytes shifting from the interstitial fluid into the plasma. (Recall that the volume of edema fluid in a burn may equal the total normal plasma volume.)

The nurse should be alert for signs of circulatory overload and pulmonary edema:

venous distention
shortness of breath
moist rales
cyanosis
coughing of frothy fluid

Parenteral Fluid Therapy

Once the fluid remobilization phase is reached, parenteral fluids should be sharply curtailed or discontinued; infusion of large volumes of fluids could easily cause circulatory overload with pulmonary edema. Oral fluids and food may supply adequate fluid and nutrition during this phase if tolerated; if not, moderate quantities of intravenous fluids may be necessary to meet daily needs. If possible, a high protein and high caloric diet is started by the second or third day.

Physiologic Basis for Treatment and Nursing Care During the Convalescent Period

NUTRITION   Good nutrition is of first importance for burned patients, all of whom have great nutritional needs (as a result of increased catabolism), several times those of the healthy person. Unfortunately, burned patients frequently do not eat well because of pain, generalized discomfort (frequent dressing changes, grafts, and so forth), and depression.

Frequent oral feedings of foods or commercial mixtures high in protein, calories, and vitamins should be started as soon as possible. Vitamin preparations containing at least members of the B complex and vitamin C should be administered. If the patient refuses oral feedings, tube feedings may be employed. Gastrostomy feedings often are safer because the danger of aspiration pneumonitis, associated with nasogastric tube feedings, is decreased. The nurse should examine the abdomen for bowel sounds before the nasogastric tube feeding in instilled and during the first few hours thereafter; recall that gastric atony and dilatation are common after major burns. Gastric residual should be checked before each feeding. Instillation of the tube feeding into a distended atonic stomach results in regurgitation of the gastric contents and possible tracheal aspiration. (Nursing responsibilities in administration of tube feedings are discussed in Chapter 14.) The nurse should be alert for gastric bleeding or other indications of a Curling's ulcer. Because the patient often has a poor appetite and psychologic depression, the nurse must take every opportunity to make food appealing to him.

Oral electrolyte supplements may also be given, depending upon the electrolytes needed. Serum electrolytes should be determined daily.

While providing the patient with optimal nutrition pays rich dividends, failure to meet his nutritional needs may lead to what Blocker terms "burn decompensation." This state is characterized by chronic weight loss, decreased resistance to infection, anorexia, failure of skin grafts to take, cachexia, and death.

Parenteral hyperalimentation may be necessary when the burned patient is unable to consume an adequate diet. (Parenteral hyperalimentation is described in Chapter 16.)

AMBULATION   Early ambulation, even in severely burned patients, improves appetite, helps to prevent contractures, helps correct negative nitrogen balance and sustains the patient's morale. Recall that immobilization predisposes the patient to renal calculi, particularly when there is a high milk intake. (Immobilization and renal calculi are discussed in Chapter 14.)

OBSERVING FOR SPECIFIC ELECTROLYTE IMBALANCES   The convalescent phase is often complicated by inadequate electrolyte intake from the diet; if supplemental replacements are not given, the patient may insidiously develop deficits of potassium, sodium, and calcium. The nurse should be alert for symptoms of these imbalances. (A thorough description of each is offered in Chapter 10. Observations to be made by the nurse are discussed in Chapter 13.) Plasma electrolyte levels should be checked on a regular basis.

Obviously, some of the major nursing problems have been omitted in the preceding discussion of burns, not because they are unimportant but because space does not allow.

REFERENCES

1. **Jacoby, F.:**   Nursing Care of the Patient with Burns, ed. 2. St. Louis: C. V. Mosby, 1976, p. 42.

2. **Monafo, W., et al.:**   Hypertonic sodium solutions in the treatment of burn shock. Am. J. Surg. 126, 1973, p. 779.

3. **Monafo, W., et al.:**   Control of infection in major burn wounds by cerium nitrate/silver sulphadiazine. Burns 3:1977, p. 104.

4. **Monafo, W.:**   Treatment of Burns—Principles and Practices. St. Louis: Warren H. Green, 1971, pp. 54–55.

BIBLIOGRAPHY

Beaumont, E. (ed.):   Septic shock in a burn patient—nursing grand rounds. Nursing 76, January 1976.

Berk, J., et al. (ed.):   Handbook of Critical Care. Boston: Little, Brown, & Co., 1976.

Farrow, S.:   Comparative effects of dextran and plasma protein solutions. Burns 3, April 1977.

Finley, R.:   Assessing and treating burns. Nursing 76, September 1976.

Harris, N., et al.:   Comparison of fresh, frozen and lyophilized porcine skin as xenografts on burned patients. Burns 2, January 1976.

Jones, C., and Feller, I.:   Burns—what to do during the first crucial hours. Nursing 77, March 1977.

Lamke, L., et al.:   The evaporative water loss from burns and the water-vapor permeability of grafts and artificial membranes used in the treatment of burns. Burns 3, March 1977.

Mangus, D., et al.:   The use of topical solutions in antibacterial burn wound therapy. Burns 3, 1973.

Monafo, W., et al.:   Cerium nitrate: a new topical antiseptic for extensive burns. Surgery 80, October 1976.

— 19 —

Fluid Balance in the Patient with Digestive Tract Disease

CHARACTER OF GASTROINTESTINAL SECRETIONS

The average daily volume of gastrointestinal secretions is approximately 8000 ml., as compared to a plasma volume of 3500 ml. Most of these secretions are reabsorbed in the ileum and proximal colon; only about 150 ml. of relatively electrolyte-free fluid is excreted daily in the feces.

Gastrointestinal secretions consist of saliva, gastric juice, bile, pancreatic juice, and intestinal secretions. Their average daily volume and pH are listed in Table 19-1. The electrolyte content of these secretions is presented in Table 19-2.

With the exception of saliva, the gastrointestinal secretions are isotonic with the extracellular fluid. In addition, material entering the gastrointestinal tract tends to become isotonic during the course of its absorption. Many liters of extracellular fluid pass into the gastrointestinal tract, and back again, as part of the normal digestive process. This movement of water and electrolytes is sometimes referred to as the "gastrointestinal circulation."

FLUID IMBALANCES ASSOCIATED WITH THE LOSS OF GASTROINTESTINAL FLUIDS

Loss of gastrointestinal fluids is the most common cause of water and electrolyte disturbances. This fact becomes evident when one considers the large volume of fluids in the gastrointestinal tract and the many ways in which they can be lost from the body. Vomiting, gastrointestinal suction, diarrhea, fistulas, and drainage tubes are some of the abnormal ways in which these fluids can be lost. Fluids trapped in the gastrointestinal tract, as in intestinal obstruction, are physiologically *outside* the body. Any condition that interferes with the absorption of fluids from the gastrointestinal tract can cause serious water and electrolyte disturbances.

Vomiting and Gastric Suction

The absorption of gastric secretions and ingested fluids is hindered by vomiting and gastric suction. To understand the imbalances likely to occur with these conditions, it is helpful to review the normal characteristics of gastric juice, which is the most acid of the gastrointestinal secretions. Gastric juice has a pH of from 1 to 3.5; occasionally, the pH is higher than 3.5. The main electrolytes in gastric juice are hydrogen, chloride, potassium, and sodium. Imbalances

Table 19-1. Average Daily Volume of Gastrointestinal Secretions and Their Usual pH

Secretion	Volume (ml.)	pH
Saliva	1,500	6–7
Gastric juice	2,500	1–3.5
Pancreatic juice	700	8.0–8.3
Bile	500	7.8
Small intestine	3,000	7.8–8.0

Table 19-2. Electrolyte Content of Gastrointestinal Secretions Expressed in Milliequivalents per Liter

Secretion	Na^+	K^+	Cl^-	HCO_3^-
Saliva	9	25.8	10	10–15
Gastric juice (fasting)	60.4	9.2	84	0–14
Pancreatic juice (fistula)	141.1	4.6	76.6	121
Bile (fistula)	148.9	4.98	100.6	40
Small intestine (suction)	111.3	4.6	104.2	31

Adapted from Weisberg, H.: Water, Electrolytes, and Acid-Base Balance, ed. 2. Baltimore: Williams & Wilkins, 1962, p. 143.

most often associated with the loss of gastric juice include:

Fluid volume deficit
Metabolic alkalosis (base bicarbonate excess)
Potassium deficit
Sodium deficit

FLUID VOLUME DEFICIT When a large volume of water and electrolytes is lost from the body, fluid volume deficit results. Note in Table 19-3 that 100 to 6000 ml. may be lost in 24 hours from vomiting or suction. Since the gastric secretions are greatly reduced when the stomach is at rest, the patient should receive nothing by mouth during gastric suction or persistent vomiting. If the suction or vomiting is prolonged, and fluid replacement therapy is inadequate, fluid volume deficit will result. Consequently, the

nurse should be alert for the following symptoms indicating the presence of fluid volume deficit:

dry skin and mucous membranes
longitudinal wrinkling of the tongue
oliguria
acute weight loss—in excess of 5 per cent
body temperature drop
exhaustion

METABOLIC ALKALOSIS Excessive loss of gastric juice by vomiting or gastric suction causes metabolic alkalosis, because hydrogen and chloride ions are lost from the body. Loss of chloride ions causes a compensatory increase in bicarbonate ions. The base bicarbonate side of the carbonic acid–base bicarbonate ratio is increased and the pH becomes alkaline. The nurse should be alert for symptoms of metabolic alkalosis when the patient has sustained a prolonged loss of gastric juice by vomiting or gastric suction. These symptoms include the following:

1. Slow, shallow respiration (compensatory respiratory reaction to retain CO_2 and to correct alkalosis)
2. Muscle hypertonicity and tetany (caused by decreased calcium ionization in alkalosis)
3. Changes in sensorium
   a. personality changes may be the first symptoms to appear
   b. previously placid patient may become irritable and uncooperative
   c. patient may be disoriented

Table 19-3. Possible Abnormal Fluid Exchange of Adult in 24-Hour Period

Entrances	Exits	Water (ml.)	NaCl (Gm.)
G.I. Tract	G.I. Tract		
Gastric Gavage	Saliva	500– 1,500	2–8
Duodenal Gavage	Vomiting	100– 6,000	0.5–40
Enemas	Suction Drainage, Intubation or		
	Fistula	100– 6,000	0.5–40
	Diarrhea	500–17,000	2–80
	Rectal Mucorrhea ("Pseudodiarrhea")	350– 2,000	1–9
	Primary or Secondary Malabsorption Syndrome	100–14,000	0.5–75

Adapted from Weisberg, H.: Electrolyte and Acid-Base Balance, ed. 2. Baltimore: Williams & Wilkins, 1962, p. 140.

Vomiting of alkaline duodenal fluid in addition to gastric juice can cause plasma pH to remain essentially normal or even cause metabolic acidosis if the loss of alkaline fluid exceeds loss of acidic gastric fluid. Patients with hypochlorhydria or achlorhydria are not apt to develop metabolic alkalosis after vomiting.

POTASSIUM DEFICIT   Gastric juice is rich in potassium. A prolonged loss of this fluid frequently leads to potassium deficit, particularly if potassium replacement therapy is inadequate. The nurse should be alert for symptoms of potassium deficit. These include the following:

muscular weakness
gaseous intestinal distention
soft, flabby muscles
carphologia (aimless plucking at bedclothes)
paresthesia and flaccid paralysis of extremities
weak, irregular pulse
respiratory failure
heart block and cardiac arrest (as late symptoms)

SODIUM DEFICIT   The sodium content of gastric juice is relatively high. The nurse should be aware that gastric suction or prolonged vomiting can lead to sodium deficit, especially if plain water is drunk. Symptoms of sodium deficit include:

Anorexia, apathy, sometimes great apprehension
Abdominal cramps
Hypotension (declines further when sitting or standing)
Syncope with position change
Rapid, thready pulse
Oliguria, low specific gravity of urine
Cold skin, particularly in the extremities
Decreased body temperature, unless infection is present
Hand veins fill slowly
Fingerprinting on sternum

OTHER IMBALANCES   Prolonged vomiting or gastric suction can result in magnesium deficit, an imbalance not as common as those listed above. The magnesium concentration in gastric juice is only 1.4 mEq./L. In addition, the body conserves magnesium well. However, its continued loss by suction or vomiting, plus its dilution with magnesium-free re-

placement fluids, can result in symptoms of magnesium deficit. These include the following:

hyperirritability
gross tremors (may occur in any extremity but are most common in the arms)
confusion and disorientation
tachycardia
hypertension
hallucinations, usually visual (may be auditory)
carphologia
abnormal sensitivity to sound (hyperacusis)
convulsions (usually generalized and not preceded by an aura)

Another imbalance is ketosis of starvation. Unless adequate parenteral nutrition is provided for the patient with prolonged vomiting or gastric suction, ketosis of starvation will occur. As a result of the absence of carbohydrate, the body must use fat for energy purposes. Because of increased fat utilization, ketone bodies accumulate in the blood. Because ketones are strong acids, they can convert metabolic alkalosis into metabolic acidosis. The odor of acetone on the breath indicates starvation ketosis; other symptoms of metabolic acidosis include deep, rapid respiration and weakness.

NURSING IMPLICATIONS   The nurse should be alert for symptoms of the imbalances described above, should report their occurrence to the physician, and, in addition, should attempt to minimize the loss of water and electrolytes by vomiting and gastric suction. When the nurse is in charge of patients with vomiting, she should:

1. Discourage oral intake, particularly water, if vomiting is persistent and frequent. Ingested substances stimulate gastric secretions. If the substance is hypotonic, electrolytes will move from the extracellular fluid into the stomach. When the stomach is emptied by vomiting, water and electrolytes from the gastric secretions and extracellular fluid are lost. Obviously, oral intake, while vomiting persists, promotes water and electrolyte depletion.

2. Report vomiting early so that appropriate treatment can be started before water and electrolyte losses become serious. Medications to relieve nausea may prevent further vomiting. Nutrition by the parenteral route allows the stomach to rest.

3. Administer p.r.n. medications, as prescribed, to relieve nausea.

4. Measure or estimate as accurately as possible the amount of vomitus lost from the body so that lost water and electrolytes can be replaced by parenteral fluids. All fluids lost and gained by the body should be recorded on the intake-output record. (Nursing responsibilities in measuring and recording fluid intake and output are discussed in Chapter 13.)

5. Measure body weight daily to detect significant changes in fluid balance. Daily weights are helpful in detecting fluid volume deficit, particularly if vomitus has not been measured. A patient on a starvation diet should lose about one-half pound a day, whereas a loss in excess of this amount probably implies a fluid volume deficit. A weight gain implies fluid volume excess if the patient is on a starvation diet. (Nursing responsibilities in measuring daily weights are discussed in Chapter 13.)

6. Report substantial improvement in the patient's condition early so that he can be returned to oral intake as soon as tolerated. (Dietary considerations for the patient with vomiting are discussed in Chapter 14.)

Important nursing actions in the care of the patient with gastric suction are as follows:

1. Irrigate the tube with isotonic sodium chloride solution, or as prescribed by the physician. Plain water is unsuitable as an irrigating solution because it washes out electrolytes. Some physicians prefer hourly irrigation of the tube with 30 to 50 ml. of air to prevent clogging; air does not interfere with electrolyte balance or with intake-output record keeping. However, when blood or thick secretions are occluding the tube it may be necessary to use isotonic saline.

2. Record the irrigating solution volume as intake and whatever is recovered as output.

3. Prohibit the intake of large quantities of water or ice chips by mouth, since water washes electrolytes from the stomach, causing metabolic alkalosis and loss of sodium and potassium. Sometimes the physician writes an order to permit the administration of ice chips sparingly; the term "sparingly" can readily be stretched by well-meaning but ill-advised persons to the point where the intake of plain ice is excessive. Some physicians allow approximately an ounce of plain ice chips per hour to relieve oral dryness.

4. Measure and record the amount of fluid lost by suction, as well as all other fluid gains and losses.

5. Measure daily weight variations to help detect early fluid volume deficit or excess.

Diarrhea, Intestinal Suction and Ileostomy

FLUID VOLUME DEFICIT Intestinal hypermotility shortens the opportunity for absorption of intestinal fluids and, thus, results in increased fluid loss in bowel movements. The hypermotility can be caused by a disease process, such as ulcerative colitis, or by the frequent use of an irritant cathartic. The liquid stools expelled as a result of hypermotility contain water and electrolytes derived from secretions, ingested food and fluids, and extracellular fluid brought into the bowel to render ingested substances isotonic. Note in Table 19-3 that as much as 17,000 ml. can be lost in 24 hours from diarrhea. Obviously, prolonged diarrhea is a serious threat to water and electrolyte balance. The amount of fluid lost in intestinal suction averages around 3000 ml. daily. Thus, the nurse should be alert for symptoms of fluid volume deficit when the patient has sustained large fluid losses from the intestinal tract. (Symptoms of fluid volume deficit are listed in the discussion of gastric suction and vomiting.)

METABOLIC ACIDOSIS Intestinal juice varies in composition according to the area of the intestine in which it was formed. However, the intestinal secretions are all alkaline, including pancreatic juice and bile, which are mixed with intestinal juices in the intestines. The chief electrolytes in intestinal juice include sodium, potassium, bicarbonate, and chloride.

The intestinal secretions are alkaline because of the preponderance of bicarbonate ions. Loss of bicarbonate results in a decreased pH. Symptoms of metabolic acidosis (primary base bicarbonate deficit) include the following:

shortness of breath on exertion (mild deficit)
deep, rapid breathing (moderate or severe deficit)
weakness and general malaise
stupor progressing to coma

SODIUM DEFICIT   Intestinal secretions have a high concentration of sodium; excessive loss of these secretions results in sodium deficit. (Symptoms of sodium deficit are listed in the discussion of gastric suction and vomiting.)

POTASSIUM DEFICIT   Relatively large amounts of potassium are contained in the intestinal fluid; therefore, potassium deficit occurs frequently with diarrhea, prolonged intestinal suction, and recent ileostomy. (Symptoms of potassium deficit are listed in the discussion of gastric suction and vomiting.)

NURSING IMPLICATIONS   The nurse should be alert for symptoms of fluid imbalances likely to occur in the presence of diarrhea, ileostomy, or intestinal suction.

Important nursing actions in the care of the patient with *diarrhea* include the following:

1. Discourage oral intake, particularly irritating foods apt to stimulate peristalsis. Less fluid is formed when the intestinal tract is at rest.

2. Report diarrhea early so that appropriate treatment can be started before water and electrolyte losses are severe. Medications to reduce peristalsis may relieve diarrhea. Nutrition by the parenteral route allows the intestinal tract to rest.

3. Administer p.r.n. medications as prescribed to prevent diarrhea.

4. Measure, or estimate as accurately as possible, the amount of liquid feces lost from the body so that lost water and electrolytes can be replaced by parenteral fluids. All fluids lost and gained by the body should be recorded on the intake-output record.

5. Measure body weight daily to detect significant changes in fluid balance. Daily weights are helpful in detecting fluid volume deficit, particularly if the liquid stools have not been measured.

6. Report substantial improvement in the patient's condition early so that he can return to oral intake as soon as tolerated.

(Dietary considerations for the patient with diarrhea are discussed in Chapter 14.)

Important nursing considerations and actions in the care of the patient with recent *ileostomy* include the following:

1. Measure and record the fluid lost by ileos-

tomy, as well as other fluid losses and gains by the body.

2. Be alert for symptoms of water and electrolyte disturbances in the immediate postoperative period; potassium deficit is the most frequent imbalance. Other imbalances may include sodium deficit and fluid volume deficit. Patients with ileostomies are more likely to develop water and electrolyte disturbances when their stomas first begin to function, as shown by a comparison of the amount of water and electrolytes lost in a 24-hour period in the early postoperative period, with the amounts lost in a similar period after the ileostomy has adapted. Fluid loss from a recent ileostomy may be as high as 4000 ml. in 24 hours; each liter of the fluid may contain 130 mEq. of sodium and 16 mEq. of potassium. (Potassium loss from a recent ileostomy may range from 4 to 98 mEq. per liter.) An adapted ileostomy usually loses no more than 500 ml. in 24 hours; each liter of fluid may contain 46 mEq. of sodium and 3 mEq. of potassium.

Nursing responsibilities in the care of the patient with *intestinal suction* include the following:

1. Irrigate the tube with an isotonic or hypotonic electrolyte solution, or as instructed by the physician. Plain water should never be used to irrigate intestinal suction tubes, particularly those located low in the intestines, since plain water is injurious to the mucosa of the ileum. In addition, it promotes increased secretion of intestinal juice and causes electrolytes to be washed out.

2. Record the irrigating solution volume as intake and whatever is recovered as output.

3. Prohibit the intake of large quantities of water or ice by mouth since electrolytes may be washed out by the suction apparatus. Some physicians allow approximately an ounce of plain ice chips per hour to relieve oral dryness.

4. Measure and record the amount of fluid lost by suction, as well as all fluid gains and losses by the body.

Prolonged Use of Laxatives and Enemas

The prolonged use of laxatives and enemas results in serious water and electrolyte disturbances, particularly potassium deficit. Other possible deficits include sodium deficit and fluid volume deficit.

Cathartics increase the water and electrolyte output through the fecal route, by hastening the excretion of fecal contents and, thus, reducing the absorption time. Irritant cathartics cause hypermotility of the bowel by irritating the bowel mucosa. Saline cathartics draw water from the extracellular fluid into the bowel. The distended bowel produces mechanical stimulation and the large amount of fluid is propelled out of the bowel. A large fluid volume deficit can result from continued use of saline cathartics, which interfere with electrolyte absorption from the intestines.

Enemas also deplete body water and electrolytes, particularly if plain water is used. Electrolytes from the extracellular fluid enter the bowel to make the water isotonic. Then the water and electrolytes are excreted by propulsive movements initiated by distension of the bowel with water.

The nurse should teach patients to avoid the repeated use of cathartics and enemas; when frequent bowel irrigations are indicated, an isotonic electrolyte solution should be used.

A roughly isotonic sodium chloride enema solution can be easily made by adding 1 tsp. (5 ml.) of table salt to a liter of tap water (furnishes 120 mEq. of Na and 120 mEq. of Cl).

Repeated tap water enemas can result in hyponatremia. On the other hand, use of commercial hypertonic cleansing enemas (containing sodium biphosphate and sodium phosphate) can result in some degree of sodium absorption and, thus, should be avoided in patients requiring sodium restriction. (A number of measures to help patients overcome the habitual use of laxatives and enemas are described in Chapter 14.)

Fistulas and Drainage Tubes

Gastrointestinal fluids can also be lost through fistulas, whereby deficits of sodium, potassium, chloride, or bicarbonate may result, depending on the area in which the fistula is located.

An educated guess as to the content of the fluid and imbalances likely to accompany its loss can be made by reviewing the usual electrolyte content of the fluid in the region of the fistula (see Table 19-3). For example, fluid from a pancreatic fistula has a high sodium content—as much as 185 mEq./L. Thus, one would expect a sodium deficit to result unless adequate sodium replacement is carried out. Because pancreatic juice is alkaline, one would expect metabolic acidosis to accompany its loss from the body. When in doubt, the physician may choose to test the fluid's pH and electrolyte content.

In addition to pH changes, fistulas can cause a serious contraction of extracellular fluid volume. For example, a duodenal or jejunal fistula may drain 3 to 6 L. daily; a pancreatic fistula may drain 2 L. daily.

If possible, the nurse should attempt to measure the fluid lost by way of a fistula by applying a stoma bag over its orifice. If not, she should try to estimate the volume as accurately as possible. Statements as to how much of a dressing was saturated, as well as extent of gown and linen saturation, help the physician plan fluid replacement therapy.

A large volume of bile can be lost after cholecystectomy when a T-tube is inserted. The nurse should measure this drainage the same as she does drainage obtained by gastrointestinal suction. The physician has to know the amount lost from the body in order to replace the water and electrolyte losses with parenteral fluids. The nurse should be alert for symptoms of sodium deficit when large volumes of bile are lost, especially if sodium is also being lost by gastric suction. Bile has an alkaline pH, so one would anticipate metabolic acidosis if the bile loss is prolonged.

Trapped Gastrointestinal Fluids

Fluids trapped in an obstructed bowel, or in the peritoneal cavity, are lost because they are not available for use by the body (third space effect). However, they cannot be measured directly as one measures fluid losses caused by vomiting or suction. Trapped fluids present a problem in planning fluid replacement therapy. Gastrointestinal conditions associated with fluid accumulation in the body include gastrointestinal obstruction, peritonitis, and cirrhosis of the liver.

GASTROINTESTINAL OBSTRUCTION Gastrointestinal obstruction is accompanied by serious imbalances in water and electrolytes, the nature of which depends on the site of the obstruction.

If the *pylorus* is obstructed, gastric contents cannot enter the intestines and are lost by vomiting; the patient may develop metabolic alkalosis. This imbalance occurs because excessive amounts of hydrogen and chloride ions are lost in vomiting.

If the *upper small intestine* is obstructed, the patient will vomit intestinal juices and gastric juice.

The loss of acid and alkaline fluids may be approximately equal; this prevents serious disturbances in pH.

If the obstruction is in a *distal segment of the small intestine,* the patient may vomit larger quantities of alkaline fluids than of acid fluids. (Recall that secretions below the pylorus are mainly alkaline.) Thus, metabolic acidosis can result from a low intestinal obstruction.

If the obstruction is *below the proximal colon,* most of the gastrointestinal fluids will have been absorbed before reaching the point of obstruction. Solid fecal material accumulates until symptoms of discomfort develop. Accumulation of gas and fluid behind the obstruction can lead to distention of the ileum if the ileocecal valve is incompetent. Reverse peristalsis may cause vomiting of a fecal nature (which can be severe) late in bowel obstruction.

Small intestinal obstruction traps gastrointestinal fluids and gas proximal to the obstruction. Large quantities of water and electrolytes continue to be secreted into the bowel lumen, even in the absence of oral intake. Also, the increased pressure within the distended bowel draws fluid from the plasma and the tissues. Decreased selectivity of the intestinal membrane allows plasma proteins to enter both the intestinal lumen and the gut wall. Because of distention, the mucosa of the bowel above the obstruction is greatly stimulated to secrete more fluid. The edematous bowel wall is not able to absorb the large fluid volume; thus, the distention becomes progressively greater. Ten liters or more of fluid can collect in the bowel, resulting in severe extracellular fluid volume deficit. Plasma volume is substantially reduced and hypovolemic shock often ensues. In addition to fluid, the gut is distended by gas, mostly from swallowed air. Stasis of the gut also causes accumulation of gas produced by bacterial action and diffusion from the bloodstream.

Blood loss from a strangulated hernia may be great. The volume of blood sequestered into an infarcted bowel segment may be approximately 10 per cent of the total blood volume for every 24 hours of obstruction. A reduced circulating blood volume causes hypotension, rapid thready pulse, and decreased renal blood flow with azotemia and oliguria. Death may result unless the blood volume is restored.

Nursing Implications   The nurse should frequently observe the vital signs of patients with gastrointestinal obstruction. A fall in blood pressure with an increased pulse rate indicates further contraction of the plasma volume and oncoming circulatory collapse. Such findings should be quickly reported to the physician. Fluid administration before surgery aims at stabilizing the vital signs sufficiently to withstand the stress of surgery. Balanced electrolyte solutions, plasma, and whole blood are frequently used replacement fluids. It is generally not possible to totally correct the fluid deficit prior to surgery since time is limited. Frequently, however, there is sufficient time to administer 2 to 3 L. of an electrolyte solution (such as Lactated Ringer's) over a three- to four-hour period to prepare the patient for operation. (The administration of only electrolyte-free solutions may easily induce water intoxication.) The rapidity of fluid replacement may compromise some patients' cardiovascular status; therefore, central venous pressure should be monitored in these patients. A steadily rising central venous pressure indicates too rapid fluid administration. (Nursing responsibilities in parenteral therapy are described in Chapter 16.) The hourly urinary output should be observed. Oliguria or anuria are indications of inadequate fluid replacement. Urinary specific gravity is high (above 1.025) when fluid replacement is inadequate. When possible, the urinary output should be at least 50 ml. per hour before surgery.

Recall that the volume of fluid trapped in the intestine can only be estimated. Weight measurements are also valueless in detecting the amount of fluid trapped in the bowel. *Careful observation of vital signs, the patient's appearance, urinary volume, and specific gravity are significant.* Mild tachycardia may suggest an acute fluid loss of 5 per cent of body weight; an acute fluid loss greater than 10 per cent of body weight can cause hypovolemic shock.

The nurse should carefully observe and record the nature and frequency of vomiting (such observations are helpful in determining the level of obstruction). Brownish liquid vomitus with a fecal odor is characteristic of distal ileal obstruction. Greenish watery vomitus, without abdominal distention, may suggest obstruction of the proximal jejunum. Patients with colon obstruction do not usually vomit until advanced obstruction is present or unless the ileocecal valve is incompetent. (Recall that most fluids are absorbed before reaching the colon.) Distention is most marked in patients with obstruction of the distal ileum or of the colon. On the other hand, obstruction of the proximal gut causes minimal distention since vomiting relieves the pressure.[1]

PERITONITIS   Peritonitis involves the loss of extracellular fluid into the peritoneal cavity as an inflammatory exudate, causing fluid volume deficit. Calcium deficit can also occur in generalized peritonitis and acute pancreatitis, because large amounts of calcium are immobilized in the diseased tissues and exudates, for reasons unclear.

CIRRHOSIS OF THE LIVER WITH ASCITES   Ascites results from a combination of factors: (1) mechanical obstruction to venous outflow from the cirrhotic liver; (2) increased capillary permeability; (3) hypoalbuminemia; and (4) hormonal effects. Water and electrolyte disturbances that may occur in cirrhosis of the liver are summarized in Table 19-4.

Symptoms of cirrhosis are variable but may include the following:

weakness and fatigue

anorexia, nausea, vomiting, diarrhea, or constipation (blood from the portal vein backs into the gastrointestinal organs and interferes with their normal activity)

abdominal fullness (at first due to flatulence, later to ascites)

weight loss (may be masked by excessive fluid retention)

enlarged liver (at first the liver may be enlarged with fatty tissue, later it becomes small, hard, and nodular)

enlarged spleen (spleen is engorged with venous blood from the portal system)

low grade fever

jaundice

edema owing to hypoalbuminemia

putrid, fecal odor to the breath

Table 19-4.   Water and Electrolyte Disturbances in Cirrhosis of the Liver with Ascites

Water and Electrolyte Disturbance	Cause
Sodium and water retention	Aldosterone level elevated (recall that aldosterone causes Na retention, which in turn causes water retention.) (The liver normally inactivates aldosterone and prevents its excessive buildup in the body; however, the cirrhotic liver does not perform this function well.)
Low plasma sodium level (which may occur)	Antidiuretic hormone level elevated (due to failure of the liver to inactivate ADH) (Recall that ADH causes the kidneys to retain water.) Frequent paracentesis Severe dietary Na restriction (Sometimes Na intake is reduced to less than 100 mg. daily to control ascites.) Na moves into the cells to replace K loss (K loss is the result of diuresis, malnutrition, or hyperaldosteronism.)
Decreased plasma protein level (Hypoalbuminemia results in reduced plasma osmotic pull.)	Albumin lost in ascites (1 L. of ascites contains as much albumin as 200 ml. of whole blood) (Normally, blood flowing into and out of the liver has the same volume. In cirrhosis, however, the volume of hepatic venous outflow is reduced by one half. This mechanical blockage leads to the formation of an ultrafiltrate of blood which escapes into the abdominal cavity.) Decreased protein synthesis resulting from liver dysfunction
Generalized edema	Reduced plasma protein level allows fluid to leave the plasma space and enter the tissue space Excessive aldosterone and ADH levels cause fluid retention Portal hypertension causes increased hydrostatic pressure and, thus, edema of the lower extremities

Table 19-4. Water and Electrolyte Disturbances in Cirrhosis of the Liver with Ascites (*Continued*)

Water and Electrolyte Disturbance	Cause
Potassium deficit (severe potassium deficit is often a late manifestation of liver disease.)	Aldosterone level elevated (Recall that aldosterone causes K loss.) Poor dietary intake because of anorexia and nausea Prolonged use of potassium-losing diuretics
Elevated blood ammonia level (Ammonia ties up glutamic acid which is necessary for brain tissue functioning, and it interferes with glucose oxidation, upon which the brain relies for energy.)	Failure of the diseased liver to convert ammonia to urea (The kidneys produce ammonia and, normally, the liver converts it to urea; the urea is subsequently excreted by the kidneys. Failure of the damaged liver to convert ammonia to urea causes the ammonia level to rise.) Occurrence of gastrointestinal hemorrhage causes the intestine to digest blood proteins, in turn causing the ammonia level to rise
Respiratory alkalosis (which may occur if the ammonia level is high)	A high ammonia level acts as a respiratory stimulant and may induce hyperventilation
Magnesium deficit (which occurs in some cases of alcoholic cirrhosis)	Poor dietary intake Alcohol produces magnesium diuresis
Calcium deficit may occur	Possibly a result of inadequate storage of vitamin D by the diseased liver

hypoglycemia (glycogen metabolism impaired)

spider angiomata (dilated superficial vessels resembling small bluish-red spiders may appear in the skin of the face and trunk)

palmar erythema

enlarged male breasts and atrophy of testicles (caused by the liver's inability to deactivate estrogen)

embarrassed respirations if the amount of ascites is large (however, if a high ammonia level is present, hyperventilation may occur)

enlarged abdominal veins, esophageal varices, and internal hemorrhoids caused by portal hypertension (these may be sites of profuse hemorrhage)

increased bleeding tendencies resulting from vitamin K deficiency and decreased prothrombin formation

deficiency of vitamins A, C, and K caused by inadequate formation, utilization, and storage by the liver

intensified reaction to certain medications, caused by the liver's inability to detoxify them (morphine and barbiturates should be avoided in patients with advanced liver disease)

greater susceptibility to infection, secondary to decreased formation of antibodies by the liver

elevated ammonia level at first causes dullness, drowsiness, loss of memory, slow, slurred speech, and personality changes—later these may progress to confusion and disorientation and, finally, to stupor and coma

"hepatic flap" is caused by a high ammonia level—this tremor is characterized by spasmodic flexion and extension at the wrists and fingers, as well as lateral finger twitching (hepatic flap can be elicited in susceptible patients by elevating the arms, hyperextending the hands, and spreading the fingers)

Patients with ascites are treated with low sodium diets and diuretics; accurate intake-output records, weight charts, and abdominal girth measurements are helpful to the physician in planning the degree of sodium restriction and the diuretic regimen. Dietary restriction of sodium to less than 200 mg. daily prevents additional fluid retention in most patients. Without the need for frequent paracentesis, protein is conserved and a high caloric, moderately high protein, vitamin supplemented diet may be better utilized. If dietary sodium restriction alone does not suffice, diuretic therapy may be necessary. It is best not to use furosemide, ethacrynic acid, thiazide, or mercurial diuretics daily because of the danger of potassium deficit. Potassium supplements may be given when hypokalemia is a problem. An aldosterone blocking agent may be used in conjunction with other diuretics when advanced disease causes more resistant fluid retention. (Recall that an aldosterone blocking agent, such as spironolactone [Aldactone], causes sodium excretion and potassium retention.) Bedrest often is useful in inducing diuresis in the patient with refractory ascites. Eventually, patients with ascites become refractory to diuretics and require paracentesis to relieve severe symptoms of intra-abdominal pressure and respiratory distress.

As much as 20 L. of ascitic fluid may accumulate in one week; unfortunately, its removal only causes more to form. Paracentesis further depletes the body of protein, sodium, and water. The patient should be observed for symptoms of circulatory collapse following the removal of a large volume of fluid by paracentesis, since a rapid shift from the plasma to the ascitic fluid space may follow the procedure; acute sodium depletion may also follow paracentesis. There is reaccumulation of ascitic fluid with flow of water and sodium from the interstitial fluid and secondarily from the plasma into the abdominal cavity, reducing plasma volume and sodium concentration. Water is retained in excess of sodium and further dilutes its concentration in plasma. The nurse should be alert for pallor, weak and rapid pulse, and hypotension following the removal of a large amount of fluid by paracentesis. Removal of as little as 1000 to 1500 ml. may precipitate hypotension in some patients. Sometimes salt-free albumin is administered intravenously to correct hypoalbuminemia; however, the quantity that is practical to give is often ineffective in restoring a normal plasma albumin level.

A low plasma sodium level is an indication to restrict the patient's water intake; the amount of water restriction must be prescribed by the physician. Fluids must be evenly spaced over the waking hours to avoid excessive thirst and discomfort. Severe edema may also necessitate fluid restriction.

Bleeding in the gastrointestinal tract increases ammonia formation (caused by digestion of blood proteins) and may precipitate hepatic coma. The nurse should be alert for gastrointestinal bleeding in the stool (melena) and in the vomitus (hematemesis). Sometimes enemas or cathartics are used to rid the intestine of blood and, thus, decrease ammonia formation. Ammonia formation caused by excessive bacterial growth in the small bowel can be decreased by the administration of bowel sterilizing antibiotics, such as neomycin. Constipation contributes to the accumulation of ammonia and must be prevented. (Ammonium chloride should not be used in diuretic therapy since it elevates blood ammonia level.)

Impending hepatic coma is an indication to temporarily eliminate protein from the diet. A decrease in protein intake results in decreased ammonia formation; as the patient improves, more protein can be added to the diet. Thiazide diuretics may increase ammonia formation and contribute to the development of hepatic coma. (Loss of potassium, caused by diuresis, apparently increases the tendency to ammonia accumulation.)

ANTACIDS AND ELECTROLYTE BALANCE Numerous antacid preparations are available commercially (Table 19-5) and are widely used (with or without the advice of a physician). Their purpose is to raise gastric pH to a level of at least 3.5 (to prevent pepsin activity). While effective in alleviating gastric distress, these agents are capable of disrupting electrolyte balance. Among the more common neutralizing agents are aluminum hydroxide, magnesium hydroxide, calcium carbonate, magnesium trisilicate, and sodium bicarbonate.

Aluminum hydroxide (Amphojel) frequently is used for its ability to relieve gastric acidity; however, this preparation can have a constipating effect. To counteract this effect, aluminum hydroxide is combined with magnesium hydroxide (which has a tendency to produce osmotic diarrhea). Examples of a combination of aluminum hydroxide and magnesium hydroxide include Aludrox, Maalox, and Mylanta. Aluminum hydroxide is sometimes used to bind phosphate in the intestines, causing the elimination of phosphate from the body. This effect is desirable in the treatment of certain cases of renal failure. However, excessive use may cause hypophosphatemia. Symptoms can include nausea, fatigue, muscle weakness, and osteomalacia. *All aluminum-containing antacids may prevent proper absorption of tetracyclines and, thus, should not be used when tetracyclines are prescribed.*

Magnesium hydroxide and other magnesium salts should not be used for patients with renal insufficiency since a small portion of the magnesium may be absorbed, causing hypermagnesemia. Symptoms

Table 19-5.   Antacids

Preparation	$Al(OH)_3$	$Mg(OH)_2$	$CaCO_3$	$MgCO_3$	$NaHCO_3$	Mg Trisilicate	$KHCO_3$
Alka-2			X				
Alka-Seltzer					X		X
Aludrox	X	X					
Alurex	X	X					
Amphojel	X						
Camalox	X	X	X				
Delcid	X	X					
Gelusil	X					X	
Maalox	X	X					
Marblen	X		X	X			
Mylanta	X	X					
Titralac			X				

include lethargy, coma, and impaired respiration. Magnesium trisilicate (present in Gelusil) may cause silicate renal stones after prolonged use.

Calcium carbonate is a very effective antacid, yet it should not be the sole agent for continued antacid therapy. Hypercalcemia may result since some of the calcium is absorbed; renal stones may occur secondary to hypercalcemia. Also, an acid-rebound effect results as calcium stimulates the release of gastrin. The consumption of large amounts of calcium carbonate can cause the milk-alkali syndrome with nausea, vomiting, confusion, polydipsia, polyuria, and deterioration of renal function. Plasma calcium levels should be checked periodically when calcium carbonate is used. (The dose of calcium carbonate should not exceed 8 Gm. in 24 hours.) It should be remembered that calcium preparations may also cause constipation. Examples of commercial calcium carbonate preparations include Titralac, Tums, and Alka-2.

Long-term use of sodium bicarbonate as an antacid is not recommended since it is absorbed into the bloodstream and can cause metabolic alkalosis. Patients requiring low-sodium intake should avoid sodium bicarbonate preparations since they have a very high sodium content (276 mg. of Na in each Alka-Seltzer tablet and 1000 mg. of Na in a teaspoon of baking soda). These preparations are frequently used as home remedies for "acid" indigestion even though the antacid effect is short-lived since they are rapidly emptied from the stomach.

A number of antacid preparations contain sizable amounts of sodium and, thus, should be used cautiously when sodium-restriction is necessary. Magaldrate (Riopan) has a low-sodium content (0.7 mg. per 5 ml.) and may be recommended for patients requiring a low-sodium intake.

Some physicians recommend mixing each liquid antacid dose with water to ensure that it enters the stomach rather than merely lining the esophagus; others recommend mixing the antacid with a glass of water and sipping the mixture over an hour's time. Antacid tablets should be chewed and followed by a glass of water to help them dissolve.

REFERENCES

1. **Stahlgren, G., Morris, N.:**   Intestinal obstruction. Am. J. Nurs. 77:1002, 1977.

BIBLIOGRAPHY

Boedeker, E., and **Dauber, J.** (eds.):   Manual of Medical Therapeutics, ed. 21. Boston: Little, Brown & Company, 1974.

Condon, R., and **Nyhus, L.** (eds.): Manual of Surgical Therapeutics, ed. 3. Boston: Little, Brown & Company, 1975.

Costrini, N., and **Thomas, W.** (eds.): Manual of Medical Therapeutics, ed. 22. Boston: Little, Brown & Company, 1977.

Given, A., and **Simmons, S.:** Gastroenterology in Clinical Nursing, ed. 2. St. Louis: C. V. Mosby, 1975.

Guyton, A.: Textbook of Medical Physiology, ed. 5. Philadelphia: W. B. Saunders Co., 1976.

Hogstel, M.: How to give a safe and successful cleansing enema. Am. J. Nurs. 77, May 1977.

Literte, J.: Nursing care of patients with intestinal obstruction. Am. J. Nurs. 77, June 1977.

Macleod, J. (ed.): Davidson's Principles & Practice of Medicine, ed. 11. New York: Churchill Livingstone, 1975.

McConnell, E.: All about gastric intubation. Nursing 75, Sept., 1975.

— 20 —

Fluid Balance in the Patient with Urologic Disease

Among their numerous cardinal functions, the kidneys excrete water, electrolytes, and organic materials and conserve whatever amounts of these substances the body requires. They act both autonomously and in response to blood-borne messengers, such as the mineralocorticoids and antidiuretic hormone. Failure of renal function causes a variety of water and electrolyte disturbances.

ACUTE RENAL FAILURE

Acute renal failure is of rapid onset (over days or weeks) and implies a pronounced reduction in urine flow in a previously healthy person. The condition can be caused by:

1. Severe and prolonged shock
2. Severe fluid volume deficit
3. Hemolytic blood transfusion reaction (lysis of red blood cells results in renal vasoconstriction and tubular blockage with hemoglobin)
4. Severe crushing injuries (severely crushed muscles release large amounts of myoglobin into the blood stream; myoglobin can block the tubules and might also produce vasoconstriction)

5. Nephrotoxic chemicals (such as lead, mercury, arsenic, and carbon tetrachloride)
6. Drugs (such as phenacetin, sulfonamides, streptomycin, kanamycin, radiographic contrast agents, tetracycline, and amphotericin)
7. Endotoxemia
8. Renal vascular occlusion

Patients with these conditions should be observed for the possible development of acute renal failure. The nurse should measure the urinary output carefully, as well as all other fluid losses and gains. A reduced urinary output may be due to excessive fluid loss through another route, to inadequate intake, or to acute renal failure. A urinary output under 400 ml. in the adult represents oliguria and should be reported.

Acute renal failure may be classified as either reversible or irreversible. In irreversible renal failure, kidney function does not return and uremia progresses. Reversible acute renal failure can be divided into two phases—oliguria and diuresis.

Oliguric Phase

The first manifestation of acute renal failure is decreased urinary output, usually appearing within a few hours after the causative event. Anuria is rare (except with urinary tract obstruction); instead, a 24-hour output of about 50 to 150 ml. is the rule for the first few days. After this time, the urine output gradually increases. The oliguric phase may last one day or several weeks; the average duration is 10 to 12 days in severe cases.

The nurse should be alert for symptoms of the major problems of this phase. They include potassium excess, fluid volume excess, metabolic acidosis, and uremia. Other problems include calcium deficit, sodium deficit, and anemia. Death usually is due to cardiac arrest caused by potassium excess or pulmonary edema caused by fluid volume excess.

POTASSIUM EXCESS Potassium excess usually occurs in the oliguric phase. Recall that the kidneys normally excrete 80 per cent or more of the potassium lost daily from the body. When the kidneys are not functioning, potassium excretion is greatly reduced. If no protein or potassium is ingested and if sufficient calories are supplied to prevent endogenous cellular catabolism, it is unlikely that serious potassium excess will develop during the first few weeks of oliguria. However, patients with massive crushing injuries or large quantities of necrotic tissues may have a rising plasma potassium concentration despite no intake of protein and potassium, since catabolized necrotic tissue releases potassium into the extracellular fluid. The presence of acidosis augments the intracellular to extracellular shift of potassium, thereby hastening potassium buildup in the plasma. Recall that the normal plasma potassium level is 5 mEq./L. ECG changes caused by hyperkalemia (6.5 to 8.0) may include tall tented T waves, depressed ST segments, low amplitude P waves, prolonged PR intervals, and widened QRS complexes with prolongation of the QT interval. (The typical alterations are best seen in leads V_2 and V_4.) A plasma potassium level above 9 mEq./L. may cause severe cardiac arrhythmias and cardiac standstill. Excessive potassium causes weakness, and dilatation of heart muscle and cardiac arrest in diastole.

The nurse should be alert for the symptoms of potassium excess. They include the following:

ECG changes (described above)
anxiety and restlessness
muscular weakness progressing to flaccid paralysis (primarily affects limbs and respiratory muscles)

respiration decreased as a result of respiratory muscle weakness
decreased pulse rate, finally resulting in bradycardia
cardiac arrhythmias
falling arterial blood pressure
cardiac arrest and death

Treatment
Restricted Intake. Dietary potassium intake should be sharply restricted and potassium-containing medications should be discontinued. The potassium content in certain medications is often overlooked. For example: Penicillin G contains 17 mEq. of potassium per 10 million units. Salt substitutes should not be allowed since they contain potassium also. Potassium-conserving diuretics (triamterene and spironolactone) are contraindicated since the additional potassium retention could prove lethal. Stored bank blood may contain as much as 30 mEq. of potassium per liter and should not be used to transfuse patients with renal damage.

Cation Exchange Resins. Cation exchange resins may be used to increase potassium excretion from the bowel. The resins may be taken by mouth, if tolerated, or may be instilled as a retention enema. When the resin is administered orally, the solution in which it is suspended should be recorded as part of the daily fluid allowance. While the cation exchange resins are given to remove potassium ions from the intestinal tract, they also remove other cations, such as sodium, calcium, and magnesium. It may be necessary to replace these ions if the resins are used for more than a few days. Such patients should have regular electrolyte studies.

Sodium polystyrene sulfonate (Kayexalate) is a sodium-potassium exchange resin. During its use, sodium ions are partially released by the resin in the intestine and replaced by potassium ions from the body. The bound potassium is then excreted in the feces. Hypokalemia may occur if the effective dose is exceeded; therefore, it is necessary to determine the plasma potassium level daily. Since sodium is released in the intestine during electrolyte exchange, the resin should be given with caution to patients with heart failure. Each gram of resin adds approximately 2 mEq. (46 mg.) of sodium. Signs of excessive sodium retention include hypertension and edema. The average adult oral dose of sodium polystyrene sulfonate is 15 Gm., 1 to 4 times daily in a small quantity of water or syrup. Sorbitol, a liquid that promotes osmotic diarrhea, may be mixed with the resin to increase the excretion of the bound potassium. The patient should be told that mild diarrhea is desired when Kayexalate is used. The resin may also be given as an enema; each adult dose, usually 30 Gm., is administered in 150 to 200 ml. of water. Best results are achieved when the emulsion is warmed to body temperature before use. The enema should be retained as long as possible (a rectal tube with an inflatable balloon may be necessary for some patients). The enema vehicle administered with the cation exchange resin should be measured before instillation and after expulsion of the cation resin enema. Oral administration of Kayexalate may be preferred because it allows the resin to come into contact with a greater surface area of the gastrointestinal tract than is possible with rectal administration.

Cation exchange resins are of most value as a preventive rather than an emergency measure to reduce severe potassium excess. Remember that cation exchange resins actually *remove* potassium from the body (approximately 1 mEq. of potassium per Gm. of resin).

Emergency Measures Emergency measures to temporarily relieve dangerously high hyperkalemia (>7.0 mEq./L.) may include the following:

1. The intravenous injection of $NaHCO_3$ solution (such as 44 mEq. over a 5 minute period) causes rapid movement of potassium into the cells, temporarily lowering the plasma potassium level (1 to 2 hours). This procedure may have to be repeated if the ECG still shows remarkable abnormalities or other symptoms persist. The patient should be observed for sodium overload and calcium deficit (tetany).

2. The intravenous administration of calcium gluconate (5 to 10 ml. of a 10 per cent solution) or calcium chloride acts rapidly to provide temporary myocardial protection from the toxic effects of hyperkalemia without actually lowering the plasma potassium level. (Recall that calcium antagonizes the cardiac effects of potassium.) This procedure is best done under constant ECG monitoring.

3. The intravenous infusion of hypertonic dextrose (usually 50 per cent dextrose in water) and regular insulin, temporarily reduces the plasma potassium level by forcing potassium into the cells. (Recall that insulin causes dextrose to enter the cell, taking potassium with it.) These substances are usually

given in the ratio of 1 unit of regular insulin to 5 Gm. of dextrose. (The regular insulin is sometimes given subcutaneously.) This form of treatment may take from half an hour to an hour; however, it usually is effective for several hours.[1] Once begun, insulin-dextrose therapy should not be stopped until the total body potassium has been reduced by other means since dangerous shifts of potassium from the cellular to the extracellular space may occur, with the return of hyperkalemia. Also, rebound hypoglycemia should be observed for after the administration of a concentrated carbohydrate solution since the pancreas may continue to secrete extra insulin for a short period after the carbohydrate is discontinued.

These emergency measures for treatment of hyperkalemia have only temporary effects. They serve to "buy time" for the institution of treatment measures to actually rid the body of excess potassium (such as cation exchange resins, hemodialysis, or peritoneal dialysis).

Dialysis Usually hyperkalemia can be controlled by conservative measures; however, dialysis (either hemodialysis or peritoneal dialysis) is indicated when conservative treatment is ineffective. Dialysis can also be indicated to correct serious metabolic acidosis, uremia, pulmonary edema, and deterioration in the patient's general condition. (Hemodialysis works more rapidly in relieving these disturbances.) Toxic drug ingestion (such as barbiturates, salicylates, meprobamate, and amphetamines) may also be treated by dialysis. A description of peritoneal dialysis and hemodialysis is presented here with a comparison of their advantages and disadvantages.

Peritoneal Dialysis. Because of its large surface area (22,000 sq. cm.), the peritoneum can be used as a dialyzing membrane for the removal of toxic substances, body wastes, and water and electrolytes, by the processes of osmosis, filtration, and diffusion.

Advantages of peritoneal dialysis (PD) include the following:

1. All hospitals can use PD, while hemodialysis (HD) usually is available only in larger medical centers. PD techniques are less complex and are more easily learned than those of HD. PD requires only a fraction of the personnel and equipment needed for HD.
2. Fluid and electrolyte shifts occur more gradu-

ally in PD than in HD, making hypotensive episodes and arrhythmias less apt to occur. (Nonetheless, careful attention must be given to maintaining fluid and electrolyte requirements and plasma electrolyte concentrations should be checked at regular intervals.)

3. Immediate life-threatening events (such as hemorrhage and embolism) are not as apt to occur during PD as in HD, making patients less fearful to use it (particularly in the home situation).

4. Patients in whom it is difficult to maintain the adequate vascular access necessary for HD may be treated with PD. PD also is indicated for patients with shock when arterial blood flow is insufficient for HD.

5. Infants and young children may be treated effectively with PD. (HD is technically difficult to perform on young children.)

6. Patients who refuse blood transfusions (such as Jehovah Witnesses) and those in whom anticoagulation is considered dangerous (recent surgery, gastrointestinal bleeding, or bleeding defects) may be treated with PD.

7. It has been suggested that PD more efficiently removes yet to be characterized uremic toxins in the "middle molecular" weight range (400 to 5000 daltons) than does HD because the peritoneal membrane is more permeable.[2]

8. PD may be started quickly (within minutes) while HD requires a longer period to initiate (a minimum of 45 minutes and, more often, 1 to 3 hours). Time may be a significant factor in some situations.

The following are disadvantages of peritoneal dialysis:

1. It is considerably slower than HD (urea clearance is only about 26 ml./minute with PD as compared to 70 to 170 ml./minute with HD). Patients on PD require at least four times as much dialyzing time as those on HD.

2. Bacterial or chemical peritonitis is a common complication of PD. It is evidenced by pain and tenderness of the abdomen, a sense of fullness, and the slow return of a cloudy dialysate fluid. (Recall that the dialysate should normally be returned a pale yellow color.)

3. Protein loss occurs during PD since plasma protein diffuses into the dialysate. An average of 0.5 to 1.0 Gm. of albumin is lost per exchange. Frequent plasma protein level checks should be made and dietary intake of complete proteins should be encouraged, as indicated, to correct hypoproteinemia. If dietary replacement is inadequate, albumin may be infused intravenously.

4. Certain conditions, such as gangrenous bowel, bowel perforation, localized peritonitis, ileus with abdominal distention, abdominal drains, extensive abdominal adhesions, or severe pulmonary insufficiency preclude the use of PD.

5. Use of hypertonic dextrose solutions in PD may cause hyperglycemia and hyperosmotic coma, particularly in diabetic patients and when repeated dialyses with prolonged dwell times are performed. Blood sugar levels should be monitored and insulin given as necessary. Urinary sugar should be tested at regular intervals. Sorbitol is sometimes used to render dialysates hyperosmotic; its absorption does not cause hyperglycemia but may cause hyperosmotic coma.

6. Crowding of the thoracic organs by a large volume of dialysate solution occasionally can precipitate acute pulmonary edema. Symptoms include dyspnea, tachycardia, tachypnea, rales, and orthopnea. If this situation occurs, the dialysate fluid must be withdrawn rapidly.

A solution for peritoneal dialysis must, in most instances, approach the electrolyte composition and tonicity of the plasma so that normal plasma constituents will not be altered (Table 20-1). It must be at least slightly hyperosmotic to plasma to prevent its absorption with development of fluid volume excess.

Table 20-1. Approximate Electrolyte Content of Peritoneal Dialysis Solution

Electrolytes	Usual Ranges
Sodium	140–141 mEq./L.
Potassium	0–4 mEq./L.
Calcium	3.5–4.0 mEq./L.
Magnesium	1–1.5 mEq./L.
Acetate or lactate	43–45 mEq./L.
Chloride	101–102 mEq./L.

Various concentrations of dextrose or sorbitol may be used to render the solution hyperosmotic. Dialysis solutions with 1.5 per cent dextrose are available commercially.* These slightly hyperosmotic solutions are useful in removing abnormal plasma constituents, such as barbiturates, or excessive amounts of normal plasma constituents, such as potassium or calcium. A 1.5 per cent solution usually leaves fluid balance status quo unless the dialysis rate is rapid. A stronger hyperosmotic effect can be achieved with the use of a dialysate containing a 4.25 per cent dextrose concentration,* resulting in a more rapid removal of fluid. Dialysis solutions are available with or without potassium; potassium is omitted only in cases of hyperkalemia. Solutions containing about 4 mEq. of potassium per liter are used for patients with normal plasma potassium levels. (If the patient has hypokalemia, a solution with a greater than normal potassium concentration may be employed.) Varying concentrations of potassium, depending on the patient's need, may be added to potassium-free solutions. The addition of potassium is particularly important for digitalized patients, since the plasma potassium may fall rapidly during dialysis. (Recall that potassium deficit makes the patient more susceptible to digitalis toxicity.)

It is desirable to warm the dialysis solution to body temperature before administration. Infusion of the dialysate at body temperature is more comfortable for the patient, increases peritoneal clearance by 35 per cent, and prevents hypothermia. The bottles can be warmed by immersion in a warm water bath set at 37° C. (98.6° F.) Rubber bands should be used to hold the wet labels in place; a glass marking pencil can be used to indicate the contents of the bottle. To avoid contamination of the equipment, the outside of the bottles should be dried carefully before use. A warming cabinet is sometimes used to warm the dialysis solution; care should be taken to avoid overheating. Air should be cleared from the administration tubing since air pockets in the peritoneal cavity impede drainage.

Medications should be added before the bottles are hung for infusion. Heparin is added to prevent the formation of fibrin clots (the dose is not sufficient to produce systemic heparinization). Antibiotics may be added to the dialysate if necessary. Extreme care is required to prevent contamination when medications

* Inpersol (Abbott Laboratories); Dianeal (Travenol Laboratories; Peridial (Cutter Laboratories).

are added; the most frequent serious complication of peritoneal dialysis is peritonitis. Some dialysates are available in single 2 L. bottles; because medications are added to only one container, the opportunity for contamination is reduced. If two separate 1 L. bottles are used, contamination risk can be minimized by adding medications to only one of the bottles. (Solutions from two separate bottles mix quickly in the abdomen.)

Prior to the initiation of peritoneal dialysis, the patient should be given a careful explanation of the treatment; reassurance and support are required throughout the lengthy procedure. The position of choice during peritoneal dialysis is a modified semi-Fowler's. Meperidine (Demerol) may be given one-half hour before the insertion of the catheter to achieve analgesia and sedation.

Before insertion of the peritoneal catheter, the bladder and colon should be emptied to avoid injury. Inadvertant bowel perforation with the catheter results in pain and fecal drainage in the dialysate return, or copious watery diarrhea. If the catheter is accidentally introduced into the bladder, the patient may void dialysate solution. Accidental introduction of the catheter into a blood vessel causes blood to appear in the catheter or in the first dialysate return. The patient's weight and vital signs should be checked, prior to the procedure, for later reference. Peritoneal dialysis can be done either manually (Fig. 20-1) or by machine.

After the abdomen is shaved and prepared, an abdominal paracentesis is performed and a catheter inserted into the peritoneal cavity. Two liters of solution are allowed to enter in about 10 minutes. If the patient complains of discomfort when the fluid is instilled, the flow rate may have to be reduced; the physician should be notified if the pain does not subside. Analgesics may be administered if necessary; lidocaine may be added to the dialysate to alleviate pain. If the pain persists, the physician may need to change the location of the peritoneal catheter.

The fluid is left in the peritoneal cavity about 20 minutes and then is drained into a bottle or plastic drainage bag. (Drainage of the fluid from the peritoneal cavity should not take much longer than 20 minutes.) To facilitate drainage, it may be necessary to massage the abdomen gently or adjust the patient's position.

The dialysis solution is instilled and drained at regular intervals until the patient shows definite im-

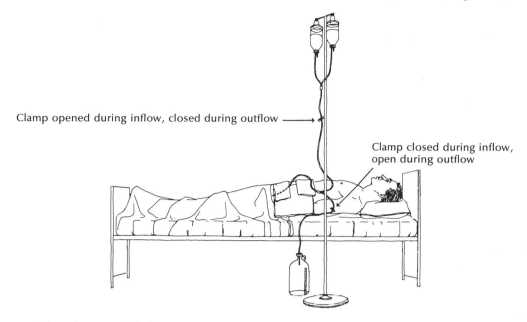

Clamp opened during inflow, closed during outflow ⟶

Clamp closed during inflow, open during outflow

Figure 20-1. Manual peritoneal dialysis setup. (Modified from Inpersol, pp. 16–17. Abbott Laboratories, North Chicago, Illinois, 1964)

provement. Peritoneal dialysis usually is performed for 24 to 72 hours in the adult patient. Some authorities state that the optimum dialysate flow rate is 2.5 L. per hour. To achieve this rate, one dialysis cycle lasts about 48 minutes.[3]

The nurse should use meticulous technique during peritoneal dialysis to prevent peritonitis. Abdominal dressings should be checked frequently for bleeding or leakage of solution; if either occurs, the physician should be notified. Wet dressings should be changed immediately to minimize the chance of wound contamination. Vital signs should be observed periodically for significant changes. The time each exchange begins and the amount of fluid instilled and removed should be recorded. When the total amount of drainage is more than the total amount of fluid infused, the patient's cumulative fluid balance is said to be negative. When the total amount of drainage is less than the total amount of fluid infused, the patient's cumulative fluid balance is said to be positive. The physician should stipulate the limits of positive and negative balance considered desirable for each patient.

A dialysis flow sheet is used to record the fluid exchange (Fig. 20-2). For each exchange, the nurse should record the starting time, amount of fluid instilled, its concentration and any added medications, finishing time of inflow, starting time of outflow,

color of outflow, finishing time of outflow, and the amount of positive or negative balance. (For example, if 2000 ml. were instilled and only 1800 ml. drained, the balance for this exchange would be +200 ml.) Vital signs should be checked frequently and the patient observed for signs of hypovolemia (particularly when a 4.25 per cent dialysate is used), peritonitis, fluid overload with respiratory difficulties (caused by dialysate pressing against diaphragm), hyperglycemia, glycosuria, and other complications.

Fluid intake and output from all routes should be measured and recorded. Finally, body weight measurements are often taken twice daily since these readings are invaluable in assessing the patient's state of fluid balance. Weight should be consistently measured at the same point during the dialysis procedure (such as immediately after the outflow is completed). Recall that 2 L. of dialysate fluid weigh approximately 2 kg. (4.4 lb). An in-bed scale is of great value in monitoring weight changes during dialysis. (See the section on weight measurement in Chapter 13.)

Hemodialysis. As mentioned earlier, hemodialysis works rapidly and effectively to control hyperkalemia and other serious fluid and electrolyte disturbances. The artificial kidney functions by allowing arterial blood to pass through numerous tiny thin membraned channels surrounded by a

PERITONEAL DIALYSIS RECORD

PATIENT_____ ROOM _____

ATTENDING PHYSICIAN _____

HOSPITAL NUMBER _____ AGE _____ SEX _____

DIAGNOSIS_____

_____

_____

WEIGHT PRIOR_____ WEIGHT ON COMPLETION_____

DATE	INPERSOL SOLUTION TYPE			MEDICATION ADDED TO SOLUTION	OTHER MEDICATION OR REMARKS	SOLUTION IN			SOLUTION OUT			DIFFERENCE PLUS OR MINUS	CUMULATIVE DIFFERENCE
	1.5%	1.5%K	4.25%			STARTING TIME	FINISH TIME	VOLUME	STARTING TIME	FINISH TIME	VOLUME		
	✔			KCl 8mEq		7$\frac{00}{A}$	7$\frac{10}{A}$	2000	7$\frac{30}{A}$	7$\frac{50}{A}$	2200	−200	−200
	✔			KCl 8mEq		7$\frac{50}{A}$	8$\frac{00}{A}$	2000	8$\frac{20}{A}$	8$\frac{40}{A}$	1900	+100	−100

97-0169/R1-1.25—APRIL. 1974   LITHO IN U.S.A.

Figure 20-2.   Peritoneal dialysis flow sheet. (Courtesy of Abbott Laboratories, North Chicago, Illinois)

dialysate bath. Unwanted substances pass through the membrane pores from an area of greater concentration to an area of lesser concentration until an equilibrium is reached. The cleansed blood is then returned to the body's venous system. Heparinization is required to prevent coagulation as the blood enters the artificial kidney. Protamine is added to the blood as it is returned to the body in order to prevent bleeding.

Hemodialysis requires highly trained personnel for safe performance. The reader is referred to more specific texts on hemodialysis techniques if detailed information is desired.

The following complications may accompany hemodialysis:

1. Accidental separation of the cannula tubing during dialysis, resulting in hemorrhage. The shunt is also subject to infection, clotting, and erosion.
2. Dialysis disequilibrium syndrome may occur as a result of the more rapid removal of urea from blood than from the brain, causing water to osmose into the brain, with resultant cerebral edema. Symptoms include mental confusion, hallucinations, nausea, vomiting, visual blurring, leg cramps, peripheral paresthesias, anxiety, hyperventilation, and convulsions. (This disturbance has occurred during PD, although much less frequently, since PD reduces the BUN more slowly than HD.)
3. Blood reactions are always a possibility when blood is administered, particularly to patients who have received multiple transfusions in the past. (Blood transfusion reactions are described in Chapter 16.)
4. Hepatitis may occur from the administration of hepatitis-contaminated blood.
5. Heparinization may result in bleeding from a recent surgical site or from an area of ulceration in the gastrointestinal tract.
6. Cardiac arrhythmias may occur for a number of reasons: electrolyte imbalances, fluid overload, hypotension, or anemia. The cause must be identified and treated appropriately. Antiarrhythmics may be administered as indicated.
7. Hypotension may result from ultrafiltration or when the blood flow from the patient to the dialyzer is rapid.

8. Hypertension may result from fluid overload, anxiety, or disequilibrium syndrome.
9. Cramping of muscles may result from rapid sodium and water removal or neuromuscular hypersensitivity.

Measures to Reduce Catabolism Factors contributing to catabolism include immobilization, infection, fever, and adrenocorticosteroid administration. Moderate activity should be encouraged as soon as possible and infections should be treated promptly with appropriate antibiotics, usually in reduced doses owing to diminished renal function. If the patient has dirty wounds, undrained pus collections, or necrotic tissue, the plasma potassium concentration rises as a result of catabolism. To prevent severe potassium excess, it is important that necrotic tissue and pus be removed. Drugs such as adrenocorticosteroids, thyroid hormones, and tetracycline increase catabolism and, thus, should be avoided or used very cautiously in renal failure. In addition to increased catabolism, steroids may cause hypertension and edema. (Anabolic steroids appear to suppress catabolism and may be used in some renal patients to help avoid negative-nitrogen balance.)

EXTRACELLULAR FLUID VOLUME EXCESS

Fluid volume excess is a frequent problem during the oliguric phase when the body is unable to excrete excess fluid. Usually it is due to the excessive administration of fluids, either orally or intravenously.

Symptoms include elevated venous pressure, distention of neck veins, edema, puffy eyelids, bounding pulse and shortness of breath. Hypertension, pulmonary edema, and congestive heart failure are complications of fluid volume excess. Pulmonary edema is manifested by severe dyspnea, moist rales and frothy sputum.

Treatment The amount of fluid administered must be carefully planned to suit the patient's needs, with the body considered as a closed system. Excessive fluid intake should be avoided. The physician calculates a fluid dose that will just replace fluid losses from the body; insensible losses are approximately 500 to 600 ml. Each degree of Centigrade (celsius) temperature elevation/24 hours necessitates adding 100 ml. to the total fluid intake. The rest of the fluid dose matches the urinary output of the previous day and other losses, such as from vomiting or diarrhea. For example: assume that an 80 kg. male excreted, during a 24-hour period, 150 ml. of urine,

200 ml. of diarrheal fluid, 100 ml. of vomitus, and sustained a temperature elevation of 2° C. His fluid allowance for this day would include 600 ml. for basic insensible loss, 200 ml. for increased insensible loss due to fever, 200 ml. for diarrheal loss, 100 ml. for loss of vomitus, and 150 ml. for urine, totalling 1250 ml. The nurse must keep an *accurate* account of all routes of fluid gains and losses, because an inaccurate record could lead to a fluid overdose and fluid volume excess with its dangerous sequelae. (Nursing considerations in measuring and recording fluid intake and output are discussed in Chapter 13.)

The nurse should let the patient decide how his limited fluid intake will be distributed over the 24-hour period. If fluid restriction is severe, it may be necessary to provide a wet cloth to suck on to relieve oral dryness. Ice chips contain only half the volume of liquid water and may be used to help stretch the fluid intake; for example: a 200 ml. glass full of ice chips really contains only about 100 ml. of water, and ice chips are well received by most patients.

Accurate daily body weight measurements are also necessary for determining the desired fluid dose. (Nursing considerations in obtaining accurate body weight measurements are discussed in Chapter 13.)

Sodium intake usually is restricted to help avoid fluid volume excess. It is sharply restricted when hypertension and congestive heart failure are present.

METABOLIC ACIDOSIS Metabolic bodily processes normally produce more acid wastes than alkaline wastes. Thus, when the kidneys fail to function, acid accumulation exceeds alkali accumulation. Metabolic acidosis is the result of the retention of these acid metabolites; their accumulation in the bloodstream causes the pH to drop. Contributing to the metabolic acidosis is the kidneys' decreased ability to reabsorb bicarbonate from the glomerular filtrate. Acidosis parallels uremia in severity. Decreased food intake causes increased utilization of body fats and the accumulation of ketonic acids in the bloodstream; these acids further decrease the pH.

Vomiting commonly occurs with the development of uremia. If vomiting occurs at the time metabolic acidosis is developing, it is possible that the metabolic alkalosis accompanying vomiting may help to counteract acidosis. However, because gastric hypoacidity frequently occurs with uremia, vomiting may not have a significant effect on the pH. Extensive diarrhea contributes to the development of metabolic acidosis.

Metabolic acidosis causes a compensatory increase in pulmonary ventilation, which causes the elimination of large amounts of carbon dioxide from the lungs with a resultant decrease in the carbonic acid content of the blood. The pH is partially corrected by this mechanism. Anorexia, weakness, apathy, and coma may also be symptoms of metabolic acidosis.

Treatment The metabolic acidosis is tolerated fairly well and usually does not require treatment unless the plasma bicarbonate level is below 16 mEq./L. (normal 26 mEq./L.) or frank Kussmaul respiration, stupor, or coma occurs. Alkalinizing agents such as sodium bicarbonate or sodium lactate may be given orally or intravenously, as indicated, to elevate plasma pH. (Sodium salts must be administered with caution to prevent fluid overload.) Patients with cardiac difficulties may be treated with sodium-free buffer solutions such as tris-hydroxymethyl aminomethane (THAM) or with dialysis.

Calcium may be indicated when alkalinizing agents are given to treat acidosis, since symptoms of calcium deficit (tetany and seizurelike movements) may be induced by an increase in plasma pH. (Calcium ionization is decreased when alkalinity of the extracellular fluid increases.) Restoration of a normal pH may disclose a calcium deficit that was not evident when the plasma pH was below normal. Usually a depressed bicarbonate is restored only gradually and partially to normal to avoid this difficulty. Since calcium acts synergistically with digitalis, it must be administered cautiously to digitalized patients.

SODIUM BALANCE The plasma sodium concentration may be normal or below normal. Contributing to sodium deficit is the administration of excessive amounts of water, which dilute the plasma sodium. Sodium deficit may also be due to a shift of sodium into the cells, particularly if acidosis is present. Occasionally, sodium deficit becomes severe as a result of excessive loss of sodium in vomiting or diarrhea. Failure of the kidneys to excrete sufficient sodium, caused by reduced glomerular filtration rate, may result in sodium retention. Sodium retention, in turn, leads to water retention with resultant fluid volume excess (described earlier).

Symptoms of sodium deficit include the following:

anorexia

apathy or apprehension

abdominal cramps

syncope on changing positions

hypotension

rapid thready pulse

cold skin

convulsions (if sodium deficit is due to excessive water intake)

Symptoms of fluid volume excess were described earlier in the chapter.

Sodium deficit usually is treated by limiting the water intake. Occasionally, hypertonic solution of sodium chloride is administered slowly intravenously in a small dose to correct a severe sodium deficit produced by excessive vomiting or diarrhea. Hypertonic solution of sodium chloride should be administered with *caution* because it can easily result in fluid volume excess with congestive heart failure and pulmonary edema.

Fluid volume excess is treated by limiting sodium and fluid intake (described earlier in chapter).

CALCIUM AND PHOSPHORUS DERANGEMENTS

The plasma calcium concentration may be below normal; calcium deficiency may be related to the increased concentration of phosphorus in the bloodstream. (Phosphorus is a constituent of one of the retained metabolic acids.) A reciprocal relationship exists between calcium and phosphorus so that an increase in one causes a decrease in the other. Decreased absorption of calcium from the gut occurs in uremia and contributes to the hypocalcemia.

The major significance of calcium deficit is that it enhances the toxic effects of potassium on the heart. (Recall that calcium and potassium have antagonistic actions on heart muscle.)

A plasma calcium level below 2 mEq./L. usually causes tetany; however, these symptoms rarely occur in renal failure since the decreased blood pH of metabolic acidosis favors calcium ionization. (Recall that calcium ionization increases in acidosis and decreases in alkalosis.) Chvostek's sign may be positive even though other symptoms of calcium deficit are not present. If metabolic alkalosis develops as a result of treatment with alkaline fluids, calcium deficit becomes manifest with the development of muscle twitching and convulsions. The ECG is usually normal but may show a prolonged QT interval.

Sustained hypocalcemia resulting from hyperphosphatemia causes the parathyroid glands to hypertrophy in an attempt to compensate for the low calcium level by production of parathormone. Calcium is withdrawn from the osteoid tissue and eventually results in bone changes if the calcium-phosphorus derangement persists. (See discussion of bone changes under chronic renal failure section.)

Calcium deficit can be treated with calcium gluconate by the oral or intravenous route—orally if nausea and vomiting are absent, intravenously in all other cases. Ten to 20 ml. of a 10 per cent calcium gluconate solution (usually given over a 20- to 40-minute period) is the recommended intravenous dose for an adult. Calcium, as mentioned earlier, can cause pronounced improvement in ECG changes produced by potassium excess, even though the plasma potassium concentration is not changed.

Some physicians administer vitamin D in the active form (25-hydroxy-cholecalciferol) in an attempt to increase calcium absorption from the gut. Measures to reduce the high phosphorus level may cause an increased calcium level. Therefore, aluminum hydroxide gels (Amphogel and Basalgel) may be administered to combine with phosphate in the gastrointestinal tract. Phosphate-binding gels may not be well accepted by patients since they can cause constipation, nausea, and vomiting. (Excessive use of these gels can cause phosphate depletion and hypercalcemia.)

MAGNESIUM EXCESS The plasma magnesium level may increase when oliguria is present as a result of decreased renal excretion of this substance. Hypermagnesemia may be intensified to a serious level when magnesium-containing drugs are administered, such as magnesium sulfate, milk of magnesia, Mylanta, Gelusil, Maalox, and Creamalin. Symptoms include weakness, drowsiness, impaired respiration, orthostatic hypotension, and coma. Magnesium excess is primarily a disorder of acute and chronic renal disease and contributes to the central nervous features associated with uremia.

URINE CHANGES The urine usually is bloody for the first few days, becoming clear about the end of the oliguric phase. If renal failure is due to hemolytic blood transfusion reaction, the urine has a port wine color. As renal failure advances, there is a tendency for the urinary specific gravity to become fixed at a low level (isosthenuria), similar to that of the glomerular filtrate (close to 1.010). A low specific gravity indicates that the renal tubules have lost their ability to concentrate urine.

ANEMIA   Anemia may develop within 48 hours after the onset of acute renal failure. The red blood cells are normal in color (normochromic) and shape (normocytic) but are decreased in number. The hematocrit usually stabilizes at a level of 20 to 25 per cent.

The inadequate production of a renal enzyme that stimulates release of erythropoietin is the probable cause of anemia. (Recall that erythropoietin normally stimulates the bone marrow to produce red blood cells—a deficit of this substance, thus, results in anemia.) Other factors that may contribute to the occurrence of anemia include high plasma levels of urea, potassium, and hydrogen ions. It has been found that the life span of red blood cells is decreased when uremia is present, further contributing to the development of anemia. The low hemoglobin level predisposes to acidosis since the buffering action of hemoglobin is diminished.

Mild bleeding, such as bruising or bleeding of gums, may occur early. Severe bleeding may occur into the gastrointestinal tract, lungs, or brain. The cause of the bleeding tendency in uremic patients is thought to be related to platelet defects resulting in impaired conversion of prothrombin to thrombin. Decreased platelet adhesiveness increases bleeding time.

The anemia of renal failure usually is tolerated well unless the hemoglobin level falls below 7 Gm./100 ml. of blood. Severe anemia may be manifested by fatigue, dyspnea on exertion, palpitations, tachycardia, and angina.

Unless symptoms are present, anemia usually is left untreated. Sometimes transfusion is absolutely necessary owing to active bleeding, angina, or hypovolemia. If so, it is best to give fresh frozen packed red cells since the risk of hyperkalemia is less than when bank blood is used; also, the risk of fluid volume overload is less. Unfortunately, the transfused cells have a shortened life span (probably a result of the abnormal constituents in the patient's blood). Transfusions depress normal bone marrow reticulocytosis, may cause hepatitis, and increase antibody levels that can later cause rejection of renal transplants. Washed cells keep the leukocyte antigenic exposure to a minimum, making rejection of a future transplant less likely to occur.

Androgenic steroids may be given for their erythropoietic effect. Administration of androgens to females causes masculinizing effects such as deepening of the voice, increased hair growth, and skin thickening.

INFECTION   Patients with acute or chronic renal failure are highly susceptible to infection; in fact, infection is a major cause of mortality in such patients. Exposure to others who are ill must be avoided; also, the patient should receive adequate rest periods and avoid chilling. Indwelling urinary catheters frequently cause urinary tract infections and should not be used in patients with renal failure unless absolutely necessary. If a catheter is required, it should be connected to a closed drainage system to minimize contamination. Scrupulous perineal and catheter care are indicated along with the application of betadine or a topical antibiotic at the catheter's point of entry into the urethra. Culture and sensitivity tests should be performed when infection does occur. Altered antibiotic metabolism in uremia may make treatment of infection difficult. The dosage of potentially nephrotoxic antibiotics must be adjusted to each patient's renal function and metabolic status. Sulfonamides should be avoided since they cause crystalluria when the urine flow rate is low.

UREMIA   Uremia is a toxic condition caused by failure of the kidneys to excrete urea, potassium, organic acids, and other metabolic waste products. It is described in the section on chronic renal failure.

DIETARY MANAGEMENT

High Carbohydrate and High Fat Intake   Liberal carbohydrate and fat intake is indicated to decrease endogenous protein catabolism and to prevent ketosis of starvation. Such catabolism is harmful, since it releases potassium and nitrogenous products into the extracellular fluid and plasma levels of these substances rise. Administered glucose forms glycogen, essential for restoration of cellular potassium stores.

Oral carbohydrate intake should be encouraged if nausea and vomiting are not present. Sometimes these symptoms can be relieved by dimenhydrinate (Dramamine) or diphenhydramine (Benadryl). (Hard candy supplies carbohydrates.)

Intravenous carbohydrate administration is necessary if oral intake is impossible. A hypertonic carbohydrate solution must be used to supply the necessary amount of carbohydrate and to avoid excessive fluid administration. A 20 per cent glucose solution may be administered by slow drip over the 24-hour period.

Fat provides less water of oxidation than carbohydrate or protein; thus, it is least likely to cause an excessive fluid volume. Frozen butter balls, ranging in size from 5 to 15 Gm., frequently are administered to achieve a high caloric intake. Some are prepared with powdered sugar to increase palatability and caloric value.

Tube feedings composed of Lipomul (a fat emulsion), glucose, vitamins, and water have been administered to patients with acute renal failure to increase caloric intake. Use of tube feedings can be hazardous, however, when frank uremia is present, because of the possibility of producing gastric bleeding. Fat emulsions are also available for intravenous use (see Chapter 16).

The aim of the diet in uremia is to give as many nonprotein, nonelectrolyte calories as possible. Unfortunately, the need for fluid restriction sometimes interferes with caloric intake.

Restriction of Potassium and Protein Intake High potassium foods should be excluded from the diet because the nonfunctioning kidneys are unable to excrete potassium. Examples of foods to avoid include bananas, citrus fruits, fruit juices, tea, coffee, legumes, and nuts. Since salt substitutes contain potassium they should not be used.

The diet should be low in protein. Four Gm. of protein furnish 1 Gm. of urea; hence, a high protein intake adds to the severity of the uremia. In addition to urea, protein foods provide potassium, sulfates, phosphates, and water. Only sufficient protein for maintenance and repair needs are given; minimum requirements in the adult approximate 10 to 20 Gm./day. Dietary protein should consist of complete proteins (eggs, milk, fish, poultry, and meat). Such proteins provide essential amino acids that cannot be manufactured by the body.

Restriction of Fluid Intake As mentioned earlier in the chapter, the amount of fluid administered must be carefully computed with the body considered as a closed system. The physician calculates a fluid dose that will just replace sensible and insensible losses, relying heavily on the nurse to supply accurate intake and output records as well as weight charts. The patient should be allowed to decide how his limited fluid intake will be distributed over the 24-hour period. It may be necessary to provide a wet cloth to suck on to relieve oral dryness when fluid restriction is severe. Ice chips help stretch the allowed intake because they contain approximately half the volume of liquid water, yet are very satisfying.

Hyperalimentation Hypertonic dextrose and essential amino acids have been administered intravenously to renal failure patients, as a modification of the Giordanno diet, to lower the blood urea nitrogen (BUN) level. The Giordanno diet primarily involves the ingestion of essential amino acids with limited intake of nonessential amino acids. Under these circumstances, the blood urea nitrogen is split to ammonia, reabsorbed, and made available for synthesis by transamination into nonessential amino acids. (Essential amino acids may also be administered orally as an elemental diet. Elemental diets are described in Chapter 14.) The essential and nonessential amino acids are then synthesized into protein.

Because the solution is hypertonic, many calories are contained in a small volume of liquid; thus, even oliguric patients may receive a substantial number of calories. Benefits of hyperalimentation in renal failure may include a somewhat lowered BUN and an improvement in the patient's ability to withstand complications. However, the hyperalimentation must be given cautiously at the prescribed rate to avoid fluid volume overload and hyperosmotic complications. Blood sugar levels should be monitored closely and insulin given as necessary. Electrolyte levels should also be closely monitored. (Hyperalimentation is described in Chapter 16.)

Diuretic Phase

The early diuretic phase begins when the 24-hour urine volume exceeds 400 ml./24 hr., usually around the tenth day after onset; in some instances, it may not occur for 14 to 21 days. The amount of urinary output depends on the treatment the patient received during the oliguric phase. If fluid overloading was allowed, the urine volume may be more than 5000 ml. daily. If the patient was well managed, the urine volume is not excessive. Urinary output usually increases in a stepwise manner, but occasionally increases rapidly.

During the early part of the diuretic phase, the partially regenerated tubules are unable to concentrate urine, and the glomerular filtrate is excreted virtually unchanged. Thus, the patient's condition does not improve in the first few days of the diuretic phase; indeed, uremia may be more severe during this period than at any other time. Convulsions, stupor, nausea, vomiting, hematemesis, bloody diarrhea, or hemorrhage may occur. The reason for the severity of the uremia lies in the rapid contraction of the total body fluid; early and prompt replacement of fluid is needed until the blood urea nitrogen level begins to fall. Dialysis may be indicated if uremia is severe. Later in the diuretic phase, metabolic wastes begin to be cleared.

Hypokalemia and hyponatremia should be watched for during this phase since potassium and sodium losses are increased when urine output is great. Urinary losses of these substances should be measured and replaced quantitatively, unless hyperkalemia is present. Body weight should be measured twice daily; if it decreases too rapidly, water and electrolytes must be supplied in sufficient amounts to prevent hypovolemic shock. Daily urine and plasma electrolyte levels should be measured in addition to daily hematocrits. Alkalinizing agents may be needed if acidosis is severe.

Prognosis is favorable for patients with little underlying disease and oliguria lasting less than ten days; it is unfavorable for those with severe underlying renal damage, prolonged oliguria, and advanced age. One fourth of the deaths that occur in acute renal failure occur during the diuretic phase as a result of infection (since the patient has extremely low resistance) or fluid and electrolyte problems.

CHRONIC RENAL FAILURE

Chronic renal failure occurs gradually over months or years and is the result of progressive irreversible loss of functional nephrons. Causes may include glomerulonephritis, pyelonephritis, polycystic kidneys, essential hypertension, or urinary obstruction. Chronic renal failure is sometimes classified into three stages:

1. Diminished renal reserve—renal function is somewhat diminished but the blood urea nitrogen level remains normal; symptoms may include nocturia and polyuria. One of the earliest regulatory functions of the kidney to fail is the maximal urine concentrating ability. It becomes necessary for the

kidneys to excrete a large urinary volume (up to 3000 ml. a day) to rid the body of wastes.

2. Renal insufficiency—renal function is impaired to the point where metabolic wastes begin to accumulate in the bloodstream; homeostasis is usually maintained sluggishly.

3. Uremia—renal function is so markedly impaired that homeostasis can no longer be maintained; the blood urea nitrogen level rises sharply and serious fluid and electrolyte disturbances occur.

Prognosis is variable, depending on the degree of irreversible renal damage. Up to 90 per cent of glomerular filtration may be lost with little overt change, indicating the kidneys' remarkable homeostatic ability. (Man is normally born with two million nephrons; he can survive, although with difficulty, with as few as twenty thousand nephrons.[4]) Death is imminent when 97 to 99 per cent of the glomerular filtration rate is lost, unless the patient can be maintained on dialysis.

POTASSIUM IMBALANCES Plasma potassium concentrations vary widely in patients with chronic renal failure. Some have normal levels until oliguria and starvation occur, causing hyperkalemia. Other causes of hyperkalemia may include severe metabolic acidosis, catabolic illnesses, excessive protein intake, administration of stored blood, and gastrointestinal hemorrhage. Use of potassium-conserving diuretics (triamterene and spironolactone) may result in fatal hyperkalemia in renal failure. As a rule, hyperkalemia doesn't usually occur until late in chronic renal failure.

In some cases of chronic nephritis with polyuria, the plasma potassium may be low. Hypokalemia may also result from anorexia, vomiting, diarrhea, and excessive aldosterone production.

Since potassium metabolism varies from patient to patient, each patient must be evaluated individually to ascertain his need for potassium restriction or replacement.

METABOLIC ACIDOSIS In late chronic renal failure, metabolic acidosis occurs as a result of the impaired renal excretion of acid metabolites and the inability of the tubules to form ammonia. (The plasma bicarbonate level usually stabilizes at approximately 18 to 20 mEq./L.) Although the respiratory mechanism partially corrects the decreased blood pH, it is sometimes necessary to treat the acidosis medically;

sodium bicarbonate tablets may be given, in dosages of several grams a day, depending on the severity of the acidosis and on the sodium intake limitations. Acidosis usually is not treated unless the plasma bicarbonate is less than 16 mEq./L. or symptoms are present (such as anorexia, weakness, apathy, and coma). Drugs that impose an exogenous acid load (such as aspirin, ammonium chloride, or methionine) worsen acidosis and are contraindicated. Calcium administration may be necessary when alkalinizing agents are given to correct acidosis, since tetany may be induced by an increase in plasma pH.

SODIUM BALANCE   Sodium is lost in the urine, but the plasma level usually remains near normal if the patient is not placed on a severely restricted low-sodium diet, or if excessive sodium loss does not occur with vomiting and diarrhea. Some patients retain sodium when it is given in average amounts; fluid volume excess, hypertension, congestive heart failure, and pulmonary edema may result from excessive administration of salt to such patients.

The need for sodium intake varies with each patient. Desired dietary sodium intake is best gauged by observing the 24-hour urinary sodium output when the patient is on a known salt intake.

CALCIUM AND PHOSPHORUS DERANGEMENTS AND BONE CHANGES   Hypocalcemia and hyperphosphatemia occur in chronic renal failure when the glomerular filtration rate falls below 25 to 30 ml./min. (normal 100 to 120 ml./min.). Phosphates are retained in excess when renal function is impaired. Since a reciprocal relationship exists between phosphorus and calcium, *hyperphosphatemia causes hypocalcemia*. Decreased absorption of calcium from the gut occurs in uremia and contributes to the hypocalcemia.

Efforts should be made to reduce the phosphate level in the bloodstream (to 5 mg./100 ml. or less); dietary intake of phosphorus is restricted; and phosphate-binding gels are given orally to increase phosphate elimination. Symptoms of hypocalcemia rarely occur in renal failure patients since acidosis allows free ionization of calcium. Should tetany occur, calcium compounds may be administered orally or intravenously. Vitamin D may also be administered to increase calcium absorption from the intestine.

The low plasma calcium level stimulates the parathyroids, causing hyperplasia and increased secretion of parathyroid hormone. Excess of this hormone eventually causes dissolution of the bone and adds both calcium and phosphorus to the extracellular fluid; decreased bone density and strength occurs. Pruritus is often associated with calcium-phosphorus derangement and may disappear after subtotal parathyroidectomy, although this procedure is performed less frequently now than in the past.

Normal serum levels of calcium (9 to 10.5 mg./100 ml.) and phosphorus (3 to 4 mg./100 ml.) have a product of approximately 30 to 40. That is, the calcium level (9 to 10.5 mg./100 ml.) multiplied by the phosphorus level (3 to 4 mg./100 ml.) equals approximately 30 to 40. Normal plasma levels of these electrolytes prevent their precipitation into soft tissues such as the blood vessels, skin, joints, and myocardium. An attempt is made to keep the Ca × P product below 70. Metastatic calcification is said to occur when calcium precipitates in such areas as the joints, cornea of the eye, heart, or lungs.

Chronic negative calcium balance produces renal osteodystrophy in about half of the adult patients and in more than half of the children with chronic renal disease. Usually the bone disease is not severe enough to cause symptoms, although pain and stiffness of the limbs and joints may occur. Demineralization of bone, most often in the hands, may be revealed by x-ray pictures; sometimes it isn't discovered until autopsy. In childhood, chronic renal failure may cause bone lesions similar to those of vitamin D deficiency rickets; efforts are directed toward early renal transplantation.

One type of osteodystrophy (osteomalacia) is due to failure of calcium salts to be deposited in newly formed osteoid tissue. Another type of osteodystrophy (osteitis fibrosa) is due to reabsorption of calcium from the bone and replacement with fibrous tissue.

Treatment of renal osteodystrophy may include phosphate-binding gels, supplemental calcium, vitamin D, and, in extreme cases, parathyroidectomy.

ANEMIA   Normocytic, normochromic anemia occurs in almost all patients with chronic renal failure. (See the discussion of anemia under the section on acute renal failure.)

CARDIOPULMONARY CHANGES   Cardiopulmonary complications of chronic renal failure include congestive heart failure with pulmonary edema, pericarditis, pleurisy, and hypertension.

Congestive heart failure and pulmonary edema may occur when excessive salt and water are administered. Treatment consists of restricting salt and water intake, administration of diuretics (such as furosemide and ethacrynic acid, in modified doses), and administration of digitalis, also in a modified dose. (The digitalis dosage must be adjusted according to the patient's level of renal function to avoid digitalis toxicity.)

Pericarditis and pleurisy usually are late symptoms; they may be associated with myocarditis, cardiac tamponade, and pneumonitis. These conditions are most apt to occur when uremia is severe and are thought to be related to poor chemical control. Frequent hemodialysis is the treatment of choice for uncomplicated uremic pericarditis. Fluid may be aspirated from the pericardial sac when effusion is present, or a pericardiectomy may be performed.

Patients with chronic renal failure usually have at least a mildly elevated diastolic blood pressure for reasons that are not always clear. Severe or symptomatic hypertension must be treated with antihypertensives such as methyldopa or with propranolol.

UREMIA   Uremia is a toxic condition that may result from acute or chronic renal failure; it is caused by failure of the kidneys to excrete urea, creatinine, uric acid, organic acids, potassium, hydrogen ions, and other metabolic waste products. Symptoms of uremia may include the following:

chronic fatigue

nocturia

insomnia

anorexia (frequently caused by sight of food)

intractable vomiting (often occurs in early morning)

gastritis, hematemesis, and hiccoughs may occur

ammonia odor to breath and unpleasant metallic taste in mouth

stomatitis (salivary urea is hydrolyzed by urease into ammonia, causing mucous membrane irritation)

pruritus—skin is dry and scaly, with excoriations caused by scratching (probably related to calcium and phosphorus disturbances)

pale sallow skin resulting from anemia and urochrome deposition in skin—discoloration most prominent on face and other body parts exposed to light

increased bleeding tendency revealed by epistaxis, bleeding gums, easy bruising, petechiae, and conjunctival hemorrhage (probably caused by platelet defects)

coarse muscular twitching, first occuring during sleep

deep, rapid respirations (a respiratory attempt to compensate for metabolic acidosis)

chest discomfort (may be caused by pericarditis or pleurisy)

involuntary leg movements (restless leg syndrome)

peripheral neuropathy (numbness, pain, and burning sensations in legs and arms; these changes begin distally and are symmetrical—they may progress to motor weakness and paralysis)

decreased libido and impotency in males; suppressed ovulation, libido, and menstruation in females

hypertensive symptoms such as headache and visual difficulties (visual difficulties caused by retinal hemorrhages)

delayed wound healing (sutures need to remain in place longer than usual) and increased susceptibility to infection

hypothermia (patients with severe uremia may have body temperatures of 95° F (35° C.) or less, even when infection is present)

decreased tolerance for all drugs that are excreted by the kidneys

gradual diminution of mental acuity over a period of time, leading to coma (resulting from toxic substances in bloodstream and acidosis)

generalized convulsions

transient episodes of agitated psychotic behavior (hallucinations and paranoid delusions) interspersed with periods of lucidity

uremic frost (urea crystals excreted through sweat glands, heaviest on nose, forehead, and neck) is rarely seen today because of improved management of uremic patients

Treatment

Pruritis may be relieved by starch or vinegar baths. Nails should be kept short and clean to avoid skin trauma and infection caused by scratching. Application of lotions or aquaphor ointments help to relieve dry, cracked skin. Antipruritic medications should be given as necessary.

Good oral hygiene is essential to prevent oral infections and alleviate oral irritation caused by ammonium hydroxide; a 0.25 per cent acetic acid solution is beneficial as a mouthwash to help neutralize this substance. (Recall that ammonium hydroxide is formed in the mouth as a result of hydrolysis of oral urea.) Chewing gum, hard candy balls, and cold liquids are helpful in alleviating the unpleasant metallic taste caused by uremia.

Since the uremic patient is subject to disorientation and convulsions, his bed should remain in the low position with the side rails up. A padded tongue blade, suction apparatus, and oxygen equipment should be immediately at hand. An anticonvulsant (such as Dilantin or Phenobarbital) may be necessary.

Food should be served in small attractive servings since anorexia and vomiting are frequent problems. The patient should be encouraged to eat and drink as much of the prescribed diet as he is allowed. (Renal patients often under-eat since they find the food unpalatable and they frequently have anorexia and other gastrointestinal problems.) Gastrointestinal bleeding may necessitate the use of enemas to remove blood from the intestine and, thus, prevent elevation of the blood urea nitrogen.

DIETARY MANAGEMENT Patients with symptoms of chronic renal failure should have their protein intake reduced, a measure which alone may improve symptoms greatly. A caloric intake high enough to prevent endogenous protein catabolism is also indicated. Oral intake may be discouraged by the presence of nausea and vomiting; medication, such as chlorpromazine, may be required. The nurse should seek such an order when necessary to relieve the patient's nausea. Attractive small frequent feedings may encourage eating. Encouraging activity may also stimulate appetite, provided congestive heart failure requiring bedrest is not present.

Sodium restriction may be necessary for some patients and harmful to others. Those retaining excessive sodium and water require a low-sodium diet. On the other hand, patients who excrete large quantities of sodium in the urine require a normal diet to prevent sodium deficit. The physician has to determine sodium needs according to test diets and clinical observations, such as excessive weight gain. (Low-sodium diets are described in Chapter 14.) If

the plasma potassium level is elevated, foods containing potassium should be eliminated.

Patients with chronic renal failure should be urged to drink from 2000 to 3000 ml. of water daily to aid in the elimination of urinary waste products. *If the patient is unable to excrete large volumes of water, however, fluid intake should be limited to his needs.* In the final stages of chronic renal failure, patients may experience extreme thirst, probably a result of cellular dehydration produced by the increased osmotic effect of the high urea level. Such patients may drink themselves into dilutional hyponatremia. Thirst is an unreliable guide to the uremic patient's state of hydration.

(See the discussion of dietary management of acute renal failure presented earlier in the chapter.)

CHRONIC PERITONEAL DIALYSIS It has been estimated that the number of potential new patients requiring treatment for end-stage renal failure in the United States each year is at least 70 to 80/one million of population; it has been suggested that peritoneal dialysis may be the treatment of choice for 10 to 30 per cent of these patients.[5] Although chemical control in peritoneal dialysis is not as good as in hemodialysis, patients seem to do equally well clinically. Maintenance peritoneal dialysis has been made more feasible for selected patients with chronic renal failure by two technical advances: (1) automated peritoneal dialysis equipment and (2) bacteriologically safer peritoneal catheters.

A closed, automated dialysate delivery and drainage system offers several advantages over manual dialysis in that there is a reduction in cost for dialysate and nursing time and the incidence of peritonitis is reduced. Also, patients may be trained to use these machines at home more easily than hemodialysis equipment.

One kind of an automated peritoneal dialysis machine sterilizes tap water by the reverse osmosis water treatment process. (Incoming water is forced through a semipermeable membrane and is then deionized to produce pure water.) The purified water is mixed with a concentrated peritoneal dialysate in a 19:1 ratio via proportioning pumps. The dialysate is pumped into the peritoneal cavity at a variable rate, remains there for the specified dwell time, and is then drained passively by a siphon effect. Adjustable timers control the duration of each step and alarms are activated when preset limits are violated. The incidence of peritonitis is less with automated peritoneal dialysis than with the manual method since breaks in the sterile system by repeated manual exchange of bottles of dialysate are not necessary. Some patients start dialysis at bedtime and disconnect themselves in the morning, allowing more free time to be active during waking hours. Usually peritoneal dialysis is performed three or four times a week, for 8- to 12-hour periods. (See the discussion of peritoneal dialysis in the section on acute renal failure for a review of the manual procedure, advantages, and disadvantages of this method of dialysis.)

Some researchers report that long-term peritoneal dialysis alleviates uremic symptoms and controls the incidence of renal osteodystrophy and uremic neuropathy to a level comparable to that found in patients undergoing hemodialysis.

The Tenckhoff peritoneal catheter is made of silastic tubing and has two attached dacron felt cuffs; one to fit in the subcutaneous tissue above the peritoneum and the other below the skin exit site. The tip of the catheter has many openings and rests in the pelvic gutter. If the catheter is too long, the patient complains of a poking sensation in this area, particularly when sitting down. Tissue grows into the cuffs in 10 to 14 days with complete healing in 2 to 4 weeks; the cuffs anchor the catheter, acting as infection barriers (Fig. 20-3). Once healed, the patient may shower and carry on normal day-to-day activities. Self-examination for skin exit infection should be taught; only patients willing to maintain good aseptic technique should become candidates for insertion of a long-term peritoneal catheter. Daily catheter care may include the application of betadine and a light sterile dressing. The external end of the catheter is covered with a removable rubber cap when not in use. Several hundred milliliters of dialysis solution may be left in the peritoneal cavity after dialysis to prevent catheter plugging. Poor drainage from the catheter may be caused by constipation, malposition, or obstruction from infection. The catheter is removed if an infection develops in the subcutaneous tunnel or if other problems develop. Although pain may occur during the first few weeks after insertion, there should be no discomfort after this period. Average catheter life is nine months.

HEMODIALYSIS Hemodialysis is an established method for treating chronic renal failure patients. However, limitations in available facilities and trained personnel, plus the high cost of this treatment, have restricted its use to only a fraction of those in need. Long-term hemodialysis may be performed at home, in selected cases, after extensive training periods in hemodialysis centers.

The use of arteriovenous shunts has made long-term hemodialysis available to chronic patients. Before shunts were available, frequent cannulation of blood vessels rendered them useless and prevented frequent hemodialysis. Although valuable, external A-V shunts are not without problems; they are subject to infections and thrombosis, despite meticulous care. A technique has been developed by Brescia and associates for anastomosing the distal radial artery and adjacent vein side-to-side, creating a subcutaneous A-V fistula. This internal shunt has several advantages over external shunts: (1) it allows the patient more freedom; (2) it does not require maintenance care; (3) it decreases the risks of clotting and infection; and (4) it is not cosmetically undesirable. A disadvantage to the use of an internal shunt is that two venipunctures with large gauge needles are required with each dialysis treatment. (Hypertrophy of the venous side of the fistula allows access to it by repeated venipunctures.)

Blood should not be drawn from the arm with the shunt, nor should blood pressure be checked on this arm.

NEPHROTIC SYNDROME

Nephrotic syndrome refers to the concurrent occurrence of marked proteinuria, hypoalbuminemia, and generalized edema. Causes of nephrotic syndrome may include inflammatory renal disease (e.g., acute glomerulonephritis), glomerular disease associated with another systemic disease (e.g., secondary syphilis), mechanical disorders (e.g., thrombosis of a renal vein), poisons (e.g., mercury), and miscellaneous causes (e.g., renal transplant). All the causes of nephrotic syndrome involve the glomeruli, and all result in tubular degeneration with increased permeability to plasma proteins.

Owing to increased glomerular permeability, large amounts of albumin are lost through the kidney, resulting in decreased plasma osmotic pressure. (Recall that albumin provides about 90 per cent of the plasma colloid oncotic pressure). Hypoalbuminemia causes fluid to be lost from the plasma to the interstitial space and also into the potential spaces of the

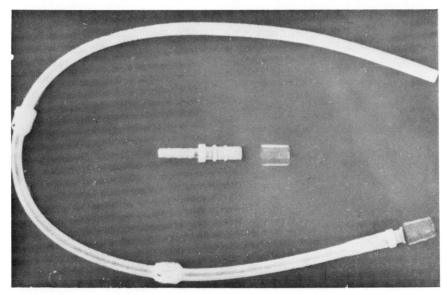

Figure 20-3. Tenckhoff silastic catheter with two attached dacron felt cuffs, connector, and cap. (From Clinical Digest, Vol. 6, March 1977. McGaw Laboratories, Santa Ana, California, with permission)

body (such as the abdominal cavity, pleural cavity, and the pericardium). Edema develops first in dependent parts and later becomes generalized. Edema may be slight or may be incapacitating.

Protein losses in the urine may amount to as much as 30 to 40 Gm. per day; the high protein losses result in malnutrition, and this, in turn, is responsible for muscle wasting. Most of the excreted protein is albumin and the albumin blood level is usually reduced to about 2.5 Gm./100 ml. (normal is 3.5 to 5.5 Gm./100 ml.). Hyperlipemia (abnormally high blood lipids) is also present; the high concentration of plasma lipids results from failure of the tissues to remove lipoproteins from the plasma, a condition especially apt to occur in nephrotic children.

Sodium retention is also a factor in nephrotic edema; it may be due to decreased glomerular filtration, increased tubular reabsorption, or both. Large quantities of aldosterone may be found in the urine when edema is present.

For extremely edematous patients, intravenous administration of albumin temporarily increases the protein osmotic effect of blood and draws the edema fluid into the intravascular space, increasing blood volume, and stimulating urine excretion. The patient should be observed carefully during this treatment to avoid cardiovascular overload. Unfortunately, the effects of albumin administration are only transient because the kidneys continue to leak this

substance. A high protein diet will be of some benefit.

Sodium restriction helps relieve nephrotic edema. Adrenal corticosteroids may be used to decrease proteinuria and increase urine output. Although it is thought that steroids may affect glomerular permeability and inhibit the secretion of ADH, their exact actions in relieving edema are not known.

Severity of symptoms in nephrotic syndrome are variable; some patients feel well and others are debilitated. Children tend to recover while some adults go on to develop renal insufficiency.

URETERAL TRANSPLANT INTO THE INTESTINAL TRACT

Electrolyte Imbalances

Ureteral transplants can be made into the sigmoid colon (ureterosigmoidostomy), terminal end of the ileum (ureteroileostomy), or into a segment of the ileum isolated from the intestinal tract (ileal-conduit). Patients with ureteral transplants into the intestinal tract may develop metabolic acidosis and eventually potassium deficit. Patients with ureterosigmoidostomies are much more apt to develop these disturbances than are those with ileal-conduits because the urine is exposed to a larger surface of bowel and the time of stagnation is longer.

Metabolic acidosis occurs when urine is re-absorbed from the intestinal tract. Recall that urine is usually acid (average pH of 6) and has a high chloride content. Absorption of urinary chloride into the bloodstream causes a compensatory decrease in bicarbonate. The decrease in the bicarbonate side of the carbonic acid–base bicarbonate balance causes the blood pH to drop.

Potassium deficit occurs, largely as the result of excessive renal chloride excretion. This can be explained in the following way: urinary chloride is absorbed from the intestine into the bloodstream and must eventually be re-excreted by the kidneys. A cation, such as potassium or sodium, is excreted with chloride. The continued absorption of urinary chloride by the intestine can deplete the body of potassium. Other factors contribute to potassium deficit. Patients with ureteral-intestinal transplants often have diarrhea, a common cause of potassium deficit. Also, it is possible that the dilute (hypotonic) urine stimulates intestinal secretions to achieve isotonicity. (Recall that all substances entering the gastrointestinal tract assume the tonicity of the area of the tract in which they are located, provided they remain there long enough.)

Intestinal secretions are rich in potassium; if the urine is excreted from the intestine before absorption can take place, the potassium of the intestinal secretions is lost with the urine, further depleting the body's potassium stores. In addition to pH decrease, potassium deficit, and perhaps mild sodium deficit, the blood urea nitrogen level is elevated, resulting from the absorption of urinary urea from the intestine into the bloodstream. The patient with electrolyte disturbances following ureteral transplants may have weakness, intense fatigue, anorexia, nausea, and vomiting. When acidosis is severe, hyperpnea is noted.

CONTRIBUTING FACTORS TO DEVELOPMENT OF ELECTROLYTE IMBALANCES   Electrolyte disturbances do not occur in all patients with ureteral-intestinal transplants. Persons with normal renal function can withstand the absorption of urine without changes in pH or electrolyte levels. Some degree of renal damage must be present for patients with such implants to develop electrolyte imbalances. Unfortunately, many patients with good kidney function

develop renal damage as a result of urinary tract infections caused by intestinal organisms, and *then* begin to develop electrolyte imbalances.

Absorption of urine is increased when the urine remains in the intestine for a prolonged period. Thus, the likelihood of metabolic acidosis is greater in patients with ureteral-sigmoid transplants than in those with implants into the intact ileum since the sigmoid is larger than the ileum and can accommodate larger volumes of urine before peristalsis in initiated. Since exposure of a large area of the intestinal mucosa is associated with a higher urinary absorption than is the exposure of a small area, it is often better to transplant the ureters into an ileal conduit.

Prolonged periods of inactivity, as when the patient is bedfast during an illness, favor unsatisfactory urinary drainage. Stricture of the ileal-conduit stoma can also cause urinary retention.

TREATMENT   Treatment of the electrolyte disturbances usually consists of the administration of potassium and sodium, as gluconate, lactate, or citrate salts. Patients with ureteral transplants into the intact bowel may require the insertion of a rectal catheter to drain urine when they are confined to bed for a prolonged period. A low acid-ash diet may also be helpful. (See Chapter 14.) The success of treatment is inversely proportional to the degree of renal damage present.

NURSING IMPLICATIONS   To prevent or minimize electrolyte disturbances in patients with ureteral transplants into the intestine, the nurse should:

1. Encourage the patient to drink approximately 3000 ml. of fluids daily, unless intake is restricted. This amount of fluids ensures frequent emptying of the intestine.

2. Encourage the patient to walk; activity favors emptying of the intestines.

3. Encourage the patient with ureteral transplant into the intact bowel to evacuate every few hours. This practice limits the absorption time of urine.

4. If the patient has an ileal-conduit, see that the ileostomy bag is emptied before it is completely full so that urine drainage will not be hindered or back up into the ureters.

5. Look for and report symptoms of electrolyte disturbances, such as weakness, intestinal distention, soft flabby muscles, deep rapid respiration, and disorientation.

REFERENCES

1. **Maxwell, M.,** and **Kleeman, C.:** Clinical Disorders of Fluid and Electrolyte Metabolism, ed. 2. New York: McGraw-Hill Book Co., 1972, p. 755.

2. **Babb, A., et al.:** Bi-directional permeability of the human peritoneum to middle molecules. Proc. Eur. Dial. Trans. Assoc. 19:247, 1973.

3. **Harrington, J.,** and **Brener, E.:** Patient Care in Renal Failure. Philadelphia: W. B. Saunders Co., 1973, p. 90.

4. **Maxwell** and **Kleeman:** Clinical Disorders of Fluid and Electrolyte Metabolism, p. 697.

5. **Blumenkrantz, M.:** Maintenance peritoneal dialysis as an alternative for the patient with end-stage renal failure. Clinical Digest, McGaw Laboratories, Santa Ana, Calif. Vol. 6, March 1977, p. 1.

BIBLIOGRAPHY

Bennett, W., et al.: A guide to drug therapy in renal failure. J.A.M.A. 230, December 1974.

Cattran, D., et al.: Defective triglyceride removal in lipemia associated with peritoneal dialysis and hemodialysis. Ann. Intern. Med. 85:29, 1976.

Leaf, A., and **Ramzi, C.:** Renal Pathophysiology. New York: Oxford University Press, 1976.

Macleod, J. (ed.): Davidson's Principles and Practice of Medicine, ed. 11. New York: Churchill Livingstone, 1975.

O'Connor, P., et al.: Renal failure and peritoneal dialysis. Nursing 75, July 1975.

Sachs, B.: Renal Transplantation—A Nursing Perspective. Flushing, N.Y.: Medical Examination Publishing Co., 1977.

— 21 —

Fluid Balance in the Patient with Cardiac Disease

ALTERATIONS IN ELECTROLYTE CONCENTRATIONS: EFFECTS ON THE HEART

Electrolytes Affecting the Myocardium

Potassium, calcium, magnesium, and hydrogen ions influence neuromuscular irritability; therefore, deficient or excessive quantities of these ions can alter heart contractions.

POTASSIUM Potassium influences both impulse conduction and muscle contractility; alterations in its concentration may change myocardial irritability and rhythm. The normal plasma potassium concentration is from 4.0 to 5.6 mEq./L. ECG changes produced by plasma potassium level variations are illustrated in Figure 21-1.

   Hypokalemia A deficit of potassium causes increased myocardial irritability; a pronounced deficit may produce cardiac arrest in systole. Adverse effects may appear at a plasma level of 3 mEq./L. ECG abnormalities include the following:

   flat or inverted T waves
   prominent U waves
   depressed ST segments

QT interval often appears prolonged because of the superimposed U waves on T waves

   Hypokalemia potentiates the action of digitalis and may result in arrhythmias. Therapy for hypokalemia is aimed at replacing the lost potassium, usually in the form of potassium chloride. Replacement must be made slowly, over a period of several days. (See Chapter 16 for a discussion of nursing responsibilities in the administration of intravenous potassium solutions.) A number of potassium supplements are available for oral use.

   Hyperkalemia Potassium excess, on the other hand, has a depressant action on the heart, causing the heart to become dilated and flaccid and slowing of the heart rate. Cardiac manifestations may occur at a level of 6 mEq./L. but are uncommon when the plasma potassium level is less than 7.0 mEq./L. They commonly are present when the concentration is greater than 8.0 mEq./L. ECG abnormalities include the following:

   tall tented T waves
   widened QRS complexes
   diminished to absent P waves
   depressed ST segments
   ventricular fibrillation at high levels

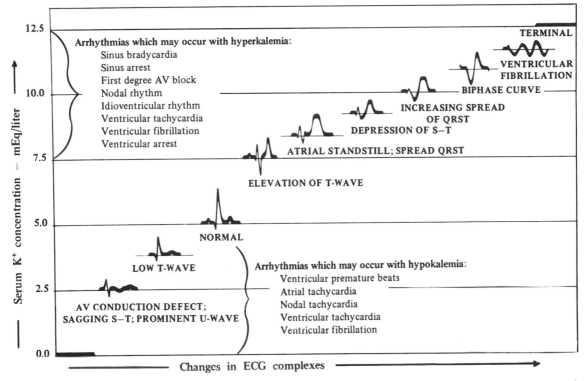

Figure 21-1. ECG changes at various levels of serum potassium concentration. (Reproduced, with permission, from Krupp, M. A., and Chatton, M. J. (eds.): Current Medical Diagnosis and Treatment. Los Altos, Calif: Lange Medical Publications, 1974, p. 24)

Elevation of the plasma potassium level to two to three times normal usually causes death through cardiac arrest during diastole (see Fig. 21-1). Severe hyperkalemia requires prompt and vigorous treatment. Objectives of treatment include:

1. Restriction of potassium intake in all forms (food, fluids, medications)
2. Elimination of excess potassium from the body (such as with cation exchange resins, peritoneal dialysis, or hemodialysis—these forms of treatment are discussed in Chapter 20)
3. Prevention of tissue catabolism (such as providing sufficient calories to prevent endogenous catabolism of body tissues and debriding necrotic tissues)
4. Depolarization of cardiac muscle by the slow intravenous administration of calcium gluconate (such as 5 to 10 ml. of a 10 per cent solution)—this form of treatment temporarily protects the myocardium from the cardiotoxic effects of hyperkalemia without actually lowering the plasma potassium level (the infusion should be stopped immediately at the first sign of bradycardia)
5. The forcing of potassium into the cells to "buy time" until excess potassium can actually be removed from the body—methods to force potassium into cells include:
   a. intravenous administration of hypertonic dextrose and regular insulin to promote the deposition of intracellular glycogen—usually effective for several hours (see page 521)
   b. intravenous administration of sodium bicarbonate (such as 44 mEq. over a 5-minute period) causes rapid movement of potassium into the cells, temporarily lowering the plasma potassium level for 1 to 2 hours

CALCIUM The effects of calcium on the heart are almost opposite those of potassium. Thus, calcium deficit depresses the heart in much the same way as does potassium excess. Because the actions of calcium and potassium are antagonistic, the two ions must be present in the proper ratio if normal heart action is to continue. For example, a deficit of calcium renders the myocardium more susceptible to potassium excess. (Conversely, the administration of a calcium solution helps alleviate the cardiotoxic effects of potassium excess.)

Calcium abnormalities are not seen often in the heart patient unless there is an associated noncardiac disease. A decrease in calcium ion concentration is rarely severe enough to alter cardiac function markedly since severe hypocalcemia will usually cause death from tetany before cardiac changes become pronounced. Hypocalcemia can produce the following cardiac changes:

> decreased contractility
> prolonged QT interval
> prolonged ST segment
> cardiac arrest in diastole

An elevation of calcium great enough to significantly affect the heart rarely occurs since calcium precipitates in bone or other tissues before such a level can be reached.[1] However, the rapid administration of calcium intravenously can have profound effects on the myocardium. Hypercalcemia can produce the following cardiac changes:

> increased contractility
> shortening of the QT interval (not diagnostic)
> cardiac arrest in systole

MAGNESIUM   A deficit of magnesium may cause ventricular premature beats; ventricular tachythmia may follow. Hypomagnesemia predisposes to digitalis toxicity. Magnesium excess can cause atrioventricular and intraventricular conduction abnormalities. A plasma magnesium level above 12 mEq./L. can cause cardiac changes (prolonged PR interval, prolonged QT interval, and widened QRS complex); heart block and death may occur.

SODIUM   An excess of sodium in the extracellular fluid can depress cardiac function. A very low sodium level (such as in water intoxication) can produce cardiac fibrillation. Hyponatremia increases the cardiotoxic effects of hyperkalemia.

pH CHANGES   Acid-base disturbances influence cardiac activity. Acidosis causes an increased heart

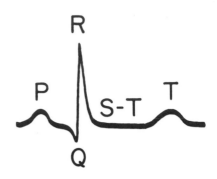

Figure 21-2. ECG changes produced by hypocalcemia. (From Sharp, L., and Rabin, B.: Nursing in the Coronary Care Unit. Philadelphia: J. B. Lippincott, 1970, p. 93, with permission)

rate because it stimulates the cardioaccelerator center, whereas alkalosis causes a slowed heart rate because it stimulates the vagus nerve. Acidosis in the range of 7.2 to 7.25 depresses cardiac output; at a pH of 7.1 the heart is not able to react normally to catecholamines.[2]

High concentrations of carbon dioxide in the blood can cause cardiac arrhythmias, both atrial and ventricular. Alkalosis promotes entry of potassium into the cells and, thus, lowers the plasma potassium concentration. Acidosis, on the other hand, promotes exit of potassium from the cells and may cause an elevated plasma potassium level (particularly if renal excretion of potassium is delayed). The effects of an excess or a deficit of potassium ions on the myocardium are described at the beginning of the chapter.

Electrocardiograms

The electrocardiogram (ECG) reflects the sum of all ionic influences on the myocardium. Therefore, disturbances in the concentrations of electrolytes alter ECG tracings. The ECG provides important diagnostic help in detecting disturbances in electrolyte concentration, especially of potassium and calcium (Fig. 21-2). Specific changes in the ECG are often associated with particular electrolyte disturbances, but these changes may also be produced by cardiac disease or certain medications. Also, it must be remembered that *not all* patients with electrolyte disturbances display the characteristic ECG changes. When these changes do occur, they do not necessarily occur at the expected level of concentration.

Evidence of an electrolyte disturbance on the ECG should be confirmed by plasma electrolyte studies. Changes resulting from myocardial damage tend to be localized, while changes caused by electrolyte disturbances often appear in all leads.

CONGESTIVE HEART FAILURE*

Heart failure is said to exist when the heart fails to discharge its contents adequately. The normal heart has the ability to adapt itself from second to second to widely varying amounts of venous return—from as low as 5 to 6 liters/minute at rest to as high as 15 liters/minute with vigorous exercise. Thus, the normally compliant ventricle is able to stretch and accommodate itself to increasing amounts of venous return without increasing the normal pressure at the end of the filling cycle—VEDP (ventricular end-diastolic pressure). The diseased heart, entering decompensated failure, loses its compliance or ability to stretch and accommodate venous return. Causative factors involved in congestive failure include inadequate ventricular filling (as in arrhythmias, mitral stenosis, or cardiac tamponade); increased work load of the heart muscle (as in vasoconstriction or anemia); and myocardial deterioration caused by infarction or cardiomyopathy.

With the development of increasing failure of the ventricular muscle, the pressure at the end of the filling cycle increases—increased VEDP. Heart failure may be the result of failure of the left ventricle, right ventricle, or, more commonly, both. Failure of one side of the heart eventually leads to failure of the other.

Left-Sided Heart Failure

Left-sided heart failure is primarily a backward failure which causes damming of blood back from the left side of the heart to the pulmonary vessels. Symptoms of pulmonary vascular congestion include dyspnea, orthopnea, dry cough, and pulmonary edema. Pulmonary capillary pressure above 30 mm. Hg. causes transudation of fluid into the alveoli and diminished oxygen-carbon dioxide exchange.[3] Acute pulmonary edema is characterized by severe dysp-

---

* This section on congestive heart failure was prepared with the assistance of Catherine A. Smith, R.N. M.S.N. Clinical Specialist in Cardiovascular Nursing, St. Louis, Missouri.

nea, profound anxiety, cyanosis, noisy respirations, and pink frothy sputum.

Physical signs associated with left-sided heart failure may include 3rd and 4th heart sounds (ventricular gallop and atrial gallop respectively) and fine moist rales in the lungs. Ventricular gallop in adults is almost never present in the absence of significant heart disease. Rhythms associated with left-sided failure may include sinus tachycardia, atrial premature contractions, paroxysmal atrial tachycardia, and ventricular premature beats. Other signs of left ventricular failure may include pulsus alternans (an alternating greater and lesser arterial pulse volume), expiratory wheezing breath sounds, and Cheyne-Stokes respirations.

Right-Sided Heart Failure

In unilateral right-sided heart failure, blood is not pumped adequately from the systemic circulation into the lungs; back pressure of the right heart causes systemic edema. Right-sided heart failure may result from stenosis of the pulmonary or tricuspid valve, cor pulmonale (chronic bronchitis, emphysema, bronchiectasis), or massive pulmonary embolism. Acute right-sided failure rarely occurs alone; when it does, symptoms are related to a low cardiac output. In rare conditions where the right heart fails acutely, cardiac output may be so low that death occurs rapidly. Chronic right-sided failure leads to progressive development of peripheral congestion, hepatosplenomegaly, and ascites. Failure of the right ventricle causes a rise in the right atrial and vena caval pressures. Neck veins will appear distended when the patient is lying in bed with the head of the bed elevated between 30 and 60 degrees (see Fig. 13-1). As with left-sided failure, sinus tachycardia and other rhythms associated with pump failure may be present. Right ventricular 3rd and 4th heart sounds may be heard.

Usually, right-sided heart failure is the result of left-sided failure; in this case, symptoms of both right- and left-sided failure are present.

Hemodynamic Monitoring in Heart Failure

It is possible to measure pressures on a continuing basis directly within the heart chambers and great vessels and to monitor cardiac output.

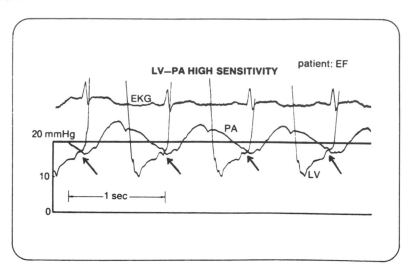

Figure 21-3. Simultaneous pressures are recorded from the pulmonary artery (PA) and left ventricle (LV) in a patient with acute myocardial infarction. At end-diastole the PAEDP and LVEDP are quite similar. Note arrows. (Reprinted with permission of the American Heart Association from Coronary Care—Invasive Techniques for Hemodynamic Measurement, 1973, p. 20. Arrows have been added by the author.)

FLOW-DIRECTED CATHETER   Left-ventricular function can be monitored indirectly by measuring pulmonary artery and pulmonary capillary wedge pressures with a flow-directed catheter. The catheter in the pulmonary artery provides an indication of the left ventricular end-diastolic pressure (LVEDP).

Consider that during left ventricular diastole the mitral valve is open and the pressures become equalized in the left ventricle and left atrium. This pressure is reflected retrogradely into the pulmonary veins, pulmonary capillary bed, and pulmonary artery. Thus, the pulmonary artery end-diastolic pressure (PAEDP) is a reflection of the left ventricular end-diastolic pressure (LVEDP) (Fig. 21-3). Monitoring PAEDP provides a guide to early changes in LVEDP—also known as left ventricular filling pressure. Increase in LVEDP in acute cardiac disease indicates failure of the left ventricle as a pump. The increased pressure is due to the diminished ability of the left ventricle to empty its contents.

Assessment of the LVEDP by means of the pulmonary artery pressure along with assessment of the RVEDP by means of the central venous pressure is a valuable guide to fluid deficit or overload. These two pressures must be evaluated together with the clinical status of the patient. Low pressures may indicate hypovolemia which may be corrected by increasing fluid administration.

Measurement of the PAEDP is useful also in monitoring the effectiveness of diuretics and other cardiovascular drugs.

The similarity between LVEDP and PAEDP would not be valid in persons with mitral disease, chronic obstructive pulmonary disease, or pulmonary hypertension.

One type of flow-directed catheter (Swan-Ganz) is illustrated in Figure 21-4. The catheter is used as a diagnostic tool to obtain hemodynamic pressures and to determine cardiac output via a cardiac output computer (Fig. 21-5). The 7F thermodilution catheter body is a quadruple-lumen design with a balloon at the distal end.

Lumen 1—terminates at the tip of the catheter. Chamber pressures, pulmonary artery pressure, capillary wedge pressures, as well as blood samples, can be obtained through this lumen.

Lumen 2—terminates 30 cm. from the catheter tip, placing it in the right atrium when the distal lumen opening is in the pulmonary artery (allowing simultaneous measurement of CVP and pulmonary artery pressure). This lumen carries the injectate necessary for cardiac output computation. An exact amount of dextrose solution of known temperature (such as 0 to 5° C. or 32 to 41° F.) is injected into the right atrium or superior vena cava and the resultant change in blood temperature is detected by the thermistor in the pulmonary artery. Cardiac output is inversely proportional to the integral of temperature change (the cooler the blood, the less is cardiac output, and vice versa).

Lumen 3—contains the electrical leads for the

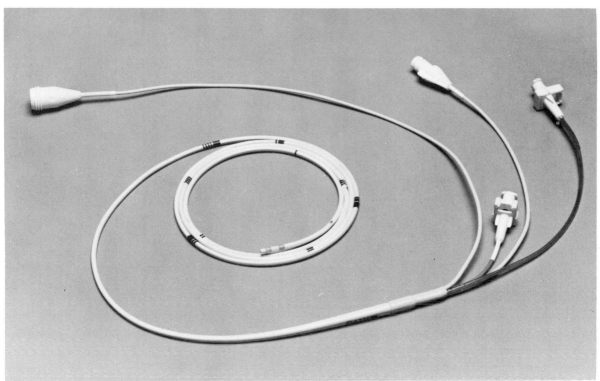

Figure 21-4. Swan-Ganz Flow-Directed Thermodilution Catheter (Model 93A-131-7F). (Courtesy of Edwards Laboratories, Division of American Hospital Supply Corporation, Santa Ana, Calif.)

thermistor, which is positioned at the catheter surface 4 cm. proximal to its tip.

Lumen 4—used to inflate and deflate the 1.5 cc. capacity balloon.

Insertion and Complications The flow-directed catheter is inserted by means of a cutdown or by percutaneous technique through a suitable needle or sheath. The catheter, connected to a transducer and monitoring system, is advanced into the vena cava near the right atrium; at this point, the balloon is inflated to the recommended volume. Filtered carbon dioxide is the inflation medium of choice since it is rapidly absorbed should the balloon accidentally rupture; however, air is sometimes used for reasons of convenience. The risk of balloon rupture and the possibility of air embolus entering the arterial system (as in the presence of intracardiac shunts) must be assessed by the physician prior to substituting air for carbon dioxide. The balloon must never be inflated with liquid (fluid interferes with balloon deflation and "flotability" of the catheter). The inflated balloon serves two purposes in the insertion procedure. First, it allows the catheter to be moved with the flow of

blood through the heart chambers; secondly, the inflated balloon covers the catheter tip, minimizing the occurrence of premature ventricular contractions during passage of the catheter. Care should be taken not to overinflate the balloon since rupture may occur.

The catheter is carefully advanced under continuous pressure and ECG monitoring. Usually it will pass within 10 to 20 seconds through the right atrium, through the right ventricle, into the pulmonary artery, and into the pulmonary wedge position (Fig. 21-6). Pulmonary artery pressure is observed as soon as the balloon passes through the pulmonary valve. Once the balloon becomes lodged in the wedge position, as noted on the pressure monitor, the balloon is quickly deflated. (Wedge position refers to lodging of the catheter in a small branch of the pulmonary artery.)

Lengthy balloon inflations during pulmonary wedge pressure recordings should be avoided since this is an occlusive maneuver and may cause infarction in the area of the lung supplied by the involved branch of the pulmonary artery. The balloon should be deflated as soon as the wedge pressure is recorded;

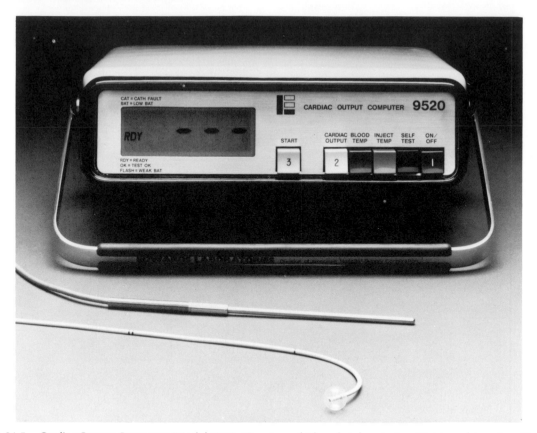

Figure 21-5. Cardiac Output Computer (Model 9520). (Courtesy of Edwards Laboratories, Division of American Hospital Supply Corporation, Santa Ana, Calif.)

it should never remain inflated more than 30 to 60 seconds.[4] After balloon deflation, the pulmonary artery contour pressure wave should return. Pulmonary infarction may be manifested by the sudden occurrence of hemoptysis.

Because the possibility of thromboembolic and infectious complications increases with the length of time of catheterization, the duration of catheterization should be limited to the minimum required by the patient's condition. Prophylactic antibiotics and anticoagulation protection should be considered when the catheter remains in place for more than 48 hours. Thrombus formation at the tip of the catheter can be prevented by the continuous infusion of a heparinized intravenous fluid. Care should be taken to maintain proper aseptic technique.

Pulmonary artery perforation may rarely occur; it can be prevented by keeping the balloon inflation time to a minimum and never using fluid as the inflation medium. Also, reinflation of the balloon should be done very slowly and stopped as soon as the wedge pressure is recorded. (The balloon should never be inflated beyond the capacity recommended by the manufacturer of the catheter.)

PRESSURE PARAMETERS Mean pulmonary artery wedge pressure should be less than 12 mm. Hg. Elevation above normal is seen in mitral stenosis, mitral insufficiency, and left ventricular heart failure.

Pressures may also be measured in the right atrium and right ventricle by the flow-directed catheter. Right atrial mean pressure should be less than 6 mm. Hg., right ventricular systolic pressure should be less than 30 mm. Hg., and right ventricular end-diastolic pressure should be less than 5 mm. Hg. Pulmonary artery systolic pressure, in the absence of pulmonary valvular disease, should be the same as right ventricular systolic pressure, i.e., 30 mm. Hg. or less. Pulmonary artery diastolic pressure should be less than 10 mm. Hg. Causes of increased right atrial pressure include hypervolemia and increased vascular tone; conversely, decreased right atrial pressure is caused by hypovolemia and by loss of systemic venous tone. Failure of the right ventricle causes a

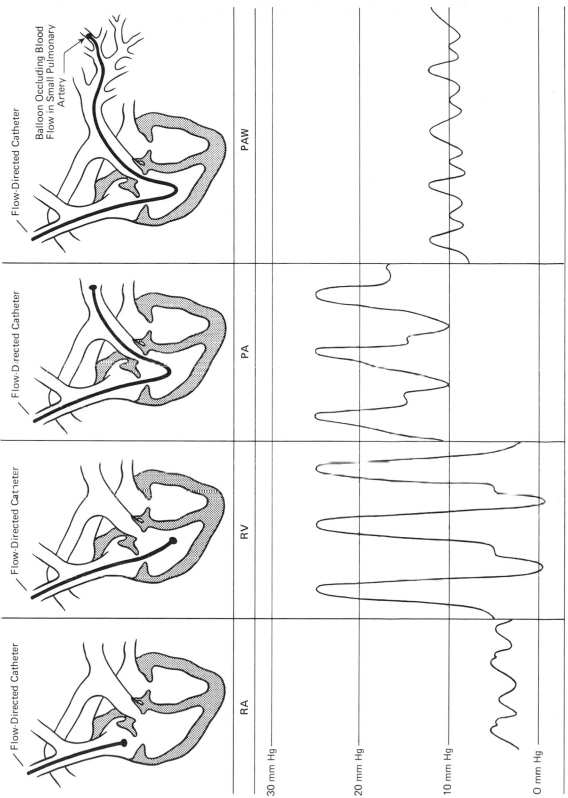

Figure 21-6. Flow-directed catheter positions with corresponding pressure tracings: right atrium (RA, right ventricle (RV), pulmonary artery (PA), and pulmonary artery wedge (PAW).

rise in right atrial pressure, as does tricuspid stenosis and pericardial tamponade. Abnormal right ventricular pressures are caused by right ventricular failure, pulmonary hypertension, pulmonary stenosis, pulmonary insufficiency, and untreated left-ventricular failure.

Right-sided heart performance can also be monitored by an ordinary CVP (central venous pressure) catheter. However, this is not a reliable procedure in assessing left heart function since left heart pressures are unpredictably transmitted to the right side of the heart. (The procedure for measuring CVP is described in Chapter 16.)

Compensatory Mechanisms in Heart Failure

The nurse should have a basic understanding of the pathologic and compensatory mechanisms involved in congestive heart failure so that nursing care can be based on sound physiologic principles.

ADRENAL CORTEX   Decreased arterial volume apparently stimulates increased secretion of aldosterone which, in turn, causes the retention of sodium and water, thus producing an increase in total blood volume. In fact, the secretion of aldosterone may increase to two or three times the normal level in patients with chronic congestive heart failure. Because of the hormone's potent sodium-retaining action, much attention has been focused on it as one of the major causes of edema in congestive heart failure. In addition to promoting sodium retention, aldosterone in excess causes excessive potassium excretion.

CENTRAL NERVOUS SYSTEM   Stimulation of the sympathetic nervous system occurs in congestive heart failure and apparently is an attempt to maintain circulation by causing increased heart rate, increased cardiac contraction force, and increased venous return to the heart.

Lowered arterial blood pressure causes increased antidiuretic hormone (ADH) secretion from the posterior pituitary. ADH acts on the distal renal tubules, causing water retention. Thus, patients with congestive heart failure frequently retain water in excess of sodium.

VASCULAR SYSTEM   Widespread vasoconstriction tends to compensate for the decreased circulating blood volume caused by weak heart action. The vasoconstriction affects both venous and arterial vessels and probably is due to sympathetic stimulation and the release of norepinephrine. Vasoconstriction is particularly pronounced in the kidneys and causes a further reduction in renal blood flow.

KIDNEYS   Renal perfusion is decreased as a result of low cardiac output and peripheral vasoconstriction. (Almost complete anuria can occur when the cardiac output falls to one half to two thirds of normal.[5]) The kidneys respond by retaining sodium and water; additional erythropoietin may be secreted in an attempt to increase the number of red blood cells and, thus, the oxygenation of body tissues.

LIVER   The increase in the venous blood volume may, in time, cause liver congestion or cirrhosis, with decreased hepatic function. Normally, aldosterone and ADH are inactivated by the liver. It is possible that the liver congestion of congestive heart failure contributes to edema by preventing the inactivation of these hormones.

Summary of Water and Electrolyte Disturbances Accompanying Congestive Heart Failure

A multitude of water and electrolyte disturbances are associated with congestive heart failure. The probable causes of these disturbances and the disturbances themselves are itemized in Table 21-1.

It is important that the nurse be aware of the water and electrolyte disturbances that can occur with congestive heart failure and with therapy. Such understanding is necessary for meaningful nursing observations. Knowledge of which fluid imbalances may occur enables the physician to institute suitable preventive measures.

Symptoms of Congestive Heart Failure

As mentioned earlier, congestive heart failure can be caused by a variety of conditions, including hypertension, myocardial infarction, disease of the valves, arteriosclerosis, and thyrotoxicosis. Although these conditions differ widely, they produce much the same clinical picture. Characteristic symptoms and their probable causes are listed in Table 21-2.

Table 21-1. Water and Electrolyte Disturbances in Congestive Heart Failure

Cause	Water and Electrolyte Disturbance

Excessive aldosterone secretion
 	
Decreased renal blood flow secondary to cardiac failure and vasoconstriction
	Increased retention of sodium and water by the kidneys resulting in:
	  Increase in total sodium content of body
	  Increase in total extracellular water volume

Excessive secretion of ADH causes increased retention of water	Relatively greater retention of water than sodium May depress serum sodium to abnormally low levels, even though the total body sodium is above normal
Hydrostatic pressure is increased by the excessive venous blood volume	Shift of fluid from the intravascular compartment to the interstitial compartment with edema
Excessive aldosterone secretion promotes potassium excretion Excessive use of potassium-losing diuretics or prolonged loss of potassium by vomiting or diarrhea represent typical causes of potassium deficit	Potassium deficit
Slowing of the circulation interferes with the excretion of metabolic acids and carbon dioxide Increased liberation of lactic acid from anoxic tissues and failure of the body to metabolize it rapidly	Mild metabolic acidosis
Pulmonary congestion interferes with the elimination of carbon dioxide from the lungs	Respiratory acidosis
Mercurial and thiazide diuretics cause a greater excretion of chloride ions than sodium ions; loss of chloride ions causes a compensatory increase in bicarbonate ions, hence alkalosis	Metabolic alkalosis if mercurial or thiazide diuretics are used extensively
Extensive use of potent diuretics plus severely restricted sodium intake Excessive loss of sodium from other routes, such as repeated paracentesis, vomiting, or diarrhea	Sodium deficit

Additional symptoms may be caused by the various water and electrolyte disturbances that can occur with congestive heart failure and its treatment; these disturbances include sodium deficit, potassium deficit, respiratory acidosis, metabolic alkalosis, metabolic acidosis, and fluid volume excess. (Descriptions of these imbalances are given in Chapters 8, 9, and 10.)

Clearly, congestive heart failure is a complex illness, demanding highly skilled nursing care. Because fluid imbalances represent a major problem in congestive heart failure, the nurse must make meaningful observations relating to these disturbances; such observations are of great help to the physician as he plans therapy. The major areas of concern to the nurse are pointed out in the following section.

Treatment of Congestive Heart Failure: Nursing Implications

When possible, treatment involves elimination of the underlying disease producing the heart failure. For example, surgical correction of a valvular disorder or removal of a calcified pericardium may restore cardiac function to normal and produce a spontaneous diuresis. Unfortunately, most persons with congestive heart failure have irreversible cardiac damage, such as that caused by myocardial infarction. When the primary disease cannot be eliminated, the only alternative is to make the most efficient use possible of remaining cardiac function.

REST   Rest causes a reduction in the tissue's oxygen need and lightens the burden on the circulatory sys-

Table 21-2. Symptoms of Congestive Heart Failure and Their Causes

Symptom	Cause
Fatigue with little exertion or at rest	Tissue anoxia due to decreased cardiac output
Troublesome cough producing noncharacteristic sputum, although it may at times be brownish or blood-tinged	Transudation of serum into the alveoli causes pulmonary congestion
Dyspnea on exertion	Cardiac output is inadequate to provide for the increased oxygen required by exertion
Elevated venous pressure	Increase in total blood volume
	Accumulation of blood in the venous system results from incomplete emptying of the heart
Decreased urinary output	Decreased cardiac output and renal blood flow
	Sodium and water retention caused by excess aldosterone secretion
	Increased water retention caused by excess ADH secretion
Visible distention of peripheral veins, most noticeable on face, neck, and hands	Elevated venous pressure
Edema first appears in dependent parts	Hydrostatic pressure is greatest in dependent parts of the body
Edema later becomes generalized	Progressive cardiac failure causes substantial increase in hydrostatic pressure in all parts of the body
Fever	Complications accompanying congestive heart failure, such as bronchopneumonia, thrombophlebitis, or myocardial infarction
	Fever may be present even in the absence of complications (the cutaneous vasoconstriction occurring with CHF may interfere with normal heat loss from the skin)
Tachycardia	Effort to compensate for decreased cardiac output
Engorgement of the liver and other organs	Decreased cardiac output causes damming of venous blood
	Increase in total blood volume and interstitial fluid volume
Nausea and vomiting	Edema of the liver and intestines
	Impulses arising from the dilated myocardium in acute CHF
	Digitalis toxicity
Anorexia	Potassium deficit
	Digitalis toxicity
Constipation	Poor nourishment and inadequate bulk in diet
	Lack of activity
	Depression of motor activity by hypoxia
Increased respiratory difficulty Dyspnea even at rest Orthopnea	Increased tissue hypoxia caused by progressive failure of the heart as a pump
Cyanosis, particularly of lips and nail beds	Venous distention
	Inadequate oxygenation of blood
Pulmonary edema with severe dyspnea, coughing of pink frothy fluid, cyanosis, shock, and death	Increased venous pressure may cause serum and blood cells to transudate into the alveoli

tem. It also produces a physiologic diuresis. Sometimes rest alone is sufficient to alleviate the symptoms of congestive heart failure. The amount of rest required varies with the individual and may range from complete bedrest to only slight restriction of activity.

The prescription of physical rest by the physician must be specific enough to have meaning to the patient. Too often, patients are given ambiguous directions to "rest" or to "take it easy." Such vague statements are not only useless; they may actually be harmful, because each person interprets rest differently. The nurse can help by encouraging the patient to ask the physician specific questions regarding the activity permitted.

Another important nursing responsibility consists in observing such responses of the patient to exercise as pulse and respiratory rate changes. Careful reporting of these observations helps the physician determine the desired amount of activity. Because the patient's condition may fluctuate widely from day to day, the nurse must often use her own judgment in controlling his activity. For example, assume that a patient has been allowed up in a chair for 30 minutes in the morning. Even though this period is permitted, the appearance of dyspnea, chest pain, or a substantially increased pulse rate before the 30 minutes are up indicates that the patient should be put back to bed.

Emotional rest is also important in the management of congestive heart failure. Periods of tension are associated with increased sodium and water retention, while periods of emotional relaxation are associated with diuresis. Nursing efforts should, therefore, be directed toward avoiding emotional problems and achieving a relaxing environment. A major nursing responsibility is emphasizing the importance of emotional rest to the patient's family and to nonprofessional personnel giving direct patient care. At times, judicious use of sedatives may help promote needed rest and relaxation.

LOW-SODIUM DIET   Restriction of sodium ions in the diet is a valuable aid in the management of congestive heart failure. In general, the fewer number of sodium ions in the body, the less water is retained.

The degree of sodium restriction necessary to control edema varies with the severity of the heart failure. Many patients can achieve a sufficiently low intake of sodium simply by not adding salt in cooking or at the table and by avoiding high sodium foods, such as salted crackers, bacon, ham, salted nuts, foods with sodium salt preservatives, and so on. As a rule, restriction of the intake of salt to from 2 to 5 Gm. daily instead of the usual 10 Gm. or more in an average diet is sufficient to control edema. But more drastic sodium restriction to less than 1 Gm. a day—even 250 mg. a day or less—may be required for some patients.

The degree of sodium restriction necessary to control edema also varies with other facets of treatment, such as rest and the use of diuretics. For example, an ambulatory patient requires more severe sodium restriction than a patient at bedrest, because rest in itself encourages diuresis. A patient receiving potent diuretics has much less need of severe sodium restriction than a patient not receiving diuretics. Indeed, drastic restriction of sodium intake can be dangerous in the patient receiving a potent diuretic.

Although dietary sodium restriction is simple in theory, it frequently is difficult to achieve. Many patients fail to adhere to low-sodium diets because they believe them to be unpalatable; others lack an understanding of the foods allowed and to be avoided. All too often, the only diet instruction given to the patient consists of handing him a copy of his diet on the day of his discharge from the hospital.

The nurse should make every effort to make the diet acceptable to the patient. First of all, she should give him an explanation of why he must be on the diet. Secondly, the dietitian should discuss the diet with the patient and learn what his food preferences are. The possible use of salt substitutes should be discussed with the physician. All of these contain potassium and, thus, should not be used in the presence of oliguria and severe kidney disease. Additional sessions should be held while the patient is in the hospital in order to increase his knowledge and acceptance of the diet. The nurse should support the dietitian's efforts. In instances where a dietitian is not available, the nurse should carry the full responsibility of diet instruction; for this reason, she should have a working knowledge of low-sodium diets. (See Chapter 14 for a more thorough discussion of sodium restricted diets.) Literature concerning these diets is available from the American Heart Association at the request of the patient's physician. Excellent books on the preparation of attractive low-sodium diets are available.

Patients on severe sodium restriction should be observed for symptoms of sodium deficit, especially if they are receiving potent diuretics, or if they are losing sodium through such routes as vomiting, diarrhea, excessive perspiration, or repeated paracentesis.

DIGITALIS   Function of the failing heart frequently is improved by the administration of digitalis, which acts by increasing the strength of the heartbeat and the cardiac output. Edema fluid is mobilized by the improved cardiac function, and diuresis results. Usually the physician attempts to give enough digitalis to reduce the resting apical pulse to 60 to 80 beats per minute.

Excessive doses of digitalis may result in the following toxic symptoms:

Aversion to food (which usually precedes other symptoms by 1 or 2 days)
Nausea
Excessive salivation
Vomiting
Abdominal pain
Diarrhea
Headache
Confusion (particularly in elderly patients with arteriosclerosis)
Blurred vision, diplopia, optic neuritis
Yellowish-green "halo" vision, or presence of white dots (frost) on objects
Bradycardia (caused by A-V block)
Variety of arrhythmias, including ventricular tachycardia, in which the heart beats rapidly and irregularly (arrhythmias may precede extracardiac manifestations)
Bigeminal pulse (coupled pulse beat)

It is important to differentiate between the combined anorexia and nausea of heart failure and that produced by digitalis toxicity. Patients receiving digitalis should have periodic electrocardiograms to detect early the development of digitalis toxicity. Before administering the drug, the nurse should check the apical-radial pulse for a full minute, noting rate, rhythm, volume, and pulse deficit. Unless otherwise ordered, the drug should be withheld, and the physician notified when:

1. The apical pulse is below 60
2. A marked change in regularity occurs (premature ventricular contractions, bigeminy, atrial fibrillation, etc.)

An overdose of digitalis may have a depressant action, causing conduction disturbance and excessive slowing of the heart. It may also cause increased myocardial irritability, producing extrasystoles or tachycardias. The nurse should be alert for a coupled pulse beat (bigeminy) in which the regular beat is followed almost immediately by a weak beat and a pause. A bigeminal pulse is a common sign of digitalis toxicity in adults; bigeminal pulse, and other irregularities, should be reported to the physician. The nurse should also report pulse deficit, caused by failure of the extrasystoles to produce a pulse at the wrist. If digitalis is not discontinued, the premature beats can take on the rhythm of ventricular tachycardia and progress to ventricular fibrillation.

Calcium ions enhance the action of digitalis; thus, decreasing the plasma calcium concentration is helpful in counteracting the cardiotoxic effects produced by digitalis. The plasma calcium level can be reduced by the intravenous infusion of disodium edetate (Endrate); this drug ties up excess calcium and removes it from the body. (Conversely, calcium should never be administered intravenously to a digitalized patient.)

Symptoms of digitalis toxicity may be induced by potassium deficit, since this deficit sensitizes the heart to digitalis. The patient maintained on digitalis without toxicity can, in the presence of potassium deficit, exhibit arrhythmias typical of digitalis intoxication. An irregular pulse caused by digitalis toxicity can sometimes be corrected by the administration of a potassium salt, either by mouth or, if necessary, parenterally. Magnesium has also been reported to correct the toxic rhythms produced by digoxin.

Patients prone to develop potassium deficit (such as those receiving furosemide, mercurial, or thiazide diuretics, or those with vomiting, diarrhea, or poor food intake) should be observed with especial care for signs of digitalis toxicity.

DIURETICS   A valuable aid in the symptomatic treatment of congestive heart failure, the primary purpose of diuretics is to promote the excretion of sodium and water from the body. In varying degrees, most diuretics tend also to promote the excretion of potassium. Diuretics that are associated with hypokalemia include the thiazides, the mercurials, furosemide (Lasix), ethacrynic acid (Edecrin) and the carbonic anhydrase inhibitors, such as acetazolamide

(Diamox). Mercurial diuretics are used less frequently than the other diuretics because many of them require intramuscular administration and they have more side effects, including cramps, diarrhea, skin rashes, and local pain at the injection site. (See Chapter 14 for a more thorough discussion of diuretics.)

Excessive loss of potassium ions during diuretic therapy can be either prevented or corrected by the administration of a suitable potassium supplement, such as K-Lyte, Kaon Elixir, Potassium Triplex, or K-Lor. The use of diuretics should be decreased when sodium loss is occurring from another route; a low-sodium diet can take the place of diuretic therapy in many persons.

Ethacrynic acid (Edecrin) and furosemide (Lasix) are potent diuretics that are effective even after their action has produced hypochloremic alkalosis. They are unusually potent and have a rapid onset. Patients receiving these diuretics should be observed closely for signs of too vigorous diuresis, such as lethargy, weakness, dizziness, anorexia, vomiting, leg cramps, mental confusion, and circulatory collapse.

Potassium conserving diuretics are capable of producing diuresis in congestive heart failure. Spironolactone (Aldactone) is an aldosterone antagonist, which acts by blocking the potent sodium retaining effect of aldosterone on the renal tubules. Aldactone should not be given in conjunction with a potassium supplement because of the danger of potassium excess. (Recall that aldosterone causes potassium loss; therefore, its antagonist permits potassium retention.) Triamterene (Dyrenium) also promotes sodium loss and potassium retention although it has a different mode of action. (It interferes with the exchange of sodium ions for potassium and hydrogen ions.) Again, potassium supplements should not be given because hyperkalemia may result; symptoms of hyperkalemia include paresthesia of the extremities, nausea, weakness, and intestinal cramping with diarrhea. If hyperkalemia is severe, cardiac arrest can occur. Only patients with adequate renal reserve should receive potassium conserving diuretics.

Primary nursing responsibilities in the care of the patient with congestive heart failure include keeping an accurate account of fluid intake and output and measuring the weight daily. (See the discussion of both of these procedures in Chapter 13.) The data obtained from these measurements are of inestimable use to the physician as he regulates the dose of diuretics and the degree of dietary sodium restriction for each patient.

VASODILATORS   Management of acute or chronic heart failure may include the administration of nitrates (either sublingually, orally, topically, or intravenously). Nitrates cause peripheral vasodilatation and, thus, reduce peripheral resistance to left ventricular ejection. In so doing, left ventricular output is increased and cardiac performance is improved. Pulmonary venous pressure usually decreases significantly owing to the peripheral venous pooling effect evoked by nitrates. Myocardial oxygen consumption is decreased.

A vasodilator (such as sodium nitroprusside) may be given intravenously in low dosage (via an infusion pump) to treat acute pump failure complicating myocardial infarction. Careful monitoring of arterial pressure, cardiac output, and left ventricular filling pressure should be done when parenteral vasodilator therapy is employed in the management of such patients. A major possible complication of vasodilator therapy is a pronounced drop in arterial pressure which could increase myocardial ischemia by restricting coronary blood flow.

CORRECTION OF ACID-BASE IMBALANCES   Acidosis, hypoxia, and electrolyte imbalance can precipitate or prolong cardiac failure. Because of this, arterial blood gases and electrolyte levels should be monitored closely in the acutely ill patient. Sodium bicarbonate should be given as necessary to correct metabolic acidosis. Adequate ventilation is mandatory to prevent hypoxia and respiratory acidosis; if necessary, intubation and artificial ventilation should be employed.

FLUID ADMINISTRATION

Oral Intake   Water intake is usually not restricted in congestive heart failure unless there is a body sodium deficit or dilution of the serum sodium by the excessive retention of water.

Undue loss of sodium may be caused by the excessive use of diuretics, vomiting, diarrhea, severe diaphoresis, or repeated paracentesis. A drastically reduced sodium intake may predispose to sodium depletion, although persons on low sodium intake for prolonged periods usually develop remarkable sodium conservation, something that does not happen in the case of patients on low potassium intake, since there is no true body conservation of potassium. If the water intake of patients in a mild state of sodium depletion is not reduced, the depressed serum sodium level may become further depressed; a frank state of sodium deficit may then develop. Symptoms of this condition include the following:

weakness
abdominal cramps
anorexia
nausea
vomiting
inexplicable feeling of impending doom
prostration
collapse

The operation of abnormal routes of sodium loss should alert the nurse to search for these symptoms, especially if the sodium intake is low and diuretics are being given. Although the total sodium content of the body is elevated in congestive heart failure, water retention caused by excessive ADH hormone secretion may dilute the serum sodium concentration to below normal levels. Moreover, part of the sodium in the extracellular fluid moves into the cells to replace the potassium loss which so often occurs with congestive heart failure. There is no characteristic clinical picture accompanying this state. When it is well developed, however, the usual therapeutic measures fail to reduce the edema that accompanies it.

One of the chief features of intractable heart failure is the inability of the kidney to respond to the usual diuretics. Treatment may consist of sodium restriction, restriction of water intake to 1000 ml. per day, and the use of more potent diuretics. It has been found that patients refractory to other diuretics often respond successfully to ethacrynic acid (Edecrin) and furosemide (Lasix).

Intravenous Fluids   The intravenous route for fluid administration may be necessary in critically ill patients with congestive heart failure. Many physicians are hesitant to administer fluids to such patients for fear of causing circulatory overload and pulmonary edema. While there is little doubt that intravenous administration of fluids to a cardiac patient carries some risk of causing circulatory overload, the fear of this complication has been exaggerated to the point that many cardiac patients receive inadequate fluid therapy. The recent increase in the use of venous pressure monitoring devices has done much to alleviate the problem. Frequent checks of venous pressure during fluid administration give early warning of circulatory overload and serve as guides to the safe administration of needed water and electrolytes.

The nurse should pay careful attention to the volume, speed, and composition of fluids administered to the patient with congestive heart failure. The response to fluids should be observed frequently and the flow rate adjusted accordingly. (See Chapter 16 for a more detailed discussion of venous pressure monitoring and nursing responsibilities in intravenous fluid administration.)

Pulmonary Edema   The following are symptoms of acute pulmonary edema:

restlessness
severe dyspnea
gurgling respirations
cyanosis
coughing up of frothy fluid

Welt has pointed out possible causes of pulmonary edema other than administering excessive quantities of fluid or too rapid administration of fluid. Inadequate fluid administration can result in peripheral vascular collapse with tissue anoxia; this condition in itself can precipitate an acute attack of pulmonary edema. Some patients develop pulmonary edema during venipuncture or shortly after fluids have been started before there has been time for expansion of the circulatory volume. Pulmonary edema in these instances can be explained as a reaction to fear related to the venipuncture. The following illustrative case was related by Welt[6]:

> A patient with chronic renal insufficiency and hypertensive and arteriosclerotic heart disease with failure despite complete digitalization was admitted to the hospital. It was decided to improve her severe anemia with blood transfusion. The nature of the procedure was not explained to her, she had not been sedated, there was a little difficulty with the venipuncture, and when the needle was successfully introduced into the vein she developed severe acute pulmonary edema. The procedure was discontinued and she recovered from this episode in a few hours. Later that day the nature of and indications for the transfusion were explained to her, she was sedated, and tolerated the administration of 1000 ml. of whole blood with no untoward reaction whatsoever.

In addition to fear of venipuncture, the patient may interpret the need for intravenous fluids as a grave prognostic sign. This is but another reason to take time to explain to the patient what the intravenous administration consists of and why it is being used.

Occasionally, a small volume of hypertonic solution of sodium chloride is administered to the cardiac patient to correct a profound sodium deficit. Great care should be taken to infuse the solution slowly in accordance with the order of the physician. A too-rapid administration of hypertonic saline results in a dangerous overloading of the circulatory system.

Acute pulmonary edema constitutes a medical emergency that requires quick, intelligent action by the nurse and the physician. The patient should be quickly placed in a high Fowler's position and oxygen should be started while the physician is being summoned. Best results are achieved when oxygen (100%) is given under positive pressure, since this helps prevent further escape of fluid into the lungs. Some authorities favor bubbling the oxygen through antifoaming agents to decrease respiratory obstruction from the mechanical interference of edema fluid. Preparation should be made for intravenous administration of morphine. The primary physiologic usefulness of morphine may be achieved through its peripheral vasodilating effect. A peripheral pool of blood is formed and, thus, venous return and cardiac work load are decreased. Morphine also decreases work of the heart by decreasing arterial blood pressure and resistance. The great anxiety associated with severe dyspnea is allayed by morphine. Morphine should be used with great caution in patients with severe hypotension or chronic lung disease.

Alternating tourniquets may be used to obstruct venous return to the heart; they can remove up to 700 ml. of blood from the circulating volume. The removal of 200 to 500 ml. of blood by phlebotomy may be tried in order to relieve the work load on the heart and to reduce venous pressure. Rapid digitalization improves cardiac function and, thus, helps relieve pulmonary edema. Either sodium ethacrynate (Sodium Edecrin) or furosemide (Lasix) may be used to treat acute pulmonary edema; they are effective rapidly when given intravenously and produce an intense diuresis.

ELECTROLYTES IN CARDIAC RESUSCITATION

SODIUM BICARBONATE   Metabolic acidosis occurs in cardiac arrest; the lack of available oxygen causes cellular processes to automatically shift to anaerobic metabolism, which yields lactic acid as the end product. The drop in plasma pH interferes with the normal functioning of many enzyme systems. Sodium bicarbonate, an alkali, is often used to correct metabolic acidosis; 50 ml. of a 7.5 per cent solution (containing 3.75 Gm. or 44.6 mEq.) may be administered by direct venous injection. This amount can be repeated every 5 to 10 minutes, as indicated, until spontaneous cardiac function is restored and blood gas studies indicate the pH is normal. (The administration of a large amount of sodium bicarbonate could conceivably cause metabolic alkalosis and fluid volume excess as a result of sodium loading; thus, the arterial pH should be monitored and the patient observed closely for fluid retention.) Vigorous treatment of acidosis is mandatory since it inhibits cardiac resuscitation. Lack of respiration causes respiratory acidosis to be superimposed on the metabolic acidosis; the excess CO_2 must be removed by effective ventilation.

CALCIUM CHLORIDE   Calcium chloride may be given intravenously or intracardially to strengthen the cardiac contraction; the dose is usually 10 ml. of a 10 per cent solution. Calcium is especially helpful in treating patients with potassium excess. Recall that calcium and potassium have antagonistic effects; thus, raising the plasma calcium level decreases the cardiotoxic effects of hyperkalemia. (Calcium should not be administered intravenously to the digitalized patient because calcium ions enhance the cardiotoxic action of digitalis.)

POTASSIUM CHLORIDE   Potassium chloride may be given intravenously to correct arrhythmias caused by digitalis; 40 mEq. of KCl in 500 ml. of 5% D/W may be given over a 2- to 3-hour period.

> If the serum potassium level is above 2.5, no more than 10 mEq. per hour or 200 mEq. per day should be given. If the serum potassium level is less than 2.0 and electrolyte changes are evident in the ECG, 40 mEq. may be given per hour with no greater concentration than 60 mEq. per liter of I.V., up to 400 mEq. per day.[7]

REFERENCES

1. **Guyton, A.:** Textbook of Medical Physiology, ed. 5. Philadelphia: W. B. Saunders Co., 1976, p. 173.

2. **Foster, W.:** Principles of Acute Coronary Care. New York: Appleton-Century-Crofts, 1976, p. 143.

3. **Guyton, A.:** Textbook of Medical Physiology, ed. 5. Philadelphia: W. B. Saunders Co., 1976, p. 316.

4. **Berk, J., et al.:** Handbook of Critical Care. Boston: Little, Brown & Co., 1976, p. 125.

5. **Guyton, A.:** Textbook of Medical Physiology, ed. 5. Philadelphia: W. B. Saunders Co., 1976, p. 334.

6. **Welt, L.:** Clinical Disorders of Hydration and Acid-Base Equilibrium, ed. 2. Boston: Little, Brown & Co., 1959, p. 131.

7. **Sharp, L.,** and **Rabin, B.:** Nursing in the Coronary Care Unit. Philadelphia: J. B. Lippincott Co., 1970, p. 185.

BIBLIOGRAPHY

Aspinall, M.: Nursing the Open-Heart Surgery Patient. New York: McGraw-Hill Book Co., 1973.

Boedeker, E., and **Dauber, J.** (eds.): Manual of Medical Therapeutics, ed. 21. Boston: Little, Brown & Co., 1974.

Chow, R.: Cardiovascular Nursing Care—Understandings, Concepts, & Principles for Practice. New York: Springer Publishing Co., 1976.

Condon, R., and **Nyhus, L.** (eds.): Manual of Surgical Therapeutics, ed. 3. Boston: Little, Brown & Co., 1975.

Conover, M., and **Zalis, E.:** Understanding Electrocardiography—Physiological and Interpretive Concepts, ed. 2. St. Louis: C. V. Mosby, 1976.

Edwards Laboratories—Product Manual. Edwards Laboratories, Division of American Hospital Supply Corporation, Santa Ana, Calif., 1977.

Gahart, B.: Intravenous Medications. St. Louis: C. V. Mosby, 1977.

Hudak, C., et al.: Critical Care Nursing. Philadelphia: J. B. Lippincott Co., 1977.

Kempe, C., et al (eds.): Current Pediatric Diagnosis & Treatment, ed. 4. Los Altos, Calif.: Lange Medical Publications, 1976.

Sweetwood, H.: The Patient in the Coronary Care Unit. New York: Springer Publishing Co., 1976.

Wade, J.: Respiratory Nursing Care, ed. 2. St. Louis: C. V. Mosby, 1977.

— 22 —

Fluid Balance in the Patient with Endocrine Disease

ROLE OF ENDOCRINE GLANDS IN FLUID BALANCE HOMEOSTASIS

The endocrine homeostatic controls include the adrenals, the parathyroids, and the anterior and posterior pituitary gland.

ADRENAL GLANDS The adrenal mechanism is closely associated with retention and excretion of sodium, potassium, and water. These effects are exerted through the action of the adrenocortical hormones on the renal tubules.

The primary adrenal cortex secretions are mineralocorticoids and glucocorticoids. Aldosterone is the most important mineralocorticoid; cortisol is the most important glucocorticoid.

The chief function of aldosterone is the control of sodium concentration in the body. Its effect on potassium and sodium is 50 times stronger than cortisol's effect on these electrolytes.

The chief action of cortisol is to promote gluconeogenesis and to deposit glycogen in the liver. It also influences protein catabolism. Other effects of the glucocorticoids include control of inflammation, maintenance of gastric acidity, and a mild mineralocorticoid influence on sodium and potassium concentrations.

Androgenic adrenocorticoids (17-ketosteroids) also are produced by the adrenal cortex. These hormones favor a positive nitrogen balance and they oppose the catabolic effects of the glucocorticoids. Sexual effects of these hormones include promotion of hair growth in the pubic and axillary areas.

PARATHYROID GLANDS Parathyroid hormone (parathormone) causes an increase in the plasma calcium concentration, primarily by increasing the rate of bone resorption. Any *decrease* in the plasma calcium concentration causes stimulation of the parathyroid glands; conversely, any *increase* in the plasma calcium level causes parathyroid activity to decrease.

Another function of parathormone is to increase the renal excretion of phosphate ions and, thus, to lower the plasma phosphate concentration. The plasma phosphate concentration indirectly influences parathyroid activity, since a reciprocal relationship exists between calcium and phosphate ions —a rise in the concentration of one causing a decrease in the other. Thus, when an increase in phosphate concentration causes a reciprocal decrease in the calcium concentration, the decreased calcium concentration causes parathyroid stimulation.

Evidence exists that the thyroid gland produces a hormone, calcitonin, which has an effect opposite that of parathormone; instead of elevating low levels of serum calcium, calcitonin serves to decrease high calcium levels.

PITUITARY GLAND   The anterior pituitary gland secretes several hormones. Some of these, such as the growth hormone, exert a direct effect on the metabolism of water and electrolytes. Others exert an indirect effect by stimulating other endocrine glands whose hormones directly influence metabolism; these include thyroid-stimulating hormone (TSH), adrenocortical stimulating hormone (ACTH), and the gonadotrophic hormones.

The posterior pituitary gland releases a water-conserving hormone referred to as the antidiuretic hormone, or ADH. As the name implies, it inhibits diuresis. (It seems more direct to think of it as conserving water.) The release of ADH is influenced by the "osmostat," an auxiliary control located in the plexus of the internal carotid artery. The osmotat is sensitive to changes in osmolarity (electrolyte concentration) of the extracellular fluid.

ENDOCRINE DISORDERS THAT CAUSE FLUID BALANCE DISTURBANCES

It is not within the scope of this chapter to discuss all of the endocrine disturbances causing fluid balance disturbances. A brief discussion of adrenocortical disorders and parathyroid disorders is presented. (Diabetes insipidus is discussed in Chapter 23.) Much emphasis is placed on diabetic ketoacidosis because this condition is more commonly encountered by the nurse.

Adrenocortical Insufficiency

Adrenocortical insufficiency may be caused by destruction or suppression of the adrenals, or it may be secondary to hypofunction of the pituitary gland. The disease can be either acute or chronic; symptoms are due primarily to decreased aldosterone and cortisol secretion.

WATER AND ELECTROLYTE CHANGES   Water and electrolyte disturbances occurring with adrenocortical insufficiency include the following:

Sodium deficit
Potassium excess
Extracellular fluid volume deficit
Mild metabolic acidosis
Hypercalcemia

Decreased aldosterone secretion is largely responsible for the increased urinary excretion of sodium and retention of potassium, although decreased cortisol secretion undoubtedly contributes to these changes as well. Water loss accompanies the increased urinary excretion of sodium and results in extracellular fluid volume deficit. Sodium is lost in addition to water. Hypercalcemia may also occur with adrenocortical insufficiency.

Decreased cortisol secretion causes a delay in water excretion; decreased glomerular filtration rate contributes to this effect. A loss of bicarbonate ions accompanies the sodium loss and a mild metabolic acidosis may result.

OTHER METABOLIC CHANGES   Carbohydrate, protein, and fat metabolism are impaired by adrenocortical insufficiency. Lack of cortisol causes decreased glyconeogenesis and depletion of the liver glycogen; thus, hypoglycemia can occur. Negative nitrogen balance results from the decreased secretion of 17-ketosteroids. Fat metabolism is slowed because of the reduced secretion of cortisol and corticosterone.

Other abnormalities include a reduced cellular response to injury, leukopenia, and a decreased number of neutrophils.

CHRONIC ADRENAL INSUFFICIENCY   Symptoms of chronic insufficiency (Addison's disease) may include the following:

fatigue out of proportion to activity
emotional depression and irritability
weight loss (owing to fluid volume deficit and negative caloric balance)
hypotension (particularly pronounced when patient changes from a supine position to an upright position)
chronic gastrointestinal complaints of a vague nature
alternating diarrhea and constipation
hypoglycemia, noticed several hours after meals (symptoms include hunger, nervousness, sweating, headache, and confusion)
poor resistance to infection
muscle wasting and weakness
pigmentation of skin and mucous membranes common in adults
dental caries

craving for salt

poor reaction to stress (mild adrenal insufficiency may become severe under stress and
can lead to vascular collapse)

Treatment consists of daily hormonal replacement therapy. Cortisone is given daily in a dose
usually varying between 12.5 and 37.5 mg. This
amount must be greatly increased when infection,
trauma, diarrhea, inability to eat, or other complications occur. Patients should be advised to consult
their physician *immediately* when such conditions
occur.

A mineralocorticoid is given in addition to cortisone to control sodium and potassium concentrations
in the body. Although cortisone causes sodium retention, its effect is too weak to prevent sodium loss during periods of stress. Desoxycorticosterone is available in a long-acting form, Percorten pivalate, that
may be given intramuscularly every four weeks.

Dietary sodium chloride intake should be consistent with the patient's taste and usually differs
little from the average salt content of a normal diet.
Salt tablets should be carried to repair sodium loss
caused by unusual circumstances, such as excessive
heat exposure and sweating. Frequent carbohydrate
feedings may prevent symptoms of hypoglycemia.

Overtreatment with cortisone may produce unfavorable symptoms such as acne, moon facies, diabetes mellitus, peptic ulcer, bleeding tendencies, and
hypertension. Overtreatment with mineralocorticoids may cause excessive fluid retention with
weight gain and hypertension. The nurse should be
alert for these symptoms. Careful recording of fluid
intake and output and daily weight measurement
are necessary to detect early fluid retention.

The patient should be made aware of the need
for systematic medical follow-up in the control of his
disease. He should be taught to avoid excessive
physical and emotional stress and infections. In addition, he should be aware of the symptoms accompanying under- and over-treatment of adrenocortical
insufficiency. (A discussion of adrenocorticosteroid
therapy is presented in Chapter 14.)

Acute Adrenocortical Insufficiency

The nurse should be alert for acute adrenocortical
insufficiency, sometimes termed "adrenal crisis,"
when patients with decreased adrenal function are
exposed to stress, such as surgery, trauma, emotional
upset, or prolonged medical illness. Such a crisis
may occur when a patient with chronic adrenocortical insufficiency fails to take his prescribed hormones. (Adrenal crisis as a result of surgical procedures in patients on prolonged adrenocortical hormone therapy is discussed in Chapter 17.)

Symptoms of acute adrenocortical insufficiency
include hypotension, thready pulse, nausea, vomiting, confusion, and circulatory collapse. The body
temperature may rise as high as 105° F. (40.5° C.).

Treatment consists of the intravenous administration of hydrocortisone as soon as possible. The
blood volume should be expanded by the administration of isotonic solution of sodium chloride and
glucose, dextran, or blood. Vasopressor drugs may be
necessary to raise the blood pressure. Sodium deficit
should be corrected over a period of several days with
hypertonic saline infusions. Glucose should be administered to prevent or correct symptoms of hypoglycemia. Intravenous hydrocortisone replacement
therapy is continued until the patient is improved
sufficiently to take cortisol intramuscularly, or cortisone when oral intake is tolerated.

The nurse should keep a close watch for changes
in the vital signs. A fall in blood pressure and a rapid,
thready pulse may indicate inadequate hydrocortisone and fluid replacement therapy. She should also
protect the patient from physical and emotional
stress, when possible.

Hyperadrenalism

One type of hypersecretion of the adrenal cortex results in a condition referred to as Cushing's disease.
It usually results from hyperplasia of both adrenal
cortices; often the hyperplasia is secondary to increased production of ACTH by the anterior pituitary. Abnormal quantities of cortisol and androgens
produce the symptoms characteristic of Cushing's
disease:

1. some degree of sodium retention (may lead
   to hypertension and congestive heart failure)
2. buffalo torso (extra deposition of fat in the
   thoracic region)
3. moon facies (edematous facial appearance)
4. hirsutism (excessive growth of facial hair
   caused by androgenic effect of excess hormones)

5. elevated blood sugar (may be as high as 200 mg./100 ml. of blood; probably a result of excessive gluconeogenesis; may actually "burn out" beta cells if present for many months and produce diabetes[1])
6. emotional changes (apathy, depression, or anxiety)
7. loss of libido (impotence in males, absence of menses in females)
8. gastric ulcers (may occur secondary to increased production of pepsin and hydrochloric acid)
9. increased plasma cortisol level
10. increased urinary level of 17-hydroxysteroids

Treatment is directed at removing the cause of ACTH hypersecretion (such as removal or radiation of hypertrophied pituitary gland) or total or partial adrenalectomy if the cause of ACTH hypersecretion cannot be corrected. Following adrenalectomy, adrenal steroids must be administered to correct any insufficiency.

Aldosteronism

Aldosteronism may be primary or secondary in nature. Primary aldosteronism usually is associated with an adrenal adenoma (resulting in overactivity of the zona glomerulosa) or with hyperplasia of one or both adrenal glands. Symptoms include the following:

episodic muscular weakness and paralysis (resulting from hypokalemia)
polyuria and polydipsia (caused by hypokalemia and impaired renal tubular reabsorption of water)
tetany, occasionally, caused by metabolic alkalosis associated with hypokalemia
moderately elevated blood pressure (probably resulting from the slight increase in body sodium content)

Treatment of primary aldosteronism is directed at removing the affected adrenal tissue, or, if this is not feasible, at medical therapy.

Secondary aldosteronism occurs in the nephrotic syndrome, cirrhosis of the liver, and severe cardiac failure. These conditions are discussed in their respective chapters.

Hypoparathyroidism

Underproduction of parathyroid hormone occurs in primary hypoparathyroidism and in the accidental removal of parathyroid tissue during thyroidectomy. Renal tubular damage can interfere with the action of parathyroid hormone and produce symptoms of hypoparathyroidism (pseudohypoparathyroidism). Decreased parathyroid activity results in the following:

decreased plasma calcium concentration
increased plasma phosphate concentration

Symptoms of hypoparathyroidism are primarily those of neuromuscular irritability produced by a decrease in the serum concentration of ionized calcium. Included in the symptoms are:

numbness of extremities
tingling of hands, feet, and circumoral region
mood changes
voice changes caused by spasms of vocal cords
muscular spasm, induced by compressing blood supply to area
abdominal cramps
diarrhea
carpopedal attitude of hands
facial spasm, induced by tapping over nerve course in front of the ear (Chvostek's sign)
laryngeal spasms
convulsions

Other symptoms of hypoparathyroidism are influenced by the duration of the parathyroid hormone deficiency and the age at which it developed. For example, cataracts or calcification of various body parts such as the basal ganglia of the brain may occur when hypoparathyroidism has long been present. Formation of new teeth is restricted when hypoparathyroidism occurs in a child, although the degree of hypoplasia depends upon the age at which hypoparathyroidism began.

The danger of the accidental removal of parathyroid tissue during thyroidectomy is always present because the parathyroids are small and resemble fatty tissue. Removal of half of the parathyroid glands usually doesn't present symptoms. (Most persons have four parathyroid glands; some have less and some have as many as seven.) However, removal of three out of four causes symptoms of hypoparathyroidism, until the fourth gland is able to hypertrophy sufficiently to fulfill the function of all the glands. Tetany also may be produced by temporary interference with the parathyroid blood supply following thyroidectomy.

The nurse should be alert for symptoms of deficit of ionized calcium during the postoperative care of patients who have undergone thyroidectomy. Such symptoms usually appear a few days after the operation. Early complaints are of numbness and tingling in the hands and feet. Compression of circulation to the hand while checking the blood pressure may cause spasm of the forearm muscles and palmar flexion of the hand. Other symptoms of deficit, such as general irritability or "jumpiness," may also be noted. It is crucial to detect calcium deficit early so that appropriate hormonal therapy or calcium replacement or both can be started before the onset of laryngeal spasms and convulsions.

Hypocalcemia caused by hypoparathyroidism may be treated by the administration of calcium salts. Calcium gluconate given intravenously may control tetany; calcium gluconate or lactate may be administered orally for the same purpose. An increased dietary intake of high calcium foods will also be beneficial.

Dihydrotachysterol is a substance having an action similar to that of parathyroid hormone (parathormone). It increases calcium absorption from the bone and, thus, causes an increased plasma calcium concentration. It is given daily until symptoms subside, then weekly until symptoms disappear. The patient may then be maintained on vitamin D.

Hyperparathyroidism

Overproduction of parathyroid hormone occurs in primary hyperparathyroidism and in tumors of the parathyroid gland. Increased parathyroid activity results in the following:

increased plasma calcium concentration
decreased plasma phosphate concentration

Secondary hyperparathyroidism may be found in patients with renal disease; poor renal function interferes with excretion of phosphate ions and causes the plasma phosphate concentration to rise. Owing to the reciprocal action of phosphate and calcium, the plasma calcium concentration drops. The low plasma calcium level causes stimulation of the parathyroids

and eventually produces parathyroid hyperplasia, which causes progressive decalcification of the skeleton, sometimes referred to as renal rickets.

Symptoms of hyperparathyroidism produced by the diminished neuromuscular irritability stemming from calcium excess include the following:

mental confusion
loss of memory or mental acuity
lethargy
weak, sluggish muscles
constipation
vomiting
anorexia
abdominal pain (may be the most striking symptom)
prolonged cardiac systole

Other symptoms of hyperparathyroidism are produced by the excess filtration of calcium through the glomeruli. Calcium sediment deposits in the kidneys and produces tubular damage. Polyuria occurs, owing to the increased renal solute load and to the damaged renal tubules. Polydipsia (excessive thirstiness) follows excessive water loss through the kidneys. Uremia and hypertension may eventually follow the renal damage imposed by calcium excess.

An early finding in many patients with hyperparathyroidism is x-ray evidence of subperiosteal resorption of the cortex, most clearly seen in the phalanges. Severe hyperparathyroidism causes excessive bone absorption and eventually produces extensive skeletal decalcification. Decalcified bones are easily broken; on x-ray pictures they show "punched out" areas. The bone disorder produced by hyperparathyroidism is sometimes called von Recklinghausen's disease. There is an increased incidence of pancreatitis and gastric ulcers in patients with hyperparathyroidism.

The treatment of hyperparathyroidism consists of surgical removal of the overactive parathyroid tissue. More than one parathyroid tumor may be present and require the excision of several parathyroid glands. Following surgery, hypoparathyroidism may be present until the remaining parathyroid tissue hypertrophies.

Bone recalcification is rapid following removal of parathyroid tumors; symptoms of calcium excess recede. However, irreversible renal damage and skeletal deformities may have developed.

SEVERE DIABETIC KETOACIDOSIS

Severe diabetic ketoacidosis is a condition that occurs with relative infrequency. It results when an insulin lack prevents normal glucose metabolism, and body energy needs are met with the catabolism of fats and proteins. Events often associated with the onset of diabetic ketoacidosis include the following:

Failure to increase insulin dosage during times of increased need (infections, thyrotoxicosis, trauma, surgery, pregnancy, and periods of undue stress, including emotional stress)
Omission, or inadequate dosage, of insulin
Overeating
Treatment with steroids or thiazide diuretics
Acute myocardial infarction

Diabetic ketoacidosis is a serious condition presenting several water and electrolyte disturbances. The nurse must be aware of the causes and manifestations of these imbalances so that she can detect their early occurrence and cooperate intelligently in their treatment.

Water and Electrolyte Disturbances Prior to Treatment

Insulin must be present for glucose to pass through the cell to participate in cellular metabolism. When insulin secretion is decreased, glucose cannot be utilized; its concentration in the blood stream rises (hyperglycemia). With glucose unavailable, the body must utilize fats and proteins; as the result of catabolism of fats, ketone bodies accumulate. This leads to ketoacidosis (metabolic acidosis).

CELLULAR AND EXTRACELLULAR FLUID VOLUME DEFICIT Hyperosmolarity of the extracellular fluid is produced by the high glucose concentration. Water is drawn from the cells to maintain osmotic equilibrium. When the glucose concentration in the blood exceeds 180 mg. per 100 ml., glucose is excreted in the urine (glycosuria). Because 10 to 20 ml. of water are required to excrete each gram of glucose, water loss through the kidneys is increased. Since sodium and chloride reabsorption are hindered by the osmotic diuresis, excessive amounts of these ions are excreted in the urine. The metabolic end products of protein and fat increase the renal solute load, thus

increasing the water loss. (Recall that materials must be in solution before the kidneys can excrete them.)

Insensible water loss by way of the lungs may be doubled as a result of the deep, rapid respiration accompanying ketoacidosis. Although both water and electrolyte loss are increased in diabetic ketoacidosis, water loss predominates. In severe diabetic ketoacidosis, there is a deficit of approximately 100 ml. of water per kg. of body weight. For example, a patient weighing 154 lb. may have a water deficit of 7 L.; water is lost both from cells and from extracellular fluid.

KETOACIDOSIS The increased utilization of fat for energy needs causes accumulation of the ketone bodies: acetoacetic acid, beta-hydroxybutyric acid, and acetone. The usual ketoacid plasma level is 1 mEq./L.; it may reach as high as 20 mEq./L. in diabetic ketoacidosis. As a result of the increased ketoacid concentration in the blood stream, ketones are excreted by the kidneys (ketonuria). The accumulation of an excessive number of H^+ stemming from the ketoacids causes the blood pH to drop, sometimes to as low as 6.9 or even 6.8. The increase in the number of ketonic anions (negatively charged ions) causes a compensatory decrease in the number of bicarbonate anions (also negatively charged), representing the body's attempt to maintain electrical equilibrium. The bicarbonate level may drop as low as 5 mEq./L.

EFFECT OF FLUID VOLUME DEFICIT ON RENAL FUNCTION Plasma volume is decreased because of excessive fluid loss; the subsequent decrease in renal blood flow interferes with glomerular filtration. Organic acids, sulfates, phosphates, potassium, magnesium, and nonprotein nitrogen waste products are retained by the kidneys, intensifying the metabolic acidosis. The increased retention of potassium, plus its liberation from the cells (owing to fluid volume deficit and starvation), elevates the plasma potassium level. Oliguria eventually results when the plasma volume is decreased sufficiently to produce circulatory shock; it is associated with increased blood levels of potassium, urea, uric acid, creatinine, ketones and nonprotein nitrogen products.

CHANGES IN ELECTROLYTE CONCENTRATIONS Destruction of cells releases protein, glycogen, water, and potassium; large quantities of potassium pass from the cells to the extracellular fluid. A cellular potassium deficit exists even though the potassium level of the extracellular fluid may be normal or even elevated. In severe diabetic ketoacidosis, a 154 lb. man may develop a total potassium deficit of approximately 500 mEq.

Deficits of sodium and chloride may develop even though hemoconcentration is present; in addition to their loss with glucose diuresis, these electrolytes may be lost because of vomiting, gastric dilatation, and paralytic ileus. Because sodium combines with ketonic anions, its excretion is increased. In severe diabetic ketoacidosis, a 154 lb. man may develop a total sodium deficit of approximately 500 mEq., and a total chloride deficit of approximately 440 mEq.

Magnesium and phosphorus are chiefly cellular electrolytes, having actions related to potassium. Cellular deficits of these electrolytes probably develop in the same way as does cellular potassium deficit. A 154 lb. patient with severe diabetic keto-

acidosis may develop a total magnesium deficit of approximately 56 mEq. and a total phosphorus deficit of approximately 260 mEq.

Recognition of Diabetic Ketoacidosis

The nurse should be thoroughly familiar with the symptoms of diabetic ketoacidosis. She should be alert for their occurrence in any diabetic patient, but particularly in those with poor diet habits who are careless in their administration of insulin and those with infections or other illness. One of the nurse's greatest responsibilities to the diabetic patient and his family is to teach them the early recognition of diabetic ketoacidosis.

Diabetic ketoacidosis is characterized by a number of readily recognizable signs and symptoms. These signs and symptoms with their probable causes are listed in Table 22-1.

Table 22-1. Signs and Symptoms of Diabetic Ketoacidosis and Their Probable Cause

Sign or Symptom	Probable Cause
Polyuria	Osmotic diuretic effect of hyperglycemia (Renal solute load greatly increased because of presence of high glucose concentration and the increased concentration of metabolic end products of fat and protein)
Polydipsia	Cellular dehydration causes thirst (Water loss causes hyperosmolarity of the extracellular fluid; water is drawn from the cells)
Glycosuria	Blood glucose level exceeds renal threshold (usually 100 mg./100 ml.)
Acetonuria	Excessive accumulation of ketones in the blood causes increased excretion of ketones in the urine (acetone is a ketone body)
High specific gravity of urine	High renal solute load
Tiredness, muscular weakness	Lack of carbohydrate, potassium deficit; loss of protein from muscles
Face appears drawn and flushed	Fluid volume deficit (sharpening of facial features) Acidosis (flushed color)
Dry tongue and mucous membranes, cracked lips	Fluid volume deficit
Deep, rapid respiration (Kussmaul)	Compensatory mechanism to increase extracellular fluid pH by the elimination of large amounts of CO_2 from the lungs with the resultant decreased carbonic acid content in blood
Nausea and vomiting (Vomitus may be dark brown, owing to blood)	Atony of the stomach Bleeding from stretched gastric mucosa
Brownish particles on teeth, lips, and gums	Deposited there when vomitus is expelled

Table 22-1. Signs and Symptoms of Diabetic Ketoacidosis and Their Probable Cause (*Continued*)

Sign or Symptom	Probable Cause
Weight loss	Fluid volume deficit, inability to metabolize glucose
Acetone breath odor (odor similar to that of over-ripe apples)	Acetone content of body increases; acetone is volatile and is vaporized in the expired air
Gastric dilatation and paralytic ileus	Neuropathy Water and electrolyte loss
Abdominal pain, rigid abdomen (can simulate appendicitis, pancreatitis, or other acute abdominal problem)	Apparently related to fluid volume deficit (condition improves when deficit is repaired)
Chest pain (may simulate pain of pleurisy)	Apparently related to fluid deficit (condition improves when fluid deficit is repaired); may be due to overactive respiration caused by acidosis
Moaning	Usually associated with abdominal or chest pain
Soft eyeballs, wrinkled cornea	Fluid volume deficit
Low blood pressure	Fluid volume deficit severe enough to decrease plasma volume significantly
Cold extremities, may have purplish appearance	Decreased peripheral blood flow secondary to fluid volume deficit
Body temperature below normal or normal (If fever is present it is almost always associated with the precipitating factor of the diabetic ketoacidosis, such as an infection)	Fluid volume deficit
Oliguria	Fluid volume deficit causes decreased renal blood flow with decreased glomerular filtration rate Atonic urinary bladder may become greatly distended with urine
Rapid, shallow, gasping respiration replacing Kussmaul breathing	Drop in blood pH below 7.0 or significantly decreased blood flow to the respiratory center
Coma	Sharp fall in plasma pH (to 7.0 or 6.9) and dehydration of cerebral cells (secondary to osmotic diuresis induced by hyperglycemia)

Laboratory Findings

Blood sugar:

   (Normal is 80–120 mg./100 ml.)

   Elevated above normal, usually 400–600 mg./100 ml.; may be as high as 2,000 mg./100 ml.   Faulty glucose metabolism causes glucose to accumulate in the blood

Bicarbonate:

   (Normal plasma bicarbonate level is 25–29 mEq./L. for adults; 20–25 mEq./L. for children)

   Decreased below normal; may be as low as 5 mEq./L.   Ketonic anions cause a decrease in the bicarbonate level

Others:

   BUN elevated   Impaired metabolism and glomerular function

   White count elevated, but differential normal

Treatment of Diabetic Ketoacidosis

INITIAL EVALUATION A patient with symptoms of diabetic ketoacidosis should be admitted to the hospital for immediate evaluation and treatment. Often the emergency room nurse spends a brief time with the patient before the physician arrives. She should utilize this time to the fullest advantage to expedite diagnosis and treatment.

While obtaining a voided urine specimen for sugar and acetone tests, the nurse should try to get an account of the events leading to the development of symptoms. If the patient is confused and nonresponsive, the information often may be obtained from an accompanying family member. The nurse should also ask if any treatment for ketoacidosis was given prior to hospital admission. (Sometimes the physician may instruct the family by phone to give a fast-acting insulin if symptoms of ketoacidosis are present.) The patient should be kept warm with blankets. (If a voided urine specimen cannot be obtained, the physician may later request a catheterized specimen.) The patient may have a dilated atonic urinary bladder; failure to void should not be attributed to renal failure until the bladder is catheterized to check for this disorder. The nurse should use meticulous technique while performing this procedure; infections are particularly dangerous in the diabetic patient.

The nurse should check and record the vital signs at frequent intervals. A low blood pressure and a rapid thready pulse may indicate severe fluid volume deficit with circulatory failure. A change from deep, rapid respiration to rapid, shallow gasping respiration may indicate a severe drop in blood pH (below 7.0) or impaired blood flow to the respiratory center because of fluid volume deficit and circulatory collapse. A temperature elevation probably indicates the presence of an acute infection; the temperature usually is subnormal in the patient with diabetic ketoacidosis. The patient's level of consciousness should be evaluated at frequent intervals; progressive loss of consciousness indicates increasing severity of acidosis. Other symptoms of ketoacidosis should be searched for and noted (see Table 22-1).

The nurse should notify the laboratory to draw blood; the physician usually requests tests for blood sugar, electrolytes, blood gases, acetone and blood urea nitrogen. Intravenous water and electrolytes such as hypotonic saline or a balanced hypotonic electrolyte solution (Butler type) may be ordered.

Initial fluids are given to improve the blood volume and blood pressure. Insulin is not usually administered until the blood sugar and urine test results are available. When acetone is found in the blood or urine, or when other pronounced signs of ketoacidosis are present, a dose of quick-acting insulin may be given before the blood sugar test result is obtained. It is imperative that the presence of hypoglycemia be ruled out before insulin is given. Hypoglycemia is characterized by anxiety, sweating, hunger, headache, dizziness, double vision, twitching, convulsions, nausea, pale wet skin, dilated pupils, normal breathing, and normal blood pressure.

When in doubt, the physician may administer 50 ml. of 50 per cent dextrose/water intravenously. If hypoglycemia is the problem, the patient's condition will quickly improve; if ketoacidosis is the problem, this amount of dextrose will do no harm. (See Table 22-2 for a comparison of symptoms in diabetic ketoacidosis versus hypoglycemia.)

INSULIN ADMINISTRATION Since the lack of insulin initiates diabetic ketoacidosis, insulin administration is required to correct it; however, there is some disagreement as to how much, when, and how it should be given.

Some physicians give half of a large initial dose of regular insulin intravenously and the other half either intramuscularly or subcutaneously; subsequent doses are given I.M. or S.Q. A newer method of treatment involves the administration of small doses of regular insulin either by continuous intravenous infusion or by frequent I.M. injections. In any event, insulin administration is closely guided by clinical observations and studies of blood and urinary glucose and acetone levels. Only regular insulin is used in the treatment of ketoacidosis; as mentioned above, it may be given I.V., I.M., or S.Q. The intravenous route is most dependable when there is some question of absorption from I.M. or S.Q. sites because of the presence of shock.

Regular insulin can be given undiluted by intravenous push (no faster than 50 units over one minute).[2] It may also be given in an infusion (regular insulin is stable in 5 per cent and 10 per cent dextrose in water with and without electrolytes).[3] It has been reported that up to 20 per cent of the insulin added to an infusion becomes bound to the flask and administration tubing; after the first infusion, when binding sites in the set have become saturated, the dose of in-

Table 22-2.   Differential Diagnosis of Diabetic Coma and Hypoglycemic Reactions

	DIABETIC COMA	HYPOGLYCEMIC REACTIONS	
		REGULAR INSULIN	MODIFIED INSULIN OR ORAL AGENTS
	Clinical Features		
Onset	Slow—days	Sudden—minutes	Gradual—hours
Causes	Ignorance Neglect of therapy Intercurrent disease or infection	Overdosage Omission or delay of meals Excessive exercise before meals	
Symptoms	Thirst Headache Nausea Vomiting Abdominal pain Dim vision Constipation Dyspnea	"Inward nervousness" Hunger Sweating Weakness Diplopia Blurred vision Paresthesia Psychopathic behavior Stupor Convulsions	Fatigue Headache Nausea Sweating (sometimes absent) Dizziness
Signs	Florid face Air hunger (Kussmaul's respiration) Finally, respiratory paralysis Dehydration (dry skin) Rapid pulse Soft eyeballs Normal or absent reflexes Acetone breath	Pallor Shallow respiration Sweating Normal pulse Eyeballs normal Babinski's reflex often present	Skin may be dry Pulse not characteristic
	Chemical Features		
Urine			
Glucose	Positive	Usually absent, especially in second voided specimen	
Acetone	Positive	Negative	
Diacetic acid	Positive	Negative	
Blood			
Glucose	>250 mg./100 ml. ordinarily	60 mg. or less/100 ml.	
CO_2 combining power	<20 volumes/100 ml.	Usually normal	
Leukocytosis	Present; may be very high		
Response to treatment	Slow	Rapid; occasionally delayed	May be delayed

Reprinted from Diabetes Mellitus, ed. 7. Eli Lilly and Co., Indianapolis, Indiana, 1976, page 167, with permission.

fused insulin approaches that added to the container.[4] The rate of the infusion should be ordered by the physician, depending on the patient's need for insulin and fluid.

The nurse should observe the patient for signs of hypoglycemia, which might occur when large doses of insulin are used to correct ketoacidosis. Other nursing responsibilities include performing urine sugar and acetone tests accurately, checking insulin orders with great care, and measuring the insulin dosage carefully. The orders for insulin are based on the blood sugar and acetone levels and on the quantities of sugar and acetone in the urine. Orders for insulin may be confusing in the early treatment of ketoacidosis; the nurse should take sufficient time to be certain she carries them out accurately.

In a sense, urine values for glucose and acetone tell the attendant less about the patient's current status than about past events. With aggressive treatment one can produce hypoglycemia in the presence of glycosuria and ketonuria.

The large doses of insulin sometimes needed to correct severe ketoacidosis may be frightening to the nurse if she is unaware that in severe ketoacidosis an abnormal serum globulin is present which antagonizes the action of insulin. As acidosis is relieved, the patient becomes less refractory to insulin and subsequent doses must be reduced. (Patients with mild acidosis or simple ketosis show only slight resistance to insulin and should not be given large doses.)

FLUID REPLACEMENT THERAPY

Early Phase (First 4 Hours). After the initial insulin dose has been given, emphasis is placed on reestablishing the blood volume and repairing extracellular and cellular fluid volume deficits. Repair of the deficient blood volume causes improved renal function and allows the excretion of excess organic acid wastes and metabolic end products. This may be accomplished by the administration of 2 to 3 L. of isotonic solution of sodium chloride or hypotonic electrolyte solutions during the first 2 to 6 hours.

Isotonic solution of sodium chloride (0.9 per cent) is readily available and is commonly used in the treatment of diabetic acidosis. It expands the extracellular fluid volume and helps replace losses of sodium and chloride. The first 2 L. can be given in 2 to 4 hours if the patient has satisfactory cardiac and renal status. It does not, however, provide free water for cellular hydration and the establishment of urine flow. Moreover, its chloride content exceeds that normally found in plasma; therefore, if used extensively, it can worsen ketoacidosis by imposing a chloride excess. (An excessive number of chloride ions causes a compensatory decrease in the number of bicarbonate ions.) Usually no more than 3 L. of isotonic saline are given in the first 6 to 12 hours, to avoid making the ketoacidosis more severe.

Some authorities recommend a solution of two-thirds isotonic saline and one-third M/6 sodium lactate to avoid imposing an excess of chloride ions. In cases of severe acidosis (plasma bicarbonate level below 12 mEq./L.), it is advisable to administer a sodium bicarbonate, or lactate, solution (such as 500 ml. of 1.3 per cent sodium bicarbonate or 1000 ml. of 1/6 molar sodium lactate.)

Since the patient with ketoacidosis loses relatively more water than electrolytes, there is much to be said for the administration of hypotonic solutions; a hypotonic solution of sodium chloride with or without added sodium lactate or bicarbonate can be employed.

Authorities disagree as to the desirability of using glucose solutions in the early treatment of diabetic ketoacidosis. Some physicians use them from the onset of treatment; others wait at least 4 hours before infusing glucose solutions. Those against the early use of glucose feel that it does nothing more than to add to hyperglycemia and, thus, increases osmotic diuresis with the resultant water and electrolyte loss from the body. Others feel that glucose should be added early since insulin therapy can readily deplete body glucose stores. After the first 4 to 6 hours of treatment (when the blood sugar is less than 250 mg./100 ml.) danger of hypoglycemia exists, and glucose should be administered.

Potassium administration is contraindicated in the early phase of treatment, since the plasma potassium level usually is elevated as a result of the liberation of cellular potassium into the extracellular fluid and to poor renal excretion of potassium caused by decreased urinary output. Potassium excess may cause cardiac arrhythmias; if elevated to two or three times the normal level, cardiac arrest may occur. Potassium solutions are best withheld until the plasma potassium level is normal or below normal. The ECG is used frequently throughout therapy to detect changes in potassium concentration. Signs of potassium excess may appear during this phase (such as tall, tented T waves (Fig. 22-1) and widened QRS complexes), or the ECG may remain normal. Only very rarely does a patient show potassium deficit at this time; if so, it is almost always associated with a severe loss of potassium prior to the onset of diabetic ketoacidosis.

Second Phase (4–8 Hours). Approximately 4 to 8 hours after the onset of therapy the patient usually is much improved and the need for parenteral fluids

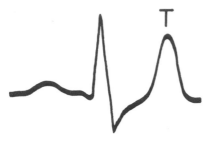

Figure 22-1. Tall, tented T wave produced by hyperkalemia. (From Sharp, L., and Rabin, B.: Nursing in the Coronary Care Unit. Philadelphia: J. B. Lippincott Co., 1970, p. 94. Used with permission)

is decreased. Usually oral fluids may be tolerated by this time. The rate of intravenous infusion can be slowed considerably. If the blood sugar has fallen substantially, glucose may be given orally to combat hypoglycemia; intravenous glucose in water may also be required.

Although potassium deficit rarely occurs this early, the plasma potassium level usually has dropped sufficiently to allow potassium to be given, by mouth or intravenously, to ameliorate the developing cellular deficit. Oral administration is preferable. Fluids of high potassium content include tomato juice, orange juice, grapefruit juice, and milk. Intravenous replacement of potassium can be accomplished by use of a Butler-type solution, or it may be added to a suitable fluid in the form of KCl. (Nursing responsibilities in the administration of potassium solutions are discussed in Chapter 16.)

Potassium supplements may also be given via nasogastric tube. Prior to administering potassium in any form, it is necessary to monitor hourly urine volumes to detect possible oliguria; potassium should be given only when adequate renal function is present (as evidenced by a urine output of at least 50 ml./hr.).

Phase of Potassium Deficit (8–24 Hours). Recall that, in the early phase of diabetic ketoacidosis, the plasma potassium level is normal or elevated, as a result of the liberation of potassium from the cells during the breakdown of glycogen and protein, and of decreased renal function with excessive retention of potassium. After administration of potassium-free fluids early in therapy, the plasma potassium decreases for the following reasons:

1. The administered fluids dilute the plasma.
2. Reestablishment of the plasma volume im-

proves renal function and increases potassium excretion.
3. Part of the extracellular potassium enters the cells as they take up glucose under the influence of administered insulin.
4. Formation of glycogen within the cells—involving utilization of potassium, glucose, and water—causes further withdrawal of potassium from the extracellular fluid.
5. Potassium reenters the cells to help repair the cellular potassium deficit.

Because of the great need for potassium during the later stages of treatment, potassium should be added to parenteral infusions during this period.

Potassium deficit becomes obvious after 8 to 24 hours of treatment, most often between the tenth and twenty-fourth hours. The plasma potassium level may fall as low as 2 mEq./L. (recall that the normal plasma K^+ level is 5 mEq./L.). The nurse should be alert for the symptoms of potassium deficit during these hours, including:

weakness
flaccid paralysis of skeletal muscles
paralysis of respiratory muscles, resulting in shallow, gasping respiration and cyanosis
abdominal distention
ECG changes (flat or inverted T waves, depressed S-T segments, Q-T intervals often appear prolonged because of the superimposed U waves on T waves—Fig. 22-2)
cardiac failure with ashen color
sudden death (most common 8 to 20 hours after therapy is started)

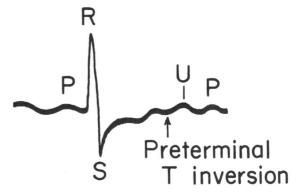

Figure 22-2. Electrocardiographic changes produced by hypokalemia. (From Sharp, L., and Rabin, B.: Nursing in the Coronary Care Unit. Philadelphia: J. B. Lippincott Co., 1970, p. 93. Used with permission)

Potassium should be given as soon as renal function improves and the plasma potassium concentration falls to normal. The cellular potassium deficit takes over a week to replace; yet, even small amounts of potassium taken regularly help ward off a severe deficit. Fluids mentioned above should be encouraged. Oral replacement of potassium is safer than intravenous replacement; if the patient tolerates oral fluids, they can be enriched with potassium additives. (K-Lyte, an effervescent potassium preparation, is palatable and well tolerated.)

Summary of Fluid Therapy Aims   In the first 24 hours of treatment of diabetic ketoacidosis, the aim is to replace 80 per cent of the total water, sodium, and chloride loss. Cellular electrolytes are not assimilated as rapidly as extracellular ones; therefore, only 50 per cent of the potassium and magnesium deficit, and 25 per cent of the phosphate deficit, are replaced on the first day. In addition to replacing past and concurrent losses, daily maintenance needs must be met.

GASTRIC LAVAGE   Some physicians routinely perform a gastric lavage on all patients with diabetic ketoacidosis since gastric atony is commonly present. Others do so only when the patient has demonstrable signs of gastric dilatation such as nausea, vomiting, and epigastric distress.

Removal of gastric contents makes the patient more comfortable; it relieves abdominal distention, vomiting, and nausea. Oral intake is made possible earlier. The danger of aspirating gastric contents is less when the distended viscus is emptied, but the hazard of inducing alkalosis should not be disregarded.

CLEANSING ENEMA   A cleansing enema may be ordered to relieve abdominal distention caused by intestinal atony.

OTHER THERAPY   The patient should be restored to his usual diet as quickly as it is tolerated. After recovery from diabetic ketoacidosis, long-acting insulin can be resumed, with supplemental doses of fast-acting insulin as indicated by urine test results. An excellent opportunity exists for teaching the patient while he is still in the hospital how to prevent future bouts of ketoacidosis.

INSULIN ADMINISTRATION   The omission of insulin injections or inadequate insulin doses are common causes of diabetic ketoacidosis. It is not unusual to admit a patient in diabetic ketoacidosis who comments, "I've been vomiting and unable to eat for the past few days and didn't need my insulin." He has assumed that when he does not eat he should omit insulin injections. This common assumption is not true. The body needs insulin, although in modified doses and perhaps a different type, even when the patient is not eating. The nurse should make it clear that insulin should never be omitted without specific direction from the physician. When unable to eat, the patient should contact his physician for instructions. The once-daily injection of long-acting insulin may be temporarily reduced or discontinued, until the patient is able to eat again; instead, frequent doses of quick-acting insulin may be given as indicated by findings of urine sugar and acetone tests. If food intake is decreased for a prolonged period, the patient should be admitted to the hospital for parenteral fluid therapy and observation. It must be remembered that the nausea and vomiting experienced by the patient may be signs of developing diabetic acidosis. If so, failure to take insulin accelerates the development of acidosis.

A number of factors can result in the administration of too little insulin. An inadequate insulin dose may be due to failure to properly mix protamine zinc, NPH, or Lente insulin vials prior to drawing up the insulin. Insulin that is too old or has been spoiled by freezing or overheating is ineffective. Continued injection at the same site may produce inflammation, hypertrophy, or atrophy of the local tissue. Additional insulin injected into these areas is not well absorbed and results in an inadequate insulin dosage. The diabetic with poor vision may draw up an inadequate amount of insulin because of difficulty in reading the insulin scale. (Sometimes such a patient may draw up, undetected, a large air bubble which decreases the amount of insulin contained in the syringe.) Drawing up insulin on the wrong scale also causes an inaccurate dosage; for example, drawing up U-40 insulin on a U-80 scale results in half the desired dose. (Of course, poor vision and faulty technique can also cause insulin overdosage.) The diabetic who is poorly controlled at home should be observed for faulty technique in drawing up and administering his insulin.

DIABETIC DIET   Eating more than permitted by the prescribed diet is a frequent cause of diabetic acidosis. While this may be due to poor emotional acceptance of the disease, it may also be due to lack of adequate understanding of the diet.

When possible, the diabetic patient should receive his diet instructions during frequent sessions with a dietitian. The nurse should have sufficient understanding of the diet to supplement the dietitian's instructions. Sometimes, in the absence of a dietitian, the nurse must carry the entire responsibility of diet instruction. Few nurses are so well acquainted with diabetic diets that they will not profit from a review prior to teaching the patient.

Urine Testing

Physicians rely heavily on urine sugar and acetone tests to serve as guides in prescribing insulin. The time and frequency of urine tests, as well as the method to be used, should be indicated on the order sheet. Some physicians order "spot checks" (tests of individual urine specimens) at regular intervals. These are usually done on arising, before lunch, before the evening meal, and at bedtime; sometimes they are done two hours after meals. Other times the physician may prefer fractional, or group, urine testing. Fractional urines are usually collected in four parts according to the time of day: before breakfast to just before lunch; before lunch to just before the evening meal; before the evening meal to bedtime; from bedtime until the next morning. Testing of fractional urines helps the physician find the time of day glucose excretion is highest. This information is helpful in prescribing the appropriate type and amount of insulin.

If the tests are performed improperly, or reported incorrectly, the physician will receive false information and the insulin dose is likely to be incorrect.

GENERAL CONSIDERATIONS

1. It is best to use the second of double-voided specimens, particularly when the patient has severe diabetes. After the first specimen is obtained, the patient is encouraged to drink a glass of water; after 30 to 45 minutes, a second specimen is collected. The second specimen is desirable for urinary sugar testing, because it reflects the glucose spill-over into the urine at that time (while the first specimen reflects an indefinite accumulation).

2. Directions given by the manufacturers of the various tests should be followed closely. Although this sounds simple, recent studies have shown that hospital personnel commonly perform urine tests inaccurately. This is a matter of concern for two reasons: (a) control of the hospitalized diabetic is difficult to achieve without the aid of accurate urine testing and (b) personnel performing urine tests inaccurately are hardly in a position to teach patients to perform these same tests.

3. The record used for charting urine test results should indicate the test method used. Unless instructions are clear, various nurses on the unit may use the method they like best; the use of different testing methods for the same patient leads to much confusion. Some nurses use plus marks interchangeably between tests—this, of course, is not accurate. For example: a two-plus on Tes-Tape indicates a sugar concentration of ¼%, while a two-plus on Clinitest indicates a sugar concentration of three times this amount (¾%). (See Table 22-3 for a comparison of results in some of the more commonly used tests for urinary sugar content.) When regular insulin is ordered on a sliding scale, based on urinary sugar content, the physician should indicate the specific test he wants used. For example, a typical order might read:

Give 5 units of regular insulin if Clinitest is one-plus
Give 10 units of regular insulin if Clinitest is two-plus
Give 15 units of regular insulin if Clinitest is three-plus
Give 20 units of regular insulin if Clinitest is four-plus

4. Clean receptacles should be used to collect the specimen; failure to thoroughly rinse out the urinal or bedpan between voidings can cause inaccurate results.

5. It is wise to check the material in the test apparatus for changes from its normal appearance. For example, Clinitest tablets that are disintegrating and have changed to a dark color are not suitable for use and should be discarded. When in doubt, materials can be tested for effectiveness with a nondietetic cola beverage; ordinary table sugar will not produce a positive reaction.

6. Good lighting is necessary for reading test results; this is particularly important when eyesight

Table 22-3.   Comparison of Degrees of Sugar Content Indicated by Various Urine Tests

Tes-Tape	Diastix	Clinitest (5-drop method)	Clinitest (2-drop method)	Clinistix
0% Negative	0% Negative	0% Negative	0% Negative	"Light" generally indicates
	$^1/_{10}$% Trace	¼% Trace		¼% or less
$^1/_{10}$% (+)	¼% (+)	½% (+)	Trace	"Medium" generally indicates
¼% (++)	½% (++)	¾% (++)	½%	¼ to ½%
½% (+++)	1% (+++)	1% (+++)	1%	"Dark" generally indicates
2% (++++)	2% (++++)	2% (++++)	2%	½% or more
			3%	
			5%	

is impaired. Diabetics with extremely poor vision should have someone else read the test results for them. The color comparison chart should be in good condition—faded charts can lead to inaccurate readings.

7. The test results should be compared with the appropriate color comparison chart. Patients switched to a different form of testing may be unaware that each test method has its own chart; unless instructed otherwise they may continue to use the old chart with the new test.

8. The nurse should be aware that the amount of sugar spilled into the urine depends on the blood sugar level and the renal threshold. Most individuals spill sugar into the urine when the blood sugar content exceeds 180 mg. per 100 ml. of blood. However, some persons have an elevated renal threshold; that is, the blood sugar may be above normal while the patient continues to have negative tests for sugar in the urine. On the other hand, some have a low renal threshold and spill sugar into the urine while the blood sugar level is near normal or is within the normal range. A urine-glucose value is significant only when the patient's renal threshold for glucose is known. It is helpful to check an occasional blood sugar at the same time as a urine sugar.

TESTS FOR URINARY SUGAR   Various tests are available to detect and measure urinary sugar content. Among these are Clinitest, Tes-Tape, Clinistix, and Diastix.

Clinitest   Clinitest* reagent tablets utilize the copper-reducing reaction to measure the amount of sugar in the urine. The method for testing with Clinitest tablets is as follows:

---

* Ames Company, Division of Miles Laboratories, Inc., Elkhart, Indiana.

1. Place 5 drops of urine and 10 drops of water in a clean test tube.
2. Drop in one Clinitest tablet.
3. Observe the reaction carefully for the rapid pass-through phenomenon. (If the solution passes through orange to some shade of brown, it indicates that more than a 2 per cent sugar concentration is present, and this should be recorded without reference to the color chart.)
4. Wait 15 seconds after the boiling stops; shake the tube gently and compare the solution with the color chart provided with test (Clinitest's color reaction ranges from blue, no sugar, through shades of green and brown to orange, 2 per cent sugar).

Because the pass-through phenomenon is not well understood, it is a common source of error. To help decrease the frequency of this error, a variation of the Clinitest method has been devised. Two drops of urine, instead of five, are mixed with 10 drops of water; the resulting solution is less concentrated and the urinary sugar content must exceed 5 per cent before the pass-through phenomenon can occur. (Although it is possible to observe the pass-through reaction using the two-drop method, it isn't very likely.) Even though the two-drop method is superior to the five-drop method for patients who commonly run high urine sugars, it may present some problems. A special color chart must be obtained from the manufacturer because the results are different from those of the five-drop method. The two charts appear similar and may be easily confused unless one is aware of their differences. A two-drop chart is available separately or as part of a specially marked two-drop Clinitest kit.

A one-drop Clinitest method can be used for severe juvenile diabetics if the two-drop method shows a 5 per cent reading or if the solution passes from orange back to greenish brown within 15 seconds. The one-drop method will measure up to a 10 per cent urinary sugar content.

Clinitest tablets are extremely hygroscopic and, thus, should not be exposed to moisture; tablets wrapped in foil should be used immediately upon opening. Glass bottles containing Clinitest tablets should be kept tightly closed; after opening, tablets in glass bottles should be used on a regular basis and not stored for an extended period of time. Tablets with a dark-blue color should be discarded.

Clinitest registers a color change in response to other reducing agents besides glucose when they are present in concentrations of ¼% or more. However, such substances are generally not present in sufficient quantities to cause false positives or elevated readings. A partial list of medications that may produce false positive results with Clinitest includes these:

ascorbic acid (in large doses)
probenecid (Benemid®)
penicillin
isoniazid
sodium cephalothin (Keflin®)
cephalexin monohydrate (Keflex®)
nalidixic acid (NegGram®)
para-aminosalicylic acid

Clinitest is not the method of choice for urine testing in patients with tuberculosis because the antituberculosis drugs are reducing agents.

Clinitest detects not just glucose, but all sugars in the urine (lactose, galactose, fructose, maltose, and pentose). Therefore, it should not be used for urine testing in the last trimester of pregnancy when lactosuria may be present. (Lactose has no effect on Diastix, Clinistix, or Tes-Tape.)

Tes-Tape Tes-Tape* is a roll of yellow test paper impregnated with a dye and an enzyme, glucose oxidase. In the presence of sugar, this enzyme reacts and releases the dye. Tes-Tape is considered specific for glucose determination. The method used for testing with Tes-Tape is as follows:

1. Collect the urine specimen in a clean container.
2. Tear off about 1½ inches of the test paper and moisten it uniformly with urine. (The tape held between the fingers should be kept dry because the hands may carry traces of sugar.)
3. Remove the test strip from the urine and wait one minute; the tape should be held during this period (laying the tape down could result in its contamination if the surface contains traces of sugar).
4. Compare the darkest area on the test strip with the color chart on the Tes-Tape dispenser (if the tape indicates ½% or higher, wait an additional minute and make a final comparison).

The tape remains yellow if the test is negative; intermediate amounts of sugar produce various shades of green, and a concentration of 2 per cent causes the tape to turn blue. Note that this color reaction is very different from that of Clinitest. Tes-Tape is more convenient than Clinitest, but Clinitest is probably more accurate in showing the precise amount of sugar present in the urine. The expiration date on the Tes-Tape package should be checked. Once opened, Tes-Tape cannot be made airtight and should be kept in a dry place. It should be discarded after being open for four months or longer.

Diastix Diastix* reagent strips are used for the semiquantitative determination of glucose in urine. The method for testing with Diastix is as follows:

1. The urine specimen should be freshly voided and well mixed—the container should be absolutely clean and free from cleansers and disinfectants. (Refrigerated urine specimens should be allowed to reach room temperature before testing.)
2. Dip the reagent end of the strip in the urine specimen for two seconds, or pass it through the urine stream.
3. Tap the edge of the strip against the side of the urine container or sink to remove excess urine.
4. Exactly 30 seconds after removing the strip from the urine, compare the reagent side of

* Eli Lilly and Company, Indianapolis, Indiana.

* Ames Company, Division of Miles Laboratories, Inc., Elkhart, Indiana.

the strip to the closest matching color block (disregard color changes that occur after 30 seconds).

This test may detect minute quantities of glucose in the urine (as low as $^1/_{100}$% to $^1/_{10}$%). It, then, may show a trace of sugar when the Clinitest is negative. (Recall that Clinitest shows trace at ¼%).

Diastix is designed primarily for use at home by late-onset diabetic patients who are unlikely to encounter ketonuria. This test is not recommended when there is a likelihood of ketonuria because moderate to large amounts of acetoacetic acid may depress the color response.

Diastix reagent strips should be kept in a cool, dry place, but not in the refrigerator; the bottle should be kept tightly closed. Prior to use, the test area on the strip should match the negative color block on the color chart; if it doesn't, the strip should be discarded.

Clinistix Clinistix* reagent strips undergo a color change when moistened with urine containing glucose. The method for urine testing with Clinistix is as follows:

1. Moisten the red end of the Clinistix by passing it once through the urine stream or by dipping it in a fresh urine specimen collected in a clean container.
2. Remove immediately from the urine (prolonged immersion may cause leaching of the reagents).
3. Exactly 10 seconds after wetting, compare the test area with the color block on the Clinistix bottle label.

Clinistix is a specific for glucose. "Light" generally indicates ¼% glucose concentration or less. (The minimal concentration of glucose detectable by Clinistix ranges from as little as $^1/_{100}$% to $^1/_{10}$%.) "Medium" generally indicates glucose in amounts of ¼% to ½%. "Dark" generally indicates ½% glucose concentration or more. Large amounts of ascorbic acid or acetoacetic acid have definite inhibitory effects on the color development.

Clinistix should be stored in a cool, dry place and protected from exposure to direct light, excessive heat, or humidity. Discolored strips should not be used. The test end of the strip should not be handled, nor should it be laid on the work surface with the reagent area downward.

TESTS FOR KETONURIA All diabetics should be taught how to test for ketonuria. It is a good practice to test for ketones periodically regardless of the urinary glucose concentration, but the consistent presence of large amounts of sugar in the urine is an indication to test for ketones regularly. Ketonuria tests should especially be performed in diabetic children, difficult to control adult diabetics, the pregnant diabetic, and in the conversion from insulin to oral hypoglycemic agents.

The ketones present in the urine of the uncontrolled diabetic include acetoacetic acid, acetone, and beta-hydroxybutyric acid. Ketonuria may provide the clue to the early diagnosis of diabetic ketoacidosis. Two common tests used to detect ketonuria include Acetest and Ketostix.

Acetest Acetest* detects both acetone and acetoacetic acid in the urine. The colorimetric chart provided with this test has three colors ranging from lavender to deep purple, representing small, moderate, or large amounts of ketones. If the test is negative, the tablet remains buff colored. The method for testing is as follows:

1. Place an Acetest tablet on a clean surface, preferably a piece of clean white paper.
2. Put one drop of urine on the tablet.
3. Read the reaction at 30 seconds against the color chart (failure of the drop of urine to completely absorb within this period indicates that the tablet has been exposed to moisture and may give a faulty reading).

Ketostix Ketostix* reagent strips are also used to test for acetoacetic acid and acetone in urine. The method for testing is as follows:

1. Dip the test area of the strip in fresh urine or pass it briefly through the urine stream and remove it immediately.
2. Tap the edge of the strip against the container to remove excess urine.

---

* Ames Company, Division of Miles Laboratories, Inc., Elkhart, Indiana.

* Ames Company, Division of Miles Laboratories, Inc., Elkhart, Indiana.

3. Fifteen seconds after wetting, compare the color of the test area with the color chart. (The shade of lavender or purple developed at 15 seconds indicates the concentration of ketones in the urine.) Ignore color developing on the test area after 15 seconds.

Ketostix strips should be protected from moisture, direct sunlight, and heat. Discoloration of the test area of the strip is an indication to discard it.

Prevention of Severe Diabetic Ketoacidosis

The best treatment of ketoacidosis is prevention through patient teaching. The nurse should stress the importance of being alert for symptoms of ketoacidosis, particularly when an infection, disease, or emotional upset is present. She should also point out that when such symptoms occur, the attending physician should be notified immediately. Manufacturers of insulin preparations provide excellent literature for diabetics; many useful facts are contained in these booklets. For example, symptoms of ketoacidosis and hypoglycemia are described in a clear and simple fashion. The patient should be given copies of such literature for use during teaching sessions and for reference at home. A member of the patient's family should also be taught to recognize symptoms of ketoacidosis.

Because the nurse is actively involved in teaching diabetic patients, she is in a splendid position to help prevent diabetic ketoacidosis. She should keep the basic learning principles in mind when teaching self-care to diabetics. The rate of learning of the individual must be considered; so must the knowledge he already possesses concerning the disease. Physicians sometimes present explanations far beyond the patient's comprehension. Rather than risk the embarrassment of asking for a more simplified explanation, the patient may pretend to understand—this can lead to serious difficulties.

It is important for the patient to gain a clear understanding of his condition and of his responsibilities to himself. Time and effort devoted to effective teaching of the diabetic patient pays off handsomely when it helps prevent complications.

Failure to teach the diabetic the importance of (1) taking the prescribed amount of insulin daily, (2) reporting conditions that may alter the need for insulin, (3) adhering to the prescribed diet, (4) performing urine sugar and acetone tests accurately, and (5) seeking medical follow-up as indicated, predisposes to diabetic ketoacidosis and other complications.

Failure of the patient to recognize the early symptoms of uncontrolled diabetes and early diabetic ketoacidosis leads to delay in instituting treatment. The longer the patient goes without treatment, the less are his chances for recovery.

Mortality is also influenced by the precipitating factor of ketoacidosis (such as trauma, infection).

NONKETOTIC HYPEROSMOLAR COMA

Nonketotic hyperosmolar coma tends to occur in mild (ketosis-resistant) diabetics over the age of 60; in fact, in a substantial number of reported cases, the diagnosis of diabetes had not yet been established.[5] This condition is characterized by marked plasma hyperosmolarity without significant ketoacidosis. Plasma osmolarities have ranged from 330 to 460 mOsm./kg. of body water (normal 275 to 295).[6]

Precipitating factors are profound hyperglycemia (blood sugar often exceeds 1000 mg./100 ml.), hypernatremia (plasma sodium usually exceeds 150 mEq./L.), and azotemia. Osmotic force pulls water out of the cells (including cerebral cells) and can produce pronounced dehydration and coma. The body's water deficit may be as great as 10 or more liters. Usually, both inadequate water intake and inadequate renal solute excretion are present. (Preexisting vascular disease usually is a problem in the older diabetic and predisposes to renal and cerebral dysfunction.)

Treatment consists of the administration of hypotonic fluids to expand plasma volume and promote solute excretion; a frequently used solution is 0.45 per cent sodium chloride (half-strength saline). Since fluid replacement volume is large, it may be necessary to monitor CVP in patients with compromised cardiac function. Also, regular insulin is given as indicated to correct hyperglycemia; the insulin dosage usually is less than that required to correct ketoacidosis (remember that in ketoacidosis an abnormal serum globulin is present which antagonizes the action of insulin).

Prognosis of nonketotic hyperosmolar coma is not good (mortality approaches 44 to 50 per cent). Contributing to the poor prognosis is the patient's age and underlying vascular disease.

LACTIC ACIDOSIS

Lactic acidosis can occur in both diabetics and non-diabetics. It is associated with serious illnesses in which tissue hypoxia exists (such as acute hemorrhage, hypotension, heart failure). Anaerobic metabolism causes excessive lactic acid formation and a drop in plasma pH. Lactic acidosis is an often fatal form of metabolic acidosis.

Since coma in lactic acidosis may be confused with the coma of ketoacidosis, particularly in growth-onset diabetics, it is important to be able to differentiate the two. Ketoacidosis is characterized by the following laboratory findings:

> high blood sugar
> high plasma acetone level
> high urinary sugar content
> high urinary ketone content
> low plasma bicarbonate level

Lactic acidosis is characterized by the following laboratory findings:

> blood sugar is variable (depending upon state of diabetic control)
> negative or slight elevation of plasma acetone level
> negative or slight urinary sugar content
> negative urinary ketone content
> decreased plasma bicarbonate level

The presence of an unexplained fall in pH associated with a condition producing hypoxia should lead one to suspect lactic acidosis; this type of acidosis is characterized by a widening anion gap.[7] An anion gap is said to exist when the sum of plasma bicarbonate and chloride anions is less than the plasma sodium level minus twelve ($[HCO_3^- + Cl^-] < [Na^+ - 12]$).

Generally, lactic acidosis can be distinguished from ketoacidosis by the absence of severe ketosis and hyperglycemia.[8] Treatment is directed at correcting the cause of hypoxia and administration of sufficient alkaline fluids (usually sodium bicarbonate) to correct the acidosis.

Phenformin was removed from the general market* in October 1977 because of the unacceptably high risk of lactic acidosis associated with its use. It was found that lactic acidosis could occur in patients taking phenformin at doses of 100 mg. or less, even when there were no underlying risk factors predisposing to lactic acidosis (such as cardiovascular or renal disease.)[9]

REFERENCES

1. **Guyton, A.:** Textbook of Medical Physiology, ed. 5. Philadelphia: W. B. Saunders Co., 1976, p. 1034.
2. **Gahart, B.:** Intravenous Medications, ed. 2. St. Louis: C. V. Mosby, 1977, p. 104.
3. Diabetes Mellitus, ed. 7. Eli Lilly and Co., Indianapolis, Ind., 1976, p. 89.
4. Ibid., p. 90.
5. Ibid., p. 176.
6. Ibid.
7. Ibid.
8. Ibid.
9. Phenformin: removal from general market. FDA Drug Bull. Vol. 7, No. 3, August 1977, p. 14.

BIBLIOGRAPHY

Boedeker, E., and **Dauber, J.** (eds.): Manual of Medical Therapeutics, ed. 21. Boston: Little, Brown & Co., 1974.

Guthrie, D., and **Guthrie, R.** (eds.): Nursing Management of Diabetes Mellitus. St. Louis: C. V. Mosby, 1977.

Macleod, J. (ed.): Davidson's Principles & Practice of Medicine, ed. 11. New York: Churchill Livingstone, 1975.

* Phenformin may still be made available to a small group of maturity-onset nonketotic diabetics in whom the benefits of phenformin outweigh the risks.

23

Fluid Balance in the Patient with Neurologic Disease

REGULATION OF FLUID BALANCE BY THE CENTRAL NERVOUS SYSTEM

RESPIRATORY CENTER AND pH REGULATION The amount of carbon dioxide given off by the lungs is controlled by the respiratory center in the medulla. Recall that carbon dioxide is crucial in the carbonic acid–base bicarbonate buffer system. Pathologic conditions can cause depression or stimulation of the medullary respiratory neurons and, thus, can alter plasma pH. (See the section dealing with changes in pulmonary ventilation, pp. 329–330.)

INFLUENCE OF CENTRAL NERVOUS SYSTEM ON OSMOTIC BALANCE The central nervous system influences water loss from the kidneys, skin, and lungs. It controls the desire to drink as well as the motor ability to do so. Emotions influence water balance by affecting the drinking pattern; for example, neuroses sometimes cause compulsive water drinking.

Hyperosmolarity stimulates the hypothalamus to release ADH, the secretion of which is also influenced by volume receptors in the left atrium and pulmonary veins.

CLINICAL CONDITIONS

Brain infections, tumors, or trauma can cause a diversity of fluid balance problems, depending on the area of the brain involved. Injury to the hypothalamus and the brain stem presents the most problems, because many metabolic functions are controlled in these areas. Many brain injuries interfere with the patient's ability to recognize thirst, as well as his ability to drink. The desire to eat and the ability to do so may also be affected. Recall that inadequate intake of food and fluids is responsible for a number of fluid imbalances.

Often, water and electrolyte balance is the most critical factor in determining the survival of the neurologic patient. For this reason, the nurse should become acutely aware of common problems so that she can aid in their early detection and correction.

HYPERTHERMIA The heat control center is located in the hypothalamus. Direct injury to this area, or pressure exerted by edema or masses in other areas of the brain, can cause a body temperature elevation. A rise in temperature in a neurologic patient often is an ominous sign. However, fever may be due to other causes such as pneumonia, urinary tract infection, or dehydration (sodium excess).

Patients who have recovered from encephalitis, or those with cerebral damage from birth injuries, may have faulty temperature regulation. Sometimes multiple sclerosis is associated with low, irregular fever. In addition, an injury to the upper cervical spinal cord often results in high, irregular fever. Finally, surgical operations in the area of the third ventricle sometimes cause pronounced hyperthermia.

Fever should be reduced by pharmacologic or physical means. An automatically regulated hypothermic blanket can be most helpful in reducing temperature; sponging with ice water or alcohol is less effective. Fever speeds up body metabolism. (See the discussion of fever in Chapter 14.) Because of the increased energy expenditure, the patient needs more calories and water. Yet, as mentioned above, a neurologic patient is often unable to recognize thirst and hunger. Moreover, impaired motor function may interfere with the mechanics of drinking and eating. Thus, at a time when the need for food and fluids is great, the patient may be unable to respond with increased intake. Because fever resulting from brain lesions may continue for weeks or even months, careful attention must be paid to meeting the patient's need for food and fluids.

Fever often occurs in a patient with cerebral edema and presents the physician with a difficult problem: the patient needs fluid replacement, yet the danger of increasing cerebral edema may contraindicate such therapy.

CONFUSED OR UNCONSCIOUS PATIENTS The nurse falsely assumes, too often, that all patients experience normal thirst and appetite and are capable of reacting to their needs for fluids and food. She should remember that confused or unconscious patients do not have this capacity. Thus, she must help assess and meet their nutritional needs.

If the patient is unable to take oral fluids, other routes of intake are available. For example, a patient with difficulty in swallowing may not be able to drink sufficient fluids, yet his fluid requirement can easily be met with tube feedings. A patient with nausea and vomiting can neither take fluids orally nor by gastric tube, but he can be provided with parenteral fluids. Keen observations by the nurse help the physician determine which replacement route is best and, thus, minimize the duration of the period of inadequate intake.

All confused or unconscious patients should be placed on careful intake-output measurements. Fluid loss by all routes, such as sweating, vomiting, or diarrhea, should be carefully recorded. Body temperature checks should be made every four hours—oftener if indicated—to detect elevations. Evaluation of fluids lost from the body serves as a basis for fluid replacement; inadequate fluid replacement eventually results in fluid volume deficit.

It is often difficult to determine the urinary output of neurologic patients, since many of them are incontinent. Because of time-consuming bed changes, the nursing staff is often misled into thinking that incontinent patients have large urinary outputs. The amount of incontinent voidings should be estimated as closely as possible. Failure to assess the urinary output accurately may lead to inadequate fluid replacement. To avoid guesswork, seriously ill patients should have indwelling urinary catheters or external devices to catch urine. The insensible water loss can be assessed by accurate daily weight measurements. (See Chapter 13 for further discussion of nursing responsibilities in fluid intake-output records and body weight measurements.)

Efforts should be made to assure maximal ventilation in order to prevent hypoxia and hypercarbia (elevated pCO_2). (Recall that severe hypoxia and hypercarbia cause a rise in intracranial pressure.) Frequently, an airway is necessary to prevent the tongue of the comatose patient from obstructing air flow; dentures and dental plates should be removed since they can obstruct the airway. The patient with a prognosis of prolonged complete unconsciousness usually requires intubation and mechanical ventilation. Great care should be taken to prevent hypoxia during suctioning (that is, avoid tracheal suctioning longer than 15 seconds; provide extra oxygen, as allowed, immediately prior to tracheal suctioning).

Pathologic Conditions Affecting the Respiratory Center

Pathologic conditions of the central nervous system can cause stimulation or depression of the respiratory neurons, thus altering plasma pH.

HYPERVENTILATION Neurologic conditions associated with overstimulation of the respiratory center include:

Meningitis
Encephalitis
Brain tumor
Fever

Hyperventilation results from the overstimulation of respiratory neurons. Increased pulmonary ventilation causes excessive elimination of CO_2 resulting in respiratory alkalosis. A mixture of 5 per cent CO_2 and 95 per cent O_2 helps relieve the symptoms of respiratory alkalosis when breathed for a short period by the patient with cerebral damage. (See the discussion of hyperventilation as a possible treatment for patients with elevated intracranial pressure later in this chapter.)

HYPOVENTILATION Neurologic conditions associated with depression of the respiratory center include:

1. Direct trauma to the respiratory neurons in the medulla
2. Pressure on the respiratory neurons secondary to tumor, hemorrhage, or brain abscess
3. Bulbar poliomyelitis

Hypoventilation results from the depression of respiratory neurons. Retention of excessive amounts of CO_2 causes respiratory acidosis. Hypoventilation, which is far more dangerous than hyperventilation, presents these hazards:

1. Hypoxia with dilation of cerebral blood vessels and subsequent increased intracranial pressure (particularly with a profoundly low arterial pO_2 of less than 50 mm. Hg.)[1]
2. Increased CO_2 retention (hypercarbia) with dilation of the cerebral blood vessels and subsequent increased intracranial pressure (particularly when arterial pCO_2 is greater than 60 mm. Hg.)[2]
3. Respiratory acidosis

Hypoventilation due to medullary depression may necessitate the use of a mechanical respirator. Treatment should also be aimed at eliminating the cause of respiratory center depression.

Nursing Implications The nurse should be alert for changes in respiration. She should check the respiratory rate, depth, and rhythm and should watch for symptoms of respiratory acidosis when breathing is suppressed. These include:

Disorientation
Weakness
Coma, if acidosis is severe

The nurse should also watch for symptoms of respiratory alkalosis when the rate and the depth of respiration are increased. These symptoms include:

Light-headedness
Numbness, tingling of fingers and toes
Circumoral paresthesia
Tinnitis
Blurring of vision
Convulsions
Unconsciousness

Some of the symptoms, such as disorientation, weakness, convulsions, coma and blurred vision, may be caused by other conditions, such as brain tumors or cerebral vascular accidents. Such symptoms should be evaluated in the light of the patient's history and neurologic status.

The physician usually orders frequent blood gas analyses to help evaluate the patient's acid-base status.

SODIUM EXCESS FOLLOWING BRAIN INJURY
Sodium excess is the most frequent electrolyte disturbance following brain injury. It is usually caused by inadequate water intake. Recall that thirst and the motor activities necessary to respond to it are often affected by neurologic trauma. Since elderly persons, young children, and unconscious patients are least able to make thirst known, hypernatremia occurs most frequently among these groups.

High protein tube feedings (which are average in sodium content) are contraindicated during the first week after trauma to the brain. Because of the stress response that follows trauma, the patient is unable to anabolize protein normally. The renal solute load is increased, resulting in excessive water loss, which eventually produces sodium excess. Fever and hyperventilation cause additional water loss and further contribute to sodium excess.

The neurologic patient with respiratory depression may require prolonged mechanical ventilation. Even with humidification, there may be a tendency for the ventilator to remove water and produce hypernatremia. If this occurs, the increased water loss must be replaced; the actual amount required is determined by the clinical condition, urine volume, urine specific gravity, and accurate body weight measurement. Sometimes the converse will occur; the common use of nebulizers with respirators has increased the hazard of water retention. A recent study showed that approximately 20 per cent of the patients treated with prolonged mechanical ventilation developed water retention, hyponatremia, and pulmonary edema. (See Chapter 24.) The nurse should keep accurate intake-output records (including the water contribution from nebulizers). Accurate daily weight measurements should also be made to help detect water deficit or water overloading.

Nursing Implications The nurse should be alert for symptoms of sodium excess when the water intake is deficient or when excessive water loss occurs. Symptoms of sodium excess (water deficit) include the following:

> severe thirst (if the patient is conscious)
> dry, sticky mucous membranes
> flushed skin
> oliguria
> irritability (particularly in children)
> urine specific gravity above 1.030
> fever
> plasma sodium above 147 mEq./L.
> delirium and hallucinations
> depressed level of consciousness

Fever after neurologic trauma calls for a check of the serum sodium level. The central nervous system symptoms may be caused by altered cerebral electrolyte concentrations and changed volume (shrinkage) of the cells. Hypernatremia may cause cerebral vascular damage (petechial and subarachnoid hemorrhages).

Efforts should be made to supply adequate water, by mouth if possible. If tube feedings are necessary, the nurse should carefully record the amount of water given, plus the total volume of the tube feeding mixture. Few tube feeding mixtures supply adequate water; additional amounts should be given between feedings. The nurse should consult with the physician to determine the desired total intake and to learn of necessary restrictions. The physician may order a specific volume for the 24-hour period in order to prevent or minimize cerebral edema and elevation of the intracranial pressure. If a specific fluid intake is not established, the nurse should give fluids in amounts sufficient to keep the tongue moist and the skin turgor normal.

It may be necessary to use the intravenous route to supply water if the patient is vomiting or has diarrhea.

Too rapid rehydration may cause further damage to a brain rapidly swelling because of osmosis. Usually several days are necessary for safe rehydration.

SODIUM DEFICIT FOLLOWING BRAIN INJURY
Brain injury may be followed by hyponatremia as a result of inappropriate ADH secretion which causes water retention, water overloading, or a combination of both. Inappropriate ADH secretion may result from brain injury that results from trauma, inflammation, neoplasia, or other causes.

The diagnosis of the syndrome of inappropriate secretion of ADH (SIADH) is based on the symptoms and these findings:

1. Urinary excretion of a significant amount of sodium in spite of the low serum sodium concentration. (Usually, in sodium deficit (hyponatremia) one would expect a low specific gravity of the urine, perhaps 1.002 to 1.004. But in SIADH the S.G. may rise above 1.012).
2. Decreased serum sodium concentration, below 130 mEq./L., even less than 115 mEq./L. Symptoms usually occur when sodium reaches 125 mEq./L.
3. Normal adrenal and renal function with normal or low NPN concentration.
4. Absence of fluid volume deficit or hypotension.
5. Absence of peripheral edema. But cerebral edema may occur.
6. Improvement in the low serum concentration and in the urinary loss of sodium when fluids are withheld.

The basic physiologic disturbance appears to be an excessive secretion of ADH, resulting in water retention and ECF volume expansion. This causes secretion of aldosterone to be suppressed. Sodium ions, therefore, are lost through the kidneys and the osmolality of urine tends to be higher than that of the plasma.

Treatment In addition to any possible treatment of the precipitating condition, the following measures have been employed:

1. Restriction of water to the extent that negative water balance is induced. This may require as little as 500 to 700 ml./24 hr.
2. When there are symptoms of severe water intoxication, intravenous administration of 3 or 5 per cent solution of sodium chloride may be successful in increasing the osmolality of the body fluids and in controlling the CNS disturbance.
3. Intravenous administration of phenytoin has been shown to improve water excretion in some neurologic patients with SIADH.
4. Administration of furosemide plus salt replacement has accomplished increase in the plasma concentration of sodium.

Essential to effective therapy is the frequent measurement of serum and urine electrolytes and osmolality.

The nurse should be alert for symptoms of water intoxication (hyponatremia) in patients with brain injury, particularly when water intake is excessive. Symptoms may appear at a plasma sodium level of 115 to 127 mEq./L. and can include the following:

nausea and vomiting
irritability
personality changes (uncooperative, hostile, and confused)
muscular twitching
positive Babinski's sign (particularly if Na level below 100 mEq./L.)
stupor and convulsions
a transient hemiparesis or aphasia

An important nursing responsibility in caring for patients with cerebral injury is the recording of all routes and types of fluid intake and output (including water used in nebulizers during artificial mechanical ventilation).

DIABETES INSIPIDUS   Diabetes insipidus results from interruption of the hypothalamohypophyseal tract by a variety of lesions, so that the posterior pituitary gland no longer secretes ADH adequately. Causes include brain tumors, head injuries, encephalitis, and vascular disease. It may occur as a complication of surgery in the region of the third ventricle. Sometimes the disease is of an idiopathic origin (no demonstrable etiologic factors).

Symptoms of diabetes insipidus include polyuria and polydipsia; polyuria is caused by the decreased secretion of ADH. (Recall that antidiuretic hormone causes the body to conserve water; a deficiency of this hormone results in an abnormally high water loss into the urine.) Urinary output is usually 4 to 6 L. per day, although it may be as great as 12 to 15 L. The large urinary loss of water causes the body fluid osmolarity to rise and produces thirst; as a result, a large volume of water is consumed. Urinary specific gravity is low, remaining between 1.002 and 1.006.

The polyuria of diabetes insipidus must be differentiated from that caused by chronic renal disease, diabetes mellitus, and compulsive water drinking. Chronic renal disease is characterized by a low urinary specific gravity, in addition to other urine abnormalities. The urine of the patient with diabetes insipidus is normal except for the large volume and low specific gravity. In diabetes mellitus, the urine volume is large but has a high specific gravity (owing to the presence of sugar). The differential diagnosis presenting the most trouble is between diabetes insipidus and compulsive water drinking.

Compulsive water drinking usually is caused by a neurosis. It is most frequent in women from 40 to 60 years of age, while diabetes insipidus is more common in younger men. The primary disturbance in compulsive water drinking is excessive water intake; polyuria occurs secondarily. Recall that polyuria occurs first in diabetes insipidus; excessive water drinking follows to prevent dehydration. In compulsive water drinking, intake depends largely upon the emotional state of the individual and, therefore, fluctuates greatly from day to day. Water intake in diabetes insipidus remains rather constant from day to day.

Several tests have been devised to help diagnose diabetes insipidus. For example, if water can be withheld long enough to cause concentration of the urine to a specific gravity of 1.010, the patient probably doesn't have diabetes insipidus. However, it is difficult to withhold fluids from the patient with diabetes insipidus, even temporarily, without causing a water deficit or even peripheral vascular collapse. Another test consists of the administration of hypertonic solution of sodium chloride. In the normal individual, this procedure stimulates ADH secretion and, thus, decreases urinary volume. The individual with diabetes insipidus is unaffected by extracellular osmolar changes; the only mechanism capable of decreasing urinary volume in such patients is the administration of pitressin (vasopressin). The administration of pitressin produces a more concentrated urine in the patient with diabetes insipidus than can be achieved with water restriction.

Posterior pituitary extracts or vasopressin are used to conserve about 90 per cent of the water which would otherwise be lost by way of the kidneys of the patient with diabetes insipidus. A small amount of powdered pituitary gland or synthetic vasopressin may be insufflated into the nose several times daily, or vasopressin tannate in oil (0.3 to 1 ml.) may be injected intramuscularly every two to three days. (The vial should be shaken thoroughly and warmed prior to administration to ensure adequate dispersion of the active agent throughout the medium; otherwise, the injection may be ineffective.) A potential complication of the administration of pitressin, either diagnostically or therapeutically, is water intoxication (excessive retention of water with subsequent sodium dilution). Although the patient with diabetes insipidus usually decreases his water intake when the polyuria is controlled, the compulsive water drinker may not. The patient who has received an overdose might be unable to rid his body of water that he had drunk, resulting in water overload. Urinary volume and fluid intake should be measured and compared to detect excessive water retention. Early symptoms of water intoxication include listlessness, drowsiness, and headache; convulsions and coma may develop later.

Nursing Implications The nurse should be alert for polyuria and polydipsia in patients with brain tumor, head injury, vascular disease, or cerebral infection. An accurate intake-output record is helpful in detecting these symptoms. Sometimes the neurosurgeon will leave orders to report large hourly urine outputs in the postoperative period (such as more than 200 ml. in each of two consecutive hours or more than 500 ml. in any two-hour period).[3] Also, a low urinary specific gravity (below 1.002) should be reported.

If diabetes insipidus is present, provision should be made for an easily accessible water supply. In addition, the patient should be as close to the bathroom as possible. Fluid balance is remarkably well maintained in the patient with diabetes insipidus, as long as his thirst mechanism is intact and he has access to as much water as he wants. Hypernatremia

will result if the output of water is not balanced by intake of water.

NONKETOTIC HYPERGLYCEMIA HYPEROSMOLAR COMA This condition may result from massive osmotic diuresis in the diabetic neurosurgical patient (particularly in the older, mild or undiagnosed diabetic). Medications frequently used in neurosurgical patients that may precipitate this disorder include hyperosmotic agents (such as urea), corticosteroids, and phenytoin. Clinical signs may include the following:

> visual hallucinations
> mental confusion
> hyporeflexia
> unilateral Babinski's sign
> nystagmus
> focal motor seizures
> aphasia
> hemiparesis
> coma

This condition may be overlooked because the symptoms may be mistaken for a worsening of the original neurologic disorder. Treatment is aimed at the intravenous replacement of the fluid loss and administration of insulin.

ELEVATED INTRACRANIAL PRESSURE

Causes Elevated intracranial pressure (ICP) occurs when the rate of cerebrospinal fluid formation is increased or when the rate of absorption of cerebrospinal fluid is decreased. Brain tumors may produce either or both of these effects. Any irritation to the meninges, such as an infection or tumor, causes large quantities of fluid and protein to pass into the cerebrospinal fluid system; the added volume causes a rise in intracranial pressure. A large hemorrhage can increase intracranial pressure directly by compressing the brain. The formation of arachnoidal granulation, caused by hemorrhage or infection, can interfere seriously with cerebrospinal fluid absorption and, thereby, increase intracranial pressure.

Cerebral blood flow is affected by carbon dioxide concentration, hydrogen ion concentration, and oxygen concentration. It has been shown that cerebral blood flow increases as the arterial pCO_2 increases; in fact, doubling the arterial pCO_2 by breathing carbon dioxide causes blood flow in the cerebrum to approximately double.[4] Danger of high intracranial pressure, thus, is greatest when the pCO_2 is high (such as an arterial pCO_2 greater than 60 mm. Hg). The mechanism involved is the increased formation of carbonic acid and dissociation of hydrogen ions; hydrogen ions then cause vasodilatation of the cerebral vessels.[5] Any substance that increases the acidity of brain tissue (such as lactic acid or pyruvic acid) can also cause increased intracranial pressure. Hypoxia can cause increased cerebral blood flow and, thus, elevated intracranial pressure. Danger of a high intracranial pressure is greatest when the pO_2 is very low (such as an arterial pO_2 less than 50 mm. Hg).

Symptoms   The nurse should be alert for the symptoms of elevated intracranial pressure in all patients with cerebral abnormalities. Symptoms of elevated intracranial pressure include these:

changes in level of consciousness
progressive rise in blood pressure (usually there is a greater rise in the systolic blood pressure than in the diastolic pressure, resulting in an increased pulse pressure)
slowed bounding pulse
slowed respiratory rate
persistent headache, increasing in intensity
projectile vomiting (may or may not be preceded by nausea)
dimming of vision, owing to papilledema (edema of the retina surrounding the region of exit of the optic nerve)
hyperthermia (resulting from pressure on the thermoregulatory center)

Treatment   Ideally, treatment of elevated ICP is directed at removing the basic cause of the pressure increase (such as removing a tumor or draining a hematoma). However, the ideal treatment might not be possible, necessitating other modes of therapy.

Hypertonic Urea. *   The intravenous administration of a hypertonic solution of urea produces a significant and well-sustained decrease in intracranial pressure in patients with cerebral injury or space-occupying lesions. Not metabolized, urea is rapidly excreted by the kidneys, carrying with it large quantities of water and sodium. It can be pre-

* Ureaphil (Abbott Laboratories, North Chicago, Illinois).

pared in concentrations of 4 or 30 per cent. The 30 per cent solution is usually employed for the reduction of intracranial pressure.

The usual adult dose ranges from 1 to 1.5 Gm./kg. body weight. One hundred ml. of a 30 per cent solution is usually given over a 1- or 2-hour period. After the solution has been prepared it should be used immediately; unused portions should be discarded. Intravenous urea should be administered slowly; the rate should not exceed 3 to 4 ml. per minute. The effect becomes maximal one hour after administration. Because urea has a pronounced diuretic effect, an indwelling urinary catheter should be used in comatose patients to assure bladder emptying; the catheter also facilitates accurate measurement of urinary output. Headache, nausea and vomiting, syncope, and disorientation have been reported after intravenous administration of urea.

Since urea in a 30 per cent concentration is an irritating hypertonic solution, it may cause phlebitis and pain. Extravasation of the solution causes sloughing of the surrounding tissues. Because venous thrombosis may occur, the infusion should be started in a large vein, with the needle carefully anchored. Because of the danger of thrombosis, veins in the lower extremities of the aged should not be used.

Contraindications to the use of urea include severe renal or hepatic damage, pronounced extracellular fluid volume deficit or active intracranial bleeding. If the solution is given to patients with kidney disease, the BUN should be checked frequently to determine if renal function is adequate to eliminate the infused urea as well as that produced endogenously. Urea should be administered with great caution to patients with liver impairment since there may be a significant rise in the blood ammonia level. Intracranial bleeding may be reactivated when cerebral edema is reduced by the use of urea.

Adrenal Corticoids.   Adrenal corticosteroids may be used to reduce cerebral edema. At first they may be given intravenously in large amounts and then either by mouth or intramuscularly. The effect is less rapid than that achieved with urea but is more prolonged.

Mannitol.   Mannitol is an osmotic diuretic capable of relieving elevated intracranial pressure when given intravenously as a 20 per cent solution. The relatively high total dose is 1.5 to 2 Gm./kg. of body weight. This amount may be given over a period of 30 to 90 minutes, provided the patient has normal cardiac and renal function. Because of the diuretic effect of mannitol, a catheter should be inserted into the bladder before the mannitol is administered. Although 20 per cent mannitol is chemically stable, it may crystallize when cooled excessively. If this occurs, the bottle should be warmed to 50° C. in a water bath, then cooled to body temperature before being administered.

Mannitol should be given via a blood infusion set to filter any undissolved crystals; it should not be administered through the same infusion set with blood. The nurse should obtain a specific order concerning the rate of administration of the solution. Urine output should be observed continuously and should exceed 30 to 50 ml./hr. If hourly output is less then this amount, the drug should be stopped and the physician notified. If a large amount of mannitol is given rapidly, the patient may complain of headache, a sensation of chest constriction, and chills. The increased intravascular fluid volume, caused by the drawing of water into the bloodstream, may cause pulmonary edema or symptoms of water excess (sodium deficit). (Symptoms of pulmonary edema are described in Chapter 21; those of water excess are described in Chapter 17.) The nurse should make every effort to observe the patient closely during the administration of mannitol, especially when it is given at a rapid rate. The site of injection should be observed frequently, since extravasation of mannitol can cause swelling and thrombophlebitis.

Hyperventilation. Hyperventilation with resultant hypocarbia (low pCO_2) decreases cerebral blood flow and, thus, reduces intracranial pressure; it also tends to decrease the likelihood of intracranial bleeding. Respiratory alkalosis has been induced in some clinical situations for *short* periods of time to lower intracranial pressure (pCO_2 lowered to a level of 25 to 35 mm. Hg).[6]

Fluids. Some physicians avoid the administration of free water (such as D_5W) and prefer the administration of Ringer's lactate or 0.9% sodium chloride in any condition likely to be associated with cerebral edema and increased intracranial pressure. In general, hypotonic I.V. fluids should be avoided. Fluid restriction is believed to be important in the control of increased intracranial pressure. It is important that the nurse carefully monitor the volume and rate of administration of parenteral fluids given to patients with elevated ICP; an excessive volume or accidental rapid administration of the correct volume can cause a rise in intracranial pressure.

Hypertonic Glucose. Once commonly used to reduce intracranial pressure, hypertonic glucose solutions are now used sparingly in most hospitals. Infusion of hypertonic glucose increases the intravascular osmotic pressure, withdrawing water from the edematous brain and from the cerebrospinal fluid space. Although the intracranial pressure is reduced, the reduction is not sustained and the pressure rises again. The reason for this lies in the fact that hypertonic glucose increases the osmotic pressure of the cerebrospinal fluid, causing it to attract water by osmosis. Some authorities feel that hypertonic glucose does more harm than good.

Position. Unless contraindicated, a body position with 30 degree head elevation is recommended to decrease intracranial pressure. Flexion of the neck should be avoided; sharp flexion of the neck can increase intracranial pressure by interfering with venous outflow and, thus, increasing the amount of blood in the cranial cavity. Extreme flexion of the hips should also be avoided since it has been found that this position can cause a rise in intracranial pressure; the prone position during cranial surgery consistently increases baseline pressure and thus should be avoided in patients with known or highly potential increased ICP.[7] Although intermittent use of the Trendelenberg position is useful in draining the tracheobronchial tree, it should not be used when the patient has an elevated intracranial pressure.

REFERENCES

1. **Mitchell, P.,** and **Mauss, N.:** Intracranial pressure: fact and fancy. Nursing 76. June 1976, p. 57.

2. **Boedecker, E.,** and **Dauber, J.** (eds.): Manual of Medical Therapeutics, ed. 21. Boston: Little, Brown & Co., 1974, p. 158.

3. **Howe, J.:** Patient Care in Neurosurgery. Boston: Little, Brown & Co., 1977, p. 206.

4. **Guyton, A.:** Textbook of Medical Physiology, ed. 5. Philadelphia: W. B. Saunders Co., 1976, p. 373.

5. Ibid.

6. **Boedecker** and **Dauber:** Manual of Medical Therapeutics, p. 396.

7. **Mitchell and Mauss:** Intracranial pressure, p. 57.

BIBLIOGRAPHY

Berk, J., et al. (eds.):   Handbook of Critical Care. Boston: Little, Brown & Co., 1976.

Core Curriculum for Critical-Care Nurses. American Association of Critical Care Nurses, Los Angeles, Calif. 1975.

Gahart, B.: Intravenous Medications. St. Louis: C. V. Mosby, 1977.

Luckman, J., and Sorenson, K.:   Medical-Surgical Nursing. Philadelphia: W. B. Saunders Co., 1974.

Maxwell, M., and Kleeman, C. (eds.):   Clinical Disorders of Fluid and Electrolyte Metabolism, ed. 2. New York: McGraw-Hill Book Co., 1972.

— 24 —

Fluid Balance in the Patient with Respiratory Disease

The primary function of the lungs is to provide the body tissues with proper amounts of O_2 and to excrete correct quantities of CO_2. Another critical role is that of H^+ control (acid-base balance) and water balance. Alveolar ventilation is responsible for the daily elimination of about 13,000 mEq. of H^+, as opposed to the 40 to 80 mEq. excreted daily by the kidneys. It is obvious that pulmonary dysfunction can produce a rapid change (matter of seconds) in the plasma H^+ concentration. In contrast, the H^+ excess of renal failure may not be evident until several hours after onset.

The lungs can be regarded as organs of body homeostasis, since they regulate the carbonic acid level of the extracellular fluid through exhalation or retention of carbon dioxide.

Under the control of the medulla, the lungs act promptly to correct systemic hydrogen ion changes, which are synonymous with acid-base disturbances. Thus, when the ketosis of starvation produces metabolic acidosis, the medulla signals the lungs to exhale carbon dioxide by means of deep, rapid respiration. When loss of hydrochloric acid through prolonged vomiting produces metabolic alkalosis, the medulla orders the lungs to retain carbon dioxide by means of slow, shallow respiration.

The disruption of normal pulmonary function can produce water and electrolyte imbalances. For example, blockage of the bronchi and of the alveolar-capillary membrane in bronchiectasis results in the inadequate elimination of carbon dioxide from the lungs, with increased carbonic acid concentration in the extracellular fluid and respiratory acidosis. High fever, with its associated hyperventilation, causes an excessive elimination of carbon dioxide from the lungs and a decreased carbonic acid concentration in the extracellular fluid, which results in respiratory alkalosis.

The lungs remove large quantities of water from the body as water vapor. (Recall that the daily insensible water loss from the lungs is about 300 ml., varying with the environmental humidity and the depth and the rate of respiration.) Abnormal conditions, such as sustained hyperpnea, excessive formation of mucus or of purulent secretions, or continued coughing greatly increase the water loss.

EFFECTS OF pCO_2, pH, AND pO_2 ON ALVEOLAR VENTILATION

A rise in pCO_2 is a powerful stimulant to respiration. In fact, an increase of alveolar pCO_2 to 63 mm. of Hg (from the normal of 40) causes a tenfold increase in alveolar ventilation.[1] The maximal effect of pCO_2 on

337

ventilation is reached at approximately a 9 per cent CO_2 concentration. Whenever the arterial pCO_2 is chronically above 50 mm. Hg, the respiratory center becomes relatively insensitive to its stimulatory effect.[2] A sudden further increase in arterial pCO_2 can render the respiratory center completely insensitive to this stimulus (leaving hypoxemia as the primary respiratory stimulus). The relationship between arterial pCO_2 and alveolar ventilation is almost linear, making arterial pCO_2 the most important single measurement to guide the adequacy of ventilation.

Plasma pH also affects ventilation. Acidosis stimulates respiration; for example: a pH of 7.1 can increase alveolar ventilation four-fold. Alkalosis depresses respiration; for example: a pH of 7.6 can decrease ventilation to about 80 per cent of normal.[3]

Arterial pO_2 influences respiration; however, its effect is not as marked as those produced by pCO_2 and pH. A fall in arterial pO_2 to below 65 mm. of Hg (from the normal of 95 to 100) usually is necessary before a marked effect on ventilation occurs.

STUDY OF ARTERIAL BLOOD GASES

Blood gas analysis includes measurement of hydrogen, oxygen tension, and carbon dioxide tension in arterial blood. The measurements are expressed as pH, pO_2, and pCO_2 respectively (Table 24-1).

pO_2 The normal partial pressure of oxygen (pO_2) in arterial blood usually is considered to be between 95 and 100 mm. Hg. However, any reading above 80 mm. Hg in adults and children is usually considered as acceptable (on room air at sea level). On room air, in patients under 60 years old, a pO_2 less than 80 mm. Hg is indicative of mild hypoxemia, a pO_2 less than 60 is indicative of moderate hypoxemia, and a pO_2 less than 40 is indicative of severe hypoxemia.[4] Hypoxemia leads to hypoxia and anaerobic metabolism; lactic acid formation results and causes metabolic acidosis.

An acceptable arterial pO_2 for the newborn breathing room air varies between 40 and 70 mm.

Hg.[5] Aged patients develop degenerative lung changes and, thus, lose some degree of ventilatory function; a general guideline is to subtract 1 mm. Hg from the minimal 80 mm. Hg for every year over the age of 60 (up to the age of 90).[6] For example: a 70-year-old patient breathing room air could conceivably have a pO_2 of 70 mm. Hg and still not be considered hypoxemic (80 mm. Hg minus 10 mm. Hg).

pCO_2 The normal partial pressure of carbon dioxide (pCO_2) in arterial blood varies between 38 and 42 mm. Hg. Acute hyperventilation causes the arterial pCO_2 to decrease and the plasma pH to increase (for example: pCO_2 30 mm. Hg↓, pH 7.5↑). Acute hypoventilation causes the arterial pCO_2 to increase and the pH to decrease (for example: pCO_2 60 mm. Hg↑, pH 7.2↓).

pH As mentioned earlier, normal arterial pH varies between 7.38 and 7.42. Acidosis stimulates respiration; alkalosis depresses respiration.

Astrup Method and Siggard-Andersen Nomogram

This method used by these workers of analyzing acid-base disturbances is ingenious but complicated. Indeed, most American authorities regard the system as needlessly complicated and as presenting what would happen if acid-base disturbances occurred in a test tube rather than in the human body. (Therefore, most centers have abandoned use of the system.) For those who have interest in the terms that the system has introduced, the following information is provided.

Standard Bicarbonate Standard bicarbonate is the bicarbonate concentration in the plasma of blood that has been adjusted so that its pCO_2 is 40 mm. Hg. Moreover, its hemoglobin has been fully saturated with oxygen. The normal value of standard bicarbonate is 24 (22 to 26) mEq./L., the same as the figure usually regarded as normal for the CO_2 combining power, which is a measure of bicarbonate, not of CO_2 as the name implies. The reason: as HCO_3 is broken down by addition of a strong acid, the CO_2 gas emitted is a measure of the HCO_3 originally present.

Base Excess Base excess indicates the presence in the blood of an excess of alkali or a deficit of fixed acid (which does not include carbonic acid), or a deficit of alkali or an excess of fixed acid. Positive values indicate alkalinity of the body fluids; negative

Table 24-1. Arterial Blood Gas Values

pH	pCO_2	pO_2	HCO_3^-	Base Excess
7.38–7.42	38–42 mm. Hg	95–100 mm. Hg	23–25 mEq./L.	−2 to +2

values indicate acidity. The normal value of base excess is 0 (+2.5 to −2.5) mEq./L. It would appear more forthright to call an excess of base "base excess" and a deficit "base deficit" rather than speaking of a positive base excess and a negative base excess. Base excess cannot be derived from the bicarbonate value alone. Rather, it is arrived at by multiplying the deviation of standard bicarbonate from normal by the factor of 1.2, which represents the buffer action of red blood corpuscles.

Methods for Obtaining Arterial Blood Samples

Arterial blood samples usually are obtained by repeated single arterial punctures. However, in the cardiopulmonary unstable patient, an arterial catheter may be inserted to provide immediately available blood samples and to allow continuous arterial pressure monitoring.[7] Complications of cannulated arteries include tissue necrosis (secondary to diminished arterial blood flow) and infection. Tissue necrosis is most likely to occur when the involved artery has inadequate collateral circulation to supply distal tissue. Some patients have lost lower limbs or required femoral endarterectomy; loss of toes and fingers have also been reported.

ARTERIAL PUNCTURE PROCEDURE   The following is the procedure used in arterial puncture.

1. *Explanation to patient.* The procedure for obtaining blood for analysis should be explained to the patient. It is important to prevent unnecessary pain and anxiety which may cause hyperventilation, resulting in a temporary change in blood gases.

2. *Selection of site.* The radial artery (at the wrist) is frequently used for arterial puncture since it is superficially located, has collateral circulation, and is not adjacent to a large vein. Some authorities feel that arterial punctures by nonphysicians should be done only in radial arteries. The brachial artery (in the antecubital fossa) is also used for arterial puncture since it has appreciable collateral circulation. The femoral artery is not used as frequently since it has certain disadvantages. For example, there is no adequate collateral flow if the femoral artery becomes obstructed. Obstruction, therefore, threatens the entire lower limb.[8] Also, it is more difficult to stop bleeding in the large femoral artery than in the

smaller radial and brachial arteries. Sometimes the femoral vein is mistaken for the femoral artery since it has a high pressure. Sites for pediatric use include the radial, temporal, brachial, and femoral arteries. The radial artery often is the preferred site since there is no associated vein (may be used in the newborn as well as in older children). If frequent arterial samples are required, an indwelling catheter may be inserted percutaneously in children over 5 years of age; the umbilical artery can be catheterized in the newborn.

3. *Positioning.* If the radial site is to be used, a rolled towel should be placed under the wrist and the hand should be pushed down to obtain wrist extension (Fig. 24-1). If the brachial site is to be used, the arm should be extended and supported with a towel under the elbow. The maximum point of pulsation in the artery should be identified.

4. *Cleansing the site.* Usually the area is cleansed with either betadine or alcohol wipes. Some operators wear sterile gloves to perform an arterial puncture; the hands, at least, should be thoroughly washed.

5. *Local anesthetic.* Some physicians favor the use of a local anesthetic prior to arterial punch; others do not. Usually the local anesthetic is not necessary if the operator is skilled in obtaining arterial samples and can do so on the first attempt with minimal pain to the patient. A strong argument for the use of a local anesthetic is that it reduces pain, particularly when more than one attempt is necessary. Also, infiltration of the anesthetic around the arterial wall reduces the likelihood of arterial spasm.

6. *Heparinized glass syringe.* A 5 ml. glass syringe (with a 19 or 20 gauge needle) should be flushed with 0.5 ml. of 1:1000 heparin solution and then emptied, leaving heparin in the needle to prevent clotting of the blood sample. (For small pediatric patients, a heparinized glass tuberculin syringe with a 25 gauge needle may be used.) It should be remembered that too much heparin left in the syringe will affect the pH of the blood sample and, thus, cause false results. The syringe should be free of air bubbles. A glass syringe is preferred to a plastic syringe since a glass syringe has freer movement and, thus, fills more easily. Use of a plastic syringe may necessitate "pulling back" on the plunger to obtain the blood sample. Also, air bubbles adhere more tenaciously to plastic syringes, making them less desirable in this situation.

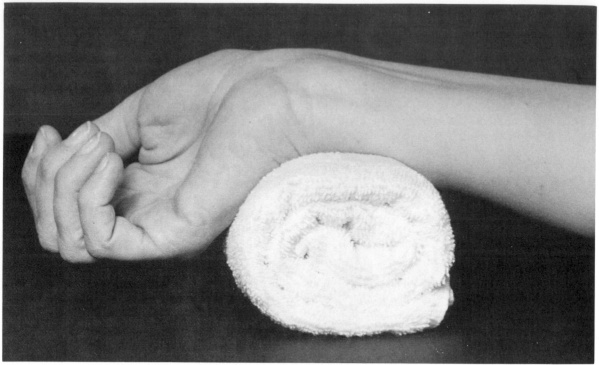

Figure 24-1. Position of wrist for radial artery puncture.

7. *Obtaining the sample.* The needle should be inserted at an angle (to enter the artery obliquely) while the artery is stabilized with the free hand. An oblique entrance into the artery minimizes the formation of a hematoma since the hole in the artery seals better when the needle is removed. Usually the initial thrust of the needle will bring a pulsating flow of blood into the syringe without pulling out on the plunger; this spontaneous pumping of blood into the syringe is proof of entry into an artery. If blood does not enter the syringe, the needle must be redirected; if the needle has gone through the artery, it must be slightly withdrawn until blood flows again. From 2 to 5 ml. of blood should be obtained (depending on individual laboratory requirements).

8. *Aftercare of the site and preparation of the specimen.* After the sample is obtained, pressure should be applied over the site with a gauze sponge and the needle removed. (Pressure should be continuously applied to the puncture site for a period of five minutes; a longer time may be necessary if the patient is on anticoagulants.) After the needle is withdrawn from the artery, the syringe should be handed immediately to a second person who at once plunges the needle into a cork or rubber stopper to seal the syringe from air. Should air accidentally enter the syringe, the specimen should be discarded. Gentle rotation of the syringe is required to mix the blood with the heparin to prevent clotting. The syringe should quickly be placed in a basin of ice slush to slow down oxygen metabolism. Failure to do so causes the gas analysis to yield inaccurate results since oxygen metabolism of blood continues even after it is drawn from the body. The specimen should be taken immediately to the lab after it is properly labeled. The label on the specimen should state the patient's name, the time of the puncture, body temperature at time of puncture, and the inspired oxygen level.

Body Temperature. It is important that the patient's body temperature be recorded accurately since arterial pO_2 and pCO_2 increase as body temperature increases; conversely, they decrease as body temperature decreases. A 6 per cent change in arterial pO_2 occurs with each degree of centigrade body temperature change.[9] Blood gas analyzers are controlled for normal body temperature; thus, the technician must correct the results to the patient's actual temperature (by use of the appropriate nomogram) if severe hypothermia or hyperthermia is present.

Inspired Oxygen Level. It is important to state on the requisition the patient's inspired oxygen level. (For example: Is the patient breathing room air? Is he breathing 40 per cent oxygen? Or, is he receiving oxygen by nasal prongs at a rate of 2 L. a minute?) This information is important in interpreting blood gases. If blood gases are obtained to measure the effectiveness of a new oxygen level, the patient should receive that level of oxygen continuously for at least 20 minutes prior to obtaining the arterial sample.

Conclusions To Be Drawn from Blood Gas Levels

The levels of pCO_2 and pO_2 provide considerable insight into what is happening to the patient. Theoretically, pCO_2 and pO_2 can be high, normal, or low (Fig. 24-2). Let us consider various combinations of these six variables.

First, of course, the pO_2 and the pCO_2 can fall within the limits of normal, in which case no deduction concerning disease can be made.

What if the pO_2 is normal and the pCO_2 is elevated? This is impossible unless oxygen is being given to the patient.

Suppose the pO_2 is normal and the pCO_2 is de-

pressed. Then the patient must be compensating successfully for a lung disorder. We say he is compensating because the low pCO_2 indicates hyperventilation and the normal pO_2 indicates a healthy state of oxygenation of the blood.

Now suppose the pO_2 is high and the pCO_2 is normal. We can only deduce from this that the patient is receiving oxygen—indeed, he must be.

Now let us move on to a high pO_2 and a high pCO_2. Such a situation is clearly impossible.

How about an elevated pO_2 and a low pCO_2? This indicates that hyperventilation is going on.

What if the pO_2 is low and the pCO_2 is normal? Here we have poor oxygenation of the blood but without compensatory activity on the part of the lungs. (There is no overbreathing, otherwise the pCO_2 would be depressed, not normal.)

Suppose the pO_2 is low and the pCO_2 is high. Here we have a condition in which pulmonary ventilation is inadequate. This might occur with any obstructive lung disease. It is not unusual for patients with COPD (chronic obstructive pulmonary disease) to have a "sixty-sixty" reading; that is, an arterial pO_2 of 60 mm. Hg (normal 95 to 100) and an arterial pCO_2 of 60 mm. Hg (normal 40). Posttraumatic injuries of the chest commonly show a low pO_2 and a mild to moderate elevation of pCO_2.

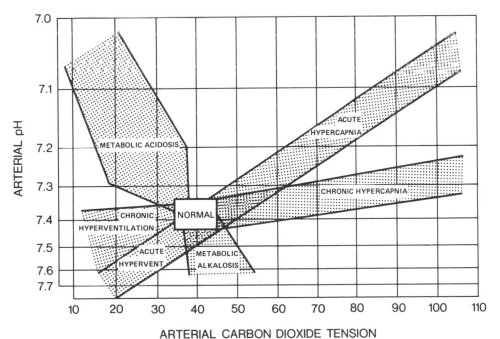

Figure 24-2. Blood gas interpretation graph. (From Burrows, B., Knudson, R. J., and Kettell, L. J.: Respiratory Insufficiency. Chicago: Year Book Medical Publishers, 1975. Used by permission)

What if the pO_2 is low and the pCO_2 is low? Here we have apparent efforts on the part of the lungs to compensate for a low oxygen saturation of the blood, but the efforts of the lungs are unavailing. We can see this in the syndrome known as "stiff lung" or in pulmonary embolism. Although acute pulmonary embolism usually is accompanied by hypoxemia and a decreased pH, blood gases may be within an acceptable range. Hypoxemia occurs in pulmonary edema as oxygen diffusion is impaired by transudation of fluid into the alveolar spaces. Thus, arterial pO_2 is below normal. The pCO_2 may range from low to high, depending on the severity of pulmonary edema and the patient's ability to breathe. Hyperventilation caused by hypoxemia can lower the pCO_2; and profound ventilatory failure can cause the pCO_2 to rise.

Expected blood gas changes for acute, partially compensated, and compensated acid-base disturbances are listed in Table 24-2.

HYPOVENTILATION

Alveolar hypoventilation always results in hypercarbia (elevated pCO_2) and hypoxemia (reduced pO_2) when the patient is breathing room air.

Hypercarbia

Hypercarbia, which is increased CO_2 concentration in arterial blood, signals the medulla to increase respirations. (Another term for hypercarbia is hypercapnia.) Symptoms that may occur with the sudden development of hypercarbia include increased pulse and respiratory rate, increased blood pressure, dyspnea, dizziness, sweating, feeling of fullness in the head, palpitation, mental clouding, muscle twitching, convulsions, and unconsciousness. However, patients with chronic pulmonary disease who gradually accumulate CO_2 over a prolonged period (days to months) may not develop these symptoms because compensatory changes have time to occur. An example is an emphysematous patient, kept alive with oxygen therapy for more than a year, who was mentally alert even when his arterial pCO_2 was 140 mm. of Hg (recall that the normal arterial pCO_2 is 38 to 42 mm. Hg). Yet a rapid rise of arterial pCO_2 to 140 mm. Hg would surely produce unconsciousness.

An elevated pCO_2 increases cardiac rate and force of contraction, whereas sudden reduction of pCO_2 from very high levels may lead to ventricular fibrillation. Carbon dioxide excess (particularly a pCO_2 greater than 60 mm. Hg) can produce cerebral vasodilation and increased cerebral blood flow. The increased blood volume in the rigid cranium may produce increased cerebrospinal fluid pressure and papilledema. Extremely high pCO_2 levels result in total anesthesia and death.

Excessive CO_2 retention, of course, produces respiratory acidosis. The plasma pH drops below normal because the increase in CO_2 causes the carbonic acid content of the blood to increase. (See the discussion of respiratory acidosis in the next section of this chapter.)

Hypoxemia

Acute hypoxemia (reduced oxygen content in the arterial blood) causes an increase in pulse rate as the heart attempts to compensate for inadequate tissue oxygenation by supplying more blood. An O_2 test may be helpful in assessing the patient's oxygen need; that is, pulse rate usually decreases by 10 or more beats per minute within the first few minutes after O_2 administration if the patient was indeed hypoxic. Other signs of hypoxemia include confusion, agitation, and an anxious facial expression.

Some observers regard cyanosis as the most characteristic clinical sign of hypoxemia. The term "cyanosis" means blueness of the skin; it is caused by an excessive amount of deoxygenated hemoglobin in the skin blood vessels. Deoxygenated Hb. has a strong blue color that is readily visible when present in a large concentration. Cyanosis only becomes discernible when the arterial oxygen saturation drops below 80 per cent. (Normal arterial oxygen saturation is 95 per cent.) A number of factors influence the degree of cyanosis: one such factor is the thickness of the skin; for example, cyanosis is readily observable in newborn babies because they have thin skin. Cyanosis is often noted first in the lips and fingernails where the capillaries are numerous and the tissues over them are thin and transparent. Another factor influencing the ability to observe cyanosis is the rate of blood flow through the skin. The presence of cyanosis demands careful clinical evaluation for the possibility of tissue hypoxia; however, the ab-

Table 24-2. Blood Gas Disturbances

Imbalance	Primary Disturbance	pH	pCO₂	HCO₃⁻
Acute respiratory acidosis (early)	Hypoventilation	↓	↑	N
Partially compensated respiratory acidosis	"	↓	↑	↑
Compensated respiratory acidosis	"	N	↑	↑
Acute respiratory alkalosis (early)	Hyperventilation	↑	↓	N
Partially compensated respiratory alkalosis	"	↑	↓	↓
Compensated respiratory alkalosis	"	N	↓	↓
Metabolic acidosis (early)	Gain of acid or loss of base (causing base deficit)	↓	N	↓
Partially compensated metabolic acidosis	"	↓	↓	↓
Compensated metabolic acidosis	"	N	↓	↓
Metabolic alkalosis (early)	Gain of base or loss of acid (causing base excess)	↑	N	↑
Partially compensated metabolic alkalosis	"	↑	↑	↑
Compensated metabolic alkalosis	"	N	↑	↑
Mixed respiratory acidosis and metabolic acidosis	Hypoventilation plus gain of acid or loss of base	↓	↑	↓
Mixed respiratory acidosis and metabolic alkalosis	Hypoventilation plus gain of base or loss of acid	? (depends on which is more severe)	↑	↑
Mixed respiratory alkalosis and metabolic acidosis	Hyperventilation plus gain of acid or loss of base	? (depends on which is more severe)	↓	↓
Mixed respiratory alkalosis and metabolic alkalosis	Hyperventilation plus gain of base or loss of acid	↑	↓	↑

sence of cyanosis does not mean than adequate tissue oxygenation is present. In fact, a severe state of tissue hypoxia may be present without cyanosis.

In shock, cyanosis may not be noted because the surface vessels are constricted and contain little blood. It is difficult to detect cyanosis in patients with severe anemia because there is sufficient oxygen available to saturate the small amount of Hb.

present. Patients with severe anemia and shock may suffer fatal tissue anoxia without the warning of cyanosis; such patients may display only skin pallor. Recognition of cyanosis also involves a subjective component of color perception. There is apt to be inconsistency among observers describing the same patient, or even in a single individual watching the same patient over a period of hours.

OXYGEN ADMINISTRATION Even though O_2 is required to correct hypoxemia, only as much as is needed should be given. The inordinate elevation of arterial pO_2 can produce pulmonary edema (resulting from damage of the linings of the bronchi and alveoli) and inactivate production of pulmonary surfactant. (Decreased production of surfactant causes the lungs to be less elastic and necessitates an increase in muscular work to bring about ventilation.) Exposure to 100 per cent O_2 at normal atmospheric pressure for a period of over six hours can produce substernal distress. The same symptom may result from the administration of 60 per cent O_2 for a period of 36 hours.[10] These effects are most profound when the oxygen is administered by mechanical ventilation. (Animals exposed for days to 80 to 100 per cent O_2 die of pulmonary edema.) Breathing 50 per cent O_2 for long periods does not seem to cause pulmonary damage.

Frequent measurement of arterial blood gases is necessary to ensure that only enough O_2 is administered to maintain a satisfactory pO_2. It is generally considered safe to give as much O_2 as is necessary to keep arterial pO_2 at 80 mm. Hg. *Dangerous levels of hypoxia must be avoided;* it is unsound to expose a patient to severe hypoxia for fear of developing oxygen toxicity.

Various methods are available for O_2 administration. Nasal prongs supply an O_2 concentration of 28 per cent at a flow rate of 2 L. a minute and a concentration of 40 per cent at 6 L. a minute. When nasal prongs are used for patients with chronic alveolar hypoventilation, the rate of O_2 flow should not exceed 1 or 2 L. a minute until blood gases are available. A nonrebreathing oxygen mask supplies an O_2 concentration of up to 90 to 95 per cent. The Ventimask is a specially constructed device that delivers a low concentration of O_2 (24, 28, 35, or 40 per cent) and is used for administering O_2 to emphysema patients.

The danger of administering a high O_2 concentration to a patient with an elevated pCO_2 is discussed later in this chapter under CO_2 narcosis.

Dyspnea

Dyspnea refers to difficult breathing. Patients with pulmonary disease often complain of shortness of breath or of being "unable to get their breath." It is a subjective symptom that cannot be measured objectively. Several factors enter into the development of dyspnea: one such factor is an abnormality of the respiratory gases in the body fluids, particularly hypercarbia, and, to a lesser extent, hypoxemia; other factors include the patient's state of mind and the degree to which the respiratory muscles must work to achieve adequate ventilation. When one consciously controls breathing rate and depth, the sensation of dyspnea is apt to occur.

Nursing Implications

In summary, hypoventilation results in a decreased pO_2 (while breathing room air), an elevated pCO_2, and a decreased plasma pH (respiratory acidosis). These blood gas changes are indications for the nurse to try to improve pulmonary ventilation. Depending on the circumstance, such actions may include:

1. Turning the patient from side to side at frequent intervals to allow for gravitational drainage of mucus from the various lung segments.
2. Placing the patient in Fowler's or semi-Fowler's position to allow for greater chest expansion.
3. Suctioning the patient as necessary to rid the respiratory tract of excessive secretions.
4. Increasing activity, as outlined by the physician, to promote ventilatory and circulatory improvement.
5. Performing other functions as prescribed by the physician, such as O_2 administration, postural drainage, chest tapping, and intermittent positive pressure breathing treatments.

RESPIRATORY ACIDOSIS

Pathologic Mechanism and Symptoms

Respiratory acidosis is caused by any clinical situation that interferes with pulmonary gas exchange, thus producing primary retention of carbon dioxide with a resultant increase in carbonic acid concentration of the extracellular fluid (Table 24-3).

Respiratory acidosis may be associated with no obvious clinical signs except dyspnea out of proportion to effort. (Hyperpnea at rest may be another

Table 24-3. Conditions Likely To Be Associated with Respiratory Acidosis

Emphysema
Pneumonia
Asthma
Cardiac failure with pulmonary edema
Partial airway obstruction
Partial respiratory paralysis
Opiates or sedatives in excessive doses
Tight abdominal binders or dressings
Abdominal distention from ascites and bowel obstruction
Pain in the chest or upper abdomen, resulting in splinting of the diaphragm
Semicomatose states, as in cerebrovascular accidents
Improperly regulated respirator, causing too shallow or too slow breathing
Pneumothorax
Prolonged open-chest and open-heart operations

sign.) Other indications of inadequate pulmonary ventilation include cyanosis and tachycardia, although respiratory acidosis can occur without cyanosis. The hydrogen excess of acidosis leads to loss of cellular potassium. The serum potassium level increases; conduction blocks and ventricular fibrillation may follow.

The symptoms of respiratory acidosis may be difficult to detect. The nurse should be alert for their occurrence when the patient has a condition prone to be associated with respiratory acidosis.

Chronic Pulmonary Diseases Associated with Respiratory Acidosis

Chronic pulmonary diseases such as bronchiectasis, asthma, pulmonary fibrosis, or emphysema may cause respiratory acidosis. A factor common to all these conditions is chronic interference with gas exchange, resulting in primary retention of carbon dioxide with an increase of carbonic acid in the extracellular fluid.

BRONCHITIS-EMPHYSEMA SYNDROME

Pathologic Mechanism and Symptoms Chronic bronchitis and emphysema so frequently occur in the same patient that the term bronchitis-emphysema syndrome has been coined. Chronic bronchitis causes mucous gland hyperplasia and mucosal inflammation with the production of abnormal amounts of mucus. Emphysema involves chronic obstruction to the flow of air into and—even more important—out of the lungs. The chronic airway obstruction causes overdistention of the lungs with air. As a result, the

alveoli become enlarged and eventually rupture and coalesce. There may be no symptoms until 20 to 30 per cent of the lung tissue has been destroyed.

Conditions that may contribute to airway obstruction include respiratory infections, smoking, and breathing polluted air. The disease is most common in older persons, particularly males who have done manual labor. Poor ventilation and interference with gaseous exchange at the alveolar level produce hypoxia and hypercarbia.

Retention of carbon dioxide causes a weighting of the carbonic acid side of the carbonic acid–base bicarbonate balance. As a result, this ratio becomes more than 1 to 20, and the balance is tipped in favor of acidosis. The pH of the blood is more acid than normal; the bicarbonate level is increased since the body retains bicarbonate ions to balance the excessive quantity of carbonic acid. Thus, both the carbonic acid content and the bicarbonate content of the blood increase. If the ratio of carbonic acid to base bicarbonate becomes stabilized at 1 to 20, the pH of the extracellular fluid will be normal. This condition is sometimes referred to as compensated respiratory acidosis. However, if the body compensatory mechanisms fail and the 1 to 20 ratio is upset, the extracellular fluid pH will drop below normal. The condition is then referred to as uncompensated respiratory acidosis. In compensated respiratory acidosis, the plasma pH will be normal; in uncompensated respiratory acidosis, the plasma pH will drop below normal.

The emphysematous patient may fluctuate between compensated and uncompensated acidosis. For example, a respiratory infection may tip his delicate state of balance and precipitate uncompensated respiratory acidosis.

The symptoms of bronchitis-emphysema syndrome with respiratory acidosis may include the following:

> chronic fatigue
> dyspnea, first noted on exertion
> moderate cyanosis, early
> respiration with a prolonged expiratory phase accompanied by wheezing or a blowing sound (decrease in elasticity of lung tissue causes terminal bronchioles to collapse when the patient exhales at normal speed)
> large barrel-shaped chest
> chest that appears to be held in permanent in-

spiration, so that the shoulders appear elevated and the neck shortened

use of accessory respiratory muscles in breathing

chronic productive cough

dull headache

severe cyanosis in the terminal stages

coma, if acidosis is severe

Treatment   Ideally, the treatment of respiratory acidosis should consist of eliminating the underlying pulmonary disease. Unfortunately, this is not possible in emphysema. For this reason, treatment is directed toward maximal relief of pulmonary obstruction and the improvement of pulmonary ventilation.

Bronchodilators, such as isoproterenol (Isuprel), help to reduce bronchial spasms and, thus, improve pulmonary ventilation. Best results are obtained when the patient first exhales completely and then inhales the medication directly into the respiratory tract. Bronchodilators may be administered by means of a positive pressure device, such as the Bennett or Bird respirator, or by means of a hand nebulizer.

Sputum may be thick in the emphysematous patient and difficult to expectorate. For this reason, an expectorant may be given to liquefy the sputum and make it easier to cough up.

An absolute increase in the number of circulating red blood cells occurs in emphysematous patients as a result of hypoxia. Total blood volume also increases. For this reason, phlebotomy may be useful as a therapeutic measure.

Patients with excessive respiratory secretions may be helped by postural drainage, which brings secretions up high enough so that they can be eliminated by coughing. Breathing exercises that utilize the abdominal muscles help the lungs empty and aid in the elimination of carbon dioxide. The nurse should supplement the educational efforts of the physical therapist and the physician and encourage the patient to practice these exercises.

Antibiotics may be necessary when a respiratory infection occurs. Unfortunately, the patient with chronic obstructive pulmonary disease is highly susceptible to such infections, particularly during the winter. Although, ideally, the patient should move to a mild climate during the fall and winter seasons, this is rarely possible. Hence, the patient should be taught to avoid exposure to respiratory infections, sudden chilling, and unnecessary exposure in damp or cold weather. If, in spite of these precautions, he develops a respiratory infection, he should immediately report that fact to his physician. The secretions of respiratory infections cause further obstruction to pulmonary ventilation in the emphysematous patient. Respiratory acidosis can occur readily, and the patient may become seriously ill in a short time.

ACUTE RESPIRATORY ACIDOSIS   The development of acute respiratory acidosis demands special measures. Bronchial aspiration may be necessary to rid the respiratory tract of mucus and purulent secretions. A mechanical respirator, used cautiously, may improve pulmonary ventilation. Overzealous use of a mechanical respirator may cause such rapid excretion of carbon dioxide that the kidneys will be unable to eliminate the excess bicarbonate ions with sufficient rapidity to prevent alkalosis and convulsions. For this reason, the elevated carbon dioxide concentration should be decreased slowly.

Fluid volume deficit accompanying respiratory acidosis may be treated by the intravenous administration of a Butler-type solution containing balanced quantities of extracellular and cellular electrolytes, plus carbohydrate, or with sixth molar lactate. Oxygen can be administered cautiously to relieve severe hypoxia. (Frequent arterial blood gas studies are needed to guide O_2 therapy.) It should be remembered that patients with hypoxemia ($\downarrow pO_2$) and hypercarbia ($\uparrow pCO_2$) may display confusion, anger, and noisy behavior (caused by neurologic manifestations of the abnormal blood gases). It would be *dangerous* to sedate these patients to quiet their behavior; instead, methods should be instituted to improve ventilation.

**PREVENTION OF CARBON DIOXIDE
NARCOSIS DURING OXYGEN THERAPY**

Carbon Dioxide Narcosis   *Carbon dioxide narcosis produced by excessive oxygen administration to a patient with chronic respiratory acidosis is still a common complication encountered in clinical practice.*

Chronic elevation of the carbon dioxide content of the extracellular fluid causes the respiratory center to become insensitive to carbon dioxide. (Recall that while the respiratory center normally is extremely sensitive to changes in carbon dioxide concentration and that a slight elevation causes respiratory stimulation, arterial carbon dioxide concentration of over 9 per cent causes respiratory depression.) Hypoxia becomes the main stimulus to respiration when the carbon dioxide mechanism is not functioning. A reduction in arterial oxygenation stimulates respiration, and an elevation of arterial oxygenation removes the stimulus. Thus, if oxygen is administered in sufficient quantities to raise arterial oxygenation significantly, respiration will decrease. Decreased respiration favors carbon dioxide retention. Eventually, carbon dioxide narcosis will result unless the situation is reversed.

The nurse should be alert for the occurrence of carbon dioxide narcosis when oxygen is administered to a patient with respiratory acidosis. The following are symptoms:

drowsiness
irritability, depression, or euphoria
warm, flushed skin
respiratory depression
tachycardia (arrhythmias may develop)
hallucinations
muscular tremors of face or extremities
normal or elevated blood pressure
convulsions
paralysis of extremities
deep coma

Safe Oxygen Administration   Oxygen therapy should be used cautiously in patients with chronic respiratory acidosis. It is important to give no more than a 30 or 40 per cent concentration of oxygen in air; a higher concentration may produce serious respiratory depression.

Continuous oxygen therapy is dangerous and should be avoided; oxygen is best given intermittently to patients with chronic respiratory acidosis. A common device for low-flow oxygen delivery to patients with chronic airway obstruction is the two-pronged nasal cannula. As mentioned earlier, the rate of O_2 flow should not exceed 1 or 2 L. a minute until blood gases are available to guide O_2 therapy. Advantages of this method are that the patient may talk, cough, and eat without removing the device. Also used for such patients is the Ventimask, a device that delivers a predetermined low O_2 concentration (24, 28, 35, or 40 per cent). Intermittent positive pressure breathing (IPPB) treatments are administered frequently during an acute exacerbation to increase carbon dioxide elimination and to fully aerate the

alveoli. To avoid impending CO_2 narcosis, the physician may order frequent checks of arterial blood gases; an inordinate rise in pCO_2 is an indication to decrease the oxygen concentration.

Acute Pulmonary Conditions Associated with Respiratory Acidosis

MECHANICAL OBSTRUCTION WITH A FOREIGN OBJECT   Mechanical obstruction of the respiratory tract with a foreign object prevents air flow into the lungs and results in severe anoxia. In addition, air flow from the lungs is interrupted. The sudden retention of carbon dioxide causes acute respiratory acidosis; it can also cause a mild rise in blood pressure.

Ventricular fibrillation and potassium excess are common causes of death in patients with acute respiratory acidosis. Treatment consists of the intravenous administration of a sixth molar sodium lactate solution.

Sudden relief of the obstruction, such as may be produced by tracheotomy, causes hyperventilation and may result in alkalosis and tetany, as carbon dioxide is rapidly eliminated from the lungs. The bicarbonate level remains temporarily high. (Recall that the kidneys cannot excrete bicarbonate ions as rapidly as the lungs excrete carbon dioxide.) Rapid correction of acidosis may cause ventricular fibrillation.

Apnea also may follow the sudden release of a respiratory obstruction through tracheotomy, possibly because of hypotension and decreased blood flow to the respiratory center. The blood pressure should be checked immediately before and also after tracheotomy to detect hypotension. If hypotension occurs, the physician may request that a vasopressor be given.

Other acute pulmonary conditions that may be associated with respiratory acidosis include pulmonary edema, atelectasis, open chest wounds, and severe pulmonary infections.

OTHER CONDITIONS ASSOCIATED WITH RESPIRATORY ACIDOSIS
Overdoses of Drugs   Overdoses of morphine, meperidine, or a barbiturate result in depression of respiration and increased retention of carbon dioxide. Before administering a drug of this class, the nurse should check the dose carefully, as well as the

time when the drug was last given. In addition, the rate and depth of respiration should be observed before and after administration of the drug.

Pain   Severe pain, particularly in the abdomen or thorax, results in splinting of the chest and shallow respiration. Carbon dioxide is retained and respiratory acidosis may develop. Judicious use of analgesics is indicated to relieve pain and to allow the patient to breathe more efficiently.

Weak Respiratory Muscles   Weakening of the respiratory muscles may be caused by such conditions as poliomyelitis or spinal cord injuries. Adequate pulmonary ventilation is not possible; an excessive amount of carbon dioxide is retained by the lungs, and respiratory acidosis may develop.

Inaccurate Regulation of Mechanical Respirators   Inaccurate regulation of a mechanical respirator may result in excessively shallow and slow respiration. Excessive carbon dioxide is retained by the lungs, causing respiratory acidosis.

Inhalation Anesthesia   The use of inhalation anesthetics, such as cyclopropane or ether, may be associated with hypoventilation and carbon dioxide retention. Mild carbon dioxide retention may be well tolerated for a while, particularly if hypoxia is not present. However, respiratory acidosis may develop as soon as 15 minutes after the start of inhalation anesthesia; it is most likely to occur in patients with chronic pulmonary disease, such as emphysema.

A patient may have normal color and still develop respiratory acidosis, particularly during an operation when the anesthetized patient is given oxygen. While the use of oxygen therapy to produce tissue oxygenation is good, if measures are not taken to increase the exhalation of carbon dioxide (such as with a positive pressure breathing device), an excessive amount of carbonic acid may form in the extracellular fluid and cause respiratory acidosis. The first indication of acidosis may be the development of ventricular fibrillation, probably caused by potassium excess. Carbon dioxide retention potentiates vagus nerve activity so that minor stimuli, such as tracheal suction, may cause cardiac arrhythmias. Positioning the patient on the operating table in such a way that normal respiratory excursions are prevented contributes to the development of respiratory acidosis.

Orthopedic Deformities   Restriction of respiratory excursions by spinal deformities may result in carbon dioxide retention and acidosis, even though the lungs are normal.

HYPERVENTILATION

Hyperventilation causes an excessive loss of CO_2 and, thus, a decrease in the carbonic acid content of the blood. Unless the kidneys can eliminate bicarbonate (HCO_3) sufficiently to maintain a normal carbonic acid–base bicarbonate ratio, respiratory alkalosis will result. (See the discussion of respiratory alkalosis in the next section.) In addition to an excessive loss of CO_2, hyperventilation causes an increased insensible water loss, a fact that must be considered in supplying an adequate fluid replacement.

RESPIRATORY ALKALOSIS

Pathologic Mechanism and Symptoms

Respiratory alkalosis may be caused by any condition that causes an increased excretion of carbon dioxide through the lungs, with a resultant decrease in the carbon dioxide concentration of the extracellular fluid. Hence, a decrease in the carbonic acid side of the carbonic acid–base bicarbonate ratio occurs.

Symptoms vary in respiratory alkalosis. They may be only those of the underlying disease process, or they may be absent. Sometimes the patient may appear to be short of breath. He may use his upper chest muscles and accessory respiratory muscles during respiration; he may complain of pain and tenderness of the left side of his chest. Alkalosis may cause increased neuromuscular excitability because of the decreased ionization of calcium. (Recall that calcium ionization is decreased in alkalosis.) Anoxia may occur because alkalosis inhibits the release of oxygen from oxyhemoglobin. The most characteristic clinical picture of respiratory alkalosis is represented by the hyperventilation syndrome:

dizziness or light-headedness
inability to concentrate
numbness and tingling of hands, feet, mouth, and tongue
tinnitus
blurred vision
palpitation of the heart
sweating
dry mouth
stiffness, aches, and cramps of muscles
positive Chvostek's sign (tapping the facial nerve in front of the ear causes the facial muscles about the mouth to contract)

positive Trousseau's sign (compression of the brachial artery for one to five minutes causes the muscles of the hand and wrist to go into spasm)

twitching and convulsions

loss of consciousness (fainting may occur without symptoms of tetany)

Hyperventilation causes decreased cerebral blood flow; light-headedness, convulsions, and unconsciousness may be due partly to cerebral ischemia. Symptoms of alkalotic tetany are more likely to occur if the respiratory alkalosis developed rapidly. The nurse should be alert for these symptoms in any patient having a condition likely to be associated with respiratory alkalosis.

Conditions Associated with Respiratory Alkalosis

A number of conditions may be associated with respiratory alkalosis (Table 24-4).

The most common cause is the hyperventilation that accompanies emotional upsets. Treatment consists of making the patient aware of his abnormal breathing practices; he should be made to realize that this breathing pattern causes his symptoms. He can be shown how to relieve his symptoms by holding his breath or breathing into a large paper bag. Such measures cause an accumulation of carbon dioxide in the lungs and relieve the alkalosis. A sedative may be required to relieve hyperventilation in very anxious patients. If alkalosis is severe enough to cause fainting, the increased ventilation will cease and respirations will revert to normal.

Hyperventilation can result from hypersensitivity of the respiratory center, such as occurs with meningitis and encephalitis. Respiratory alkalosis

Table 24-4. Conditions Likely To Be Associated with Respiratory Alkalosis

Anxiety
Lack of oxygen
Pulmonary embolism
Pregnancy (high progesterone level sensitizes respiratory center to CO_2)
Hyperventilation resulting from inaccurately regulated mechanical respirators
Early salicylate intoxication
High fever
Neurologic conditions associated with overstimulation of respiratory center (such as meningitis or encephalitis)
High environmental temperature

develops because excessive amounts of carbon dioxide are blown off by the lungs. The inaccurate regulation of a mechanical respirator, causing too deep and too rapid respiration, results in excessive carbon dioxide elimination—hence, respiratory alkalosis.

Overdoses of salicylates cause excessive stimulation of the respiratory center and hyperventilation. Alkalosis may occur early in salicylate intoxication; later, by the time the patient arrives at the hospital, metabolic acidosis may predominate (particularly in young children). Other causes of hyperventilation include high fever, exposure to high environmental temperatures, and oxygen lack. If the hyperventilation is prolonged, respiratory alkalosis may supervene.

WATER BALANCE IN PROLONGED MECHANICAL VENTILATION

WATER EXCESS A study conducted at Massachusetts General Hospital reviewed 100 patients treated with prolonged continuous mechanical ventilation.[11] Nineteen of the 100 patients developed a positive water balance, associated with weight gain and a significant drop in the plasma sodium concentration and in the hematocrit. The water retention existed primarily as pulmonary edema rather than as peripheral edema. It appears to be in no way connected with the patient's original diagnosis and is not affected by the type of respirator used. Water overloading may be associated with the use of efficient nebulizers providing an additional 300 to 500 ml. of water per day. Positive pressure ventilation produces changes in the dynamics of flow in the pulmonary vessels; possibly this causes excess water to move into the interstitial spaces. The water retention, with its associated weight gain and dilutional hyponatremia, may be associated with an elevated ADH level.

To avoid the dangerous complications that can result from water overloading in ventilated patients, careful monitoring of intake and output is essential. The water contribution from nebulizers should be included in the intake column. Daily body weight measurement is valuable in detecting weight gain from water loading, particularly when a sensitive in-bed scale is used. The actual weight gain may appear small, but one must consider that immobilized patients with low caloric intake would normally lose about 200 to 500 Gm. daily. Any gain in weight, or even maintenance of a steady weight under these conditions, may be caused by water retention.

An increase in pulmonary extravascular water may be detected by x-ray pictures. Treatment consists of water restriction and the use of diuretics. Failure to notice pulmonary water loading encourages progressive difficulty in ventilation.

CARE OF THE NEAR-DROWNED PATIENT

Drowning has increased as water sports have become more popular. Today accidental drowning is a common cause of death in the United States. Drowning is also a common method of suicide. The following factors may contribute to accidental drowning: (1) fatigue; (2) hyperventilation with prolonged breath-holding in order to swim long distances underwater; (3) muscle cramps; (4) hysteria; (5) currents or underwater obstacles; and (6) intoxication.

The nurse should be acquainted with the physiologic changes occurring with drowning and with the treatment of these changes, since she may be called upon to care for near-drowned patients in the hospital or at the scene of the accident.

Most submersions are fatal after two to three minutes; respiratory arrest occurs by the third minute and cardiac arrest occurs during the fourth minute.[12] Rescue before the third minute may result in spontaneous resuscitation.

Treatment of Near Drowning Immediate treatment of the near-drowned patient is very important. The following procedures are important.

1. Immediate treatment at the scene consists of clearing the airway and giving mouth-to-mouth ventilation, cardiac massage if necessary, and 100 per cent oxygen by mask (as soon as available). Recent recommendations of the American Heart Association and the American Red Cross include pressing on the upper abdomen to expel water from the lungs, in a modification of the Heimlich Maneuver.

2. If no pulse is palpable at the time of hospital admission, 1 ml. of 1:1000 epinephrine solution should be given into the heart.

3. Electrical defibrillation should be performed if ventricular fibrillation is present.

4. Sodium bicarbonate may be used to rapidly correct metabolic acidosis (secondary to hypoxemia).

5. The trachea should be intubated and suctioned, then ventilation provided by a volume-cycled respirator.

6. Frequent blood gas studies are indicated to guide oxygen administration.

7. A gastric tube should be inserted to remove swallowed water.

8. Electrolyte and hematocrit studies should be done and replacements made as indicated (initially, fluid administration is kept low until it is clear that pulmonary edema is not a problem). Urine output and central venous pressure should be closely monitored (as well as standard vital signs). There is a tendency toward hypernatremia in saltwater drowning (since sea water is strongly hypertonic) and a tendency toward hyperkalemia in freshwater drowning (since hemolysis of red blood cells may result from hemodilution, releasing potassium into the extracellular fluid). Low sodium-plasma or dextran in 5 per cent dextrose/water may be used to treat shock in saltwater drowning. Low potassium-plasma, packed cells, or dextran in saline may be used to treat shock in freshwater drowning.

9. Postural drainage may be utilized following administration of a bronchodilator aerosol.

10. Antibiotics may be necessary since the inhaled water frequently is contaminated; however, they should not be used until specific organisms have been identified by culture.

11. Corticosteroids may be used as indicated.

CHEST DRAINAGE

The pleural cavity is a "potential" space in the body. Normally it is empty, except for a few milliliters of fluid present to lubricate the pleural surfaces. In abnormal conditions this potential space can enlarge and contain large quantities of fluid, blood, or air. A chest tube may be inserted to empty the cavity after chest surgery, chest trauma, or in the presence of pleural effusion. Pleural effusion may be due to a variety of medical conditions (such as congestive heart failure, bronchial cancer, breast cancer, tuberculosis, pulmonary infarction, leukemia, and subdiaphragmatic abscess).

Frequently the nurse is required to observe the quantity and nature of chest drainage and, thus, must

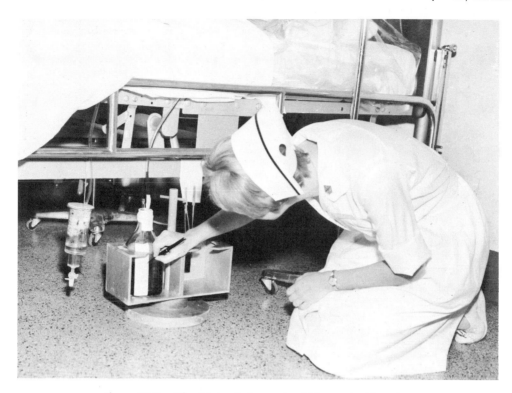

Figure 24-3.   Chest tube drainage should be marked hourly.

have an understanding of the principles of water-seal drainage. With a clear understanding of the mechanics of respiration, one can feel perfectly at ease with the water-seal drainage system. The purpose of the system is to drain excess fluid from the pleural cavity and to reestablish normal intrapleural pressure.

The chest tube must be kept patent by regular milking; this should be done every hour, more frequently if necessary. Milking should begin near the patient's chest and continue down the tubing to the bottle, clearing the tubing of any clots. The tubing should be kept free of any kinks, and care should be taken to prevent looping of excess tubing on the floor.

The nurse must make certain that the bottle *always* rests below the lowest level of the patient's chest. If the bottle is raised to chest level, negative pressure may suck water into the intrathoracic space. The chest bottle should either be kept in a holder or taped securely to the floor; this will prevent accidentally knocking the bottle over and breaking the water-seal system.

All connections must be secure and well taped. If the drainage bottle should be broken or if the water-

seal fails for any reason, the tube should be clamped immediately, near the chest. Two clamps should be kept at the bedside for each chest tube at all times.

The water-seal setup should be observed for the amount and character of drainage. Bright red drainage is expected immediately postoperatively following thoracotomy, gradually becoming darker, then more serosanguineous. Any sudden change should be reported immediately. To record the amount of drainage, a piece of adhesive tape should be vertically applied to the bottle so that hourly marks can be made, thus giving an accurate account of fluid loss (Fig. 24-3). A commercially available pleural drainage set is pictured and described in Figure 24-4.

The nurse should keep in mind the importance of determining how much the patient has lost in an hour-by-hour pattern. For instance, consider these contrasting records in a postoperative thoracotomy patient:

300 ml.	First hour	400 ml.
50 ml.	Second hour	50 ml.
50 ml.	Third hour	50 ml.
25 ml.	Fourth hour	25 ml.
50 ml.	Fifth hour	25 ml.

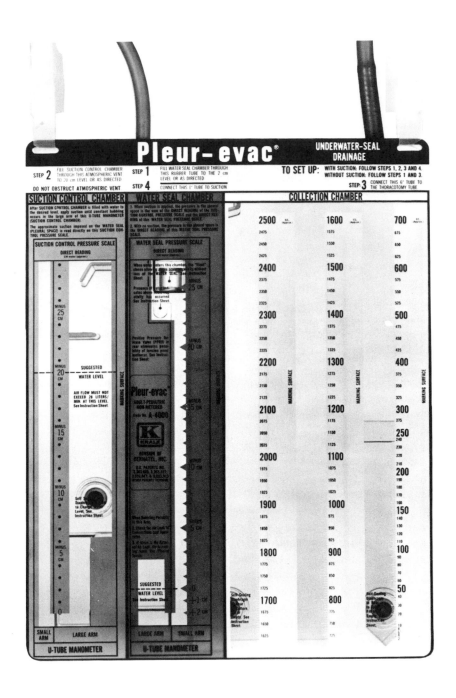

Figure 24-4. Pleur-evac®. A disposable pleural underwater-seal drainage set with three chambers: left—suction control chamber; center—water-seal chamber; right—collection chamber. (Courtesy of Deknatel, Inc., Queens Village, L. I., New York)

100 ml.	Sixth hour	0 ml.
100 ml.	Seventh hour	10 ml.
150 ml.	Eighth hour	5 ml.
Cause for		No Cause
Concern		for Concern

Oscillation of the fluid in the tubing should also be noted. When this ceases, it may indicate that the lung has reexpanded or that a clot obstructs the tubing. The tubing should be checked for patency at this time.

There should be adequate tubing to allow the patient to turn freely in bed; he should be turned every one to two hours. Turning to the affected side will facilitate drainage. Care must be taken that the patient does not occlude the chest tube.

REFERENCES

1. **Guyton, A.:** Textbook of Medical Physiology, ed. 5. Philadelphia: W. B. Saunders Co., 1976, p. 561.
2. **Boedeker, E., and Dauber, J.** (eds.): Manual of Medical Therapeutics, ed. 21. Boston: Little, Brown & Co., 1974, p. 158.
3. **Guyton:** Textbook of Medical Physiology, p. 562.
4. **Shapiro, B.,** et al.: Clinical Application of Blood Gases, ed. 2. Chicago: Year Book Medical Publishers, 1977, p. 140.
5. Ibid., p. 130.
6. Ibid.
7. Ibid., p. 151.
8. Ibid.
9. **Wade, J.:** Respiratory Nursing Care, ed. 2. St. Louis: C. V. Mosby, 1977, p. 74.
10. Ibid., p. 133.
11. **Sladen, A., Laver, M.,** and **Pontoppidan, H.:** Pulmonary complications and water retention in prolonged mechanical ventilation. New Eng. J. Med. August 1968.
12. **Graef, J.,** and **Cone, T.:** Manual of Pediatric Therapeutics. Boston: Little, Brown & Co., 1974, p. 54.

BIBLIOGRAPHY

Kempe, C., et al.: Current Pediatric Diagnosis and Treatment, ed. 4. Los Altos, Calif.: Lange Medical Publications, 1976.

Petty, T.: Intensive and Rehabilitative Respiratory Care, ed. 2. Philadelphia: Lea & Febiger, 1974.

— 25 —

Water and Electrolyte Disturbances from Heat Exposure

Although heat disorders occur most often in tropical zones, the temperate climate of North America can cause heat stress. Many persons living in a temperate climate withstand heat stress poorly, hence the increased number of deaths during heat waves. Another common source of heat disorders is the heat stress imposed by certain occupations.

Industry is often associated with artificially created hot climates, resulting from or deliberately designed for some industrial process. For example, persons working in the textile weaving and processing industry are often subjected to an artificially induced, warm, humid climate, because these conditions are best suited to textile processing. Certain segments of the glass, rubber, steel, and mining industries are also associated with high environmental temperatures. Laundry, construction, and agricultural workers and firemen are often exposed to heat stress.

Athletes are prone to heat disorders. A survey made by a group of football coaches showed that from 1931 through 1971 there were fifty football deaths resulting from heatstroke. This figure probably is low because such deaths may be inaccurately attributed to heart failure or other causes. Heat exhaustion and heat cramps are common occurrences on the football field, as well as in other strenuous sports. They are particularly common in athletes training vigorously in the late summer for fall sports.

Because so many persons in our society may be subject to heat disorders, the nurse should become familiar with their prevention, recognition, and treatment.

A brief review of body thermoregulation mechanisms will promote a more thorough understanding of the section concerning specific heat disorders.

THERMOREGULATION IN THE BODY

Mechanisms of Thermoregulation

To maintain thermoequilibrium in the body, the amount of heat lost must be equal to the amount of heat gained. Heat is lost when the environmental temperature is less than body temperature. It is gained when the environmental temperature exceeds body temperature and when body energy expenditures are high. Fortunately, the body has a sensitive and efficient thermoregulation system. Let us consider its elements.

HYPOTHALAMUS The heat control center, located in the hypothalamus, has two anatomically separate subcenters: one is responsible for conserving heat and the other for giving off heat. The heat control center is made aware of body temperature variations directly from local brain temperature changes (secondary to variations in the temperature of blood supplying the brain), and reflexly from afferent fibers of the many cutaneous nerve endings sensitive to hot and cold. Efferent fibers of these nerves are chiefly involved with vasomotor activity and the functioning of the sweat glands.

CIRCULATORY SYSTEM   The circulatory system bears much of the burden of thermoregulation. The constriction of cutaneous blood vessels occurs when the environmental temperature is lower than the body temperature and when energy expenditures are low. Cutaneous vasoconstriction decreases the amount of blood brought to the surface for cooling and, thus, conserves body heat. Dilatation of the cutaneous blood vessels occurs when the environmental temperature exceeds the body temperature and when energy expenditures are high. Because more blood is brought to the surface for cooling by radiation and conduction, body temperature is lowered.

Sweating is initiated when the environmental temperature exceeds 82.4 to 86° F. (28 to 30° C.). The evaporation of sweat from the body surface causes cooling of peripheral blood. The cooled blood is returned to core parts of the body and serves to reduce body temperature.

SWEAT GLANDS   Of the body's sweat glands, approximately two million have thermoregulation as their chief function. Sweat is normally a hypotonic fluid containing several solutes, the chief of which is sodium chloride. The concentration of sodium chloride in sweat depends largely on the dietary intake; thus the amount per liter of sweat is highly variable. For example, 5 L. of sweat may contain from 2 to 20 Gm. of sodium chloride. A high salt intake causes an increased excretion of salt by the kidneys and sweat glands. Decreased salt intake, or excessive salt loss, causes renal conservation of salt; the sweat glands similarly conserve salt. The retention of needed salt by the kidneys, and possibly by the sweat glands, occurs in response to increased aldosterone secretion.

Other solutes in sweat include potassium, ammonia, and urea. The potassium concentration in sweat may be as high as 9 mEq./L.; excessive sweat losses can lead to potassium deficiency.

The *maximal* sweating rate for most persons is roughly 2 L./hour; obviously, this rate cannot be

maintained for long periods. Individuals accustomed to high heat stress may sweat as much as 3 or more L. per hour. As much as 20 Gm. of sodium chloride has been reported lost in one day's sweat during high heat stress.

SUMMARY OF BODILY RESPONSES TO HEAT STRESS   Exposure of the body to heat stress elicits the following responses:

1. Increased peripheral vasodilatation, to allow more blood to come to the surface for cooling by radiation and conduction.
2. Increased sweating, to allow for cooling by evaporation.
3. Increased blood volume and venous tone, to improve venous return to the heart.
4. Increased cardiac output and pulse rate.
5. Increased secretion of antidiuretic hormone, to allow the conservation of body water (the 24-hour urinary output may drop to as little as 300 ml.).
6. Increased aldosterone secretion, to allow the conservation of body salt (aldosterone causes sodium retention by the kidneys and may exert a similar effect on the sweat glands). Unfortunately, this mechanism increases potassium loss.

Acclimatization to Heat

It has long been known that individuals accustomed to high temperature, either in a natural hot climate or in their work, tolerate heat stress much better than those accustomed to cool temperatures. Yet, the latter can gradually develop a tolerance for heat when repeatedly exposed to it. This process of physiologic adaptation is called *acclimatization*. It is accomplished by a series of physiologic changes, which serve to ameliorate the effects of heat stress.

PHYSIOLOGIC CHANGES   Individuals exposed repeatedly to heat stress gradually experience fewer of the disagreeable sensations induced by heat, such as lassitude and general discomfort, because of the physiologic changes induced by acclimatization. The sweat contains a lower concentration of sodium chloride and a higher quantity of potassium than normal, as a result of increased production of aldosterone. (Recall that aldosterone causes sodium retention and potassium loss.) Retention of sodium causes water retention and, thus, an increased plasma volume. Other specific changes include a progressive decrease in rectal and skin temperatures, a decreased pulse rate, and increased sweating ability.

RATE OF ACCLIMATIZATION Most of the changes brought about by acclimatization occur in the first four to seven days of heat exposure; they usually attain their maximum after two weeks of daily heat exposure. A person does not have to be subjected to heat stress 24 hours a day in order to become acclimatized. According to Leithead and Lind,[1] the best way to induce acclimatization is to engage in repeated, uninterrupted periods of 100-minutes work under heat stress. Even a daily heat exposure period of 50 minutes is sufficient to induce an important measure of acclimatization. Short exposures to heat will not induce acclimatization because they present no threat to the body's thermoregulation mechanisms.

PLASMA pH CHANGES Respiratory alkalosis occurs at first during exposure to heat stress (a result of hyperventilation) and probably is responsible for the heat-induced tetany seen in some patients. (No actual change in total body calcium occurs; apparently the tetany is caused by the rapid rise in plasma pH, causing decreased ionization of calcium.) This condition is resolved when heat stress and hyperventilation are relieved.

Metabolic acidosis is superimposed on respiratory alkalosis as the subject exercises in the heat, possibly due to an increased buildup of acid metabolites.

HEAT DISORDERS

There are several classifications of heat disorders. The classification used in this chapter was derived chiefly from *Heat Stress and Heat Disorders* by Leithead and Lind.[2]

Prolonged exposure to heat can produce several reactions:

Heat syncope
Heat cramps
Heat exhaustion
  Primary water depletion (sodium excess)
  Primary salt depletion (sodium deficit)
Heatstroke

The clinical picture of each disorder is related to the length of exposure to heat and the individual's peculiar response.

Heat Syncope

Heat syncope is also referred to as heat collapse. It is characterized by a sharp reduction in vasomotor tone after heat exposure, which causes peripheral vasodilatation and a tendency to venous pooling. There are no underlying water or electrolyte disturbances.

SYMPTOMS The pooling of venous blood in the peripheral vessels in heat syncope causes hypotension and cerebral anoxia. Symptoms may include fainting, lightheadedness, or fatigue. Fainting most often follows an additional stress, such as sudden postural changes, heavy lifting, or prolonged standing. Other symptoms may include pallor, nausea, weakness, blurring of vision, numbness, and sensations of hot and cold. The pulse rate is increased at the onset of syncope and then decreases. Breathing is low and sighing. The systolic blood pressure is greatly decreased, the diastolic pressure only moderately. The temperature may be above normal; if the patient was engaged in strenuous activity before fainting, the temperature may reach 102° F. Usually the muscles are flaccid. Perspiration, most evident on the forehead, is present.

TREATMENT Symptoms subside when the patient is placed in the recumbent or head-low position; consciousness is regained in a few minutes. Rest for one or two hours in a cool environment is indicated.

Although diagnosis usually is not difficult, the patient should be examined for more serious illnesses associated with fainting. Other causes of sudden fainting may include epilepsy, heart disease, depletion of sodium or water, and heatstroke. The patient should be checked for urinary incontinence and a bitten tongue; both are indicative of an epileptic seizure. The presence of an arrhythmic pulse rate may indicate heart disease. The specific gravity and salt content of the urine should be measured; both are usually normal in heat syncope because there are no major water and electrolyte changes accompanying this disorder. The presence of a high urinary specific gravity may indicate the presence of heat exhaustion caused by sodium excess rather than heat syncope.

PREVENTION   Persons not accustomed to high temperatures should gradually expose themselves to heat, as described earlier in the section dealing with acclimatization to heat. Strenuous activities in a hot environment should not be attempted until maximal heat tolerance is achieved. Patients with cardiac disease should be cautioned against excessive heat exposure, particularly when exercising.

Heat Cramps

Sometimes heat cramps are called miner's, fireman's, or stoker's cramps. They are painful spasms of voluntary muscles of the legs, abdomen, back, and forearms that follow strenuous exercise in hot surroundings, either climatic or industrial, coupled with consumption of plain water. The basic pathophysiologic process in this disorder is related to a low plasma osmolality, caused by water excess; this, in turn, causes movement of water into the cellular space.

Good health does not preclude their occurrence; even workers well accustomed to their jobs can develop them. Workers in some occupations accept heat cramps as an occupational hazard of no serious consequence; they seldom seek medical help unless severe cramps develop.

There is some doubt in classifying heat cramps as a separate entity rather than including it as a manifestation of heat exhaustion caused by sodium deficit. Both are due to a depletion of sodium chloride. However, heat exhaustion is more severe and has a broader symptomatology than heat cramps.

SYMPTOMS   The only symptom in heat cramps is the intermittent cramping of voluntary muscles. Usually the muscles involved are the ones most exercised. Cramps may be preceded by a twitching in the affected muscles, which tighten into a hard lump. They vary in intensity from mild to severe. Pain is excruciating during severe heat cramps and subsides as the spasmodic contractions cease. Many cramps last less than one minute; the patient is comfortable between cramps.

The time of onset is almost invariably toward the end of a day's work. *Heat cramps are always preceded by several hours of strenuous exercise, heavy sweating, and liberal plain water intake.* (Patients on hemodialysis or on strict low-sodium diets sometimes develop the type of cramps here described.)

TREATMENT   Analgesics offer little or no relief for the spasms. The specific treatment is salt replacement; one fourth of a teaspoon of salt may be added to a glass of water and repeated at intervals of 5 to 30 minutes. Severe cramps may require an infusion of one-half to 1 L. of isotonic saline to relieve immediate symptoms; when cramps have subsided, salt can be given orally. The patient should rest for 24 hours after the cessation of cramps. Muscles are stiff and sore after heat cramps, and several days' rest may be necessary before the patient can return to work.

PREVENTION   The prevention of heat cramps includes increasing the salt intake or decreasing the plain water intake. The former is much to be preferred. Decreasing the water intake predisposes to more serious heat disorders, such as heat exhaustion resulting from sodium excess and heatstroke. Acclimatization is helpful.

In addition to the normal dietary salt intake, some workers may need 2 or 3 Gm. of extra salt daily to prevent heat cramps; others require as much as 5 Gm. extra. Tablets of salt are often provided at drinking fountains in factories where excessive sweating is a problem. Some workers can sweat profusely and drink water liberally without developing heat cramps. This unexplained fact sometimes causes others to ignore medical advice to take supplemental salt tablets.

Heat Exhaustion Caused by Sodium Deficit

Heat exhaustion (sodium deficit) stems from the inadequate replacement of the sodium chloride lost in sweat during prolonged heat exposure. It is often associated with the performance of hard work in high environmental heat.

Even though sweat is hypotonic, a sizable amount of salt can be lost when sweating is excessive. If plain water is drunk freely, without salt replacement, symptoms of sodium deficit become pronounced. Unacclimatized persons are more apt to develop sodium deficit than those accustomed to high heat stress. Sweat glands of acclimatized persons have a greater ability to conserve salt when the body's supply is low. This adaptation process takes place after an exposure period to heat of about five to six days. The phenomenon may explain why some men, accustomed to working and sweating in hot industries, can pay little attention to salt replacement and drink plain water freely without developing symptoms of sodium deficit. However, it should not be forgotten that anyone exposed to high heat stress is vulnerable to salt-depletion heat exhaustion.

SYMPTOMS Although both sodium and chloride are lost in heat exhaustion caused by sodium loss, the symptoms are primarily those of sodium deficit. Because sodium is the chief extracellular ion, its depletion causes a fall in the osmolarity of the extracellular fluid. As a result, water enters the cells, diluting their electrolytes, and causing them to swell. Equally important, water diuresis occurs and causes a pronounced decrease in the extracellular fluid volume. The decrease of extracellular fluid volume and the increase in cellular fluid volume seems to be at least partly related to all of the symptoms of this form of heat exhaustion. Plasma volume is progressively decreased as sodium deficit becomes more severe. In some cases the volume has been reduced by half.

Symptoms of heat exhaustion caused by sodium deficit develop insidiously over three to five days and include:

> fatigue
> headache
> muscle cramps
> giddiness
> vomiting
> nausea
> anorexia
> syncope
> listlessness
> constipation or diarrhea
> circulatory collapse (in last stages)

In early sodium deficit, the complaints are of apprehension, weariness, muscle weakness, headache, and giddiness. These symptoms persist and later are accompanied by nausea, cramps, and vomiting. Painful muscle cramps lasting up to two or more minutes frequently occur in heat exhaustion; usually the cramps occur in muscles fatigued by exercise. In severe sodium deficit, the legs, arms, and abdominal muscles may be involved.

Thirst is not a striking feature, as it is in heat exhaustion caused by sodium excess. The body temperature usually is subnormal or normal; occasionally it may rise to 101° F. (38.3° C.). The urine is not highly concentrated and contains negligible amounts of sodium chloride. The plasma sodium and chloride levels are reduced. The hematocrit percentage is high, often about 60 per cent.

Only badly neglected persons reach the stage of profound circulatory collapse. The hypotension, oliguria, and shock that result may cause death. Clinically, it is sometimes difficult to distinguish between heat exhaustion resulting from sodium deficit and that caused by water depletion. Table 25-1 lists a comparison of symptoms to help differentiate the two.

TREATMENT The treatment consists of bedrest in cool surroundings, and a high salt and water intake. The daily salt intake should be approximately 20 Gm. until sodium deficit is corrected. Unlike some animals, man does not crave salt when sodium deficit is present; therefore, a natural drive to consume enough salt to repair the deficit cannot be relied on.

Salt can be palatably replaced by adding it to liquids such as tomato juice or broth. It can also be supplied in oral isotonic saline if nothing else is at hand. Enteric-coated salt tablets should not be used for treatment because they take hours to dissolve in the intestines; they should be used only as a prophylactic measure.

PREVENTION Persons working in a hot environment should consume an adequate amount of salt. Most diets contain approximately 10 Gm. of salt; acclimatized men generally need no supplement to their normal dietary salt intake. Unacclimatized men working in hot surroundings may require as much as 5 Gm., and rarely 10 to 15 Gm., of extra salt daily to prevent salt depletion. This amount can be reduced after acclimatization has been achieved. The occurrence of other abnormal losses of salt, such as in vomiting or diarrhea, is an indication to increase salt intake.

Since it is difficult to add more than 10 Gm. of table salt to the daily diet without making it unpalatable, salt tablets are used to supplement dietary salt intake. Some salt tablets are merely compressed salt and are designed to add to drinks or food; their only advantage over table salt is that they require less storage space. The most widely used salt tablets are enteric coated; these tablets are available in 5 grain

Table 25-1. Distinction Between Heat Exhaustion Caused by Sodium Deficit and That Resulting from Water Depletion (Sodium Excess)

Features	Sodium Deficit	Water Depletion (Sodium Excess)
Duration of symptoms	3 to 5 days	Often much shorter
Thirst	Not prominent	Prominent
Fatigue	Prominent	Less prominent
Giddiness	Prominent	Less prominent
Muscle cramps	In most cases	Absent
Vomiting	In most cases	Usually absent
Thermal sweating	Probably unchanged	Diminished
Hemoconcentration	Early and marked	Slight until late
Urine chloride	Negligible amounts	Normal amounts
Urine concentration	Moderate	Pronounced
Plasma sodium	Below average	Above average
Mode of death	Oligemic shock	High osmotic pressure, oligemic shock, heatstroke

Adapted from Leithead, C., and Lind, A.: Heat Stress and Heat Disorders. Philadelphia: F. A. Davis Co., 1964, p. 165.

(0.33 Gm.) and 10 grain (0.65 Gm.) sizes. Other tablets are chocolate coated and disintegrate quickly when swallowed.

Patients receiving diuretic therapy should be observed closely for salt depletion during the hot summer months; physicians sometimes deem it necessary to curtail the use of diuretic drugs during this time. Recall that most diuretics cause an increased urinary excretion of sodium, water, and potassium.

Heat Exhaustion Resulting from Sodium Excess

This form of heat exhaustion is due to inadequate water replacement during prolonged heat exposure and sweating. A high price is paid in sweat to allow successful thermoregulation in hot surroundings. Because sweat is hypotonic, relatively greater amounts of water than salt are lost. This is particularly apt to occur after acclimatization when the body has decreased its sodium loss in sweat, causing an even more hypotonic sweat loss. Failure to adequately replace the water loss leads to water depletion (sodium excess). This form of heat exhaustion, if uncorrected, predisposes to heatstroke.

SYMPTOMS Thirst occurs early, and the patient will respond to it unless circumstances prevent. These may include an inadequate or unpalatable water supply or the inability of infants and extremely enfeebled persons to respond to thirst.

Symptoms of heat exhaustion caused by sodium excess depend upon the degree of water loss; three clinical grades can be described, as shown in Table 25-2.

Generally speaking, a man can survive in a tem-

Table 25-2. Heat Exhaustion Caused by Water Depletion (Sodium Excess)

Clinical Grade	Symptoms
Early	Thirst Loss of 2% body weight (equivalent to 1.5 l. in a man weighing 70 kg.)
Moderately severe	Intense thirst Dry mouth, difficulty in swallowing Scanty urine of high concentration Rapid pulse Increase in rectal temperature to about 102° F. Poor skin turgor Loss of 6% body weight (equivalent to 4.2 L. in a man weighing 70 kg.)
Very severe	Intense thirst Dry mouth, difficulty in swallowing Scanty urine of high concentration Rapid pulse Poor skin turgor Marked impairment of mental and physical capacities High rectal temperature Cyanosis, circulatory failure, extreme oliguria, or anuria Rapid breathing (hyperventilation may cause tetany) Loss of more than 7% body weight (equivalent to 5 to 10 L. in a man weighing 70 kg.) Coma and death when 15% of body weight is lost

Adapted from Leithead, C., and Lind, A.: Heat Stress and Heat Disorders. Philadelphia: F. A. Davis Co., 1964, p. 148.

perate climate for seven to ten days without water; he can survive only one or two days without water when exposed to the extreme heat of the desert.

TREATMENT   The patient should rest in bed in a cool environment. Sponging with cool water may be necessary if the body temperature is greatly elevated. The feet should be elevated to improve blood return to the heart; the arms and legs should be rubbed to stimulate blood flow.

A high fluid intake is indicated. If the patient can tolerate water by mouth, cool fluids should be given at frequent intervals to achieve an intake of 6 to 8 L. in the first 24 hours.

Intravenous infusion of 4 or more liters of 5 per cent dextrose in water may be necessary if the patient is unconscious or otherwise unable to take fluids orally. Renal function should be assessed before a large volume of intravenous fluids is given. The presence of severe oliguria or anuria could cause circulatory overload. Water intoxication can result if large volumes of 5 per cent glucose in water are given to a patient with renal damage. Daily body weight and fluid intake-output records should be kept; further fluid replacement is made as clinical findings indicate.

The plasma sodium level and urinary sodium chloride content are measured daily. Recall that sodium chloride is also lost in sweat, even though the water loss is more pronounced. If a sodium deficit is present after water replacement, isotonic saline may be given.

PREVENTION   An adequate supply of cool water should be made easily accessible to men working in hot surroundings. Infants exposed to heat should be offered water frequently; aged or otherwise enfeebled persons should also be offered fluids frequently. Inadequate oral intake should be reported so that another replacement route can be used.

Heatstroke

Heatstroke is the most serious heat disorder and is associated with a high mortality rate. It is characterized by the sudden cessation of sweating following exposure to high heat stress. Its distribution is worldwide, either in naturally occurring hot climates or in artificial hot surroundings, such as occur in some industries. Heat waves in usually temperate climates

account for a large number of heatstroke victims, especially among the elderly, many of whom are receiving diuretics.

The exact pathologic cause of heatstroke is not understood—the production of sweat seemingly fails. So long as sweating continues, with water and salt losses replaced, the body can withstand heat stress well.

According to Guyton,[3] an individual can tolerate, with no apparent ill effects, several hours of exposure to a temperature of 150° F. (65.5° C.) if the air is completely dry and if air currents are flowing in order to promote rapid evaporation of sweat from the skin surface. However, if the air is 100 per cent humidified, evaporation cannot take place and the body temperature begins to rise when the environmental temperature exceeds approximately 94° F. (34.4° C.).

Central nervous system symptoms, failure of sweat formation, and high body temperatures (above 105° F. or 40.5° C.) are characteristically present in heatstroke.

PREDISPOSING FACTORS   Certain factors predispose individuals to heatstroke:

Inadequate acclimatization
Obese body build
Preexistent acute or chronic illness
Recent use of alcohol
Inadequate water and salt intake
Recent use of atropine-like drugs
High relative humidity
Extremes in age
Strenuous physical activity in hot surroundings
Failure to appreciate the dangers of heat exposure and to take adequate precautions

DISCUSSION   Much evidence supports the thesis that lack of acclimatization predisposes to heatstroke. Malamud, Haymaker, and Custer, in 1946, studied the heatstroke deaths of 125 soldiers undergoing intensive training in the southern United States. They found that one fourth of the men who died had been in camp less than two weeks, and about half had been there less than eight weeks.

An obese person has less body surface in proportion to body weight than does a person of slight build; thus, he has greater difficulty in dissipating heat. Conditions such as myocardial ischemia, arteriosclerosis, and hypertension seem to predispose to heatstroke.

Recent use of alcohol prior to heat exposure may predispose to heatstroke. According to Leithead and Lind,[4] there probably are several reasons why this is true: alcohol causes an increased metabolic load and steps up internal body temperature; it dulls judgment and critical thinking; and it causes increased water loss from the body.

Atropine-like drugs cause decreased sweating and, thus, interfere with the dissipation of body heat. The administration of atropine before surgery has been implicated as a predisposing factor in heatstroke of heavily draped surgical patients in hot operating rooms.

A high relative humidity predisposes to heatstroke because it interferes with the evaporation of sweat from the body. Failure of sweat to evaporate causes inefficient body cooling. As mentioned earlier, body temperature begins to rise when the relative humidity is 100 per cent and the environmental temperature is above 94° F. (34.4° C.).

The high incidence of cardiovascular disease in the aged predisposes this age group to heatstroke. Infants are also predisposed to heatstroke; they have an unstable thermoregulatory mechanism, in addition to immature renal function. The infant's renal function, particularly during the first month of life, does not allow concentration of urine when excessive water loss by other routes has occurred. Sodium excess results because of the kidneys' inability to conserve needed body water, when perspiration losses are great.

Strenuous activity increases the metabolic rate and, thus, elevates the body temperature. The addition of a hot external temperature subjects the body to two sources of excessive heat and predisposes to heatstroke. Heatstroke has been observed in persons doing heavy manual labor when the environmental temperature was as low as 84.2° F. (29° C.). Of 159 heatstroke patients studied by Gauss and Meyer (1917),[5] the majority were manual laborers, including some firemen or laundry workers. However, it should be remembered that even mild activity in extremely hot surroundings may result in heatstroke.

Failure to appreciate the dangers of heat exposure is often related to the development of heatstroke. The nurse should become familiar with the preventive measures listed at the end of the chapter so that she can offer sound advice about heat disorders to lay persons.

SYMPTOMS Persons mildly afflicted with heatstroke may have no prodromal symptoms. Others may experience symptoms for a few minutes to one to two hours before loss of consciousness. These symptoms may include euphoria (associated with a rise in body temperature), headache, dizziness, faintness, numbness, drowsiness, aggressiveness, mental confusion, and incoordinated movements.

Usually the onset of heatstroke is sudden and heralded by disturbances of the central nervous system. Symptoms of heatstroke include the following:

disorientation
absence of sweating
complaint of feeling hot
involuntary limb movements
skin dry and hot to touch (skin turgor is usually good unless heatstroke is preceded by water depletion)
rectal temperature of at least 105° F. (40.5° C.)
convulsions, either localized or generalized
projectile vomiting
rapid pulse (may be as high as 150 beats per minute)
rapid respiration (may be as high as 60 per minute)
systolic blood pressure elevated
red, blotchy appearance of face (patient may look as if he has been strangled)
incontinent liquid feces
circulatory collapse
petechial hemorrhages in the brain, heart, kidney, or liver (if the patient survives, residual damage to these organs, particularly the brain, may become evident)
coma

Most persons suffering with heatstroke are comatose at the time they receive medical attention. Many times the comatose heatstroke patient is mistaken for a stroke victim; the presence of neurologic symptoms resembling those of stroke accounts for this confusion.

Rapid breathing in heatstroke may cause respiratory alkalosis, owing to the excessive blowing off of CO_2, and result in hypokalemia. This imbalance is less threatening, however, than hyperkalemia, which occasionally occurs. Potassium excess is associated with cellular breakdown caused by heat. Potassium leaves the cells and enters the extracellular fluid, where it remains because of poor renal function owing to circulatory collapse and the cessation of sweating. (Recall that sweat contains potassium.) Potassium excess can cause sudden death in heatstroke victims.

TREATMENT   *Quick and effective reduction of the high body temperature is essential.* Even a few hours delay may leave the patient with severe neurologic deficits. The longer the temperature remains high, the greater the possibility of irreversible brain damage. When the body temperature is above 106° F. (41.1° C.), damage to the parenchyma of cells throughout the entire body occurs. Especially devastating is the loss of neurons, since neuronal cells, once destroyed, cannot be replaced. When the body temperature reaches 110 to 114° F., (43.3 to 45.5° C.), the patient can live only a few hours unless the temperature is reduced rapidly. (Once the body temperature has reached 110° F. or 43.3° C., the body metabolism has doubled.) Regardless of the degree of temperature elevation, it should be reduced to 102° F. (38.9° C.) within the first hour of treatment. Recovery from heatstroke depends largely on reducing the degree and duration of fever.

A highly effective method of cooling is immersion in a tub of water to which ice is slowly added. This measure may seem drastic, yet the temperature must be rapidly lowered to 102° F. (The use of a bathtub filled with ice can usually lower body temperature to this level within one hour.) Since the patient may be comatose, or at least disoriented, he must be protected from drowning. The trunk and extremities should be massaged during the bath to bring blood to the periphery for cooling. The body temperature should be checked every three to five minutes. When it reaches approximately 102° F., the patient should be removed from the ice water bath since, as a rule, the body temperature continues to fall another 3 to 4° F. Reduction of the temperature to 102° F. causes the patient to feel better; slight paralysis is sometimes relieved by the temperature reduction. After removal from the tub, the body temperature should be measured at frequent intervals so that any rise can be noted early. (It may be necessary to repeat hypothermic treatment.) The patient should next be placed in a cool room with low humidity.

Some industries with a high risk of heat disorders are equipped with a latticelike bed to suspend the patient while he is sprayed with cold water and exposed to air movement supplied by an electric fan. A less effective cooling method includes sponging the patient with alcohol or cool water; this method is made more effective when good air movement is insured, as with an electric fan. Electrically-controlled hypothermic mattresses have been used successfully in the treatment of heatstroke. Antipyretics are too slow and do not lower the body temperature sufficiently to be of value in the initial treatment of heatstroke.

In the presence of shock, fluids must be administered carefully while the central venous pressure is being monitored. Care should be taken to avoid precipitation of pulmonary edema by too rapid fluid replacement. The initial status of body water and electrolytes depends upon the state of hydration prior to the onset of heatstroke. Some patients have no water or salt loss; others have a severe depletion of salt or water or both. Hypernatremia is present in a large number of the cases and requires treatment with dextrose and water, or hypotonic electrolyte solutions, or both. Usually metabolic acidosis is present and may be treated with an isotonic sodium bicarbonate solution. (It is not clear whether or not the metabolic acidosis is the result of vasomotor collapse, anoxia, or disordered lactic acid metabolism; elevated lactic acid levels have been found in some patients.)[6] Vasopressors are contraindicated initially since they cause vasoconstriction and, therefore, interfere with heat dissipation.

A decrease in plasma potassium has been observed in about half of the reported cases of heatstroke. Some authorities account for this by speculating that heatstroke patients may be depleted of potassium. Hypokalemia is unusual when metabolic acidosis is present. (Recall that acidosis usually causes a shift of potassium from the cells into the plasma, and a decreased secretion of potassium into the tubular urine, resulting in *hyper*kalemia.)

Sometimes a phenothiazine derivative (chlorpromazine) is used intravenously for its hypothermic and metabolism-lowering effects and for its sedative action; however, a significant drop in blood pressure may occur with its use, so the blood pressure should be monitored closely.

Usually an indwelling catheter is inserted into the bladder to monitor hourly urine output. If the hourly output is consistently less than 20 ml./hr., mannitol or another diuretic, such as furosemide or ethacrynic acid, may be used in an effort to prevent the development of acute tubular necrosis. Acute renal failure is reported to occur in 5 to 20 per cent of heatstroke patients.[7]

Disturbances in blood coagulation factors have been described in many severe cases of heatstroke; a prolonged prothrombin time (caused by decreased activity of factors V and VII) and a reduced plasma content of fibrinogen often develop within 12 to 36 hours.[8] These coagulation defects may play a major role in the mortality of heatstroke patients since petechial hemorrhages in the heart, brain, skin, and skeletal muscles are prominent features in fatal cases. Fresh blood may be given as indicated. Other complications include arrhythmias, myocardial infarction, and cerebral vascular accident.

After one to three days of intensive treatment, the sweat glands should become functional again, although it may be as long as six months before they begin to secrete normally. The patient should continue to rest in bed and avoid exposure to sunlight for one to two weeks after temperature reduction.

EMERGENCY MEASURES BEFORE MEDICAL AID IS AVAILABLE   Because time is so vital in preventing fatalities from heatstroke, one should take every measure to reduce body temperature as soon as possible. Unfortunately, heatstroke may occur in an area some distance from medical aid; furthermore, facilities for ice water baths or even sponging may not be available. *The following points should be kept in mind to care for the heatstroke victim before medical aid is available:*

1. Move the patient out of the sun to the coolest, best ventilated spot available.

2. Remove most of the patient's clothing.

3. Summon medical aid; if necessary, move the patient to medical aid. The transporting vehicle should have all of its windows opened so that a draft can blow on the patient to promote cooling. If moving the patient entails further exposure to high heat stress, it is better to wait until a more suitable means of transportation is available. Additional heat stress could cause death.

4. Investigate surroundings for *any* immediate means of reducing the patient's temperature until more effective measures can be made available. For

example, if heatstroke occurs during an outing near a body of water, the patient may be partially immersed to promote cooling. Or, if a water hose is available, the patient can be sprayed continuously with water. If nothing but a drinking water supply is available, the patient can be sponged with it.

5. Massage the patient's skin vigorously; this maintains circulation, aids in accelerating heat loss, and stimulates the return of cool peripheral blood to the overheated brain and viscera. Body heat may be lost rapidly in this manner.

Summary of Measures to Prevent Heat Disorders

The nurse has a responsibility to the public to offer sound advice about heat disorders and their prevention. In addition, she should be alert to the prevention of heat disorders in hospitalized patients. The following should be remembered:

1. All persons exposed to high heat stress should increase their daily salt, potassium, and water intake. Heat resistance is developed by replenishing water and salt losses as they occur. Infants should be offered water frequently during hot days, as should enfeebled adults. Salt tablets, preferably with potassium incorporated, should be taken to supplement dietary salt intake when excessive sweating occurs, except in acclimated persons and those on low-sodium diets.

2. Strenuous activity should be curtailed as much as possible during hot days.

3. Persons customarily exposed to heat stress should maintain good physical condition. (Sufficient rest and proper food and fluid intake help prevent heat disorders.) They should take supplemental potassium, perhaps 25 or 50 mEq. or more daily, provided renal function is normal. (Bear in mind that prolonged heat stress can cause potassium deficit and impaired renal concentration.)

4. Persons moving from a temperate to a hot climate, or those subjected to heat stress in their work, should gradually build up a tolerance to heat through planned acclimatization. Sudden exposure of an unacclimatized person to high heat stress predisposes to heat disorders. (See section dealing with acclimatization to heat.)

5. Prickly heat should be prevented as much as possible, because it interferes with sweating and dis-

sipation of heat from the body. Persons exposed to heat should wear loose, porous clothing, take frequent cool baths, and keep their rooms well ventilated.

6. Persons particularly susceptible to heat disorders should be protected from hot, unventilated places. Such persons include infants, the aged, persons with cardiovascular disease, and those under the influence of alcohol.

7. Persons taking atropine-like drugs should be protected from excessive heat exposure; atropine causes a decrease in sweating and an increased susceptibility to heat disorders. Such persons should be urged to keep their rooms well ventilated during hot weather, take frequent cool baths, and wear loose, porous clothing.

8. Persons taking diuretics should avoid excessive heat exposure and sweating. Recall that diuretics cause an increased excretion of sodium and potassium from the body; if the sodium and potassium levels are further depleted by excessive sweating, the patient may develop sodium and potassium depletion.

9. Persons confined to bed should be protected from excessive bedclothing and hot, poorly ventilated rooms.

10. Potassium deficit has been shown to help cause some heat disorders. Hence, persons prone to develop potassium deficit—those taking diuretics, for example—should guard against potassium deficit in hot weather. Food intake, i.e. potassium intake, usually decreases in hot weather; at the same time, more potassium than normal is lost in heavy sweating. Thus, potassium supplements are indicated. A decrease in the requirement for digitalis, caused by hypokalemia, may render the management of cardiac patients more difficult during their stay in a hot environment. (Recall that hypokalemia potentiates the action of digitalis on the heart.)

REFERENCES

1. **Leithead, C.,** and **Lind, A.:** Heat Stress and Heat Disorders. Philadelphia: F. A. Davis Co., 1964.
2. Ibid.
3. **Guyton, A.:** Textbook of Medical Physiology, ed. 5. Philadelphia: W. B. Saunders Co., 1976, p. 967.
4. **Leithead** and **Lind:** Heat Stress and Heat Disorders.
5. **Gauss, H.,** and **Meyer, K.:** Heat stroke: report of 158 cases from Cook County Hospital, Chicago. Am. J. Med. Sci. 154:554, 1917.
6. **Gardner, D.:** Potassium metabolism and potassium therapy. J.A.O.A. 66:257–270, 1966.
7. Ibid.
8. Ibid.

BIBLIOGRAPHY

Boedeker, E., and **Dauber, J.** (eds.): Manual of Medical Therapeutics, ed. 21. Boston: Little, Brown & Co., 1974.

Coburn, J. W., and **Reba, R.:** Potassium depletion in heat stroke: a possible etiological factor. Mil. Med. 131:678–687, 1966.

Knochel, J., and **Vertel, R.:** Hypothesis: salt-loading as possible factor in the production of potassium depletion, rhabdomyolysis and heat injury. Lancet 1:659–661, 1967.

Maxwell, M., and **Kleeman, C.:** Clinical Disorders of Fluid and Electrolyte Metabolism, ed. 2. New York: McGraw-Hill Book Co., 1972.

Schamadan, J., and **Snively, W.:** The role of potassium in diseases due to heat stress. Ind. Med. Surg. 36:785–788, 1967.

Toor, M. et al.: Potassium depletion in permanent inhabitants of hot areas. Israel J. Med. Sci. 3:149–151, 1967.

26

Fluid Balance in Pregnancy

Mystery still surrounds many of the body changes that occur during pregnancy. When these changes are physiologic in nature, they are not only beneficial, but, indeed, essential. Sometimes, however, what appears to be a physiologic change really represents the early stages of a pathologic change that can be harmful, even fatal. For example, diabetes mellitus may first appear as apparently physiologic glycosuria or polyuria; pathologic dilatation of the renal calyx, pelvis, and ureter with partial ureteral obstruction may first reveal itself as mere physiologic dilatation of these structures; pernicious vomiting of pregnancy may first be regarded as the ubiquitous but harmless vomiting of pregnancy. (These examples will be enlarged upon and others introduced later in the chapter.)

Among the various transformations in pregnancy, none is more important than the changes in body fluids. Even these, forthright though they appear, pose many unanswered questions. For example, in the nonpregnant woman or in the male, excessive water retention invariably is accompanied by excessive retention of sodium. Whether or not there is excessive sodium retention in pregnancy remains controversial; however, many, perhaps most, clinicians believe that pregnant women do retain excessive sodium. They, therefore, restrict sodium intake and may even prescribe diuretics. (Diuretic drugs appear to be overused in pregnancy. One authority reports the deaths of four patients from excessive use of diuretics; three of these died from electrolyte deple-

tion, and one from hemorrhagic pancreatitis.) Other physicians believe that pregnant women are sodium wasters; they add supplemental salt to the diet to avoid preeclampsia. Both the secretion and excretion of the sodium-conserving hormone, aldosterone, increase during normal pregnancy; however, the effect of this increase on sodium homeostasis is poorly understood. Were it not, perhaps we could explain the puzzling situation in preeclampsia, in which there is apparent sodium retention, even though aldosterone secretion actually decreases.

In this chapter, we first examine changes in body fluids during normal pregnancy. Knowledge of the normal pregnant state enables the nurse to recognize the borderline between a physiologic and a pathologic change. She will know, for example, what is a physiologic increase in hydration and what is a pathologic increase. Next, we look at disorders of pregnancy closely related to body fluid disturbances. Finally, we examine the effects of pregnancy on various other ailments characterized by disruption of the body fluids.

PHYSIOLOGIC CHANGES IN BODY FLUIDS DURING PREGNANCY

Water Content

At term, the fetus, placenta, and amniotic fluid contain about 3.5 L. of water. An additional 3 L. has accumulated because of increases in the mother's blood volume, in the size of her breasts, and in the mass of the uterus. The average woman, therefore, retains at least 6.5 L. of extra water in the extracellular compartment during a normal pregnancy. Such hydration of the maternal tissues is physiologic in nature, and the body's physiologic processes handle it with equanimity.

The increase in blood volume deserves comment: it averages from 40 to 45 per cent and results from increases in plasma volume and in red cell mass. Plasma volume increases 45 to 50 per cent, or about 1200 to 1400 ml., with the maximum reached two to six weeks before term. During the last weeks of pregnancy, the rate of increase in plasma volume declines. With delivery, plasma volume rapidly diminishes, so that, by the end of the first week postpartum, it has returned to the nonpregnant value. Red blood cell volume increases during pregnancy some 20 to 40 per cent, an addition of 300 to 500 ml. The proportionately greater increase in plasma than in red blood cells results in the "hemodilution of pregnancy." (The hemoglobin level may fall to 10.5 to 12 Gm. from the nonpregnant normal of 12 to 15 Gm.; the hematocrit may fall to 30 to 33 per cent from the nonpregnant normal of 35 to 45 per cent.) In addition, there occurs a 10 per cent increment in heart rate and as much as a 40 per cent increase in cardiac output, reaching its maximum at from 28 to 32 weeks, then decreasing to term. A natural accompaniment of these phenomena is a linear increase in the consumption of oxygen, peaking at term. Because of these factors, the pregnant woman with heart disease may be hard pressed to meet the strenuous demands imposed on her cardiovascular system.

FLUID RETENTION Now let us review known factors that produce fluid retention during pregnancy:

1. An increase in venous pressure elevates the effective intracapillary hydrostatic pressure. This results from two mechanisms: first, the pregnant uterus impinges against the inferior vena cava, thus causing increased back pressure; second, the vascular congestion of the pregnant pelvis also increases pressure on the vena cava. The increased venous pressure enhances filtration from the vascular bed and often produces physiologic dependent hydrostatic edema, to be differentiated from the edema of toxemia. When the woman lies on her side, the pressures against the

inferior vena cava are relieved, and the venous pressure is not elevated. Also, when the woman lies on her side, some or all of the accumulated fluid may be mobilized and excreted (thus explaining the observation that in late pregnancy the urinary volume at night approaches that excreted during the day).

2. Plasma albumin decreases by about 1 Gm./100 ml. of plasma. This reduction in the colloidal osmotic pressure of the plasma amounts to some 20 per cent; it favors plasma-to-interstitial fluid shift.

3. Capillaries become more permeable to water and electrolytes, but not to protein. This is revealed by the fact that the protein content of edema fluid is less than 0.4 Gm./100 ml. in pregnancy.

4. Still controversial is the question of whether excessive sodium is retained by the pregnant woman. Many obstetricians now believe that salt and water restriction in the normal pregnancy is not only unnecessary but also harmful. They would confine such restriction to those patients with a pathologic process.

5. A threefold increase in aldosterone secretion may occur. Increased production of steroid hormones causes increased sodium and water retention; however, the 50 per cent increase in the glomerular filtration rate during pregnancy tends to offset fluid retention so that the normal pregnant woman has only a moderate fluid excess.

How does one go about measuring the retention of water in pregnancy? Our must useful gauge is weight gain, but water retention is also revealed by pitting edema of the ankles and legs—especially at the day's end—due to mechanical obstruction by the enlarging uterus, elevated femoral venous pressure, and the gravity effect produced by the upright position. In fact, edema of the feet and ankles occurs in about 75 per cent of all late pregnancies, especially in the summer. This edema usually disappears overnight and should be regarded as a physiologic rather than as a pathologic phenomenon. Generalized edema may be tested for by finger swelling and tightening of finger rings. Its presence may be significant in the development of preeclampsia. However, one retrospective study showed that 20 per cent of otherwise normal pregnant women displayed some degree of generalized edema.

Management of ankle edema or of weight gain slightly exceeding that normally expected can usually be accomplished by lateral recumbency plus mild sodium restriction. If the physician employs severe sodium restriction, diuretics, or both, the patient is in danger of becoming sodium depleted, perhaps potassium depleted as well. Sodium depletion is particularly unfortunate. Not only is it dangerous per se, but its signs (including oliguria, decreased glomerular filtration rate, and increased plasma concentration of uric acid) imitate preeclampsia. This may cause further sodium restriction, leading to more severe sodium depletion.

Conservation of Carbohydrate and Protein

Both carbohydrate and protein are conserved during pregnancy—carbohydrate to meet energy requirements and protein to meet structural demands. The mother appears to retain enough nitrogen (the measure of protein) to provide for the growth of the reproductive system and the fetus and for the needs of milk production. This represents an average increase of 80 Gm. of total circulating plasma protein. Five hundred Gm. of protein—about half of the additional protein retained during pregnancy—are added to the maternal blood as hemoglobin and plasma proteins, to the uterus, and to the glandular tissue of the breasts. At term, the fetus plus the placenta weigh about 4 kg., containing 500 Gm. of protein—also about half of the increase in protein caused by pregnancy.

In regard to carbohydrate, the question is often asked, "Does pregnancy produce a diabetic effect?" Certainly increased thirst, increased appetite, polyuria, and glycosuria are not uncommon during pregnancy. But normal pregnancy occasions many variables, including elevated plasma insulin and increases in various hormones, such as growth, thyroid, and adrenal hormones. Apparently there is no interference either in the use or storage of carbohydrate, nor is there any resistance to insulin or obstruction in the glycolytic cycle. Nevertheless, the glucose tolerance test is modified, with a delay in the return of blood glucose levels to normal, when glucose is given orally. Thus, instead of the two hours it usually takes for blood glucose to return to normal in the nonpregnant patient, it takes about three hours in the pregnant. This phenomenon does not occur when glucose is given intravenously.

Acid-Base Balance

There is a decrease in the concentration of total base from about 155 mEq./L. before pregnancy to some 146 mEq./L. during pregnancy. Plasma sodium falls from 142 mEq./L. to 136 mEq./L., and plasma bicarbonate from 25 mEq./L. to 22 mEq./L. The mother can be considered as having a moderate respiratory alkalosis combined with metabolic acidosis. Respiratory alkalosis is the result of hyperventilation, presumably induced by increased progesterone levels. (Progesterone increases the respiratory center's sensitivity to carbon dioxide.) Loss of carbon dioxide from the blood is compensated for by renal loss of bicarbonate. With overbreathing induced by labor, the maternal CO_2 can fall below 17 mm. Hg, resulting in a delay in the initiation of respiration in the newborn infant.

Calcium Levels

Some 30 to 40 Gm. of calcium are deposited in the fetus, chiefly during the last trimester of pregnancy. Plasma calcium levels may decrease, probably because of an increase in extracellular fluid volume. The average present-day pregnancy diet, containing from 1.5 to 2.5 Gm. of calcium, appears quite adequate to supply the needs of mother and fetus without depletion of the maternal stores. Possibly because of the high phosphorus content of milk, some patients—especially heavy milk drinkers—may suffer an imbalance in the ratio of calcium to phosphorus in the plasma. (Recall that calcium and phosphorus are antagonistic. An increase in plasma phosphorus tends to decrease plasma calcium, and vice versa.) This imbalance in the calcium-phosphorus ratio may be responsible for the leg cramps that sometimes occur in pregnancy. Indeed, some clinicians have reported that the leg cramps can be relieved by reducing the milk intake and administering supplemental calcium.

PREGNANCY DISORDERS CLOSELY RELATED TO BODY FLUID DISTURBANCES

Toxemia of Pregnancy

The syndrome of toxemia of pregnancy has no known origin. Some theorize that toxemia is the result of autoimmunity or allergic reaction caused by the fetal presence. Lending credence to this theory is the fact that symptoms disappear within a few days after delivery. Toxemia can be divided into two types, depending upon the severity: *preeclampsia*, or toxemia without convulsions; and the extremely serious *eclampsia,* or toxemia with convulsions. Patients with underlying vascular or renal disease are not included under the diagnosis of toxemia of pregnancy; yet, they are often difficult to distinguish from patients with toxemia, especially during the last trimester.

Preeclampsia occurs in from 5 to 10 per cent of all pregnancies, usually after the 24th week of gestation. Eclampsia—which, fortunately, now is rare—used to develop in approximately 0.2 per cent of pregnancies. Preeclampsia occurs chiefly in primigravidas, especially in the very young or in older patients. Sisters and daughters of patients who have suffered from toxemia are prone to develop it. A twin pregnancy or hydramnios appears to predispose to it, as may preexisting hypertension. Once a patient has had toxemia, she is a likely candidate to develop it in future pregnancies. Other factors of questionable significance include obesity, separation of upper incisor teeth, and red hair. While the cause of toxemia remains unknown, abnormal sodium retention and generalized vasoconstriction explain the signs and symptoms.

Widespread vasoconstriction of arterioles affects the placental circulation, kidneys, and eye grounds. This vasoconstriction appears to be related to the increased blood pressure and may account for the visual problems experienced in severe eclampsia. Small degenerative infarcts appear in the placenta, apparently caused by vasoconstriction; the damaged placenta may separate prematurely or may fail to nourish the fetus adequately. A slight decrease in renal blood flow and glomerular filtration rate occurs in the toxemic patient. (Recall that in normal pregnancy, both the glomerular filtration rate and the renal blood flow increase.) In addition to the above changes, the toxemia patient develops fibrinoid deposits in the basement membrane of the glomerular tufts.

It appears incorrect to think that control of weight gain and limitation of sodium intake reduces the incidence of preeclampsia; this belief confuses cause and effect. Although preeclamptic patients retain water and sodium, weight gain does not cause preeclampsia. Certainly endocrine or metabolic disorders or both may be implicated in the genesis of the disease.

The signs of the onset of toxemia include edema, not only of the ankles but also of the hands and face; hypertension; and, in some patients, proteinuria. A significant rise in blood pressure consists of an increase of 30 mm. Hg or more in the systolic pressure and 15 mm. Hg or more in the diastolic. (Thus, a patient with a normal blood pressure of 90/60 could be in difficulty with a pressure of 120/75.)

Proteinuria becomes significant when it exceeds 0.3 Gm./L. A weight gain of more than five pounds per week or a blood pressure higher than 140/90 should cause one to consider early toxemia. (However, almost half of the patients in whom toxemia develops do not display excessive weight gain.) The blood pressure in preeclampsia or eclampsia rarely exceeds 190/115.

More advanced symptoms include generalized edema, headache, visual disturbances, abdominal pain, oliguria, nausea, and vomiting—a cluster of symptoms warning of the approach of eclampsia. With eclampsia, death can occur during a convulsion, or it can result from cerebral hemorrhage, congestive heart failure, or kidney shutdown. The fetus also may be seriously threatened, either by the toxemia or by the eclamptic convulsions. Should the pregnancy be terminated either therapeutically or naturally, symptoms of toxemia promptly disappear.

Autopsies on patients who died of eclampsia reveal hemorrhagic lesions in the placenta, liver, kidneys, heart, brain, spleen, adrenals, and pancreas. In addition, necrosis, tissue infarction, fibrin deposits, and evidence of disseminated intravascular coagulation may be found. Pallor of the kidney cortex may be observed, with little blood in the glomerular capillaries.

Even the suspicion of toxemia should be the signal for therapy. Sodium chloride should be restricted to less than 2000 mg. (about 1 Gm. sodium) daily. The diet should be adequate in protein. Should diuretics be given, care should be taken to avoid sodium or potassium depletion. In addition, sedation should be adequate. If the disease has lasted more than two or three weeks, or should it become severe (regardless of its duration), the patient should be hospitalized promptly so that vital signs can be closely monitored. If the symptoms progress, and especially if eclampsia develops, surgical termination of the pregnancy or induction of labor should be considered. The danger of convulsions is not over until three or four days after delivery.

Many physicians have found intravenous or intramuscular magnesium sulfate effective in relieving eclampsia. Various antihypertensive drugs have been employed. If the airway becomes obstructed because of convulsions or coma, tracheotomy may be required.

NURSING RESPONSIBILITIES The nurse should observe all maternity patients for signs of preeclampsia. Prompt recognition and treatment are necessary to prevent the condition from progressing to eclampsia.

The hospitalized preeclamptic patient should have a private room, free from bright lights and loud noises. Nursing care should be planned to provide regular uninterrupted rest periods. Vital signs should be checked at least every four hours. An accurate intake and output record must be kept and daily body weight measurement should be recorded. (See Chapter 13 for nursing responsibilities in these procedures.) An indwelling urinary catheter usually is inserted so that output can be monitored closely. The nurse must be especially alert to report a rise in blood pressure, hyperactive reflexes, a weight increase, or a low urinary output.

Should convulsions occur, placing a padded mouth gag between the back teeth will prevent biting of the tongue. A rubber airway may be used to assure an adequate airway. Suction apparatus may be necessary to prevent aspiration of secretions. Padded siderails should be used to prevent the convulsing or heavily sedated patient from falling or otherwise injuring herself. The duration and character of each convulsion should be noted, as well as the depth of coma that follows. Fetal heart tones should be checked as often as possible. The convulsing patient should be observed for signs of rapid labor; abruptio placentae and excessive bleeding may occur. It should be remembered that a heavily sedated patient may also have a rapid labor.

MAGNESIUM SULFATE Magnesium sulfate is indicated when proteinuria increases to 5 Gm. or more in 24 hours, BP increases to 160/110 mm. Hg or more, visual or cerebral disturbances occur, urine output decreases to 400 ml. or less in 24 hours, and hyperreflexia occurs despite conservative management.[1] Magnesium sulfate's purpose is to prevent or control convulsions by blocking neuromuscular transmission. It depresses the central nervous system and produces an initial hypotensive effect because of peripheral vasodilating effect. (Hypermagnesemia may cause flushing and a sensation of heat.) Some au-

thorities feel that the desired therapeutic plasma magnesium level in convulsion-prone toxemia patients is 2.5 to 7.5 mEq./L.[2] Others feel a magnesium level in plasma of 4.2 to 5.8 mEq./L. is the desired therapeutic range. Deep-tendon reflexes may be depressed when the plasma level exceeds 4 mEq./L.— the patellar reflex disappears when the plasma magnesium level reaches 8.3 to 10 mEq./L. Respiratory paralysis occurs when the concentration reaches 10 to 12.5 mEq./L., hence the importance of frequent checks on the patellar reflex.[3] Concentrations above 12 mEq./L. can cause ECG changes (prolonged PR interval and widened QRS complex); heart block and death may occur.

Magnesium sulfate is given I.V. or I.M. to toxemia patients since oral doses fail to produce satisfactory blood levels. The action of I.V. magnesium sulfate is immediate and lasts about 30 minutes; I.M. doses do not become effective until about one hour after administration and last about three to four hours.[4] Since intramuscular doses of magnesium sulfate are painful, they should be given deep in the upper outer quadrant of the buttocks. The injection site should be massaged well to encourage absorption; large doses should be equally divided between both buttocks.

After the initial dose of magnesium sulfate, *subsequent doses should be given only if:*

1. there is no respiratory depression—as a rule, the physician should be notified if the respiratory rate decreases below 12 to 14 per minute.
2. at least 120 ml. of urine has been excreted since the last dose was given—99 per cent of the magnesium administered parenterally is excreted by the kidneys. Oliguria leads to an accumulation of magnesium in the bloodstream. Report a urinary output below 30 ml./hr.
3. the patellar reflex is present—a poor to absent patellar reflex may be indicative of hypermagnesemia and should be reported to the physician.
4. The patient is oriented to person, place, and time—excessive CNS depression can cause drowsiness, lethargy, slurring of speech, and eventually coma.
5. there has been no significant drop in blood pressure or in the maternal or fetal heart rates.

To counteract possible magnesium toxicity, an ampule of 10 per cent calcium gluconate, with a 20 ml. syringe, should be kept at the bedside. Calcium is an antidote for magnesium excess since calcium and magnesium are mutually antagonistic. (Magnesium blocks release of acetycholine at the neural endplate; calcium counteracts this effect by increasing the release of acetycholine.) The intravenous administration of 5 to 10 mEq. of calcium usually reverses respiratory depression and heart block.[5] Equipment for respiratory resuscitation should be available for emergency use. Twenty grams of magnesium sulfate in 48 hours is the maximum dose if there is renal insufficiency.[6] Magnesium blood levels of 6 to 8 mEq./L. may reduce uterine contractions and prolong labor.[7]

Hyperemesis Gravidarum (Pernicious Vomiting of Pregnancy)

Half of all pregnant women become nauseated or vomit in the first trimester of pregnancy, but true pernicious vomiting of pregnancy has decreased greatly in recent years. The diagnosis of true pernicious vomiting of pregnancy applies only to those patients who have lost large amounts of weight and suffer severe body fluid disturbances, including extracellular fluid volume deficit, acid–base disturbances, and potassium deficit.

Pernicious vomiting of pregnancy frequently—perhaps usually—is brought about by psychic factors. In some instances, however, liver disease may be associated with it.

It has been suggested that the nausea may be due to the large quantity of estrogen secreted by the placenta. Some have postulated that it is related to high levels of chorionic gonadotropin; this substance peaks at the 10th week, much as does the vomiting of hyperemesis gravidarum. Others feel it may be related to decreased gastric motility and hypochlorhydria. Characteristically, the ailment starts as simple morning sickness, in which the typical patient feels nauseated when she awakens and may be unable to eat breakfast. By noon, however, her symptoms have disappeared, and she remains symptom-free until the next morning. Morning sickness usually subsides without treatment by the fourteenth to sixteenth week but, in some patients, morning sickness may develop into nausea and vomiting lasting throughout the day. This is called pernicious vomit-

ing or hyperemesis gravidarum, which usually appears during the fifth or sixth week of pregnancy. It can last a month or two or even longer, and produce a weight loss of 10 to 20 lb. or more. Ketonuria appears as a result of starvation. (Metabolic alkalosis rarely occurs, even when vomiting is severe, since most women in early pregnancy have hypochlorhydria or achlorhydria.)

The blood urea nitrogen and uric acid rise slightly. Plasma chloride and CO_2 combining power decrease. Plasma potassium is likely to decline. Urinary output falls, but the concentration of the urine rises.

An ominous complication of hyperemesis gravidarum is hemorrhagic retinitis. With its appearance, the mortality rate reaches 50 per cent.

The patient with pernicious vomiting should be hospitalized, isolated, and sedated. The use of antinauseant preparations deserves high priority in managing the condition, although some authorities minimize the use of drugs because of the danger of teratogenicity. (Pyridoxine apparently benefits some patients.) Some physicians use gastric suction to control vomiting, while others believe it makes the condition worse. Along with therapy to control vomiting, the physician should take immediate steps to correct body fluid disturbances. Repeated ophthalmoscopic examinations should be performed to detect early retinitis. Should hemorrhagic retinitis appear, the pregnancy should be promptly terminated.

NURSING RESPONSIBILITIES The pregnant woman with severe vomiting requires hospitalization for intravenous therapy. Usually all food and fluids are withheld during the first 24 hours to permit the gastrointestinal tract to rest. Electrolyte and glucose solutions are administered intravenously, in amounts of 3 L. or more in 24 hours. An accurate record of fluid intake and output should be kept.

Rest is of primary importance. Visitors should not be permitted during the first day or so. Because psychic factors play a large role in this condition, the patient should be encouraged to verbalize her feelings. Psychologic counseling usually is instituted.

When tolerated, small dry feedings (such as toast or crackers) are alternated with small amounts of liquids. Usually, hot tea or cold gingerale are better tolerated than water; lukewarm liquids are not well accepted. Food intake is gradually increased to a full diet. Trays should be prepared carefully; portions should be small and served attractively. Unpleasant odors or sights should be avoided because the slightest stimuli can initiate nausea and vomiting. Occasionally, tube feedings may be necessary if the patient is unable to eat; the tube feeding mixture must be introduced very slowly to avoid nausea. (Nursing responsibilities in tube feeding are discussed in Chapter 14.)

Water Intoxication

Chesley states: "Probably the only feature of pregnancy that predisposes the patient to water intoxication is her exposure to physicians."[8] Obstetricians tend to avoid the use of sodium-containing solutions for pregnant women, often preferring dextrose and water solutions. For example: induction of labor is sometimes instituted by adding oxytocin to a liter of 5 per cent dextrose in water; failure of the uterus to respond is often countered by speeding the infusion rate rather than increasing the concentration of oxytocin. The problem is compounded when the patient lies on her back during the infusion; recall that the supine position in late pregnancy inhibits urinary output. Also, the pharmacologic action of oxytocin includes an antidiuretic effect, causing increased water retention. Symptoms of water intoxication (hyponatremia) include behavior changes, headache, blurred vision, nausea, vomiting, and convulsions. One case was reported in which a primigravida developed a convulsion during delivery, after receiving 4.5 l. of 5 per cent dextrose in water with oxytocin within a 3½ hour period.

The nurse should carefully monitor the amount of oxytocin and dextrose/water solution given to each patient. She should be alert for, and quickly report to the physician, signs of water intoxication. It is wise to monitor plasma sodium levels during treatment with oxytocin, particularly when it is administered in dextrose/water solutions.

PREGNANCY EFFECTS ON CERTAIN AILMENTS WITH BODY FLUID DISRUPTION

Renal Disease

The gross and microscopic structure of the kidneys of pregnant and nonpregnant women do not differ significantly; however, both the interstitial space and renal blood volume increase during pregnancy. Dilatation of the calyx, pelvis, and ureter may appear as early as the second trimester, especially on the right. X-ray studies have attested to increased kidney size.

While the above changes are physiologic in nature, they may favor overt disease. Thus, by the third trimester, the alterations combined with the woman's supine or upright posture can cause partial ureteral obstruction, and the resulting ureteral dilation can pose problems. For example, since the dilated collecting system may contain large volumes of urine, serious errors may occur in the measurement of timed urinary output of estriol, creatinine, and protein. The misreadings can be avoided if the pregnant woman is given water loads and is kept in bed, positioned in lateral recumbency, for an hour before starting and finishing urine collections.

Perhaps of greater significance, urinary dilatation and stasis may cause asymptomatic bacteriuria to progress to frank pyelonephritis. If the woman already has chronic pyelonephritis, she may regress. Such women should be restricted in their upright activity, and frequent rest periods in the lateral recumbent position should be prescribed.

Some patients whose urine is sterile at the start of pregnancy develop positive urine cultures as the pregnancy progresses. Favoring susceptibility to urinary tract infection are extracellular fluid volume deficit and loss of potassium caused by prolonged vomiting. Glycosuria, added to ureteral dilatation and stasis, provides an ideal environment for bacterial multiplication. Pregnant women with confirmed positive urine cultures should receive treatment, even though they have no symptoms.

Apparent deterioration of kidney function in pregnant patients with preexisting kidney disease can be traced to extracellular fluid volume deficit and decreased renal perfusion resulting from strict sodium restriction or administration of diuretics. Nevertheless, patients with chronic renal disease who become pregnant retain sodium abnormally. A diet restricted to 1 Gm. of sodium daily for these patients appears reasonable. Should the pregnant woman with renal disease develop azotemia, abortion should be considered because of the ominous nature of the situation.

Most women with a mild degree of functional renal impairment can complete their pregnancies, but with progression of kidney disease, the ability to sustain a viable pregnancy to term diminishes. Even so, women with severe renal impairment have completed their pregnancies with the aid of hemodialysis.

Certain complications of pregnancy (such as severe toxemia; hemorrhagic shock from abruptio placentae, placenta previa, rupture of ectopic pregnancy, or uterine rupture; and septic shock of abortion) can predispose to acute renal failure. In fact, patients from obstetric services may comprise a sizable fraction of the patients treated for acute renal failure. (Care of patients with renal failure is described in Chapter 20.)

Heart Disease

As mentioned earlier, there is a 10 per cent increment in heart rate and a 40 per cent increase in cardiac output during pregnancy. Thus, women with cardiac impairment have an increased risk of decompensation during pregnancy. The diagnosis of heart disorders during pregnancy poses problems; systolic functional murmurs, distention of veins, tachycardia, and distortions of the chest x-ray can be caused by the pregnancy per se rather than by heart disease.

Enormously helpful in managing and making a prognosis of the course of the patient with heart disease is the New York Heart Associations's Functional Status Classification:

Class 1. Ordinary activity produces no fatigue.
Class 2. Ordinary activity produces some fatigue and some signs of cardiac insufficiency.
Class 3. Physical activity is greatly limited, but patients are comfortable at rest. Extraordinary activity leads to dyspnea, palpitation, even angina.
Class 4. Symptoms of cardiac insufficiency are present at rest.

Approximately 80 per cent of pregnant women with heart disease belong to the first two groups and tolerate pregnancy with minimal trouble.

Should the woman show an abnormality of cardiac rhythm or evidence of pulmonary congestion, she should be hospitalized at bedrest. Certain crucial periods demand digitalization—from the twenty-eighth to the thirty-fourth week, during labor, and exactly at postpartum. It is at these times when the heart is placed under the heaviest load.

Most deaths from congestive heart failure in pregnancy occur in patients in Classes 3 and 4. Those in Class 3 require digitalis plus bed rest, beginning the twenty-eighth week. Therapeutic abortion should be considered for patients in Class 4.

The pregnant patient with heart disease deserves special attention during labor, particularly in respect to the use of antibiotics, anesthetics, and the method of delivery. Voluntary bearing down should be avoided. Immediately following delivery, heart failure can result from the rapid redistribution of fluids, with an increase in the volume of circulating blood, even in cardiac patients who had an uneventful pregnancy and delivery. Not only the mother, but the fetus as well, is endangered by maternal heart disease. It may die during maternal congestive heart failure or because of prematurity.

Diabetes Mellitus

From 0.2 to 0.3 per cent of pregnant women have diabetes mellitus, which may either be so mild as to require no special diet or so severe as to demand complex therapy.

The potentially damaging effects of diabetes during pregnancy are many. (Certainly it increases the risk of intrauterine fetal death.) Should the patient have had unexplained stillbirths, should the urine have been positive for glucose during pregnancy, or should the infant weigh 9 lb. or more, a glucose tolerance test should be done. A fasting blood sugar over 130 mg./100 ml. or a blood sugar higher than 170 mg./100 ml. at any time during a glucose tolerance test raises a strong suspicion of diabetes.

The pregnant patient with poorly controlled diabetes has an increased tendency to develop metabolic acidosis because of extensive production of ketone bodies; such ketoacidosis is poorly tolerated by the fetus. One should bear in mind that even the non-diabetic pregnant patient has a low renal threshold for glucose, especially in the third trimester, and may show glycosuria. This is because the increase in glomerular filtration rate that occurs in pregnancy presents more of a sugar load per unit time; the tubular reabsorption, on the other hand, is not increased. Tubular urine, therefore, contains greater amounts of glucose than normal. As a result, glycosuria occurs, even though the blood glucose may be normal.

Pregnancy changes the insulin requirement for the diabetic patient. Hypoglycemic episodes can occur during early pregnancy, and most pregnant patients with diabetes need increased insulin as they approach term. Insulin dosage is best gauged by periodic blood sugar measurements and determination of ketones in the urine rather than by urinary glucose.

Renal disease must always be considered in the diabetic patient. Kidney failure is signalled by retinopathy, elevated blood pressure, proteinuria, and edema before the 25th week of gestation. Should azotemia appear, termination of the pregnancy and sterilization of the patient is usually indicated.

The incidence of hydramnios, with the amniotic fluid exceeding 2000 ml., may be seen in as many as 20 per cent of pregnant diabetics. In order to prevent or minimize this phenomenon, Priscilla White, famed specialist in diabetes at the Joslyn Clinic in Boston, recommends restriction of sodium to 1500 mg. daily. In addition, she employs potent diuretics. Such a program has reduced the degree of hydramnios so that early rupture of the membranes simply does not occur. When patients present with hydramnios, management is difficult.

Pregnant diabetic patients suffer a mortality rate of about 0.7 per cent; death usually occurs because of a cerebrovascular accident, toxemia, or diabetic coma. For diabetic patients who have been carefully controlled, the perinatal fetal mortality rate is between 2 and 15 per cent. Many deaths occur in utero between the 36th week and term.

Frequently pregnancy is terminated in the pregnant diabetic between the 36th and 37th week, balancing the hazard of fetal deterioration against loss of the fetus from prematurity. Maternal 24-hour urinary estriol measurements provide direct physiologic information on the fetal-placental status as the pregnancy progresses. When the values are rising, danger to the fetus is minimal. Provided the mother is progressing well, delivery can be delayed until the gestational age guarantees adequate maturity. However, if two successive decreases in estriol levels are found, or if the mother deteriorates, the pregnancy should be terminated. Serial estriol determinations should be started by the 30th week and obtained at least three times a week beginning at the thirty-fourth week.

Regardless of the gestational age and birth weight of the infant of the diabetic mother, he should be treated as if he were premature. He will suffer from respiratory and circulatory problems, from excessive bilirubin retention, from difficulty in temperature regulation, and from disordered glucose and calcium levels of plasma. The newborn of the diabetic mother may suffer from hypoglycemia. This is especially likely to occur after cesarean section, during which the mother has been given an infusion of dextrose solution to prepare her for surgery. When the infant is presented with a high glucose level because of the intravenous infusion, he responds by secreting large quantities of insulin. With the withdrawal of dextrose after the cord is clamped, the following occurs: the baby continues to secrete high levels of insulin; hypoglycemia develops; blood sugar may drop to as low as 0 (instances of irreversible hypoglycemic reactions have been reported). Because of these considerations, glucose should be given to the newborn early. Oral feedings should be started as soon as possible, even though the baby is clinically premature. Such neonatal problems demand expert pediatric management.

REFERENCES

1. **Butts, P.:** Magnesium sulfate in the treatment of toxemia. Am. J. Nurs. 77: August 1977, p. 1294.

2. Ibid., p. 1295.

3. **Maxwell, M.,** and **Kleeman, C.** (eds.): Clinical Disorders of Fluid and Electrolyte Metabolism, ed. 2. New York: McGraw-Hill Book Co., 1972, p. 1018.

4. **Butts:** Magnesium sulfate, p. 1295.

5. Ibid., p. 1297.

6. **Gahart, B.:** Intravenous Medications, ed. 2. St. Louis: C. V. Mosby Co., 1977, p. 116.

7. **Butts:** Magnesium sulfate, p. 1297.

8. **Maxwell** and **Kleeman:** Clinical Disorders, p. 1009.

BIBLIOGRAPHY

Dickason, E.: Maternal and Infant Care. New York: McGraw-Hill Book Co., 1975.

Guthrie, D., and **Guthrie, R.** (eds.): Nursing Management of Diabetes Mellitus. St. Louis: C. V. Mosby Co., 1977.

Guyton, A.: Textbook of Medical Physiology, ed. 5. Philadelphia: W. B. Saunders Co., 1976.

Reeder, S., et al.: Maternity Nursing, ed. 13. Philadelphia: J. B. Lippincott Co., 1976.

— 27 —

Fluid Balance Disturbances in Infants and Children

Water and electrolyte disturbances occur more frequently in children than in adults. Although one recognizes and manages fluid imbalances in children in much the same way he does in adults, there are also important differences. The younger the child, the more pronounced are the differences. The nurse should understand the peculiar problems posed by the child with a body fluid disturbance, so that she can make meaningful observations and can cooperate intelligently in his care.

An obvious and important difference between small children and adults is size. Yet, children are *not* merely miniature adults, for the child's body composition and homeostatic controls differ from those of the adult. It is helpful to compare the child's body composition with that of the adult and to review the salient characteristics of the child's homeostatic and metabolic functioning.

DIFFERENCES IN WATER AND ELECTROLYTE BALANCE IN INFANTS, CHILDREN, AND ADULTS

BODY WATER CONTENT   The premature infant's body is approximately 90 per cent water; the newborn infant's body, 70 to 80 per cent; the adult's body

about 60 per cent. The infant has proportionately more water in the extracellular compartment than does the adult. For example, 40 per cent of the newborn infant's body water may be in the extracellular compartment, as compared to less than 20 per cent in the case of the adult.

As the infant becomes older, his total body water percentage decreases, possibly a result of progressive growth of cells at the expense of the extracellular fluid. The decrease is particularly rapid during the first few days of life, but continues throughout the first six months. After the first year, the total body water is about 64 per cent (34 per cent in the cellular compartment, and 30 per cent in the extracellular compartment). By the end of the second year, the total body water approaches the adult percentage of approximately 60 per cent (36 per cent in the cellular compartment, and 24 per cent in the extracellular compartment). At puberty, the adult body water composition is attained. For the first time, there is a sex differentiation: females have slightly less water because they have a higher percentage of body fat.

DAILY BODY WATER TURNOVER IN INFANTS AND ADULTS   The infant's relatively greater total body water content does not always protect him from excessive fluid loss. On the contrary, the infant is more vulnerable to fluid volume deficit than is the adult, because he ingests and excretes a relatively greater daily water volume. An infant may exchange half of his extracellular fluid daily, while the adult may exchange only one sixth of his in the same period. Proportionately, therefore, the infant has less reserve of body fluid than does the adult.

The daily fluid exchange is relatively greater in infants, in part because their metabolic rate is two times higher per unit of weight than that of adults. Owing to the high metabolic rate, the infant has a large amount of metabolic wastes to excrete. Because water is needed by the kidneys to excrete these wastes, a large urinary volume is formed each day. Contributing to this volume is the inability of the infant's immature kidneys to concentrate urine efficiently. In addition, relatively greater fluid loss occurs through the infant's skin because of his proportionately greater body surface. The premature has approximately five times as much body surface area in relation to weight, and the newborn, three times, as do the older child and adult. Therefore, any condition causing a pronounced decrease in intake or increase in output of water and electrolytes threatens the body fluid economy of the infant. According to Gamble, an infant can live only three to four days without water, while an adult may live ten days.

ELECTROLYTE CONCENTRATIONS AND METABOLIC ACID FORMATION

Plasma electrolyte concentrations do not vary strikingly between infants, small children, and adults. The plasma sodium concentration changes little from birth to adulthood. Potassium concentration is higher in the first few months of life than at any other time, as is the plasma chloride concentration. Magnesium and calcium are both low in the first 24 hours after birth. The serum phosphorus level is higher in infants and children than in adults. The newborn's and the child's bicarbonate levels are lower than the adult's (Table 27-1). Inability of the premature infant to regulate its calcium ion concentration can bring on hypocalcemic tetany.

Because the infant's metabolic rate is high, the rate of metabolic acid formation is also high. Thus, the infant has a tendency toward metabolic acidosis. Buffer systems are not as efficient in the newborn as they are in older infants and children. A full-term newborn infant is slightly acidotic at birth; however, the pH usually is normal by the second day of life. The premature infant is even more acidotic and may remain so for a few weeks. Because cow's milk has higher phosphate and sulfate concentrations than breast milk, newborns fed cow's milk have a lower pH than do breastfed babies.

KIDNEY FUNCTION The newborn's renal function is not yet completely developed. Thus, if infant and adult renal functions are compared on the basis of total body water, the infant's kidneys appear to become mature by the end of the first month of life. However, if body surface area is used as the criterion for comparison, the child's kidneys appear immature for the first two years of life. Since the infant's kidneys have a limited concentrating ability and require more water to excrete a given amount of solute, he has difficulty in conserving body water when it is needed. Also, he may be unable to excrete an excess fluid volume.

Table 27-1. Comparison of "Average" Blood (Serum or Plasma) Electrolyte Values (mEq./L.) at Different Ages Under Varying Conditions

Electrolyte	Prematures "Acidotic"	"Well"	First Week	Newborns On Breast Milk	On Cow's Milk	Child 5–20 yrs.	Adults Young	Over 70
Sodium	..	..	146	..	..	144	142	144
Potassium	..	6.1	5.8	..	..	4.3	4.5	4.6
Calcium	..	..	4.9	..	..	4.9	4.9	5.2
Chloride	102.6	106	107	107.7	108	103	103	105
Phosphorus	4.2	4.1	4.2	..	..	2.8	2.0	1.7
Organic Acids	20.9	17.8	6	..	..	6	5	..
Bicarbonate (CO_2 combining power)	12.1	16.8	22.1	22.3	20.2	23	26.3	25
CO_2 Content	..	20	23.4	23.6	21.4	24.5	27.6	..

Adapted from Weisberg, H.: Water, Electrolyte and Acid-Base Balance, ed. 2. Baltimore: Williams & Wilkins, 1962, p. 334.

BODY SURFACE AREA The infant's relatively greater body surface area is present until the child is two or three years old. The skin represents an important route of fluid loss, especially in illness. Since the gastrointestinal membranes are essentially an extension of the body surface area, their area is also relatively greater in the young infant than in the older child and the adult. Hence, relatively greater losses occur from the gastrointestinal tract in the sick infant than in the older child and adult. In comparing fluid losses in infants to those in adults, one might regard the baby as a smaller vessel with a larger spout.

WATER REQUIREMENTS Regardless of age, all normal individuals require approximately 100 ml. of water per 100 calories metabolized. Since infants and children have higher metabolic rates than adults, they need proportionately more water. For example, an infant expends 100 calories per kg. of body weight and an adult only 38 calories. An infant needs 100 ml. of water per kg., while the adult requires only 38. Water needs for various age groups are listed in Table 27-2.

ELECTROLYTE DISTURBANCES IN CHILDREN

Sodium Imbalances

HYPONATREMIA Recall that the normal concentration of plasma sodium ranges from 137 to 147 mEq./L. (normals may vary slightly from laboratory to laboratory). Mild hyponatremia is present when the sodium level drops to 120 to 130 mEq./L.; moderate hyponatremia with a level of 114 to 120; and severe hyponatremia with a level below 114 mEq./L. This imbalance may result from excessive loss of sodium, as occurs in gastroenteritis and renal salt-losing states. Treatment consists of oral or intravenous sodium replacement.

Hyponatremia may also result from water overloading. This situation can be caused by over-administration of electrolyte-free parenteral fluids to the pediatric patient, particularly when impaired renal function exists. Another cause is inappropriate antidiuretic hormone (ADH) secretion; recall that ADH is the water-conserving hormone. Over-secretion of ADH may result from meningitis, hydrocephalus, head injuries, pneumonia, and bronchogenic neoplasms. Certain medications, such as mor-

Table 27-2. Mean Ranges of Daily Water Requirements of Infants and Children at Different Ages Under Normal Conditions

Age	Average Body Weight (kg.)	Total H_2O Requirements per 24 Hours (ml.)	H_2O Requirements per kg. in 24 Hours (ml.)
3 days	3.0	250–300	80–100
10 days	3.2	400–500	125–150
3 months	5.4	750–850	140–160
6 months	7.3	950–1100	130–135
9 months	8.6	1100–1250	125–145
1 year	9.5	1150–1300	120–135
2 years	11.8	1350–1500	115–125
4 years	16.2	1600–1800	100–110
6 years	20.0	1800–2000	90–100
10 years	28.7	2000–2500	70–85
14 years	45.0	2200–2700	50–60
18 yeras	54.0	2200–2700	40–50

Reprinted from Nelson, W. E.: Nelson's Textbook of Pediatrics, ed. 5. Philadelphia: W. B. Saunders Co., 1969, p. 128, with permission.

phine or barbiturates, as well as the presence of extreme stress, may occasionally trigger inappropriate ADH secretion. A rapid fall in the plasma sodium level to below 120 mEq./L. may cause confusion, headache, twitching, and convulsions. A slow decrease causes milder symptoms such as anorexia, nausea, and vomiting. Treatment usually consists of merely limiting the water intake until the kidneys can correct the condition; however, the presence of severe CNS symptoms may require the cautious parenteral administration of hypertonic sodium chloride solution.

HYPERNATREMIA Hypernatremia may result from decreased intake or increased output of water or from increased intake or decreased output of sodium. Infants, very young children, and unconscious or retarded patients are unable to communicate thirst; therefore, they may develop hypernatremia, particularly if excessive water losses are sustained (as in prolonged fever, tracheobronchitis, and diabetes insipidus). Hydrocephalus or other neurologic conditions may disrupt the thirst center in the hypothalamus, causing inadequate water intake.

The accidental substitution of salt (sodium chloride) for sugar in formula preparation results in a disastrously high sodium intake. (Widespread use of commercially prepared formulas has decreased the likelihood of this problem.) A grossly hypertonic formula causes the infant to cry; if his cry is interpreted as indicating hunger, more of the hypertonic formula is given and the condition worsens. Symptoms accompanying the excessive ingestion of sodium include these:

dry, sticky mucous membranes
avid thirst
irritability when disturbed (otherwise lethargy)
tremors and convulsions
nuchal rigidity
muscle rigidity
elevation of protein and chloride concentrations
    of the spinal fluid
expansion of the extracellular fluid
visible edema
brain damage in some patients

(Hypertonic dehydration [fluid volume deficit with sodium excess] caused by severe watery diarrhea is discussed later in this chapter.)

High protein tube feedings, plus inadequate water intake, can produce hypernatremia regardless of whether or not the feeding solution contains an excessive amount of salt. High solute feedings act as osmotic diuretics and "pull" water out of the body, particularly in infants because of their immature renal function. (See the section on tube feedings later in this chapter.)

Potassium Imbalances

HYPOKALEMIA   Recall that the normal plasma potassium level ranges from 4.0 to 5.6 (normals vary slightly from laboratory to laboratory). Excessive loss of potassium-rich body fluids, such as occurs in vomiting and diarrhea, results in hypokalemia. Other causes include use of potassium-losing diuretics and adrenocorticosteroids, excessive sweating, familial periodic paralysis, and aldosterone-secreting tumors of the adrenal cortex. Potassium depletion is often associated with metabolic alkalosis.

Symptoms include apathy, abdominal distention, and muscular weakness; severe hypokalemia causes flaccid paralysis and cardiac arrhythmias. (ECG changes evoked by hypokalemia are described in Chapter 21.)

Hypokalemia is treated by potassium replacement, either orally or intravenously. Potassium-rich fruit juices include orange, tomato, prune, grapefruit, and pineapple. (See Table 14-4 for precise potassium content of various foods.) As always, great care should be exercised when potassium is administered intravenously. The concentration of potassium should not exceed 20 to 40 mEq./L.; the suitably diluted solution should be given at the precise prescribed rate. A microdrip and volume-controlled pediatric set should be used to limit the chance of accidental excessive fluid administration. (Pediatric sets are described later in this chapter.) The normal potassium requirements are approximately 2 mEq./kg./24 hr., or 50 mEq./m²/24 hr. As a rule, no more than 4 mEq./kg. of potassium should be given daily to correct hypokalemia, unless a severe deficit is present. Potassium solutions should not be administered to anuric or oliguric children since dangerous hyperkalemia can result. Suitably diluted potassium solutions should be administered evenly over the 24-hour period; they should never be given undiluted or by I.V. push. (Excessive or too rapid administration of potassium can cause cardiac arrest.)

HYPERKALEMIA   Hyperkalemia may be caused by renal failure, hemolysis, Addison's disease, and excessive, or too rapid, administration of potassium solutions. Symptoms may include muscle weakness, paresthesia, and flaccid paralysis. Cardiac changes are the principal manifestations of hyperkalemia and may prove lethal. (These changes are described in Chapter 21.) Emergency measures to alleviate toxic effects of potassium on the myocardium may include the intravenous administration of:

1. Calcium gluconate 10 per cent, 0.5 ml./kg., over a 5 to 10 min. period with ECG monitoring (too rapid administration of calcium can cause cardiac arrest)
2. Sodium bicarbonate, 2.5 mEq./kg., over 30 to 60 min.
3. Regular insulin, 0.5U/kg., may be given I.V. while infusing a 20% dextrose solution

Calcium relieves the cardiotoxic effects of hyperkalemia, temporarily, without actually decreasing the plasma potassium level. Sodium bicarbonate alkalinizes plasma and drives potassium into the cells.

Dextrose and insulin cause potassium to enter the cells by the process of glycogen formation.

Calcium Imbalances

HYPOCALCEMIA   Recall that the normal concentration of calcium in plasma ranges from 4.5 to 5.8 mEq./L. (normals may vary slightly from laboratory to laboratory). Hypocalcemia may occur in the pediatric patient for a variety of reasons. It is more apt to occur following abnormal pregnancies for reasons that are not clear; sometimes it occurs in the presence of other diseases or may be an isolated finding. Transient hypoparathyroidism, with hypocalcemia, may occur in the offspring of hyperparathyroid or diabetic mothers.

Prolonged hypocalcemia may produce a variety of symptoms in the young child. Symptoms include numbness, twitching, cramps, carpopedal spasm (see Fig. 13-6), positive Chvostek's sign, laryngospasm, positive peroneal sign (tapping the peroneal nerve over the fibular side of the leg produces abduction and dorsiflexion of the foot), irritability, convulsions, and retarded physical and mental growth. Other symptoms of prolonged hypocalcemia may include poor dentition, photophobia, conjunctivitis, and cataracts.

A disorder called "tetany of the newborn," occurring in the third or fourth week of life, is sometimes seen in infants fed a milk formula with a high phosphorus/calcium ratio. A liter of cow's milk contains approximately 1220 mg. of calcium and 900 mg. of phosphorus (a ratio of 1.35 to 1); a liter of human milk contains approximately 342 mg. of calcium and 150 mg. of phosphorus (a ratio of 2.25 to 1).[1] High phosphorus intake from large quantities of cow's milk tends to raise the phosphorus concentration in the bloodstream and, thus, to lower the calcium level. (Recall that a reciprocal relationship exists between calcium and phosphorus; a rise in one causes a decrease in the other.) It is not known why only a few babies fed cow's milk are subject to this disorder; possible reasons include immature renal function and relative hypoparathyroidism. Treatment includes lowering the solute and phosphorus loads in the formula and providing extra calcium.

Babies with low serum calcium levels usually are symptom-free; however, twitching or frank convulsions may occur. Calcium can be replaced either orally, as calcium lactate or gluconate, or intravenously. The intravenous route is used only for severe hypocalcemia since it can cause serious cardiac problems. A suitably diluted calcium preparation is infused slowly while the heart rate is being monitored; bradycardia is a sign to stop the infusion immediately. (Recall that cardiac slowing and arrest can result from rapid administration of calcium intravenously.) Calcium salts should not be added to a solution containing sodium bicarbonate since an insoluble precipitate (calcium carbonate) will form.

HYPERCALCEMIA   A brief period of hypercalcemia may cause abdominal pain, nausea, and vomiting; prolonged hypercalcemia may cause precipitation of calcium stones in the renal system. Primary hyperparathyroidism causes calcium excess but is uncommon in children.

A rare condition known as idiopathic hypercalcemia may occur in children. Although its cause is unknown, some believe it might be due to increased intake of vitamin D during pregnancy, abnormal sterol synthesis, or a defect in vitamin D metabolism. Idiopathic hypercalcemia sometimes occurs in a severe form characterized by elfin facies, prominent lips and eyes, hanging jowls, large low-set ears, motor and mental retardation, hypotonia, polyuria, polydipsia, and cardiac defects.[2] Milder forms have a favorable prognosis, but severe forms may be fatal. Treatment consists of limiting dietary calcium and vitamin D intake; if necessary, adrenocorticosteroids may be used to interfere with calcium absorption from the gut.

Magnesium Imbalances

HYPOMAGNESEMIA   Recall that the normal plasma magnesium concentration is 1.4 to 2.3 mEq./L. Hypomagnesemia may be seen in the newborn as a familial condition or with hypoparathyroidism. It may also be a problem in artificially-fed neonates. Symptoms may include positive Chvostek's sign, irritability, tremors, and, especially in the newborn, convulsions.

Magnesium deficiency simulates calcium deficiency. Magnesium sulfate may be administered either orally or parenterally as indicated to correct hypomagnesemia.

HYPERMAGNESEMIA   Hypermagnesemia may be seen rarely in the newborn after the mother has received magnesium sulfate. It is particularly apt to occur when the mother received frequent and repetitive doses of magnesium sulfate before delivery. It may also be seen in children in renal failure. (Recall that magnesium is normally excreted by the kidneys; renal failure causes magnesium buildup in the bloodstream.)

Symptoms of hypermagnesemia do not usually appear until the magnesium concentration in the plasma exceeds 4 mEq./L.; drowsiness and hypotension may be early signs. Loss of deep-tendon reflexes can occur when the plasma magnesium concentration is greater than 7 mEq./L.; respiratory failure and heart block can occur when the concentration exceeds 10 mEq./L. The newborn with hypermagnesemia has a weak or absent cry. Usually, treatment of hypermagnesemia is not necessary unless the plasma level exceeds 7 mEq./L.; in this case, dialysis may be indicated.

pH Disturbances

RESPIRATORY ALKALOSIS Respiratory alkalosis may occur in pediatric patients as a result of hysterical hyperventilation, salicylate intoxication, and abnormal irritability of the respiratory center caused by encephalitis or meningitis. Symptoms may include circumoral paresthesia, dizziness, palpitations, chest discomfort, and convulsions secondary to hypocalcemia (recall that calcium ionizes poorly in alkalosis). The patient's respirations are increased, causing excessive loss of carbon dioxide (the primary disturbance). In respiratory alkalosis, the increased respirations are the *cause* of the imbalance. Plasma pH is elevated (may be above 7.6) and the pCO_2 is decreased (sometimes as low as 10 mm. Hg). Treatment depends on the condition causing respiratory alkalosis. The hysteric hyperventilating child may be treated by rebreathing into a bag and by the administration of tranquilizers; psychologic help may also be indicated. (Salicylate intoxication treatment is described later in the chapter.)

RESPIRATORY ACIDOSIS Chronic respiratory acidosis may occur in cystic fibrosis, advanced muscular dystrophy, asthma, rickets, and bulbar poliomyelitis. The patient may be dyspneic, confused, and uncooperative. Plasma pH is slightly below normal and the pCO_2 is elevated as a result of hypoventilation. The base excess is above normal owing to renal conservation of bicarbonate to compensate for the excess carbonic acid concentration in the blood.

Acute respiratory acidosis may result from upper airway obstruction (croup or aspiration of a foreign body), hyaline membrane disease, respiratory failure, or cardiac arrest. Acute air hunger is present and the child often appears cyanotic. A severe drop in plasma pH (may be as low as 7.0) occurs along with an elevated pCO_2. Treatment depends on the underlying cause; therapy is always directed at improving ventilation. If possible, correction of an obstruction is done; artificial ventilation is used as indicated. A sodium bicarbonate solution may be administered slowly I.V. as needed to correct severe acidemia.

Respiratory distress syndrome occurs in some immature infants because of a deficiency of surface active agents, causing inadequate alveolar expansion.[3] The decreased functional lung surface area leads to a decreased pO_2, an elevated pCO_2, and a decreased pH (respiratory acidosis). Hypoxia follows and leads to metabolic acidosis as a result of excessive lactic acid formation. Acidosis causes increased pulmonary artery resistance and diminished pulmonary blood flow. Frequent arterial blood gas studies are necessary to assess the infant's condition; blood may be obtained via a catheter in the umbilical artery or from puncture of the radial, temporal, or brachial arteries. Symptoms of respiratory distress syndrome include expiratory grunting, retractions of the chest wall, rapid seesaw respirations, and cyanosis. Therapy is directed at supporting ventilation until the infant matures enough to produce surface active agents. The infant is placed in an Isolette and is given enough oxygen to keep the arterial pO_2 at a level of 50 to 70 mm. Hg; an endotracheal tube and positive pressure ventilation may be necessary if difficulty is encountered in elevating the pO_2 to the minimal level. High concentrations of oxygen must be used cautiously since they may cause retrolental fibroplasia or pulmonary oxygen toxicity; the goal of oxygen therapy is to keep the arterial pO_2 between 50 to 70 mm. Hg (it should never exceed 100 mm. Hg). A pCO_2 higher than 70 mm. Hg may necessitate use of a respirator. An arterial pH of less than 7.25 compromises pulmonary blood flow and may be treated with an alkalinizing agent, such as sodium bicarbonate.

METABOLIC ALKALOSIS Metabolic alkalosis results when the plasma bicarbonate level rises and the pH increases. A frequent cause of metabolic alkalosis is loss of gastric juice from nasogastric suction or from vomiting. This imbalance is particularly likely to occur in pyloric stenosis since only gastric juice is lost. The lungs attempt to compensate for metabolic alkalosis by conserving carbon dioxide (hypoventilation); however, this form of compensation is limited by oxygen need. Treatment of this imbalance consists of surgical correction of the stenosed pylorus and administration of chloride-containing solutions and potassium.

METABOLIC ACIDOSIS   Metabolic acidosis results when the plasma bicarbonate level falls and the pH decreases. Conditions associated with metabolic acidosis include diabetes mellitus, salicylate poisoning in children under 5 years of age, starvation, renal failure, hypoxia, and loss of alkaline intestinal secretions. Remember that infants tend toward metabolic acidosis because of their high basal metabolic rates. Hyperventilation occurs in an attempt to increase the respiratory loss of carbon dioxide, thus relieving the acidemia. Treatment is aimed at eliminating the precipitating condition; sodium bicarbonate is given, as indicated, to alkalinize the plasma.

NURSING OBSERVATIONS RELATED TO FLUID IMBALANCES IN CHILDREN

Charted nursing observations can be immensely helpful to the physician or can mean nothing, depending on whether the nurse knows what to look for and takes the time to record her observations on the nursing notes. Because small children cannot describe their problems, the pediatric nurse has to be especially observant. Some of the major areas in which observations should be made are described below.

TISSUE TURGOR   Tissue turgor is best palpated in the abdominal areas and on the medial aspects of the thighs. In a normal person, pinched skin will fall back to its normal configuration when released. In a patient with fluid volume deficit, the skin may remain slightly raised for a few seconds. Skin turgor begins to be lost after 3 to 5 per cent of the body weight is lost as fluid. Severe malnutrition, particularly in infants, can cause depressed skin turgor even in the absence of fluid depletion.

Poor nutrition can also cause poor tissue turgor. Obese infants with fluid volume deficit often have skin turgor that is deceptively normal in appearance. An infant with water loss in excess of sodium loss (sodium excess), such as occurs in some types of diarrhea, has a firm thick-feeling skin. This same phenomenon is observed in the child who has sodium excess owing to an excessive sodium intake, as occurs in salt poisoning.

MUCOUS MEMBRANES   Dry mouth may be due to a fluid volume deficit or to mouth breathing. When in doubt, the nurse should run her finger along the oral cavity to feel the mucous membrane where the cheek and gums meet; dryness in this area indicates a true fluid volume deficit. The tongue of the fluid-depleted child is smaller than normal.

BREATHING RATE, DEPTH, AND PATTERN   The nurse should observe the rate, depth, and pattern of respiration. Hyperpnea, such as occurs in metabolic acidosis resulting from diarrhea or salicylate poisoning, can double the water loss by way of the lungs. The overbreathing of metabolic acidosis is not always as obvious in the child as it is in the adult; however, children do develop a curious sign not seen in adults —namely, cherry-red lips.

Accelerated breathing should be reported so that water losses through this route can be replaced. Older children and adults with metabolic alkalosis have decreased rate and depth of respiration, with irregular rhythm. The young infant may normally have irregular respiration; thus, changes in respiratory rhythm are not dependable in detecting metabolic alkalosis.

Changes in respiratory rate and depth are significant in evaluating the child's response to therapy. For example, a change from deep, rapid respiration to slower, less deep respiration indicates improvement in the child with metabolic acidosis.

TEARING AND SALIVATION   The absence of tearing and salivation is a sign of fluid volume deficit and should be noted on the chart. It becomes obvious with a fluid loss of 5 per cent of the total body weight.

THIRST   Avid thirst indicates increased tonicity of the extracellular fluid with cellular dehydration. An infant can be tested for thirst with water, although the presence of nausea may mask the symptom.

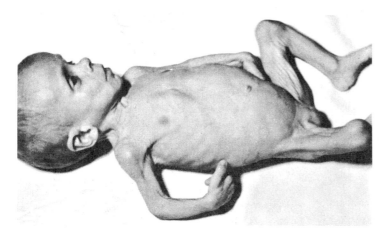

Figure 27-1. Severely dehydrated infant. (From Waechter, E., and Blake, F.: Nursing Care of Children, ed. 9. Philadelphia: J. B. Lippincott Co., 1976. Used with permission)

BEHAVIOR The child's general behavior is also significant in evaluating the response of fluid imbalances to therapy. When the very ill child begins to display appropriate responses to people, ceases to have irritable, purposeless movements, and is less lethargic, his condition has improved.

GENERAL APPEARANCE A child with a fluid volume deficit has a pinched, drawn facial expression (Fig. 27-1). A fluid volume deficit of 10 per cent of body weight causes decreased intraocular pressure and, thus, the eyes appear sunken and feel soft to the touch. Suture lines in the skull become prominent. If the anterior fontanel is still patent, it may be depressed. A grayish skin color, owing to decreased peripheral circulation, also accompanies severe fluid volume deficit. The occurrence of mottling of the skin is an ominous sign.

NATURE OF CRY The cry of an ill infant is higher pitched and less energetic than normal. With improvement in his condition, the cry becomes less high pitched and more lusty.

BODY TEMPERATURE Fluid volume deficit is often associated with a subnormal temperature because of reduced energy output. Depending on the underlying disease, however, fever can accompany fluid volume deficit. If fever is present, its height should be recorded frequently. The rate of insensible water loss is greatly increased with fever; the amount of water lost depends on the height and duration of the fever. Fever may indicate excessive water loss from the body with resultant sodium excess, or it may be caused by an infection. The extremities are cold to the touch in severe fluid volume deficit, even when fever is present; this is due to decreased peripheral blood flow.

It should be remembered that the neonate under phototherapy has increased insensible loss. The baby's temperature should be monitored since phototherapy units produce heat.

URINE OUTPUT In addition to noting the number of voidings, the nurse should estimate how much of the diaper is saturated with urine. Occasionally she would do well to weigh a dry diaper and compare its weight with that of the same diaper after the child has voided. The nurse should also note the urine's concentration, as revealed by its color. Failure to record urinary output accurately makes treatment far more difficult. When the physician requests an accurate hourly recording of urine output, and a catheter is not inserted, the nurse must devise a method to catch all the urine passed.

Some hospitals have metabolic beds, consisting of synthetic cloth mesh suspended from the bed frame with a sloping surface beneath to catch the urine from the diaperless child and divert it into a collecting device (Fig. 27-2). For male infants, a finger cot with the blind end cut off can be used to conduct urine from the penis to the drainage tube. A plastic diaper with the collecting area connected to drainage tubing may be used. The collection apparatus should be checked frequently for leakage. Good skin care is necessary to prevent irritation of the genitalia.

A child with fluid volume deficit has a decreased urinary output and an increased urinary specific gravity. If the fluid deficit is severe, he may go as long

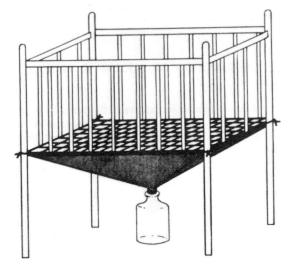

Figure 27-2. Metabolic Crib. (From Kempte, C. H., Silver, H. K., and O'Brien, D. (eds.): Current Pediatric Diagnosis and Treatment, ed. 4. Los Altos, Calif: Lange Medical Publications, 1976, p. 933. Used with permission)

as 18 to 24 hours without voiding and still not have a distended bladder. If a child with a known fluid volume deficit excretes large amounts of dilute urine, he probably has renal damage. If renal concentrating ability is impaired, or if the patient is receiving a high solute diet, the urine volume will be somewhat above normal in order to clear all the metabolic wastes. The same is true if a hypercatabolic state (such as fever or infection or both) is present.

CENTRAL VENOUS PRESSURE Central venous pressure (CVP) can be measured in the newborn by inserting an umbilical vein catheter in the superior vena cava at a level above the diaphragm. The child should be in the supine position with the zero level of the manometer at the midaxillary line (see Fig. 16-37). A pressure of 4 to 7 cm. of water is within the normal range in premature and newborn infants.[4] In infants and older children, the CVP catheter may be inserted into the external jugular vein or via a peripheral vein into the superior vena cava. A pressure of 6 to 15 cm. of water is within the normal range in children.[5] (The procedure for measuring CVP is described in Chapter 16; a rough measure of venous pressure in adults and older children is described in Chapter 12.)

Normally, the level of transition between collapse and distention of the jugular vein can be observed 1 to 2 cm. above the suprasternal notch when the patient is at a 45 degree angle. This procedure is not very helpful in infants and young children since they have short, fat necks.

STOOLS Again, it is not enough just to chart the number of stools. The quantity of the stool should be estimated as nearly as possible; its character should be described. Thus, if a stool appears normal, it should be so described on the chart. If the stool is liquid, the degree of saturation of the diaper should be noted. Any abnormal contents, such as blood or mucus, should also be recorded.

VOMITING It is important to chart the number of times the patient has vomited, when he vomited, the quantity of vomitus (approximated if necessary), and the nature of the vomitus. Merely charting the number of times the patient vomited helps little in planning fluid replacement therapy, since the amount of fluid lost can vary widely from one attack of vomiting to another. Failure to describe the vomitus may make fluid replacement therapy more difficult. For example, if the vomitus is bile stained, one can conclude that it came from below the pylorus. Since fluids from below the pylorus are chiefly alkaline, fluid therapy must be designed to replace alkaline losses, using, for example, an intestinal replacement solution.

WEIGHT CHANGES Weight loss can be caused by loss of fluid or by catabolism of body tissues. The weight loss associated with fluid volume deficit occurs more rapidly than that caused by starvation. A mild fluid volume deficit in an infant or child entails a loss of from 3 to 5 per cent of the normal body weight; a moderate fluid volume deficit, from 5 to 9 per cent; a severe fluid volume deficit, 10 per cent or more. (A loss of 15 per cent of the body weight will likely cause hypovolemic shock.)

If possible, the child's weight before the onset of the illness should be obtained from the parents, or from the family physician, who may have a record of the normal weight from a recent office visit.

If weighing is not performed accurately, it is useless. Even a minor error is important when the patient is small. The child should be weighed at the same time each day, before he has eaten, after he has voided. The same scales should be used each time, and the child should be weighed naked.

FLUID LOST BY SUCTION OR OTHER ROUTES The amount and character of fluid lost by suction, drainage tubes, or fistulas should be recorded. If the fluid loss cannot be directly measured, it should be estimated as accurately as possible.

FLUID INTAKE   The amount and type of fluids received by the patient, either orally or parenterally, should be recorded.

FLUID REPLACEMENT THERAPY IN CHILDREN

Daily Requirements

The basic requirements of water and electrolytes must be met daily. In addition, one should supply the amounts necessary to correct preexisting deficits, as well as concurrent abnormal losses, such as those that occur from diarrhea, vomiting, suction drainage, and the like. The normal water requirements per kilogram of body weight at various ages are listed in Table 27-2. Approximately 2 to 3 mEq. of sodium and potassium are required for each kilogram of body weight to meet maintenance needs. This corresponds to approximately 50 to 70 mEq. of sodium or potassium/m.^{2} of body surface/day.

Although the adult can go without food for several days without developing gross ketonuria, infants and children react quickly to the omission of calories. Ketonuria can occur within a few hours after the onset of fasting. For this reason, carbohydrate must be incorporated in fluids designed to meet daily maintenance needs.

Determination of Body Surface Area in Infants and Children

Body surface area is used increasingly as a gauge for dosage. It possesses this advantage: requirements for water and electrolytes, as well as therapeutic doses of many pharmaceutical agents, are roughly proportional to surface area (neonates and prematures excepted). In addition to its convenience, use of body surface area offers increased accuracy and safety, despite theoretical objections to its scientific validity.

Frequently used for determination of body surface area are (1) the DuBois nomogram, requiring weight and height; (2) the Sendroy nomogram, also requiring weight and height; and (3) the West table, requiring weight only. Snively and coworkers[6] have introduced a quick method for estimating body surface area of infants and children, employing a formula that requires only the crown-rump length in infants and the sitting height in children, measured in centimeters. The formula for infants six months of age or less is as follows:

Body surface area in m.^{2} = 0.00017 × (sitting height in cm.)^2

The formula for children over six months of age is as follows:

Body surface area in m.^{2} = 0.00019 × (sitting height in cm.)^2

Let's take the example of a child with a sitting height of 50 cm. and see how the formula works:

0.00019 × 50^2 (2,500) = 0.48 m.^{2}

Since none of the infants and children used in the study by Snively and others exceeded 14½ years in age, further investigation would be desirable before applying the sitting height method to older people.

A comparison of the various formulas for determining body surface area is given in Table 27-3.

Any dose determination, whether it be for water, electrolytes, or medicinals, is approximate and must be adjusted in accordance with the individual tolerance, requirement, and clinical progress of the patient. Great accuracy is not, therefore, essential. As-

Table 27-3.   A Statistical Comparison of Formulas for Estimating Body Surface Area

	Sitting-Height Formula vs. Sendroy Nomogram	West Table vs. Sendroy Nomogram	Dubois Nomogram vs. Sendroy Nomogram
No. of children in analysis	267	267	267
Mean	− 3.02%	+ 4.99%	+ 0.28%
Median	− 4.73%	+13.71%	+ 6.64%
Range (high and low extremes)	+28.57% −38.03%	+54.34% −26.92%	+23.8% −10.52%
Approximate 95% limits	+15% −20.76%	+28.57% −10.29%	+12.9% − 6.57%
Standard deviation	9.36%	11.45%	5.11%

Reprinted from Snively, W. D., Montenegro, J. L. B., and Dick, R. G.: Quick method for estimating body surface area. J.A.M.A. 197:208–209. Copyright 1966, American Medical Association. With permission.

sessment of body surface area for children up to age 14½ years is greatly facilitated by the use of the sitting height formula, particularly when nomograms or tables are not immediately available. The method requires only a centimeter measure, easily carried in the physician's bag or available in any hospital.

Oral Replacement

Water and electrolyte replacement is best accomplished by the oral route for these reasons:

1. Fluids taken into the gastrointestinal tract are slowly absorbed, while parenterally administered fluids pass directly into the circulation. The body is less adversely affected if excessive amounts of water or electrolytes are given by the oral than by the parenteral route.

2. Oral fluid replacement allows the child free movement and activity, as opposed to hours of being restrained during subcutaneous or intravenous infusions.

It should be emphasized, however, that, even in the case of the oral route, it is relatively easy to overwhelm the body's homeostatic capabilities, particularly in the case of the infant and small child. For this reason, the dose for fluids administered orally should be calculated with the same care and precision as doses to be administered parenterally. Moreover, although the oral route is far safer than the intravenous route, potassium should not be given by mouth when oliguria or anuria is present.

A suitable oral solution for providing water, electrolytes, and calories is Lytren, prepared by mixing 8 measures of Lytren and 32 oz. of water. Measures should be carefully leveled in accordance with the manufacturer's instructions. Each liter of this solution supplies 25 mEq. of sodium, 25 mEq. of potassium, 30 mEq. of chloride, 4 mEq. of calcium, 4 mEq. of magnesium, and 280 calories, plus other ingredients.

Other suitable oral solutions include Pedialyte, half-strength flavored gelatin, and decarbonated soft drinks. Homemade electrolyte solutions (made with measured amounts of salt, baking soda, or sugar) are risky since they may be incorrectly prepared, leading to serious electrolyte disturbances (Table 27-4). For this reason, parents should not be told to prepare such oral electrolyte solutions at home.

Table 27-4. Electrolyte Contents of Solutions of Table Salt

Concentration Salt / 1 Quart of Tap Water	Approximate Composition	
	Na mEq./L.	Cl mEq./L.
⅛ tsp.	10–15	10–15
¼ tsp.	20–30	20–30
½ tsp.	45–60	45–60
1 tsp.	120	120
1 tbs.	350	350

Reprinted from Statland, H.: Fluid and Electrolytes in Practice, ed. 3. Philadelphia: J. B. Lippincott Co., 1963, p. 201, with permission.

Tube Feedings

Sometimes tube feedings are used to feed unconscious children or those with swallowing difficulties. Many tube feeding mixtures contain large solute loads which, if associated with limited water intake, may increase plasma osmolarity. The nurse will do well to watch for signs of inadequate water intake, particularly when the feedings are high in protein content. Should insufficient water be provided, water will be drawn from the tissues to supply the needed volume for urinary excretion of the increased solute load. Eventually, dehydration (sodium excess) will occur, along with an accumulation of nitrogenous waste products in the blood stream.

Hypernatremia may cause the skin to feel inelastic and "doughy" and the fatty tissue to feel unusually firm. Excessive protein in relation to water causes nausea, vomiting, diarrhea, and, eventually, ileus. If the condition is allowed to go uncorrected, it will result in high fever and disorientation. Laboratory tests will reveal an elevated blood urea nitrogen (BUN) level. Early in protein overloading, the urine volume is large even though water intake is inadequate. The large urine volume can easily lead the staff to think that water intake is adequate; in such instances, however, output actually exceeds intake—the extra fluid is being withdrawn from the body tissues. Very young children and unconscious patients should be observed carefully for inadequate water intake since they are unable to express thirst.

Parenteral Fluid Therapy

SUBCUTANEOUS ROUTE Subcutaneous fluids are easier to start than are intravenous fluids, particularly in infants and small children. For this reason, the subcutaneous route is sometimes used in pediatrics, even though it has serious hazards and limitations. Subcutaneous fluids are poorly absorbed in the child with a severe fluid volume deficit because of the frequently associated peripheral circulatory collapse. The route, therefore, is not dependable in patients with severe fluid balance disturbances. Another disadvantage of the subcutaneous route is the limitation of the types of fluids that can be administered by this route with even a modicum of safety. (The reader is referred to Chapter 16 for a discussion of which fluids can be given subcutaneously.)

Fluids may be administered to an infant, using the subcutaneous tissues of the anterior or posterior axillary folds, medial aspect of the midthigh, inferior aspect of the scapula, or the lower abdominal wall. Older children may receive fluids in the outer aspect of the midthigh. Restraints must be used as necessary to prevent breakage of the needles in the hypodermoclysis sites. Flow rates should be checked frequently and adjusted as necessary to prevent painful swelling. Because fluid-logged tissues are fertile sites for infection, rigid aseptic technique must be maintained at all times. Sterile dressings should be applied after the needles are withdrawn. It must be emphasized that the subcutaneous route is erratic and less desirable than the intravenous avenue of fluid administration.

INTRAVENOUS ROUTE

Procedure Prior to performing the venipuncture, the child should be properly restrained according to the area involved. Restraints should not be so tight that they impede breathing and circulation. Venipuncture sites for the pediatric patient may include superficial veins of the scalp, wrist, hand, arm, leg, or foot. Since superficial veins of the scalp do not have valves, fluids may be infused in either direction.[7] Some physicians place a rubber band with an adhesive tag around the infant's forehead to distend the scalp veins prior to venipuncture; the adhesive tag is used to readily release the tourniquet. Special care in cleansing the skin is mandatory before venipuncture is made in superficial scalp veins since they communicate with the dural sinuses. A sandbag may be necessary to hold the infant's head in position. The scalp-vein infusion set (see Fig. 16-5) is attached to a syringe filled with sterile saline. After the needle enters the vein (as evidenced by aspirating blood into the syringe), the operator slowly injects 1 ml. of

saline while observing for swelling at the site. If no swelling is noted, the infusion set is attached to the I.V. tubing and taped into place.

Venipuncture may also be performed with an intracatheter (catheter threaded through a metal needle) or with a plastic needle (catheter mounted on a metal needle). (See Figs. 16-3 and 16-4.) A cutdown (surgical insertion of a catheter into a vein) may be performed if fluids are urgently needed and difficulty is encountered in finding a suitable vein. The internal saphenous vein can be entered at any point along its course and is easily identified.

After the venipuncture is accomplished, the designated rate of flow must be established and thereafter carefully monitored. The danger of administering an excessive fluid volume is a real one in all age groups. Infants and small children are faced with special dangers simply because of their small size and the ease of supplying fluids in adult-sized bottles. The accidental administration of an extra 500 ml. of fluid, such as 5 per cent dextrose in water or isotonic solution of sodium chloride, might mean little to the adult, but it can be disastrous to the infant or small child. This group of patients has greater difficulty excreting excessive fluid volume. Moreover, they are more susceptible to pulmonary edema than are adults. In fact, pneumonia from overhydration is thought to be one of the commonest treatment-related diseases of hospitalized children.

Measures to Assure Accurate Flow Rate Measures should be taken to avoid an overdose of intravenous fluids. The volume available in the bottle, which might run rapidly into the patient, should be limited. It has been recommended that quantities exceeding 150 ml. not be connected to children under 2 years of age, no more than 250 ml. to children under 5, and no more than 500 ml. to children under 10.

The development of special administration sets for pediatric use has added a greater margin of safety to fluid administration. (See the section on volume controlled sets in Chapter 16.) There should never be more than enough fluid for two hours in any of these volumetric sets. A microdrip adaptor may be supplied with these sets; one delivering 60 drops/ml. is particularly convenient in that the number of drops delivered per minute is also the number of milliliters delivered per hour. (For example: 60 drops/min. delivers 60 ml./hr., 20 drops/min. delivers 20 ml./hr., and so forth.)

The physician prescribes the total volume of

fluid to be given over a designated period of time, as well as the desired number of milliliters per hour or drops per minute. When the nurse knows the total volume to be administered in a fixed period of time, plus the drop factor of the set to be used, she can easily check the flow rate by her own computations. (The reader is referred to the discussion on calculation of flow rates in Chapter 16.) Great care should be taken to assure accuracy when the flow rate is calculated.

Even though drop size adaptors and small containers are used to reduce the possibility of error, the nurse must still keep a close vigil on the flow rate, as well as on the patient's response to the fluids. The flow rate should be counted every 15 minutes and adjusted as necessary. (Factors that can alter the flow rate are discussed in Chapter 16.) A pediatric parenteral fluid sheet should be kept at the bedside of infants and small children to record the observed flow rate, the amount of fluid absorbed each hour, and the amount of fluid left in the bottle. Such frequent observations and notations greatly reduce the risk of excessive fluid administration.

Occasionally, veins may be too small in some infants to allow administration of fluids by gravity (even when the container is elevated to its highest position); in these cases, a mechanical infusion pump is indicated. Because it is often necessary to administer very small volumes to pediatric patients, it is advisable to use an intravenous infusion pump whenever such an apparatus is available. Most infusion pumps can deliver a constant, exact flow rate (a definite improvement over the erratic flow of a gravity apparatus). (Infusion pumps are described in Chapter 16.)

Tubing and dressing changes should be made daily, always utilizing strict aseptic technique. Complications such as thrombophlebitis and infiltration should be observed for frequently. (See Chapter 16 for a discussion of the complications of intravenous therapy.)

Factors Influencing Fluid Intake

The child's condition should be reassessed at frequent intervals to reevaluate his fluid requirements. The clinical status of infants can improve or deteriorate remarkably in a few hours. The high humidity in an incubator or isolette minimizes insensible water loss and, thus, decreases the total amount of fluid to be given by about a third. Fever increases fluid maintenance requirements by about 10 per cent for each degree of Fahrenheit elevation. As a general rule, the fluid intake should be adequate to keep the child's urine output in the normal range for his age. The desired urine flow for a child one year old or less is approximately 5 to 10 ml. per hour. Children from one to ten years of age should excrete approximately 10 to 25 ml. of urine per hour. However, normal outputs are usually not achieved in the immediate postoperative period because of the influence of stress.

Parenteral Hyperalimentation

Parenteral hyperalimentation is a method of feeding a patient who cannot tolerate an oral feeding or in whom it is necessary to bypass the gastrointestinal tract. Sufficient nutrients can be given intravenously for prolonged periods of time to achieve weight gain and growth. Young infants with gastrointestinal anomalies have been maintained for months on parenteral hyperalimentation. Patients with dehydration and negative nitrogen balance from diarrhea and vomiting also benefit from this treatment.

The pediatric hyperalimentation solution consists of amino acids, hypertonic glucose, electrolytes, and multiple vitamins. Hypertonicity of the solution is irritating to small veins; thus, the solution must be given into a central vein which has a rapid blood flow to dilute the solution quickly. Usually the catheter is inserted via a cut down through the internal or external jugular vein and is threaded down into the superior vena cava. Rigid sterile technique is required to prevent infection. An infusion pump is used to administer the solution at a slow, constant rate, despite vigorous crying in the child. (Recall that venous pressure is elevated when the child cries; this causes resistance to the flow.) A filter is inserted in the infusion line to filter out bacteria or particulate matter that might be present in the hyperalimentation solution.

Complications of parenteral hyperalimentation can include thrombophlebitis, local and systemic infections, and hyperosmolar dehydration (electrolyte excess). If the concentrated solution is administered too fast, glucose overload will occur and produce an osmotic diuresis which can lead to severe dehydration, shock, and death. The nurse must carefully observe and record the following:

> Rate of flow of the parenteral solution
> Vital signs
> Intake and output
> Body weight
> Signs of inflammation around the infusion site
> Urinary sugar content
> Signs of dehydration

Parenteral hyperalimentation is best done in centers with specially trained hyperalimentation teams.

CLINICAL CONDITIONS COMMONLY ASSOCIATED WITH FLUID IMBALANCES IN SMALL CHILDREN

Diarrhea

Diarrhea is a common cause of water and electrolyte disturbances in infants and small children. The large loss of liquid stools can rapidly deplete the young child's extracellular fluid volume, especially when it is combined with vomiting. Usually water and electrolytes are lost in isotonic proportions (fluid volume deficit or isotonic dehydration). However, water can be lost in excess of electrolytes (fluid volume deficit with sodium excess or hypertonic dehydration), and electrolytes can be lost in excess of water (fluid volume deficit with sodium deficit or hypotonic dehydration). Because sodium is the chief extracellular ion, its excess or deficit is of primary importance in producing symptoms.

Intestinal fluids are alkaline; therefore, large losses of fluids in diarrhea may result in metabolic acidosis. Potassium deficit is another frequent accompaniment of diarrhea.

Extracellular Fluid Volume Deficit (Isotonic Dehydration)

SYMPTOMS Approximately 70 per cent of patients with severe diarrhea undergo a proportionate loss of water and electrolytes. Symptoms of fluid volume deficit due to infantile diarrhea include the following:

> history of large quantities of liquid stools

> weight loss
> dry skin with poor tissue turgor
> diminished tearing
> soft eyeballs with a sunken appearance (resulting from decreased intraocular pressure)
> depression of anterior fontanel, if it is still present
> skin ashen or gray in color and extremities cold (owing to inadequate peripheral circulation)
> depressed body temperature, unless fever accompanies the diarrhea, as in an infection
> lethargy
> signs of hypovolemic shock
> weak rapid pulse
> decreased blood pressure
> oliguria

Metabolic acidosis usually accompanies frequent liquid stools. (Recall that the intestinal secretions are alkaline because of their high bicarbonate content. Therefore, loss of alkaline secretions in diarrheal stools results in metabolic acidosis.) Decreased dietary intake contributes to metabolic acidosis; thus, in the absence of adequate food intake, the body utilizes its own fats for energy purposes. The metabolism of these fats causes the accumulation of acidic ketone bodies in the blood, further contributing to the metabolic acidosis caused by bicarbonate loss.

A major symptom of metabolic acidosis is the increased depth of respiration, a body compensatory mechanism that blows off carbon dioxide, thus reducing the carbonic acid content of the blood and influencing the carbonic acid–base bicarbonate balance in the direction of an increased pH. If ketosis of starvation is present, an acetone odor may be noted on the breath. Symptoms of severe potassium deficit include weakness, anorexia, vomiting, excessive abdominal gas, and muscles flabby, like half-filled water bottles.

TREATMENT The first goal of fluid replacement therapy is to expand the extracellular fluid volume sufficiently to prevent or correct symptoms of hypovolemic shock. A restored blood volume permits adequate renal blood flow and increased urine formation. Improvement of renal function helps the body eliminate organic acids and, thus, correct acidosis. Physicians vary in the precise fluid therapy employed. All agree that if kidney function is depressed because of extracellular fluid volume deficit, a special solution should be administered to correct renal depression. Renal depression is indicated by:

Urinary specific gravity above 1.030
Oliguria, revealed by the history of voiding less than three times during the previous 24 hours
Anuria, shown by absence of urine in the bladder

Renal depression is assumed to be present when there has been a recent fluid loss of great magnitude, such as occurs with severe infectious diarrhea of explosive onset.

When renal depression is present, the physician administers an initial hydrating or pump-priming solution for the following reasons: (1) to restore the kidneys to normal function if the cause of the depression is extracellular fluid volume deficit, or (2) to discover that the renal depression is not the result of a fluid volume deficit, but rather of serious renal impairment.

Pump-priming solutions have about one third the electrolyte concentration of extracellular fluid. A typical solution is simply a one-third isotonic solution of sodium chloride in 5 per cent dextrose. Such a solution provides 51 mEq. of sodium and 51 mEq. of chloride. All commercial companies make available such solutions.

With renal flow established, one can then administer a repair solution. Some physicians use lactated Ringer's solution with dextrose and added potassium. Doses of such solutions are usually based on ml./kg. of body weight.

The water and electrolyte requirements for infants and children, when expressed in units/kilogram, vary considerably for children of different ages and weights. For this reason, many physicians prefer to use body surface area as the dose criterion since this is independent of age and weight, except in the case of prematures.

Many physicians prefer to use Butler-type solutions, sometimes known as balanced solutions, so formulated that, when used to correct a fluid volume deficit, they provide electrolytes in such quantities that the homeostatic mechanisms can:

1. Retain those required for normalization of body fluid electrolyte composition.
2. Excrete electrolytes that are not needed.

3. Provide carbohydrate to combat ketosis and tissue breakdown.

Balanced solutions provide both cellular and extracellular electrolytes, including sodium, potassium, lactate, chloride, phosphate, and, sometimes, calcium, magnesium, citrate, and sulfate. A conventional Butler solution provides 75 cations (or anions) per liter and is designed for administration to older infants, children, and adults. A balanced solution specially designed for infants contains 48 cations (or anions) per liter. It is designed for administration to full-term or large premature to one-month-old infants. An oral balanced solution, Lytren, based originally on the formula devised by Darrow and Cooke, provides 52 mEq./L. All balanced solutions provide added carbohydrate in order to help meet the caloric requirements of the child. Balanced solutions are given at a dose level of 1500 ml./m.^{2} of body surface/day for maintenance. In the presence of a moderate fluid volume deficit, the dose level is 2400 ml./m.^{2} of body surface/day. For a severe volume deficit, the dose level is 3000 ml./m.^{2} of body surface/day.

Fluid Volume Deficit with Sodium Excess (Hypertonic Dehydration)

SYMPTOMS Approximately 20 per cent of patients with severe diarrhea have suffered a relatively greater loss of water than of electrolytes. If the infant has ingested a high solute-containing formula during his illness or has been inadvertently given an overly-concentrated electrolyte mixture, the renal water loss intensifies the sodium excess already present. Because the infant cannot concentrate urine efficiently, large volumes of water are needed to excrete solutes. The infant's need for water is intensified by the fact that his insensible water loss is great because of his large body surface area.

Symptoms of fluid volume deficit and sodium excess caused by diarrhea include these:

history of large quantities of liquid stools associated with a low water intake, high solute intake, poor renal function, or all three
weight loss
skin elasticity and turgor not lost (however, the skin has a thickened, firm feeling)

avid thirst (hypertonic extracellular fluid draws water from the cells, producing cellular dehydration)

irritability displayed when disturbed (otherwise behavior is lethargic)

tremors and convulsions

muscle rigidity

nuchal rigidity

chloride and protein concentration of spinal fluid elevated

although signs of extracellular fluid volume deficit are not present for first few days, they eventually occur with symptoms of hypovolemic shock

brain injury (may be due to intracranial hemorrhage and effusion into the subdural space)

TREATMENT Treatment principles and details are similar to those given under extracellular fluid volume deficit.

Small amounts of electrolytes are used in the repair solutions to prevent a too-rapid correction of the sodium excess, since a rapid return of the plasma sodium concentration to normal may precipitate acute sodium deficit (water intoxication).

Symptoms of sodium deficit can result from the abnormal uptake of water by the cells, secondary to the inability of the immature kidneys to maintain the normal relationship between water and solute. Convulsions can result from the too-rapid reduction of the sodium concentration in the extracellular fluid; they are less likely to occur when the correction of the sodium excess is carried out gradually. Convulsions occurring in an infant with sodium excess can also be an indication of brain damage, in which case, phenobarbital may be required to control them.

Hypocalcemia can occur during treatment, possibly caused by the loss of calcium in the stool or by the decreased ionization of available extracellular calcium, which occurs with correction of the metabolic acidosis. Symptoms of hypocalcemia occur less frequently when calcium is included in the treatment solution. The administration of 10 to 30 ml. of 10 per cent calcium gluconate added daily to one of the infusions may prevent calcium deficit from developing.

During repair of water losses, the patient with sodium excess may develop fluid volume excess with edema and, possibly, heart failure.

Fluid Volume Deficit with Sodium Deficit (Hypotonic Dehydration)

SYMPTOMS Approximately 10 per cent of patients with severe diarrhea have suffered a relatively greater loss of electrolytes than of water, usually because fluid losses have been replaced with plain water in dextrose or some other electrolyte-free solution, which dilutes the electrolyte concentration of the extracellular fluid. Because sodium is the chief extracellular ion, the primary symptoms are due to its deficit. Symptoms of fluid volume deficit and sodium deficit caused by diarrheal losses include these:

clammy skin

lethargy

hypovolemic shock, in severe cases

TREATMENT Treatment principles and details are similar to those given under extracellular fluid volume deficit.

Measures to Prevent or Minimize Water and Electrolyte Loss in Diarrhea

The following measures should be taken to prevent or minimize imbalances caused by infant diarrhea:

1. Hospitalized infants with diarrhea should be isolated so as to prevent infecting other children in the unit. Meticulous attention should be paid to isolation technique.

2. Diarrhea can be caused by infections transmitted to the infant by contaminated formula or equipment. Unless technique is impeccable, this can occur readily in the hospital. The nurse should see that the mother knows how to prepare the baby's formula safely before she goes home.

3. Water and electrolyte losses can be minimized if diarrhea is reported immediately, so that treatment can be started. Mothers should be instructed to report diarrhea as soon as it is noticed.

4. Liquid stool losses are greater if the baby continues to take oral feedings than if his gastrointestinal tract is put to rest temporarily. Mothers should be instructed to withhold formula feedings when diarrhea occurs until they have checked with the physician. Because of the high solute content of skim milk, boiled skim milk that is undiluted should not be

used in the treatment of infants with diarrhea. Because of the infant's poor renal concentrating ability, he needs large quantities of water to excrete the large renal solute load presented by undiluted skim milk. Boiled skim milk should never be used unless diluted with at least an equal volume of water, plus added carbohydrate.

5. Mothers should be encouraged to follow the physician's instructions precisely in returning the infant to full formula feedings following a bout of diarrhea. In most cases the infant with diarrhea is given initially an oral electrolyte solution with glucose. When tolerated, a little milk is added each day until full feedings are resumed.

Vomiting Caused by Hypertrophic Pyloric Stenosis

SYMPTOMS   Hypertrophic pyloric stenosis is a common cause of vomiting in small infants, usually under six weeks old. Males are reportedly affected five times more often than females.

Because of the repeated vomiting, the infants are poorly nourished. While hypertrophic pyloric stenosis can be corrected surgically, preoperative correction of the water and electrolyte disturbances caused by the prolonged vomiting is mandatory.

Vomiting causes the same imbalances in children as it does in adults. These include metabolic alkalosis, potassium deficit, sodium deficit, and fluid volume deficit. Metabolic alkalosis occurs because of the excessive loss of potassium, hydrogen, and chloride in the vomitus. Loss of chloride causes a compensatory increase in the number of bicarbonate ions; this occurs because both are anions (negatively charged ions). Total cations must always equal the total anions so that electrical equality can be maintained; if the quantity of one anion is decreased, another anion must increase in compensation. The bicarbonate side of the carbonic acid–base bicarbonate ratio is increased, and the pH increases—that is, becomes more alkaline. Sodium and potassium are plentiful in gastric juice; prolonged vomiting leads to deficits of both. Since water is also lost in the vomitus, fluid volume deficit occurs. Because the losses are sustained over a relatively long period, circulatory collapse is not prominent in hypertrophic pyloric stenosis as it is in severe diarrhea.

The infant with hypertrophic pyloric stenosis has the following symptoms:

difficulty in retaining feedings, which becomes progressively worse during the first few weeks of life; eventually, projectile vomiting follows each feeding

appearance of malnutrition

symptoms of fluid volume deficit

decreased respiration (compensatory action of lungs to retain carbon dioxide and increase the carbonic acid content of the blood)

tetany accompanying alkalosis (owing to decreased calcium ionization in an alkaline pH)

despite starvation, ketosis does not usually appear

palpable pyloric tumor

TREATMENT   Preoperative Period   To minimize fluid losses, oral feedings should be discontinued and fluids given parenterally. If gastric suction is used, the water and electrolytes lost by this procedure should be replaced. Treatment principles and details are similar to those given under extracellular fluid volume deficit. A solution of 5 per cent dextrose in 0.45 per cent sodium chloride, with added potassium, may be used as a correction fluid for metabolic alkalosis.

Postoperative Period   The young child does not retain sodium after a surgical operation, as do many adults. Sodium should, therefore, be included in the postoperative repair solution. There is excellent rationale for including potassium likewise.

Vomiting Caused by an Obstruction Below the Pylorus

Vomiting caused by an obstruction below the pylorus contains alkaline secretions from the intestines, in addition to the acid secretions from the stomach. Vomitus may be bile-stained. If alkaline secretions predominate, metabolic acidosis results. Contributing to the metabolic acidosis is the ketosis of starvation.

Bowel obstruction causes the bowel to become distended with gas and a substantial volume of fluid. Repeated vomiting leads to a loss of water and electrolytes; the vomitus should be analyzed for electrolyte content since variations occur according to the site of the obstruction and with each individual. These losses should be replaced prior to surgery unless an emergency exists. A nasogastric tube should be inserted to relieve distention; the patient

CHILD: one year

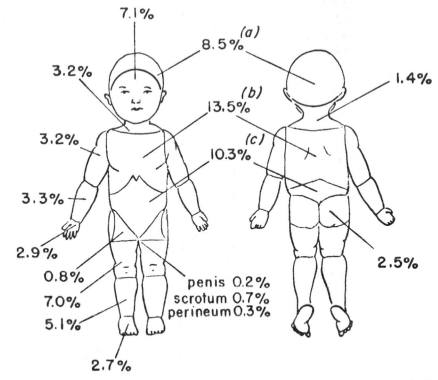

PERCENTAGE OF SURFACE
AREAS OF BODY PARTS

(a) Entire scalp
(b) Entire upper trunk,
    front and back
(c) Entire lower trunk,
    front and back

7.1%

8.5% (a)

3.2%

1.4%

(b)
13.5%

3.2%

(c)
10.3%

3.3%

2.9%

0.8%

7.0%

5.1%

penis 0.2%
scrotum 0.7%
perineum 0.3%

2.5%

2.7%

Figure 27-3. Surface diagram constructed from Meeh's data. Child of six months to three years. (From Moyer, C.: Treatment of large burns. Arch. Surg. 90:856, 1965, American Medical Association, with permission)

should be NPO until bowel sounds return after surgery. Parenteral feedings are necessary. (General care of the patient with bowel obstruction is discussed in Chapter 19.)

Burns

The treatment of children with burns is essentially the same as that described for adults in Chapter 18. The major difference lies in the calculation of the percentage of the body involved in the burn, since the child's body proportions are different from those of the adult (Fig. 27-3).

Another major difference between the child and the adult lies in the need for greater accuracy in fluid administration in children, since the child has greater sensitivity to minor errors in fluid administration. Both pulmonary edema and shock develop more quickly in children than in adults.

A second degree burn of more than 10 per cent of the body surface in a child under one year of age or of 15 per cent in an older child represents serious injury

and requires hospitalization. To evaluate the effectiveness of fluid replacement, it is necessary to measure the urinary output at regular intervals. A metabolic crib may be used (see Fig. 27-2) or an indwelling urinary catheter may be necessary. A child under one year of age should have an hourly output of from 5 to 10 ml.; a child between one and ten years between 10 and 25 ml.; or, 10 to 30 ml./m.^{2} of body surface/hour, regardless of age.

Salicylate Intoxication

Salicylate intoxication is commonly seen in children and accounts for 12 per cent of all toxic ingestions. It has resulted from leaving aspirin in the reach of the small child, particularly flavored aspirin. Recent use of safety caps, however, has decreased the occurrence of this problem. Half of the cases of salicylate intoxication now are due to parent or practitioner errors;[8] that is, some children are sensitive to theoretically permissable doses. Occasionally an older child may attempt suicide by aspirin ingestion. Salicylate poisoning can result also from ingesting sodium salicylate tablets or from drinking methyl salicylate (oil of wintergreen).

SYMPTOMS   Salicylates cause the respiratory center to be more sensitive to carbon dioxide; they cause respiration to become deep and rapid. As a result, excessive amounts of carbon dioxide are eliminated from the lungs and respiratory alkalosis develops. Symptoms of a deficit of ionized calcium caused by the alkalosis appear. They include numbness and tingling of the face and extremities, positive Chvostek's sign, muscle twitching, and convulsions.

Respiratory alkalosis is the major disturbance in adults and older children. Management consists of suitable fluid and electrolyte infusions to promote excretion of salicylates.

Children under five years of age usually develop a more complicated acid–base disturbance. Quickly following the initial respiratory alkalosis, they develop metabolic acidosis, as a result of inadequate utilization of carbohydrate caused by the toxic doses of salicylates and the resultant increased utilization of body fat. Symptoms of severe salicylate intoxication in the child consist of severe hyperpnea, vomiting, and fluid volume deficit. Hyperthermia is common and is manifested by a flushed appearance and sweating. Bleeding may occur, owing to prolonged prothrombin time and platelet dysfunction. The serum salicylate level is over 40 mg./100 ml. Hypokalemia may result from excessive loss of potassium in vomitus.

The blood pH is affected by two imbalances—respiratory alkalosis and metabolic acidosis. Sometimes the two imbalances neutralize each other and the pH remains normal. If respiratory alkalosis is more severe than metabolic acidosis, as is frequently the case in older children and adults, the pH is elevated above normal. If metabolic acidosis is more severe than respiratory alkalosis, as is frequently the case in small children, the pH is decreased below normal.

Adults and older children can cope with the impaired metabolism of salicylate intoxication better than can young children.

TREATMENT   Emergency therapy is directed at removing as much of the salicylate from the stomach as possible before it is absorbed. Syrup of ipecac may be

used to induce emesis or the stomach may be lavaged with an isotonic solution of sodium chloride.

After the stomach contents have been emptied, attention is given to supplying adequate fluids to promote excretion of salicylates by the kidneys, which account for the excretion of about 80 per cent of ingested salicylates. Carbohydrate is administered to prevent or combat ketosis. The amount of fluids required depends largely upon the length of time elapsed since poisoning occurred. Since severe hyperpnea usually accompanies metabolic acidosis, large quantities of water are lost by way of the lungs. Some patients who have not received prompt therapy suffer severe fluid volume deficit, which must be repaired. Potassium may be given as indicated to correct hypokalemia and allow alkalinization of the urine once urine flow is established.

General treatment principles and details are similar to those given under extracellular fluid volume deficit.

The urine can be alkalinized as a means of promoting salicylate excretion. This can be accomplished by the intravenous administration of lactate-containing solutions. Keeping the urinary pH above 7.5 will result in the excretion of 50 per cent of the salicylate in six hours.[9]

Calcium gluconate can be given to relieve symptoms of ionized calcium deficit, such as tetany. Vitamin K_1 can be used to prevent excessive bleeding resulting from hypoprothrombinemia. Dialysis is indicated when potentially fatal serum levels exist or when oliguria or anuria are present.

REFERENCES

1. **Graef, J.,** and **Cone, T.** (eds.): Manual of Pediatric Therapeutics. Boston: Little, Brown & Co., 1974, p. 85.

2. **Kempe, C.,** et al.: Current Pediatric Diagnosis and Treatment, ed. 4. Los Altos, Calif.: Lange Medical Publications, 1976, p. 658.

3. **Graef** and **Cone:**   Manual of Pediatric Therapeutics, p. 108.

4. Ibid., p. 35.

5. Ibid.

6. **Snively, W. D.,** et al.:   Quick method for estimating body surface area. J.A.M.A. 197:208–209, 1966.

7. **Kempe, C.,** et al.:   Current Pediatric Diagnosis and Treatment, p. 939.

8. **Waechter, E.,** and **Blake, F.:** Nursing Care of Children, ed. 9. Philadelphia: J. B. Lippincott Co., 1976.

9. **Graef** and **Cone:** Manual of Pediatric Therapeutics, p. 77.

BIBLIOGRAPHY

Dickason, E., and **Schult, M.** (eds.): Maternal & Infant Care. New York: McGraw-Hill Book Co., 1975.

Guyton, A.: Textbook of Medical Physiology, ed. 5. Philadelphia: W. B. Saunders Co., 1976.

Maxwell, M., and **Kleeman, C.:** Clinical Disorders of Fluid and Electrolyte Metabolism, ed. 2. New York: McGraw-Hill Book Co., 1972.

Plumer, A.: Principles and Practice of Intravenous Therapy, ed. 2. Boston: Little, Brown & Co., 1975.

Index

(t = table, f = figure, n = note)